REVIEW QUESTIONS IN ORTHOPAEDICS

REVIEW QUESTIONS IN ORTHOPAEDICS

Editors

JOHN M. WRIGHT, M.D.

Attending Surgeon
Department of Orthopaedics and Sports Medicine
Straub Clinic
Honolulu, Hawaii

PETER J. MILLETT, M.D., M.Sc.

Associate Surgeon
Department of Orthopaedic Surgery
Brigham & Women's Hospital
Instructor
Department of Orthopaedics
Harvard Medical School
Boston, Massachusetts

HEBER C. CROCKETT, M.D.

Attending Orthopaedic Surgeon
Trails West Sports Medicine
Good Samaritan Hospital
Kearney, Nebraska

EDWARD V. CRAIG, M.D.

Attending Orthopaedic Surgeon
Hospital for Special Surgery
Professor of Clinical Orthopaedics
Department of Orthopaedic Surgery
Cornell Medical School
New York, New York

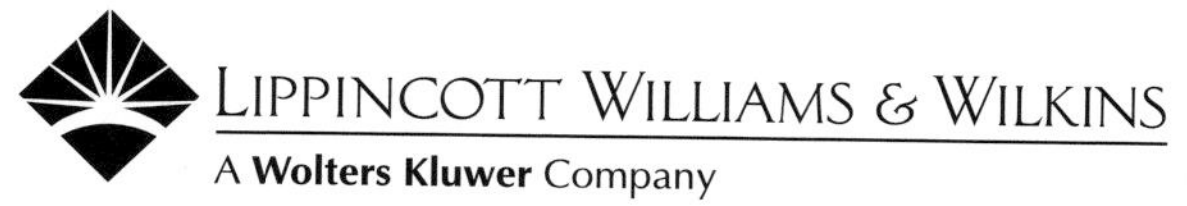

Philadelphia • Baltimore • New York • London
Buenos Aires • Hong Kong • Sydney • Tokyo

Acquisitions Editor: Robert Hurley
Developmental Editor: Pamela Sutton
Manufacturing Manager: Colin Warnock
Production Editor: Tom Wang
Cover Designer: Catherine Lau Hunt
Compositor: Lippincott Williams & Wilkins Desktop Division
Printer: Maple Press

530 Walnut Street
Philadelphia, PA 19106 USA
LWW.com

Printed in the USA

Library of Congress Cataloging-in-Publication Data
Review questions in orthopaedics /editors, John M. Wright ... [et al.] — 1st ed.
p. ; cm.
Includes bibliographical references and index.
ISBN 0-683-30243-4
1. Orthopedics—Examinations, questions, etc. I. Wright, John M., M.D.
[DNLM: 1. Orthopedics—Examination Questions. WE 18.2 R4543 2001]
RD732.6.R48 2001
616.7'0076–dc21
2001038245

Care has been taken to confirm the accuracy of the information presented and to describe generally accepted practices. However, the authors, editors, and publisher are not responsible for errors or omissions or for any consequences from application of the information in this book and make no warranty, expressed or implied, with respect to the currency, completeness, or accuracy of the contents of the publication. Application of this information in a particular situation remains the professional responsibility of the practitioner.

The authors, editors, and publisher have exerted every effort to ensure that drug selection and dosage set forth in this text are in accordance with current recommendations and practice at the time of publication. However, in view of ongoing research, changes in government regulations, and the constant flow of information relating to drug therapy and drug reactions, the reader is urged to check the package insert for each drug for any change in indications and dosage and for added warnings and precautions. This is particularly important when the recommended agent is a new or infrequently employed drug.

Some drugs and medical devices presented in this publication have Food and Drug Administration (FDA) clearance for limited use in restricted research settings. It is the responsibility of the health care provider to ascertain the FDA status of each drug or device planned for use in their clinical practice.

10 9 8 7 6 5 4 3 2 1

To all of the residents and attendings with whom we worked and from whom we learned so much during our time at the Big House.

CONTENTS

CONTRIBUTING AUTHORS

Former and current orthopaedic residents, fellows, and staff of the Hospital for Special Surgery, Cornell University Medical College, New York, New York.

Luis Alvarez, M.D.
James Bates, M.D.
Kevin Bonner, M.D.
Pamela Sherman Browne, M.D.
Struan H. Coleman, M.D.
Edward F. DiCarlo, M.D.
Gregory S. Difelice, M.D.
Shevaun Doyle, M.D.
Jeffery R. Dugas, M.D.
William J. Ertl, M.D.
Deborah A. Faryniarz, M.D.
Douglas Freedberg, M.D.
Bernard Gelhman, M.D.
Federico Girardi, M.D.
Dermot O'Farrell, M.D.
Hugh O'Flynn, M.D.
Alexandra E. Page, M.D.
Hollis G. Potter, M.D.
Adam B. Shafritz, M.D.
Daniel J. Stechschulte, M.D.
David Tate, M.D.
Karen Schneider, M.D.
Kurt V. Voelmicke, M.D.
Riley J. Williams III, M.D.

PREFACE

This book is intended to assist orthopaedic surgery residents prepare for their in-training examinations and part I of their American Board of Orthopaedic Surgery Examinations.

For most of us, an attempt to exhaustively review the topic of orthopaedic surgery prior to taking such an examination is infeasible, daunting, and unproductive. As we prepared for these joyous opportunities to yet again fill bubbles with a number 2 lead pencil, we felt that the most useful tool was to complete practice questions, and to look up the explanations for answers that we did not know. Unfortunately, existing compilations of questions either (1) provided no explanation whatsoever for the appropriate answer; (2) provided too terse an explanation; or (3) provided a decent explanation without optimizing the teaching/review potential of the question. We hope that this book accomplishes its goal of being a more user-friendly review tool.

ACKNOWLEDGMENTS

We are especially grateful to Nancy Bischoff, Dr. Bernard Gehlman, and Dr. Hollis Potter for their many contributions to this book and for their sustained genuine commitment to resident education. We would also like to thank our family and friends who put up with our whining and lost hours during residency in general and throughout this project.

1

THE HAND

QUESTIONS

1. Which of the following muscles is not innervated by the anterior interosseous nerve?
   (a) The pronator quadratus
   (b) The radial half of the flexor digitorum profundus
   (c) The flexor pollicis longus
   (d) The abductor pollicis longus
2. The proper sequence for repairing structures during replantation of a digit is which of the following?
   (a) (1) Nerves; (2) arteries; (3) bone; (4) veins; (5) extensor tendon; (6) flexor tendons
   (b) (1) Bone; (2) extensor tendon; (3) flexor tendons; (4) arteries; (5) nerves; (6) veins
   (c) (1) Bone; (2) arteries; (3) nerves; (4) veins; (5)flexor tendons; (6) extensor tendon
   (d) (1) Bone; (2) extensor tendon; (3) flexor tendons; (4) arteries; (5) veins; (6) nerves
   (e) (1) Arteries; (2) bone; (3) flexor tendons; (4) extensor tendon; (5) veins; (6) nerves
3. A 30-year-old hibachi chef sustains an accidental, self-inflicted volar laceration within zone 3 of his nondominant hand. Which of the following statements is most accurate?
   (a) The A2 pulley may need to be repaired.
   (b) The lumbrical takes origin from the flexor digitorum profundus tendon and runs along its ulnar border in this region.
   (c) It is highly unlikely that the flexor digitorum profundus tendon would be lacerated without concomitant flexor digitorum superficialis laceration.
   (d) There may likely be concomitant lacerations of the main trunks of the median and/or ulnar nerves.
   (e) After primary repair, the potential for functional recovery is relatively poor (as compared with tendon lacerations in the other flexor zones).
4. The most common type of thumb polydactyly is
   (a) Bifid distal phalanx (Wassel type I)
   (b) Duplicated distal phalanx (Wassel type II)
   (c) Bifid proximal phalanx (Wassel type III)
   (d) Duplicated proximal phalanx (Wassel type IV)
   (e) Bifid metacarpal (Wassel type V)
5. Which of the following statements regarding polydactyly is *true*?
   (a) It is one of the least common congenital musculoskeletal abnormalities of the hand.
   (b) Postaxial (ulnar) polydactyly is often associated with a generalized syndrome.
   (c) Postaxial (ulnar) polydactyly affects whites more frequently than blacks.
   (d) Polydactyly, in general, is more common in blacks than in whites.
   (e) The Bilhaut-Celoquet procedure entails excision of the least developed digit with reconstruction of the ipsilateral collateral ligament.
6. A 20-year-old collegiate rugby player presents with a focal, painful, swollen, erythematous area over the dorsum of his dominant third metacarpal head with an associated laceration, which is proximal to the metacarpophalangeal joint and radial to the extensor tendon. He gives a history of punching an opponent in the face approximately 36 hours previously (in retaliation for a bite inflicted on his ear). Examination of the ear reveals a small laceration with no missing tissue and no sign of infection. However, purulent discharge can be expressed from his hand laceration. There is no clinical evidence of tenosynovitis, lymphangitis, or axillary adenopathy. The patient has full active extension of the third ray. Radiographs reveal no fracture or foreign body. The most appropriate management of this patient is
   (a) Outpatient management with warm soaks, oral antibiotics, and daily wound reassessment
   (b) Outpatient management with oral antibiotics, windowed casting of the hand and wrist, daily wound reassessment, and strict instructions for activity modification (rugby cessation)
   (c) Admission to the hospital for warm soaks, close observation, and intravenous antibiotics, with prompt incision and drainage if no response to intravenous antibiotics
   (d) Admission for incision and drainage of the lesion and intravenous antibiotics

(e) Admission for incision and drainage of the lesion with exploration of the third metacarpophalangeal joint and intravenous antibiotics

7. The microorganism most likely to be responsible for the infection described in question 6 is which of the following?
   (a) *Staphylococcus aureus*
   (b) *Eikenella corrodens*
   (c) *Pasteurella multocida*
   (d) *Bacteroides fragilis*
   (e) Fungus (yeast form)
8. The most appropriate empiric antibiotic regimen in the management of the situation depicted in question 6 is which of the following? (You may assume that the patient has no known allergies.)
   (a) A first-generation cephalosporin
   (b) Ciprofloxacin
   (c) Trimethoprim-sulfamethoxazole
   (d) A first-generation cephalosporin plus penicillin
   (e) Vancomycin
9. Which of the following statements regarding the biomechanics of flexor tendons is least accurate?
   (a) Flexor tendons are viscoelastic structures.
   (b) Passive metacarpophalangeal motion produces no differential excursion between the flexor digitorum profundus and flexor digitorum superficialis tendons.
   (c) As a tendon passes farther from a joint's axis of rotation, the tendon has a greater moment arm across that joint.
   (d) As a tendon passes farther from a joint's axis of rotation, it will create more motion at that joint per unit of muscle contraction.
   (e) Flexor tendon moment arms are governed by the pulley system.
10. What is the most common malignant tumor of the hand?
   (a) Epithelioid sarcoma
   (b) Chondrosarcoma
   (c) Osteosarcoma
   (d) Basal cell carcinoma
   (e) Squamous cell carcinoma
11. Which of the following is most commonly acknowledged to be a risk factor for the development of avascular necrosis of the lunate bone (Kienböck disease)?
   (a) Long-term steroid use
   (b) Negative ulnar variance
   (c) Previous scaphoid fracture
   (d) Madelung deformity of the distal radius
   (e) Positive ulnar variance
12. A heavy metal drummer presents with distal radioulnar joint pain. Conservative treatment has failed, and he is to undergo wrist arthroscopy. The Lister tubercle is palpated. It lies between two dorsal wrist compartments. Which of the following correctly matches the correct two compartments and their contents?
   (a) 1 (abductor pollicis longus), 2 (extensor carpi radialis brevis)
   (b) 1 (extensor pollicis brevis), 2 (extensor carpi radialis longus)
   (c) 2 (extensor carpi radialis longus), 3 (extensor digitorum communis)
   (d) 2 (extensor carpi radialis brevis), 3 (extensor pollicis longus)
   (e) 3 (extensor pollicis longus), 4 (extensor indicis proprius)
13. The most common primary tumor that occurs in the bones of the hand is which of the following?
   (a) Intraosseous ganglion
   (b) Giant cell tumor
   (c) Chondrosarcoma
   (d) Enchondroma
   (e) Epithelioid sarcoma
14. What is the most common soft tissue sarcoma of the hand?
   (a) Alveolar rhabdomyosarcoma
   (b) Synovial sarcoma
   (c) Epithelioid sarcoma
   (d) Malignant fibrous histiocytoma
   (e) Soft tissue osteosarcoma
15. Figure 1.1 is a diagram of the digital flexor sheath of a finger. What two structures are the most important for maintaining the integrity of finger flexion?
   (a) A1 and A3
   (b) A2 and A4
   (c) A1 and A4
   (d) A2 and A5
   (e) A1 and A2
16. A 32-year-old kickboxer underwent plate fixation of fractures of his proximal radius and ulna. Postoperatively, he is unable to extend the metacarpophalangeal joints of his ulnar four digits. Interphalangeal joint extension of the thumb is also weak. Wrist dorsiflexion is accompanied by radial deviation. Sensation is intact throughout the hand. Injury to what structure is the most likely cause of the patient's problem?
   (a) The radial nerve
   (b) The anterior interosseous nerve
   (c) The ulnar nerve
   (d) The posterior interosseous nerve
   (e) The superficial radial nerve
17. A 44-year-old recreational skier falls and injures her right thumb. Examination reveals swelling about the metacarpophalangeal joint with localized tenderness along the ulnar aspect of the joint. Radiographic evaluation of the thumb reveals no fracture. Valgus stress testing with the metacarpophalangeal joint in full extension reveals 35 degrees of angulation. With the metacarpophalangeal joint in 30 degrees of flexion, there is 45 degrees of angulation. Which of the following forms of management would be most appropriate?

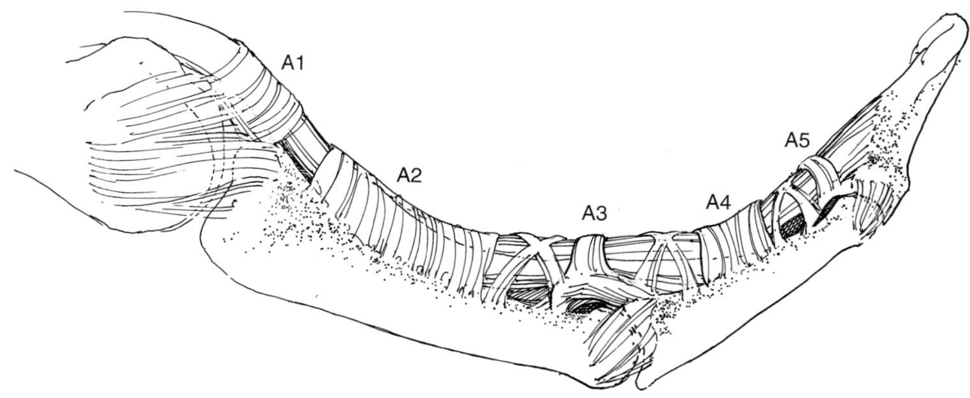

FIGURE 1.1

(a) Short-arm thumb spica cast for 4 to 6 weeks
(b) Reconstruction of the ulnar collateral ligament using palmaris longus tendon graft
(c) Repair of the torn ulnar collateral ligament
(d) Repair of the torn volar plate
(e) Repair of the avulsed adductor pollicis tendon to the base of the proximal phalanx

18. Which of the following correctly describes a Stener lesion?
(a) Displacement of the ulnar collateral ligament distal and superficial to the adductor aponeurosis
(b) Displacement of the ulnar collateral ligament distal and superficial to the adductor pollicis tendon
(c) Displacement of the ulnar collateral ligament distal and superficial to the ulnar sesamoid
(d) Displacement of the ulnar collateral ligament proximal and superficial to the adductor pollicis tendon
(e) Displacement of the ulnar collateral ligament proximal and superficial to the adductor aponeurosis

19. A 29-year-old attending pediatrician sustains a self-inflicted ring finger distal interphalangeal disarticulation while removing sutures from your patient's posterior spinal fusion wound (on postoperative day 3). The wound is débrided and closed by the attending general surgeon on call. The pediatrician presents to you 3 months later with a complaint of weak ipsilateral grip strength. The most likely explanation for this phenomenon is which of the following?
(a) The double-crush syndrome
(b) Posttraumatic adhesions within the flexor sheath
(c) Reflex sympathetic dystrophy
(d) The quadregia effect
(e) Malingering

20. A 24-year-old carpenter presents with a complaint of dorsal wrist pain and swelling. Examination reveals moderate tenderness over the dorsum of the wrist and mild swelling. Range of motion is 20 degrees of dorsiflexion and 35 degrees of palmar flexion. Radiographs reveal sclerosis of the lunate bone with subchondral lucency but no collapse. Measurements reveal 3 mm of negative ulnar variance. The physician should recommend which of the following?
(a) Lunate replacement with a silicone prosthesis
(b) Short-arm cast immobilization for 6 weeks
(c) Ulnar lengthening osteotomy
(d) Proximal row carpectomy
(e) Fourcorner arthrodesis

21. The most common muscle used as a transfer to restore wrist extension in a patient with a high radial nerve palsy is which of the following?
(a) The flexor carpi ulnaris
(b) The flexor carpi radialis
(c) The brachioradialis
(d) The pronator teres
(e) The palmaris longus

22. What nerve innervates the pronator quadratus muscle?
(a) The posterior interosseous nerve
(b) The ulnar nerve
(c) The anterior interosseous nerve
(d) The distal motor branch of the median nerve
(e) The radial nerve

23. After wrist arthroscopy and arthroscopic suture repair of a torn triangular fibrocartilage complex performed using regional anesthesia (axillary block), a patient complains of pain and paresthesias in the dorsoulnar surface of the hand and the dorsum of the ring and small fingers. The most likely cause of this patient's discomfort is which of the following?
(a) Injury to the dorsal cutaneous branch of the ulnar nerve
(b) Failure of the torn fibrocartilage complex repair
(c) Injury to the main trunk of the ulnar nerve
(d) Compartment syndrome in an interosseous compartment from arthroscopy fluid extravasation
(e) Neuritis of the posterior cord of the brachial plexus from the axillary block

24. The most appropriate position for arthrodesis of the metacarpophalangeal joint of the thumb is

(a) 10 degrees of flexion, 10 degrees of pronation, 0 degrees of abduction
(b) 10 degrees of flexion, 0 degrees of pronation, 0 degrees of abduction
(c) 30 degrees of flexion, 0 degrees of pronation, 10 degrees of abduction
(d) 30 degrees of flexion, 10 degrees of pronation, 5 degrees of abduction
(e) 30 degrees of flexion, 5 degrees of supination, 5 degrees of abduction

25. A 36-year-old man presents with a nontender nodule of 3 months' duration overlying the metacarpophalangeal joint of the middle finger. He maintains a large tropical fish aquarium in his home. The astute clinician performs a synovial biopsy and plates a culture on Lowenstein-Jensen medium at 32°C. The isolated organism is most likely to be which of the following?
(a) *Eikenella corrodens*
(b) *Sporothrix schenckii*
(c) *Mycobacterium marinum*
(d) *Pasteurella multocida*
(e) *Staphylococcus aureus*

26. Which of the following structures is the least likely to cause compression of the posterior interosseous nerve?
(a) The arcade of Frohse
(b) The leash of Henry
(c) The ligament of Struthers
(d) Fibrous bands anterior to the radial head
(e) The tendinous margin of the extensor carpi radialis brevis

27. Which of the following structures is the origin of the most common type of ganglion in the hand and wrist?
(a) The scapholunate ligament
(b) The radiocarpal ligament
(c) The extensor retinaculum
(d) The distal radioulnar joint capsule
(e) The scaphotrapezial joint capsule

28. With the thumb stabilizing the tuberosity (distal pole) of the scaphoid at the volar aspect of the carpus, the wrist is moved from ulnar to radial deviation. If pain or a clunk is elicited, then the test is positive. What is the name for this maneuver?
(a) Phalen test
(b) Sheer test
(c) Froment sign
(d) Watson test
(e) Terry Thomas sign

29. An elite ping-pong player presents with paresthesias in his median nerve distribution. What is the most radial structure within the carpal tunnel?
(a) The ulnar nerve
(b) The palmaris longus tendon
(c) The median nerve
(d) The flexor pollicis longus tendon
(e) The flexor carpi radialis tendon

30. The exposure of the proximal third of the radius using the volar approach of Henry proceeds in the interval between which two muscles?
(a) The brachioradialis and flexor carpi radialis
(b) The flexor carpi radialis and pronator teres
(c) The palmaris longus and flexor carpi radialis
(d) The brachioradialis and pronator teres
(e) The pronator teres and palmaris longus

31. Which of the following muscles is not innervated by the ulnar nerve?
(a) The first dorsal interosseous
(b) The flexor carpi ulnaris
(c) The flexor pollicis brevis
(d) The flexor digitorum superficialis to the small finger
(e) The adductor pollicis

32. A 36-year-old postal worker presents for a preemployment physical examination. He has recently moved across the country, and his past medical records are unavailable. He states that he had some sort of operation on his right (dominant) wrist for chronic, posttraumatic pain. Radiographs show a solid distal radioulnar synostosis with a more proximal ulnar pseudarthrosis. What procedure did this patient have?
(a) Darrach procedure
(b) Spinner-Kaplan procedure
(c) Hemiresection interposition arthroplasty
(d) Carroll-Imbriglia procedure
(e) Suave-Kapandji procedure

33. The patient in question 32 reports that his preoperative wrist discomfort was dramatically relieved by the procedure. His only active complaint is of wrist pain with heavy lifting. Physical examination reveals no focal wrist tenderness. There is painless, unrestricted active wrist range of motion (flexion/extension, radial/ulnar deviation, and pronation/supination). His pain is reproduced by resisted elbow flexion. Resisted elbow extension, pronation, and supination are painless. The most likely explanation for the patient's pain is which of the following?
(a) Radioulnar nonunion
(b) Radioulnar malunion
(c) Prominent hardware
(d) Radioulnar impingement
(e) Triangular fibrocartilage complex tear

34. What structure is marked by the arrow in the axial T1 magnetic resonance image of the forearm in Fig. 1.2?
(a) The flexor digitorum superficialis
(b) The palmaris longus
(c) The flexor carpi ulnaris
(d) The extensor carpi radialis longus
(e) The brachioradialis

35. Which of the following statements is correct?
(a) The deep brachial artery runs along the ulnar side of the ulnar nerve in the proximal arm.

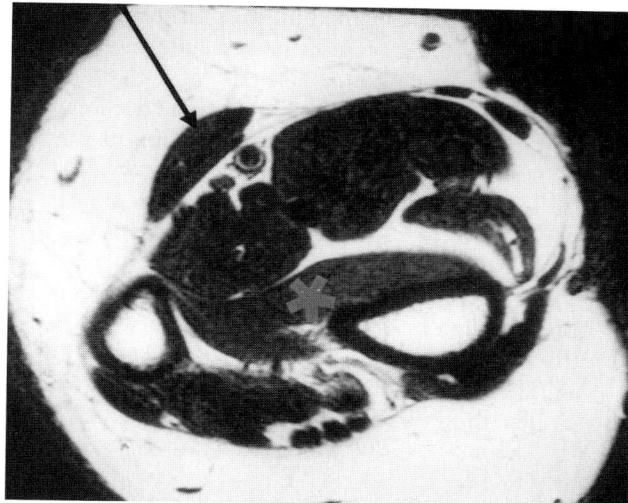

FIGURE 1.2

(b) The deep brachial artery runs along the radial side of the median nerve in the proximal arm.
(c) The deep brachial artery travels with the radial nerve in the proximal arm.
(d) The deep brachial artery exits the axilla through the quadrangular space.
(e) None of the above

36. Which of the following muscle flaps is or are most useful for reconstruction of a full-thickness shoulder defect?
(a) Latissimus dorsi and pectoralis major
(b) Trapezius and pectoralis major
(c) Latissimus dorsi and pectoralis minor
(d) Trapezius and latissimus dorsi
(e) Free gracilis

37. A 35-year-old disc jockey complains of pain on the volar surface of his proximal forearm and associated paresthesias involving the volar surfaces of his radial three digits. A radiograph of his elbow reveals a hook-shaped process of bone projecting anteromedially from the humerus 5 cm above the medial epicondyle. This process most likely represents
(a) The origin of the ligament of Struthers
(b) The origin of the arcade of Frohse
(c) The origin of the ligament of Grayson
(d) An osteochondroma
(e) The insertion of the coracobrachialis

38. Which of the following flaps would be the most appropriate for coverage of a full-thickness defect involving the distal third of the tibia?
(a) Gastrocnemius
(b) Soleus
(c) Free latissimus dorsi
(d) Rotational semitendinosis
(e) Free gracilis

39. What cell type is implicated in the pathophysiology of Dupuytren contracture?
(a) The fibroblast
(b) The macrophage
(c) The T lymphocyte
(d) The B lymphocyte
(e) The myofibroblast

40. What is the most common primary tumor that results in metastatic lesions in the hand?
(a) Lung
(b) Breast
(c) Prostate
(d) Multiple myeloma
(e) Thyroid

41. In the caput ulnae syndrome
(a) The ulnar head is dorsally subluxated; the carpus is dorsally subluxated and pronated.
(b) The ulnar head is volarly subluxated; the carpus is volarly subluxated and pronated.
(c) The ulnar head is volarly subluxated; the carpus is dorsally subluxated and pronated.
(d) The ulnar head is dorsally subluxated; the carpus is dorsally subluxated and supinated.
(e) The ulnar head is dorsally subluxated; the carpus is volarly subluxated and supinated.

42. The most common primary tumor that occurs in the bones of the hand is which of the following?
(a) Intraosseous ganglion
(b) Giant cell tumor
(c) Chondrosarcoma
(d) Enchondroma
(e) Epithelioid sarcoma

43. The vertical septa of the palm that separate the compartments are called what?
(a) Legeue and Juvara
(b) Grayson ligaments
(c) Natatory cords
(d) Lateral digital sheath
(e) Malcolm septa

44. The abnormal structures involved in Dupytren contracture involve all of the following except:
(a) Grayson ligament
(b) Cleland ligament
(c) Lateral digital sheet
(d) Pretendinous band
(e) Spiral band

45. During which stage of Dupytren disease does the collagen ratio switch, and what becomes more prevalent?
(a) Stage I: proliferative stage, increasing the ratio of type I to type III collagen
(b) Stage II: involutional stage, increasing the ratio of type III to type I collagen
(c) Stage III: residual stage, increasing the ratio of type I to type III collagen

(d) Stage III: residual stage, increasing the ratio of type III to type I collagen
(e) Stage II: involutional stage, increasing the ratio of type I to type III

46. Classic features of Madelung deformity include all of the following except:
(a) A wedge-shaped carpus
(b) Early fusion of the radial half of the distal radial physis
(c) Volar angulation of the distal radial articular surface
(d) Magnitude of the associated supination deficit greater than the magnitude of the associated pronation deficit
(e) Dorsal subluxation and enlargement of the distal ulna

47. Which pulleys should be preserved for the best function of the flexor tendons after repair?
(a) Al and A2
(b) A2 and A3
(c) A3 and A5
(d) A4 and A2
(e) Al and A5

48. Which of the following has not been shown to have a superior effect on the result of flexor tendon repair?
(a) Tendon sheath repair
(b) Increasing the number of sutures that cross the repair site
(c) Using atraumatic technique during repair
(d) Using an epitendinous suture
(e) Meticulous sterile technique

49. A patient comes into your office with a history of trauma to his ring finger approximately 3 weeks ago. He complains of difficulty bending his distal interphalangeal joint. The injury is shown in Fig. 1.3. The treatment at this time should consist of

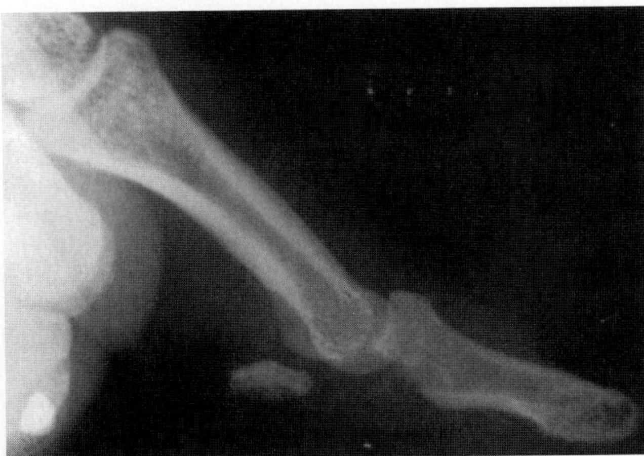

FIGURE 1.3

(a) Débridement of the bony fragment and advancement of the profundus tendon into the distal phalanx
(b) Arthrodesis of the distal interphalangeal joint
(c) Open reduction and internal fixation of the fragment to the distal phalanx
(d) Tendon graft to the distal phalanx
(e) Excision of the distal interphalangeal joint with palliative pseudarthrosis

50. Which of the following interossei muscles has only one muscle belly?
(a) The first dorsal
(b) The second dorsal
(c) The third dorsal
(d) The fourth dorsal
(e) The fifth dorsal

51. Rupture of the radial sagittal band causes the patient which bothersome complaint?
(a) A locking metacarpophalangeal joint in flexion with flexible proximal and distal interphalangeal joints and passive full extension of the metacarpophalangeal joint
(b) A clicking when reaching full extension of the metacarpophalangeal joint, with normal distal and proximal interphalangeal joint motion
(c) A tight proximal interphalangeal joint with metacarpophalangeal extension
(d) A tight proximal interphalangeal joint with metacarpophalangeal flexion

52. Which malignant tumor has a predilection for the fingers and hands?
(a) Chondrosarcoma
(b) Osteogenic sarcoma
(c) Ewing sarcoma
(d) Epithelioid sarcoma
(e) Neuroblastoma

53. Sites of ulnar nerve compression include all the following except
(a) The medial intermuscular septum
(b) The transverse fascial fibers of the cubital tunnel roof
(c) Osborne fascia
(d) The medial epicondyle
(e) The Guyon canal

54. A 35-year-old woman comes into your office with a complaint of a painful index finger just under the nail, which she notes is very tender. She denies any previous trauma and states that she is unable to wash her hands in any water that is cold and is unable to hold cold items with that hand. Her previous physician sent her to a psychologist. What would you expect to find on examination?
(a) A picture of hypersensitivity throughout her entire hand
(b) A ridging of her nail bed and discoloration

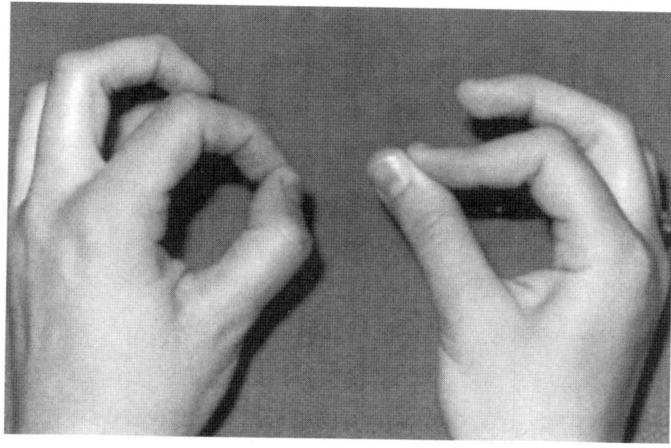

FIGURE 1.4

(c) Stiffness of her entire hand
(d) No real findings and evidence of malingering
(e) Sausage digits

55. Dorsal intercalated segment instability has
    (a) A scapholunate angle of more than 70 degrees
    (b) A scapholunate angle of less than 30 degrees
    (c) A scapholunate gap of more than 3 mm
    (d) Palmar flexion of the lunate
    (e) Dorsal rotation of the scaphoid
56. A patient with the observed deformity in the right hand of (Fig. 1.4) may present with all the following except
    (a) A positive Phalen test
    (b) Thenar weakness
    (c) Palm paresthesias
    (d) A lack of electrodiagnostic abnormalities
    (e) Pain in the forearm
57. Which of the following is not one of the four classic findings of pyogenic flexor tenosynovitis described by Kanavel?
    (a) Excessive tenderness over the course of the tendon sheath
    (b) Excruciating pain on passive extension of the finger, most markedly at the proximal end
    (c) Flexed position of the finger
    (d) Erythema along the course of the tendon sheath
    (e) Symmetric enlargement of the whole finger
58. A 2-year-old child presents with the deformity seen in the radiograph shown in Fig. 1.5. The parents state the child has had previous surgery. They are now asking for the thumb deformity to be treated. The best treatment option is
    (a) Derotational osteotomy of the proximal phalanx with stabilization of the metacarpophalangeal joint with Kirschner wires
    (b) Arthrodesis of the metacarpophalangeal joint only
    (c) Excision of the present thumb with toe-to-thumb transfer
    (d) First metacarpophalangeal fusion at 15 degrees of flexion, abduction, and pronation
    (e) Excision of the present thumb with index pollicization
59. The radiograph in Fig. 1.6 demonstrates which Wassel bifid thumb classification?
    (a) Wassel type II
    (b) Wassel type IV
    (c) Wassel type VI
    (d) Wassel type VII
    (e) Wassel type I
60. All the following are associated with a boutonniere deformity except which?

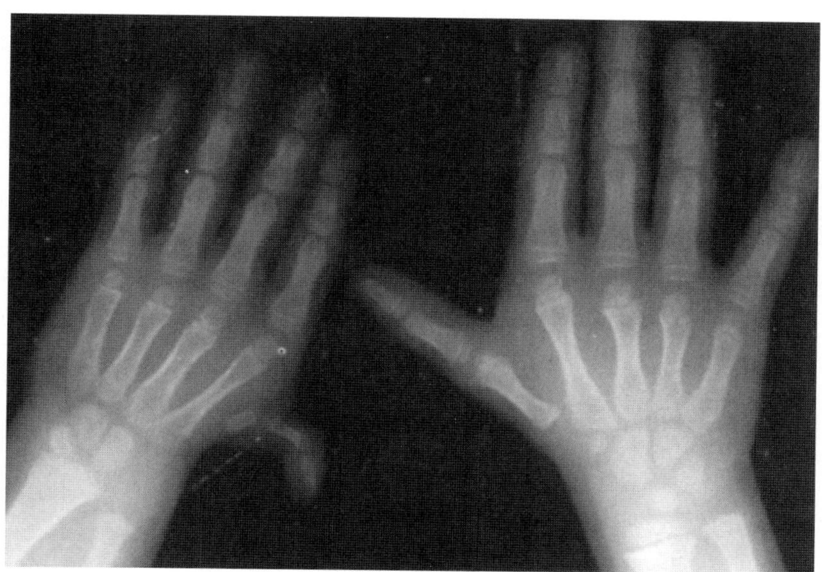

FIGURE 1.5

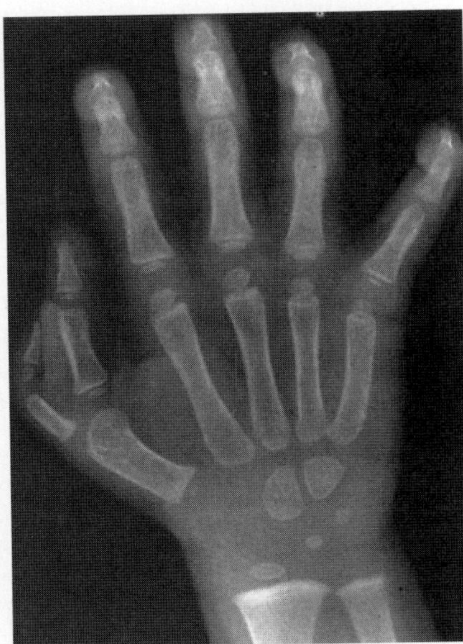

FIGURE 1.6

(a) A triangular ligament tear
(b) Lateral band volar subluxation
(c) Central slip insufficiency
(d) Volar plate injury
(e) Decreased distal interphalangeal flexion

61. Figure 1.7 shows a 32-year-old man who hit his finger while playing football approximately 6 weeks ago. This is his first visit to a physician regarding the problem. The finger is passively correctable to full extension at the proximal interphalangeal joint with full active distal interphalangeal motion. What is the most appropriate treatment in this situation?
(a) Splinting of the proximal interphalangeal joint in extension for a minimum of 6 weeks

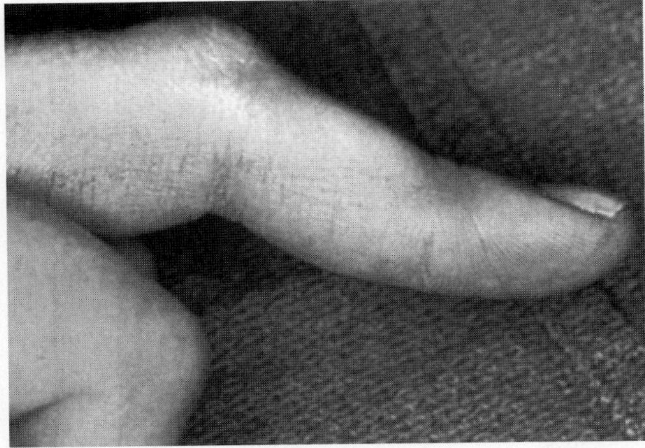

FIGURE 1.7

(b) Central slip advancement
(c) Conjoined tendon release
(d) Lateral band transfer
(e) Soft tissue release and secondary tendon reconstruction

62. A persistent medial artery contributes to the palmar blood supply in which percentage of patients?
(a) 0%
(b) 10%
(c) 25%
(d) 35%
(e) 45%

63. This muscle originates on the hook of the hamate and inserts into the ulnar shaft of the fifth metacarpal. It has which function?
(a) Flexion of the metacarpophalangeal joint
(b) Abduction the fifth digit with the metacarpophalangeal joint stabilized
(c) Flexion and adduction of the fifth metacarpal
(d) Abduction of the fifth metacarpal and extension of the distal phalanx
(e) Flexion of the fifth metacarpal and stabilization of the fifth metacarpophalangeal joint

64. A patient is brought into the emergency department with a complaint of mild hand pain. He has recently started a job as a painter in a factory using a high-pressure gun. He feels that he may have injected some paint into his nondominant left palm. On physical examination, he has a small puncture wound over his palm with some mild edema. Appropriate treatment at this time consists of which of the following?
(a) Discharge home after given a tetanus booster on antibiotics and instructions to return to your office in 1 week
(b) Admission for observation
(c) Immediate transfer to the operating room for exploration and débridement
(d) Immediate amputation of the involved area
(e) Immediate débridement in the emergency room, admission, and intravenous antibiotics

65. The scapholunate interosseous ligament, which connects the scaphoid and lunate, is composed of
(a) One dorsal ligament
(b) One palmar ligament
(c) A dorsal and a proximal ligament
(d) A dorsal and a palmar ligament, separated by the long radiolunate ligament
(e) A dorsal and a palmar ligament and proximal fibrocartilage, the latter two separated by the radioscapholunate ligament

66. Which of the following is not characteristic of scapholunate dissociation?
(a) The Terry Thomas sign
(b) A scapholunate gap of more than 3 mm
(c) The cortical ring sign

(d) A volar intercalated segment instability deformity
(e) A dorsal intercalated segment instability deformity

67. Which of the following is a carpal instability nondissociative lesion?
(a) Scapholunate dissociation
(b) Lunatotriquetral dissociation
(c) Midcarpal instability
(d) Giant cell tumor of scaphoid
(e) Scaphoid fracture

68. A 47-year-old right-hand–dominant postal worker presents with right wrist pain 5 weeks after a motor vehicle accident. He is unable to do his job without pain. On physical examination, there is tenderness over the scapholunate region with a positive Watson test. He has decreased grip and pinch on the right side as compared with the left. Radiographs reveal a scapholunate gap of more than 4 mm. Which treatment option is unacceptable?
(a) Closed reduction and pinning
(b) Blatt capsulodesis
(c) Open reduction and internal fixation
(d) Proximal row carpectomy
(e) Primary repair of ligaments

69. Which of the following statements is correct?
(a) The digital arteries lie volar to the digital nerves in the palm, but dorsal to the digital nerves in the fingers.
(b) The digital arteries lie volar to the digital nerves in the palm and volar to the digital nerves in the fingers.
(c) The digital arteries lie dorsal to the digital nerves in the palm, but volar to the digital nerves in the fingers.
(d) The digital arteries lie dorsal to the digital nerves in the palm and dorsal to the digital nerves in the fingers.
(e) The digital arteries lie ulnar to the digital nerves in the palm and ulnar to the digital nerves in the fingers.

70. What is the most radial structure in the carpal tunnel?
(a) The flexor digitorum superficialis tendon to the index finger
(b) The flexor pollicis longus tendon
(c) The flexor digitorum profundus tendon to the index finger
(d) The radial artery
(e) The radial nerve

71. Three common variations in the course of the thenar branch of the median nerve have been described. For the purposes of this question, type A is defined as branching beneath the transverse carpal ligament and having a transligamentous course to the thenar musculature. Type B is defined as a branching beneath the transverse carpal ligament, running close to the median nerve, and then having a recurrent course distal to the transverse carpal ligament. Type C is defined as an extraligamentous recurrent course from the median nerve after branching just distal to the transverse carpal ligament. Which of the following answers describes the approximate distributions of these anatomic variations in the general population?
(a) A, 30%; B, 50%; C, 20%
(b) A, 20%; B, 50%; C, 30%
(c) A, 30%; B, 20%; C, 50%
(d) A, 20%; B, 30%; C, 50%
(e) A, 50%; B, 30%; C, 20%

72. What is the normal value for twopoint discrimination in adults at the fingertips?
(a) 2 to 3 mm
(b) 3 to 4 mm
(c) 5 to 6 mm
(d) 7 to 8 mm
(e) 9 to 10 mm

73. Which of the following is not a site of potential compression in entrapment neuropathy of the median nerve?
(a) The lacertus fibrosus
(b) The arcade of Frohse
(c) The ligament of Struthers
(d) The pronator teres
(e) The arch of the flexor digitorum superficialis

74. An otherwise healthy 12-year-old, left-hand–dominant, Hispanic girl presents to your clinic with symptoms of deepaching pain in the proximal volar aspect of her forearm. She worked in a designer clothes factory in South America until last month, when she came to the United States. She states that her pain began over the past 6 months and has slowly worsened. Initially, the pain was exacerbated when only she used her arm, and it was relieved with rest. Now, she often has pain at rest and feels the need to massage her forearm, although this does not seem to relieve the pain. She also complains of some numbness and tingling in the volar aspect of the palm, index finger, and long fingers. She recalls a fall onto the elbow in the past, remote from the onset of her pain. Physical examination reveals full, painless range of motion at the elbow, a negative Phalen sign, and a negative Kiloh-Nevin sign. Anteroposterior and lateral radiographs reveal a small, hookshaped process of bone found approximately 5 cm above the medial epicondyle of the elbow. Which of the following answers would be the most likely diagnosis at this point?
(a) Pronator syndrome
(b) Carpal tunnel syndrome
(c) Anterior interosseous syndrome
(d) Heterotopic ossification
(e) Cubital tunnel syndrome

75. You order electrodiagnostic studies that reveal muscle denervation and increased nerve latencies. The most appropriate treatment at this point would be

(a) Occupational therapy and splinting
(b) Surgical excision of heterotopic ossification
(c) Surgical release of the median nerve at the wrist
(d) Surgical release of the median nerve at the elbow
(e) Surgical release of the anterior interosseous nerve

76. Which of the following muscles is not innervated by the ulnar nerve?
(a) The ring lumbrical
(b) The pronator quadratus
(c) The flexor digitorum profundus to the ring finger
(d) The deep head of the flexor pollicis brevis
(e) The adductor pollicis

77. During dorsal proximal interphalangeal joint dislocations, the volar plate and ligament box are most likely to avulse from which surface in the majority of cases?
(a) The base of the middle phalanx
(b) The radial side of the head of the proximal phalanx
(c) The ulnar side of the head of the proximal phalanx
(d) The volar aspect of the head of the proximal phalanx
(e) None of the above

78. A 35-year-old female attorney presents to your office complaining of the inability to extend her long finger for the last 2 weeks. She states that while preparing a brief, one of her assistants accidentally dropped a heavy law book onto the back of her clenched fist. Radiographs were normal at the emergency room, but several days later, the patient noted that she was unable to extend her long finger. Physical examination reveals tenderness and swelling at the metacarpophalangeal of the long finger. She is not able to initiate metacarpophalangeal extension from a flexed position, but she can keep the finger extended once passively extended. Dorsal and proximal interphalangeal joint extension are intact. What is the most likely diagnosis?
(a) Closed, zone 5 extensor tendon rupture
(b) Closed, zone 3 extensor tendon rupture
(c) Radial sagittal band rupture
(d) Ulnar sagittal band rupture
(e) Lumbrical rupture

79. What treatment would you recommend at this point?
(a) Dynamic extension splints for 6 weeks, then active range-of-motion exercises
(b) Surgical repair of the sagittal band
(c) Surgical repair of the extensor tendon
(d) Static extension splint for 6 weeks
(e) Dynamic extension splints for 6 weeks

80. Current recommendations for the repair of flexor tendon lacerations call for the use of which of the following?
(a) Four-strand core stitch
(b) Four-strand core stitch with continuous peripheral epitendinous suture
(c) Two-strand core stitch
(d) Two-strand core stitch with continuous peripheral epitendinous suture
(e) Six-strand core stitch

81. A 14-year-old boy presents to your office complaining of throbbing pain at the tip of his index finger for the last 5 days. During the course of your thorough history, you learn that he has no prior history of these symptoms and no history of recent trauma. In addition, you wisely elicit that he is not sexually active and has no current genitourinary complaints. His mother, however, complains that he still bites his nails and is convinced that this is the source of his current problem. Figure 1.8 shows the appearance of his fingertip. Recommended treatment should include
(a) Office-based irrigation and débridement
(b) Miconazole cream three times daily
(c) Warm soaks and splinting
(d) Oral acyclovir
(e) Observation

82. Which of the following is the most common pathogen attributable to dog bites in the hand?
(a) α-Hemolytic *Streptococcus*
(b) *Staphylococcus aureus*
(c) *Eikenella corrodens*
(d) *Pasteurella multocida*
(e) *Bacteroides fragilis*

83. According to the current literature, the most common hand infection that presents in human immunodeficiency virus–positive patients is
(a) Flexor tenosynovitis
(b) Herpes simplex
(c) Fungal infections
(d) Cellulitis
(e) Pulp space infections

84. A 23-year-old man has a motor vehicle accident and sustains right upper extremity fractures to the diaphyses of the humerus, radius, and ulna. The fractures are closed, and there is no neurovascular compromise. The recommended treatment for this injury is

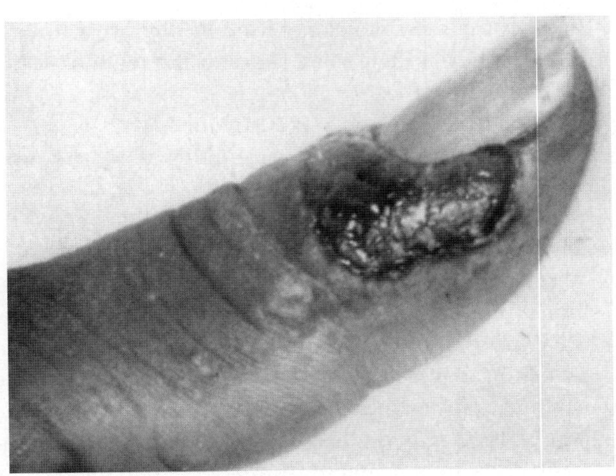

FIGURE 1.8

(a) Open reduction and internal fixation of the humerus and forearm fractures
(b) Open reduction and internal fixation of the humerus and closed reduction of the forearm fractures
(c) Closed reduction of the forearm fractures and functional bracing of the humerus
(d) Open reduction and internal fixation of the forearm fractures and functional bracing of the humerus
(e) Functional bracing of both the humerus and forearm

85. Figure 1.9 is a T1 coronal magnetic resonance image of a right shoulder of a managed care executive with an overuse injury of his right shoulder associated with an excessive golf habit. What muscle is marked by the letter O?
(a) The pectoralis major
(b) The infraspinatus
(c) The teres major
(d) The subscapularis
(e) The teres minor

86. A Stryker notch view of the shoulder demonstrates an osteochondral defect (impaction fracture) in the posterior humeral head. This is consistent with which of the following diagnoses?
(a) Posterior glenohumeral instability
(b) Rotator cuff arthropathy
(c) Subacromial impingement syndrome
(d) Anterior glenohumeral instability
(e) Rheumatoid arthritis

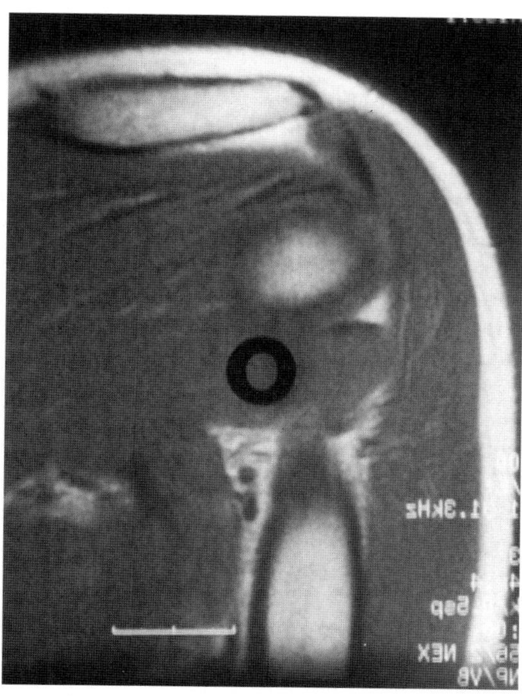

FIGURE 1.9

ANSWERS

1. **d** The anterior interosseous nerve innervates three muscles: (1) the pronator quadratus, (2) the radial half of the flexor digitorum profundus, and (3) the flexor pollicis longus. The abductor pollicis longus is innervated by the posterior interosseous nerve.
2. **b** The proper sequence for repair during digital replantation is as follows: (1) locate and tag vessels and nerves, (2) débride necrotic tissues, (3) shorten and fix the *B*one, (4) repair *E*xtensor tendons, (5) repair *F*lexor tendons, (6) perform *A*rtery anastomosis, (7) repair the *N*erves, (8) perform vein anastomosis, and (9) obtain skin coverage. BEFANV is the suggested mnemonic: *BE* a *FAN* of *V* (five fingers). Bony stability must be established before vessel repair, so the vessel anastomoses are not disrupted during bone reconstruction. Definitive bone length must be established before tendon repair, so appropriate tendon resting length can be set.

Reference

Brown ML, Wood MB: Techniques of Bone Fixation in Replantation. Microsurgery 11:255–260, 1990.

3. **c** Zone 3 consists of the region between the metacarpal neck (distally) and the distal end of the flexor retinaculum (proximally). (The five flexor tendon zones (Verdan zones) are depicted schematically in Fig. 1.10. The

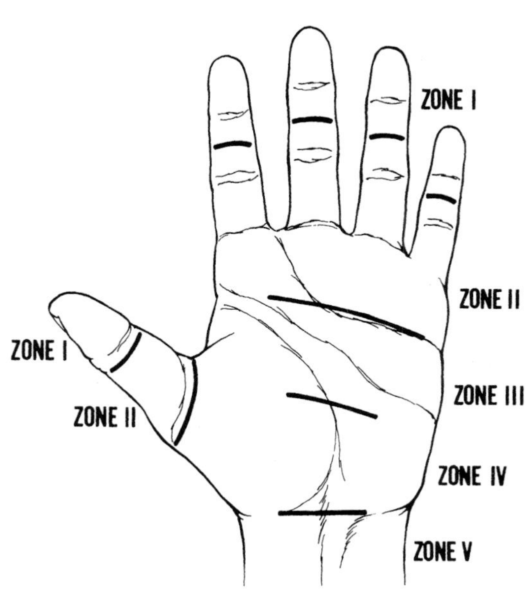

FIGURE 1.10

flexor digitorum profundus tendon runs deep (dorsal) to the flexor digitorum superficialis tendon proximal to Camper chiasma (which is in zone 2). Thus, a zone 3 laceration that penetrated deep enough to sever the flexor digitorum profundus tendon would also have to sever the flexor digitorum superficialis tendon as well (which lies directly superficial to the flexor digitorum profundus tendon).

The A2 pulley is a zone 2 structure and thus would not be injured if the laceration is contained within zone 3. The lumbrical takes origin from the flexor digitorum profundus tendon and runs along its *radial* (not ulnar) border in zone 3.

Concomitant laceration of the main trunks of the median and/or ulnar nerves is likely in zone 4 (carpal tunnel) and zone 5 (forearm). However, the main trunks divide proximal to the level of zone 3.

The potential for functional recovery is relatively good after repair of zone 3 lacerations (as compared with tendon injuries in other flexor zones). Zone 2 (no-man's-land) is notorious for being the region with the least favorable prognosis after flexor tendon repair. This relatively poor prognosis is linked to the diathesis for adhesion formation, which stems from the close proximity of the tendons in this region where they are enclosed within the tight, unyielding flexor sheath.

Reference

Leddy JP: Flexor Tendons: Acute Injuries. In Green DP, ed: Operative Hand Surgery, 3rd Ed. New York, Churchill Livingstone, pp. 1823–1825, 1993.

4. **d** The most common classification system for thumb polydactyly is that described by Wassel. This system divides thumb polydactyly into seven types: I, bifid distal phalanx; II, duplicated distal phalanx; III, bifid proximal phalanx; IV, duplicated proximal phalanx; V, bifid metacarpal; VI, duplicated metacarpal; and VII, triphalangism. In Wassel's large series, type IV was the most common (43%).The percentages of each type were as follows: I, 2%; II, 15%; III, 6%; IV, 43%; V, 10%; VI, 4%; VII, 20%.

References

Flatt AE: The Care of Congenital Hand Anomalies. St Louis, CV Mosby, pp. 99–117, 1977.

Wassel HD: The Results of Surgery for Polydactyly of the Thumb: A Review. Clin Orthop, 64:175–193, 1969.

Wood VE: Polydactyly and the Triphalangeal Thumb. J Hand Surg, 3:436–444, 1978.

5. **d** Polydactyly is the *most* common congenital musculoskeletal abnormality of the hand. Polydactyly, in general, is more common in blacks than in whites. Postaxial (ulnar) polydactyly is more common than preaxial (radial) polydactyly and is typically an isolated abnormality. Preaxial (radial) polydactyly is more common among whites and is more frequently associated with a generalized syndrome. Preaxial polydactyly is typically treated by excision of the least developed digit with attention to preservation of the ulnar collateral ligament. The Bilhaut-Celoquet procedure entails a fusion of the two bifid parts (with partial preservation of each).

Reference

Gallant GG, Dora FW: Congenital Deformities of the Upper Extremity. J Am Acad Orthop Surg, 4(3):162–171, 1996.

6. **e** Any infected wound over a metacarpal head that is sustained by a clenched fist to face mechanism should be treated as a human bite with metacarpophalangeal joint penetration. With the digits extended, the laceration will move proximally, and the unenlightened examiner may overlook the fact that the laceration lay directly over the metacarpophalangeal joint at the time that the fist contacted the offending tooth. A partially lacerated extensor mechanism may not be recognized by a nonastute examiner because the affected portion will retract proximal to the skin wound when the finger is examined in extension. Proper treatment consists of prompt incision and drainage of the lesion with concomitant exploration of the extensor mechanism and metacarpophalangeal joint. Thorough irrigation of the metacarpophalangeal joint is indicated if its capsule has been violated. The hand should be immobilized in an intrinsic-plus position.

Reference

Abrams RA, Botte MJ: Hand Infections. J Am Acad Orthop Surg, 4:219–230, 1996.

7. **a** *Staphylococcus aureus* is the most common organism responsible for human bite infections in the hand. It is also the most common pathogen in hand infections in general. α-Hemolytic *Streptococcus* is another common pathogen in human bite infections of the hand. *Eikenella corrodens* (a gram-negative species), despite its reputation as a characteristic offender in this situation, is isolated from only approximately 10% to 30% of human bite wounds. *Bacteroides* species are the most commonly isolated anaerobic species in human bite infections of the hand. *Pasteurella multocida* (a gram-negative coccobacillus) is a common pathogen in scratch and bite wounds from cats and dogs.

Reference

Abrams RA, Botte MJ: Hand Infections. J Am Acad Orthop Surg, 4:219–230, 1996.

8. **d** The recommended first-line empiric regimen for human bite infections of the hand is a first-generation cephalosporin (such as cefazolin 1g intravenously every 8 hours) plus penicillin G (2 to 4 million units intravenously every 4 to 6 hours). The penicillin is necessary to cover *Eikenella.* The same regimen has been espoused for the first-line empiric coverage of animal bite infections. Of course, intraoperative cultures should be obtained at the time of irrigation and débridement of all bite wounds, with subsequent refining of the antibiotic treatment as indicated by culture results and sensitivities.

Reference

Abrams RA, Botte MJ: Hand Infections. J Am Acad Orthop Surg, 4:219–230, 1996.

9. **d** Statement d is inaccurate. In fact, as a tendon passes farther from a joint's axis of rotation, it will create *less* motion at that joint per unit of muscle contraction. As a tendon passes farther from a joint's axis of rotation, more tendon excursion is required to produce a given angular rotation of that joint. This finding is the basis for the reason that joint motion is compromised when there is pulley incompetence and tendon bowstringing (Fig. 1.11). The four other statements (a, b, c, and e) are all correct.

Reference

Strickland JW: Flexor Tendon Injuries: I. Foundations of Treatment. J Am Acad Orthop Surg, 3:44–54, 1995.

10. **e** Squamous cell carcinoma is the most common malignant tumor of the hand. Its incidence is greater among male patients. It demonstrates a predilection for sun-exposed regions (i.e., the dorsum of the hand) and elderly persons. Subungual lesions are often overlooked or misdiagnosed. This tumor tends to spread to regional lymph nodes. Thus, regional lymph nodes should always be examined, and lymphadenectomy is sometimes indicated in addition to the mandated wide excision of the lesion itself.

Reference

American Society for Surgery of the Hand: Regional Review Course Syllabus. American Society for Surgery of the Hand, 1995.

11. **b** Ulnar variance refers to the length relationship between the articular surfaces of the distal radius and ulna. Negative ulnar variance (ulnar minus variance) implies that the ulna is shorter than the radius; positive ulnar variance implies that the ulna is longer than the radius. The relationship between ulnar minus variance and Kienböck disease was first described by Hulten,

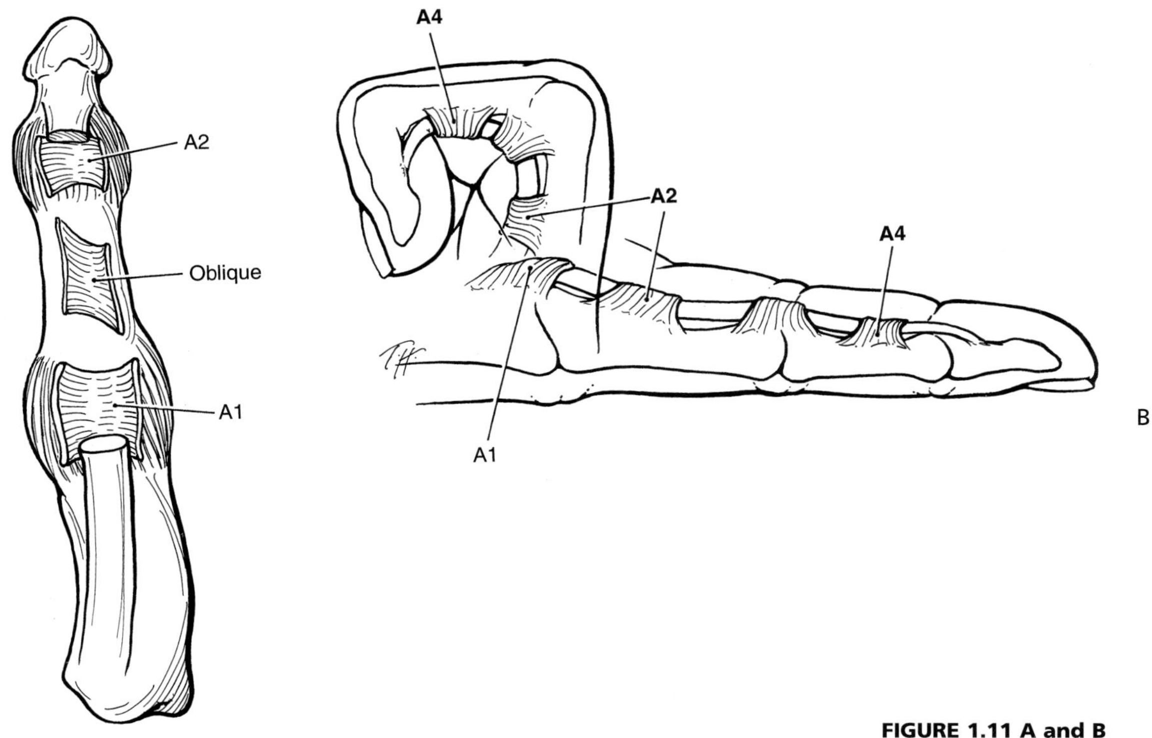

FIGURE 1.11 A and B

who noted this condition in 230 of normal wrists and in 78% of those afflicted with Kienböck disease. The relatively short ulna is thought to contribute to the development of Kienböck disease by increasing the compressive and tensile strains across the lunate from the radius and capitate. The other listed factors have not been shown to be significant in the origin of Kienböck disease.

Reference

Weiland AJ: Avascular Necrosis of the Carpus. In Hand Surgery Update. American Society for Surgery of the Hand, pp. 85–89, 1996.

12. **d** The key landmark is Lister's tubercle. There are six extensor tendon compartments across the dorsal wrist (Table 1.1): Lister's tubercle is the border between compartments II and III.

    Note: Distal to the wrist, the extensor indicis tendon travels along the ulnar side the extensor digitorum communis tendon to the index finger. The extensor digiti minimi tendon travels on the ulnar side of the extensor digitorum communis tendon to the small finger.
13. **d** Enchondroma is the most common primary neoplasm that occurs in the skeleton of the hand. Enchondromas are most commonly discovered either incidentally or when a pathologic fracture occurs through a solitary lesion in the diaphysis or metaphysis of a phalanx or metacarpal in a young adult. The proximal phalanx is the most commonly affected region. The incidence among males and females is equivalent. Intraosseous ganglia, giant cell tumors, and chondrosarcomas rarely occur in the bones of the hand. Giant cell tumors *do* commonly occur in extraosseous locations in the hand (specifically, in the flexor tendon sheath). *Giant cell tumor of tendon sheath* is the second most common soft tissue mass found in the hand (ganglia are the most common). Histologically, giant cell tumor of tendon sheath is virtually indistinguishable from pigmented villonodular synovitis.

TABLE 1.1. SIX EXTENSOR TENDON COMPARTMENTS

Compartment	Tendons Contained
I	Abductor pollicis longus Extensor pollicis brevis
II	Extensor carpi radialis longus Extensor carpi radialis brevis
III	Extensor pollicis longus
IV	Extensor digitorum communis Extensor indicis
V	Extensor digiti minimi
VI	Extensor carpi ulnaris

Reference

American Society for Surgery of the Hand: Regional Review Course Syllabus. American Society for Surgery of the Hand, 1995.

14. **c** Epithelioid sarcoma is the most common soft tissue sarcoma of the hand. Alveolar rhabdomyosarcoma and synovial sarcoma are the second and third most common, respectively. Epithelioid sarcoma tends to occur in the second and third decades, with a 2:1 male predilection. It affects the digits more commonly than the hand or forearm. Recommended treatment is wide resection or amputation. The guarded prognosis stems, in part, from the finding that this lesion is commonly misdiagnosed or inadequately treated.

Reference

American Society for Surgery of the Hand: Regional Review Course Syllabus. American Society for Surgery of the Hand, 1995.

15. **b** Figure 1.1 illustrates the flexor tendons, the flexor sheath, and the pulley system. The structures are labeled. The A2 and A4 pulleys are located at the proximal and middle phalanges. These are the most important structures for preventing tendon bowstringing during active flexion.

Reference

Strickland JW: Flexor Tendon Injuries: I. Foundations of Treatment. J Am Acad Orthop Surg, 3(1):44–54, 1995.

16. **d** This patient exhibits typical signs of posterior interosseous nerve palsy. This includes deficits of the extensor digitorum communis, extensor pollicis longus, and extensor carpi ulnaris. Wrist dorsiflexion is preserved because the radial nerve branches to the extensor carpi radialis longus and extensor carpi radialis brevis diverge from the main trunk of the radial nerve prior to the bifurcation of the main trunk of the radial nerve. Branches from the common trunk of the radial nerve supply the entire mobile wad of three (extensor carpi radialis brevis, extensor carpi radialis longus, and brachioradialis). The main trunk of the radial nerve subsequently bifurcates (at the level of the radiohumeral joint) into the superficial radial nerve, which travels distally beneath the brachioradialis, and the posterior interosseous nerve, which passes into the supinator muscle. The extensor carpi ulnaris is innervated by the posterior interosseous nerve. Thus, when the posterior interosseous nerve is injured, radial deviation occurs with active wrist dorsiflexion because the innervation to the extensor carpi ulnaris is damaged yet the innervation to the extensor carpi radialis brevis and extensor carpi radialis longus is intact.

Patients undergoing open reduction and internal fixation of a proximal radial shaft fracture are at risk of posterior interosseous nerve injury during elevation and/or retraction of the supinator muscle. Sensation in the distribution of the superficial branch of the radial nerve is preserved in this situation because this nerve originates proximal to the supinator.

Reference

Fuss FK, Wurzl GH: Radial Nerve Entrapment at the Elbow: Surgical Anatomy. J Hand Surg Am, 16(4):742–747, 1991.

17. **c** The clinical history and findings on examination are consistent with an acute tear of the ulnar collateral ligament. The positive stress test in 30 degrees of flexion (more than 30 degrees of laxity or 15 degrees more laxity than the contralateral thumb) indicates disruption of the proper ulnar collateral ligament. The positive stress test in full extension (more than 30 degrees of laxity or 15 degrees more laxity than the contralateral thumb) implies complete tears of both the proper and accessory ulnar collateral ligaments. If the accessory collateral ligament were intact, then it would confer relative stability in extension.

The accepted treatment for this lesion is direct repair of the ulnar collateral ligament. This lesion will not heal reliably with immobilization alone, particularly given the potential for an associated *Stener lesion.*

When this type of injury is initially neglected, then late ligament reconstruction with autograft tendon may be required (e.g., palmaris longus). Casting for 4 to 6 weeks would be appropriate for an incomplete ulnar collateral ligament tear.

Although the ulnar corner of the thumb metacarpophalangeal palmar plate may be detached from the metacarpal with complete ulnar collateral ligament injuries, complete ruptures of palmar plate typically occur as a result of dorsal dislocations by a hyperextension mechanism. Associated collateral ligament instability is usually less than 25 to 30 degrees and typically heals with appropriate immobilization.

Reference

Heyman P: Injuries to the Ulnar Collateral Ligament of the Thumb Metacarpophalangeal joint. J Am Acad Orthop Surg, 5(4):224–229, 1997.

18. **e** Displacement of the ulnar collateral ligament proximal and superficial to the adductor aponeurosis constitutes a *Stener lesion* (Fig. 1.12). Such interposition of the adductor aponeurosis precludes anatomic ulnar collateral ligament healing. A Stener lesion is present in more than 84% of cases when physical examination indicates complete ulnar collateral ligament disruption. A palpable lump at the ulnar aspect of the metacarpophalangeal joint suggests that a Stener lesion may be present. However, the displaced ulnar collateral ligament is not always palpable.

Reference

Heyman P: Injuries to the Ulnar Collateral Ligament of the Thumb Metacarpophalangeal joint. J Am Acad Orthop Surg, 5(4):224–229, 1997.
Stener B: Displacement of the Ruptured Ulnar Collateral Ligament of the Metacarpophalangeal Joint of the Thumb. J Bone Joint Surg Br, 44:869–879, 1962.

19. **d** The quadregia effect occurs when the flexor digitorum profundus tendons act as a single unit because

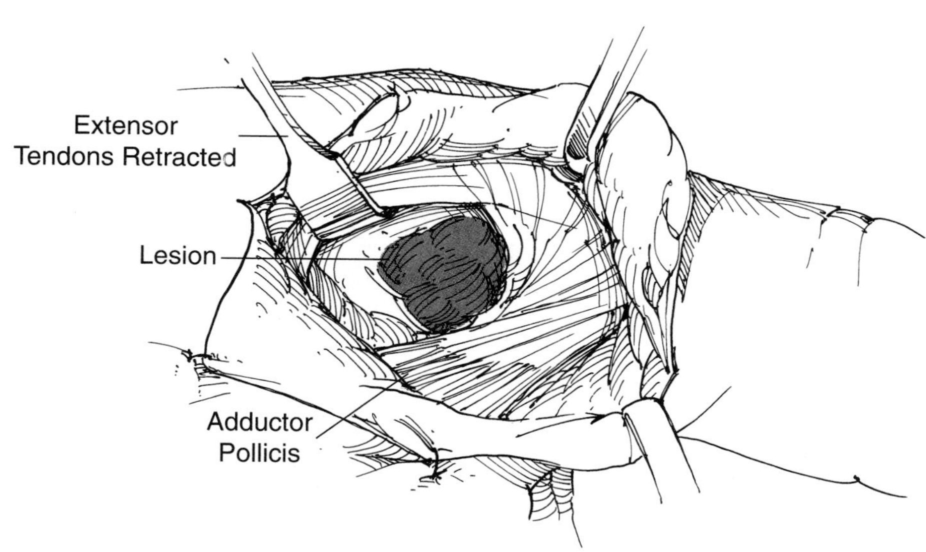

FIGURE 1.12

they share the same muscle belly. This may occur posttraumatically when the injured or avulsed flexor tendon is inadvertently reattached to the extensor tendons as with an amputation or tenodesis. The inability of this tendon to obtain its proper excursion in flexion limits the flexor digitorum profundus tendons to the other fingers and therefore decreases the overall grip strength.

20. **c** This patient has Kienböck disease. The staging system for avascular necrosis of the lunate was originally proposed by Stahl and was later modified by Lichtman. In *stage I,* there is a linear or compression fracture within the lunate with otherwise normal architecture and density. In *stage II,* the relative density of the lunate is abnormal (without collapse). In *stage III,* there is lunate collapse. In *stage IV,* osteoarthritic changes are present at the lunate articulations (radiocarpal and/or intercarpal).

    This patient has stage II disease with ulnar minus variance (the ulna is short relative to the radius at the wrist). This may be treated by unloading the forces across the lunate by performing a joint leveling procedure such as ulnar lengthening or radial shortening. Lunate implant arthroplasty has been highly unsuccessful and fraught with complications, particularly silicone synovitis. Furthermore, lunate replacement has not proven capable of preventing carpal collapse. Proximal row carpectomy is a salvage procedure that is reserved for stage IV disease. The fourcorner arthrodesis (capitate-hamate-triquetrum-lunate) is not a form of treatment for Kienböck disease. Rather, it is a form of treatment for the scapholunate advanced collapse (SLAC) wrist. The fourcorner arthrodesis is predicated on the resistance of the radiolunate joint to degenerative change in cases of SLAC wrist. *Note:* The radiolunate joint is *not* spared in cases of advanced Kienböck disease.

References

Green DP, ed: Operative Hand Surgery, 3rd Ed. New York, Churchill Livingstone, 1993.

Lichtman DM, et al.: Kienbock's Disease Update on Silicon Replacement Arthroplasty. J Hand Surg Am, 343–347, 1982.

21. **d** The patient with high radial nerve palsy has lost wrist extension, finger (metacarpophalangeal joint) extension, thumb abduction, and thumb extension. The muscles available for transfer to restore wrist extension in this situation are the extrinsic muscles that are innervated by the median and ulnar nerves. Many options exist. The pronator teres, palmaris longus, flexor carpi ulnaris, flexor digitorum superficialis, and flexor carpi radialis are all conceivably capable of restoring wrist extension. However, to restore all the deficits that result from high radial nerve palsy, the pronator teres to extensor carpi radialis brevis transfer is most commonly used to restore wrist extension. Extensor digitorum communis function is most commonly restored by transfer of the flexor carpi ulnaris, flexor digitorum superficialis, or flexor carpi radialis tendons. The palmaris longus is commonly used to restore extensor pollicis longus function.

Reference

Green DP: Operative Hand Surgery, 3rd Ed. New York, Churchill Livingstone, p. 1406, 1993.

22. **c** The pronator quadratus is innervated by the anterior interosseous branch of the median nerve. The distal motor branch exits the carpal tunnel to supply the thenar muscles.

23. **a** Injury to the dorsal cutaneous branch of the ulnar nerve may occur during arthroscopy of the wrist. Injury may occur as a result of use of the 6R or 6U portals, which are located on the radial and ulnar sides of the extensor carpi ulnaris tendon, respectively. The nerve may also be injured or entrapped during repair of a torn triangular fibrocartilage complex when sutures are tied in the subcutaneous tissues at the dorsoulnar region of the wrist.

    An axillary block can cause neuritis of the posterior cord, but the described complaints do not correspond to the cutaneous distribution of the posterior cord. The ulnar nerve arises from the medial cord of the brachial plexus.

Reference

Osterman AL: Arthroscopic Debridement of Triangular Fibrocartilage Complex Tears. Arthroscopy, 6(2):120–124, 1990.

24. **a** The correct position for arthrodesis of the metacarpophalangeal joint of the thumb is 5 to 15 degrees of flexion, 0 degrees of radial or ulnar deviation, and approximately 10 degrees of pronation to facilitate pinch.

Reference

Brockman R, Weiland AJ: Small Joint Arthrodesis. In Green DP, ed: Operative Hand Surgery, 3rd Ed. New York, Churchill Livingstone, pp. 100–101, 1993.

25. **c** *Mycobacterium marinum* is an atypical mycobacterium that inhabits aquatic environments and may cause an infection in humans as a result of minor trauma occurring in swimming pools, aquariums, or natural bodies of water. Such an infection typically presents as a nodular lesion over a bony prominence of an extremity (commonly the hand or knee). It is rarely suppurative and is frequently misdiagnosed. The diag-

nosis is established by culturing a biopsy of the lesion on LowensteinJensen medium at 30 to 32°C (rather than the standard of 37°C). The lesion typically resolves with antibiotics. Operative débridement is rarely required.

Eikenella corrodens is common in human oral flora, and *Pasteurella multocida* is common in the oral flora of domestic animals. These two organisms are typically involved in acute hand infections as a result of bite wounds. *Sporothrix schenckii* is a fungal organism that dwells in soil and may produce a chronic nodule at the site of minor trauma (stereotypically from a rose thorn). It may present similarly to *Mycobacterium marinum* infections. It grows at room temperature in simple culture media.

Reference

Abrams RA, Botte MJ: Hand Infections: Treatment Recommendations for Specific Types. J Am Acad Orthop Surg, 4(4):219–230, 1996.

26. **c** The recognized sites of potential posterior interosseous nerve compression are (1) fibrous bands crossing anterior to the radial head at the entrance to the radial tunnel, (2) the leash of Henry (the fanshaped leash of radial recurrent blood vessels that lie across the nerve and supply the brachioradialis and the extensor carpi radialis longus), (3) the tendinous margin of the extensor carpi radialis brevis, and (4) the arcade of Frohse (a ligamentous band at the entrance to the supinator muscle).

    The ligament of Struthers connects the supracondylar process of the humerus to the medial epicondyle. This ligament may sometimes be responsible for entrapment of the median nerve at the distal humerus. This clinical situation may produce symptoms that resemble those of carpal tunnel syndrome.

Reference

Fuss FK, Wurzl GH: Radial Nerve Entrapment at the Elbow: Surgical Anatomy. J Hand Surg Am, 16(4):742–747, 1991.

27. **a** The most common wrist ganglion is the dorsal wrist ganglion. This lesion typically originates from the scapholunate ligament. It accounts for 60% to 70% of all ganglia of the hand and wrist. The dorsal wrist ganglion is most commonly located directly over the scapholunate ligament and protrudes between the extensor pollicis longus and extensor digitorum communis tendons. However, multiple other locations on the dorsal wrist are also encountered. The ganglion typically remains in continuity with the scapholunate ligament through a pedicle. Even when a dorsal wrist ganglion presents at a site far from the scapholunate ligament, the two structures tend to be linked by an elongated pedicle. Failure to excise all attachments to the scapholunate ligament is commonly invoked to account for the predilection for the dorsal wrist ganglion to recur.

    The second most common type of ganglia in the hand and wrist is the volar wrist ganglion, which accounts for 18% to 20%. This type of ganglion most commonly arises from either the radiocarpal ligament or the scaphotrapezial joint capsule. Proximity to the radial artery is a potential surgical hazard.

    The third most common hand and wrist ganglion is the volar retinacular ganglion. This arises from the proximal annular ligament (A1 pulley) of the flexor tendon sheath and accounts for 10% to 12% of all ganglia of the hand and wrist.

References

Freeglar EJ: Soft Tissue Tumors: Benign and Malignant. In Hand Surgery Update. American Society for Surgery of the Hand, pp. 331–337, 1996.
Greendyke SD, Wilson M, et al: Anterior Wrist Ganglia from the Scaphotrapezial Joint. J Hand Surg Am, 17:487–490, 1992.

28. **d** This is a description of the *Watson scaphoid shift test.* A positive test result signifies insufficiency of the scapholunate ligament. Under normal circumstances, the distal pole of the scaphoid palmarflexes when the wrist is radially deviated. With scapholunate insufficiency, pressure on the volar aspect of the distal pole prevents palmarflexion of the distal pole and forces the proximal pole to subluxate dorsally relative to the radius.

    The *Phalen test* is used to aid in substantiating the diagnosis of carpal tunnel syndrome. It is performed by placing the wrist in full, unforced flexion. This maneuver increases pressure within the carpal tunnel and decreases local blood flow to the median nerve. A positive test is one that produces sensory disturbances in the median nerve distribution within 60 seconds.

    A positive *Froment sign* indicates dysfunction of the ulnar nerve. It is elicited by asking the patient to grip a piece of paper between the thumb and the radial side of the index proximal phalanx. Normally, maximal compression between the digital pulp of the thumb and the radial aspect of the index proximal phalanx is accomplished by maintaining the thumb interphalangeal joint in slight extension while contracting the adductor pollicis muscle. The adductor pollicis is innervated by the ulnar nerve. When the ulnar nerve is dysfunctional, the patient compensates for the lack of adductor strength by flexing the interphalangeal joint of the thumb (using the flexor pollicis longus to grip the paper against the index proximal phalanx). This response is a positive Froment sign.

    The *Terry Thomas* sign is a description of the radiographic finding of scapholunate diastasis. Widening of more than 3 mm is diagnostic of scapholunate dissociation. (Terry Thomas was a British actor who had a remarkably large gap between his two front teeth.)

The *Kleinman sheer test* is a test for lunotriquetral sprain. A dorsally directed force is applied to the volar aspect of the pisotriquetral mass while a simultaneous volarly directed force is applied to the dorsum of the lunate. The test is positive if pain is evoked when the lunotriquetral ligament is stressed in this manner.

Reference

Watson HK, et al.: Examination of the Scaphoid. J Hand Surg Am, 13:657–660, 1988.

29. **d** The transverse carpal ligament spans the roof of the tunnel between the hook of the hamate (ulnar) and the trapezium (radial). The carpal tunnel contains 10 structures (four flexor digitorum superficialis tendons, four flexor digitorum profundus tendons, the flexor pollicis longus tendon, and the median nerve). The flexor pollicis longus tendon is the most radial structure within the tunnel. The cross section of this tendon is relatively distinct because it is enveloped in its own discrete sheath (the radial bursa).

    The flexor carpi radialis does not travel within the carpal tunnel. It perforates the flexor retinaculum further proximally and travels in a groove on the volar aspect of the trapezium en route to its insertion on the bases of the second and third metacarpals. Likewise, the *palmaris longus tendon* lies outside the carpal tunnel. It runs along the volar surface of the flexor retinaculum.
30. **d** The volar approach to the radius (as described by Henry) may be used to expose the entire radius. This approach exploits the internervous plane between the radial and median nerves. Distally, dissection proceeds in the interval between the brachioradialis (radial nerve) and the flexor carpi radialis (median nerve). Proximally, dissection proceeds in the interval between the brachioradialis (radial nerve) and the pronator teres (median nerve).

Reference

Hoppenfeld S: Surgical Exposures in Orthopaedics, 2nd Ed. Philadelphia, JB Lippincott, 1994.

31. **d** The ulnar nerve innervates two forearm muscles: (1) the flexor carpi ulnaris and (2) the ulnar half of the flexor digitorum profundus (to the ring and small fingers). The radial half of the flexor digitorum profundus (to the index and long fingers) is innervated by the median nerve.

    The ulnar nerve innervates all the intrinsic hand muscles *except* the following (which are innervated by the median nerve): (1) *half* of the **L**umbricals (to the index and long fingers), (2) the *O*pponens pollicis, (3) the *A*bductor pollicis brevis, and (4) *half* of the *F*lexor pollicis brevis (which is also partially innervated by the ulnar nerve). A useful mnemonic for remembering these exceptions is "half LOAF half."
32. **e** A distal radioulnar joint fusion with creation of an ulnar pseudarthrosis proximal to the fusion is known as the *Suave-Kapandji Procedure.* The *Darrach procedure* is a resection of the distal end (approximately 2.5 cm) of the ulna. The *hemiresection interposition arthroplasty* is a modification of the Darrach procedure in which the articular head of the ulna is resected and the ulnar styloid is left in continuity with the shaft. An interpositional anchovy of tendon is used to fill the resultant radioulnar joint gap to prevent contact between the ends of the two bones. The *Carroll-Imbriglia procedure* is a distal radioulnar joint arthrodesis with no attempt to preserve forearm rotation.

    The *Spinner-Kaplan* procedure (unlike the other four procedures listed) is not indicated for distal radioulnar joint arthritis. Rather, it is performed to stabilize the extensor carpi ulnaris tendon. This is accomplished by mobilizing a flap of extensor retinaculum to construct a tunnel for the extensor carpi ulnaris.

Reference

Buterbaugh GA: Triangular Fibrocartilage Complex Injury and Ulnar Wrist Pain. In Hand Surgery Update. American Society for Surgery of the Hand, pp. 105–115, 1996.

33. **d** The Suave-Kapandji procedure liberates the proximal ulna from its linkage to the distal radius; hence the residual proximal fragment of the ulna is relatively mobile. Because of the insertion of the brachialis on the coronoid process of the ulna, resisted elbow flexion causes the proximal fragment of the ulna to flex relative to the radial shaft. This scissoring action causes the distal end of the proximal ulna to impinge upon the radial shaft. Isolated pain with resisted elbow flexion is not consistent with any of the other options listed.

Reference

Buck-Gramcko D: On the Priorities of Publication of Some Operative Procedures on the Distal End of the Ulna. J Hand Surg [Br], 15:416–420, 1990.

34. **c** The oblong shape of this cross section (Fig. 1.2) of the radius is a key landmark. From this, one can localize this axial image to the middistal forearm. A cross section of the ulna would not have this shape, and the radius would be more circular in cross section further

proximally. The pronator quadratus (marked with an *asterisk* on the image) runs volarly between the radius and ulna at this level; this muscle must be elevated to expose the volar aspect of the distal radius. The digital extensor tendons are located immediately deep to the subcutaneous fat at the top of this image.

Thus, the *arrow* marks the most superficial and most ulnar muscle belly on the volar aspect of the distal forearm, that is, the flexor carpi ulnaris.

Note: Observe the two circular structures that lie immediately deep to the flexor carpi ulnaris. The more radial of the two is the ulnar artery; the more ulnar of the two is the ulnar nerve. As demonstrated by this image, arteries often produce a target appearance on magnetic resonance imaging cross section as a result of laminar flow. Nerves often yield a cluster-of-grapes appearance on magnetic resonance imaging cross section because of their multifascicular composition. The flexor digitorum profundus lies directly deep to these neurovascular structures in this image. The flexor digitorum superficialis lies on the radial side of the ulnar artery in this image.

35. **c** The deep brachial artery (profunda brachii artery) travels with the radial nerve and perfuses the triceps. It exit the triangular space, the borders of which include the humerus laterally, the long head of the triceps medially, and the teres major superiorly.

36. **a** Fullthickness defects involving the shoulder pose difficult problems for the reconstructive surgeon. The two flaps that have been found to be most useful for coverage in this area are the latissimus dorsi and the pectoralis major. These muscles have long vascular pedicles that permit rotational mobilization to the shoulder region. Mobilization of local tissues is superior to free flap coverage because it avoids the potential morbidity associated with the anastomosis and the donor site.

References

Cohen BE: Soft Tissue Coverage of the Upper Extremity. In Hand Surgery Update. American Society for Surgery of the Hand, pp. 284, 1996.

White WL: Flap Grafts to the Upper Extremity. Surg Clin North Am, 40:389, 1960.

37. **a** The patient's presenting complaints are consistent with entrapment of the median nerve at the elbow *(pronator syndrome).* One of the potential sites of median nerve entrapment is beneath the supracondylar process of the humerus (when present). The ligament of Struthers runs from this process to the medial epicondyle and may serve as an accessory origin of the pronator terres. The medial nerve may be compressed by either the ligament or by the supracondylar process itself.

The arcade of Frohse is a ligamentous band at the proximal border of the supinator. The posterior interosseous nerve enters the supinator beneath the arcade of Frohse. This site is the most common source of posterior interosseous nerve entrapment.

Note: Potential sites of median nerve compression at the elbow include (1) the supracondylar process and/or ligament of Struthers, (2) the lacertus fibrosus, (3) the pronator teres (muscle belly or deep aponeurotic fascia), and (4) the arch of the flexor digitorum superficialis.

Reference

Kessel L, Rang M: Supracondylar Spur of the Humerus. J Bone Joint Surg Br, 48:765–769, 1966.

38. **c** In general, the soft tissue defects of the tibia are divided into three groups: proximal third, middle third, and distal third. Gastrocnemius flaps are generally used for the proximal third deficits. Soleus flaps are used for the middle third defects, and free flaps are used for the distal third defects.

Reference

Pederson WC: Bone and SoftTissue Reconstruction. In Rockwood CA, Green PD, eds: Fractures in Adults, 4th Ed. Philadelphia, Lippincott–Raven, 1996.

39. **a** The fibroblast. Histologically, the important cells in Dupuytren disease are the myofibroblasts. Myofibroblasts were first described in 1971 by Gabbiani and Majno. The relation of the myofibroblasts to Luck's three stages of Dupuytren contracture has been studied thoroughly. In the first stage (proliferative stage), large myofibroblasts predominate. In the second (involutional) stage, a dense myofibroblast network is present, and type III to type I collagen is increased. In the third stage (residual stage), the number of myofibroblasts decreases dramatically, and fibrocytes are the dominant cell type.

Reference

Sappino A, Schurch W, Gabbiani G: Biology of DiseaseDifferentiation Repertoire of Fibroblastic Cells: Expression of Cytoskeletal Proteins as Marker of Phenotype Modulations. Lab Invest, 63(2):144–161, 1990.

40. **a** Lung. metastatic lesions distal to the elbow are extremely rare and almost always occur in bone. Metastases to the hand arise from a primary lung tumor in most cases throughout the literature. The distal phalanx is the most common location, where the lesions are often mistaken for infections.

Reference

Kann SE, Jacquemin J, Stern PJ: Simulators of Hand Infections. Instruct Course Lect 45:69–82, 1996.

41. **e** The ulnar head is dorsally subluxed; the carpus is volarly subluxed and supinated. *Caput ulnae syndrome*

is a condition associated with the rheumatoid wrist in which the ulnar head is dorsally subluxated and the carpus is volarly subluxated and supinated. Synovitis of the distal radioulnar joint with erosion of the dorsal aspect of the ulna leaves sharp spikes on the ulna that erode through the joint capsule and eventually through the extensor tendons on the ulnar as part of the wrist (fifth and fourth extensor compartments). It is important to recognize and treat the caput ulnae syndrome before tendon rupture occurs.

Reference

Feldon P: Rheumatoid Arthritis. In Hand Surgery Update. American Society for Surgery of the Hand, pp. 173–181, 1996.

42. **d** Enchondroma is the most common primary neoplasm that occurs in the skeleton of the hand. Enchondromas are most commonly discovered either incidentally or when a pathologic fracture occurs through a solitary lesion in the diaphysis or metaphysis of a phalanx or metacarpal in a young adult. The proximal phalanx is the most commonly affected region. The incidence among males and females is equivalent. Intraosseous ganglia, giant cell tumors, and chondrosarcomas rarely occur in the bones of the hand. Giant cell tumors do commonly occur in *extraosseous* locations in the hand (specifically, in the flexor tendon sheath). *Giant cell tumor of tendon sheath is the second most common soft tissue mass found in the hand (ganglia are the most common).* Histologically, giant cell tumor of the tendon sheath is virtually indistinguishable from pigmented villonodular synovitis.

Reference

American Society for Surgery of the Hand: Regional Review Course Syllabus. American Society for Surgery of the Hand, 1995.

43. **a** The vertical septa that separate the palm into nine compartments, in the cross-sectional plane, are called the *vertical septa of Legeue and Juvara.* Five compartments contain nerves, vessels, and muscles. The remaining four contain pretendinous bands, tendons, and bone.

Reference

Benson LS, et al.: Dupuytren's Contracture. J Am Acad Orthop Surg, 6(1):24–35, 1998.

44. **b** In Dupuytren disease, Cleland ligaments are most often free of disease. The horizontal palmar fascia is also usually free of disease and assists in protecting the neurovascular bundles during dissection of palmar disease. The remaining choices are most often involved in the disease process. Other areas that may be involved in the clinical picture of Dupuytren disease include the dorsum of the proximal interphalangeal joints (knuckle pads), dorsum of the penis (Peyronie disease), and plantar fascia (Ledderhose disease).

Reference

Benson LS, et al.: Dupuytren's Contracture. J Am Acad Orthop Surg, 6(1): 24–35, 1998.

45. **b** During the involutional phase of Dupytren disease, the dense myofibroblast network aligns along the collagen bundle axis, with an increase in the ratio of type III to type I collagen formation. In the third residual stage, the fibrocytes become the predominant cell type. In stage I, the proliferative stage, the myofibroblast number increases.

Reference

Benson LS, et al.: Dupuytren's Contracture. J Am Acad Orthop Surg, 6(1): 24–35, 1998.

46. **b** Madelung deformity characteristically results from deficient growth of the *ulnar* and volar portion of the distal radial physis. As a result, the distal radial articular surface tilts in an excessively volar and ulnar direction. (*Note:* This is easy to remember because it is an exaggeration of the normal tilt of the distal radius). Associated deformities of the distal ulna include dorsal subluxation, enlargement, and displacement away from the dysplastic distal radius. The carpus is wedged between the radius and ulna, where it is forced to assume a triangular configuration (with the lunate at its proximal apex). Supination is characteristically compromised to a greater extent than pronation.

Reference

Nielsen JB: Madelung's Deformity: A Followup Study of 26 Patients and a Review of the Literature. Acta Orthop Scand, 48:379–384,1977.

47. **d** The preservation of A2 and A4 pulleys is necessary for full flexion. The absence of either the A2 or A4 pulley produces bowstringing and increases the moment arm of the force of the tendon. This necessitates greater excursion from the muscle belly to produce the same joint motion and therefore weakens overall grip strength.

Reference

Hume EL, Hutchinson, DT, Jaeger SA, Hunter JM: Biomechanics of Pulley Reconstruction. J Hand Surg Am, 16(4):722–730, 1991.

48. **a** Although tendon sheath repair theoretically may improve tendon gliding and nutrition, it has not been proven clinically to improve the results of repair. Increasing the number of core sutures across the repair

site increases the strength of the repair. Atraumatic technique decreases the damage to epitenon, which may lead to adhesions. A supplemental epitendinous repair adds additional strength to the tendon repair.

49. **c** Type III (Leddy and Packer classification) profundus injuries can be treated with open reduction and internal fixation using screw, intraosseous, or Kirschner wire fixation. The timing of treatment is not as critical, as long as joint motion remains adequate. With type I, in which the tendon has retracted into the palm and the blood supply is lost, treatment within 7 to 10 days is critical. After this time, the tendon is usually too severely contracted to advance back into the distal phalanx. With type II, the most common, the tendon is retracted to the proximal interphalangeal joint level, and it retains its blood supply and may be advanced and repaired to the phalanx at a later time than type I.

Reference

Coyle, Leddy, Stover CN: Injuries of the Distal Finger. In Primary Care, 3rd Ed. Philadelphia, WB Saunders, pp. 245–258, 1980.

50. **c** All the volar and the third dorsal interossei muscles have only one muscle belly, whereas the first, second, and fourth dorsal interossei muscles have two muscle bellies. These two bellies have similar courses, but they insert into separate sites. The superficial belly inserts into the base of the proximal phalanx. The deep inserts into the dorsal aponeurosis. There is no such thing as a fifth dorsal interossei muscle.

51. **a** A rupture of the sagittal bands on the radial side causes subluxation of the extensor tendon. The patient may present with a locking metacarpophalangeal joint, but may have full passive extension. There is no involvement of the proximal or distal interphalangeal joint. Answer c describes intrinsic tightness, and answer d describes extrinsic tightness.

References

Koniuch MP, Peimer CA, VanGorder T, et al.: Closed Crush Injury of the Metacarpophalangeal Joint. J Hand Surg Am, 12:750–757,1987.
Wrist and Hand: Trauma: Chapter 31, OKU 4,Upper Extremity, 1994.

52. **d** Epithelioid sarcoma is the most common soft tissue sarcoma of the hand and is more common in the fingers. It occurs in adolescents and young adults and is twice as common in male patients. Its origin is unknown, and treatment is controversial. All the remaining answers are very rare in the hand and fingers.

Reference

Fleegler EJ: SoftTissue Tumors: Benign and Malignant. In Hand Surgery Update. American Society for Surgery of the Hand, pp. 331–337, 1996.

53. **d** The ulnar nerve may be compressed under the transverse fibers of the roof of the cubital tunnel, as well as more proximally at the intermuscular septum. Distally, the transverse fascial fibers between the two heads of the flexor carpi ulnaris, also known as Osborne fascia, can also compress the nerve (Fig. 1.13). The Guyon canal is also a common site of distal ulnar nerve compression. A flexed elbow with dorsal cutaneous nerve findings (paresthesias) may help to differentiate between a cubital tunnel compression and a compression at the Guyon canal. Anatomically, the dorsal cutaneous nerve divides from the ulnar nerve before it enters the Guyon canal. Subluxation over the medial

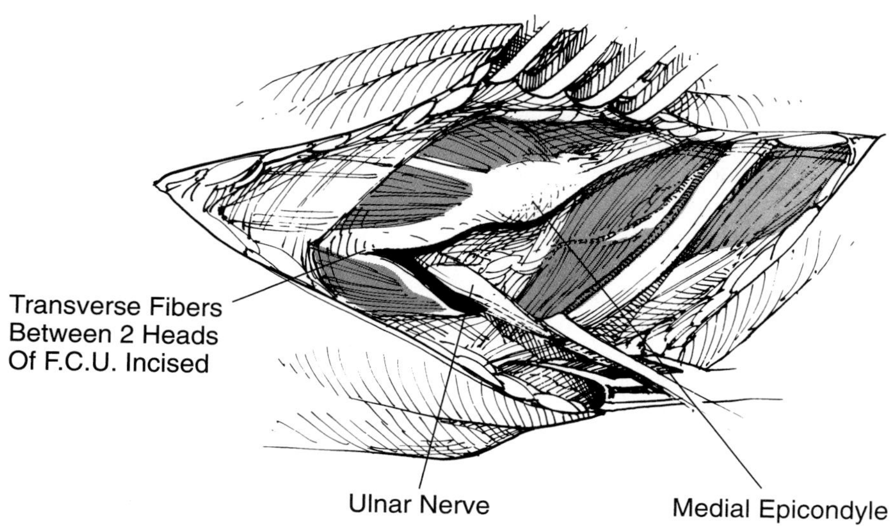

FIGURE 1.13

epicondyle can cause neuropathy symptoms, but not compression.

References

Dellon AL: Review of Treatment Results for Ulnar Nerve Entrapment at the Elbow. J Hand Surg Am, 14:688–700, 1989.

Szabo RM: Nerve Compression Syndromes. In Hand Surgery Update. American Society for Surgery of the Hand, pp. 221–231, 1996.

54. **b** The patient most likely has a glomus tumor, which can cause nail ridging and discoloration and temperature sensitivity. Often times, these people are treated by unknowing physicians who see no abnormality on examination because it can be quite subtle. It is not uncommon for the patient to have been sent for psychiatric evaluation along their treatment course. These tumors are radiolucent and can sometimes cause an erosion of the phalanx seen on the lateral radiograph. Recognition and complete excision are usually curative.

Reference

Fleegler EJ: Soft-Tissue Tumors: Benign and Malignant. In Hand Surgery Update. American Society for Surgery of the Hand, pp. 331–337, 1996.

55. **a** Dorsal intercalated segment instability is evident on lateral radiographs when the lunate rotates into dorsiflexion. The normal scapholunate angle is 30 to 60 degrees; an angle greater than 70 degrees is diagnostic of dorsal intercalated segment instability. A volar intercalatedsegment instability is characterized by palmar flexion of the lunate and a scapholunate angle of less than 30 degrees. Early treatment with closed reduction and pin fixation may avoid the need for a difficult late reconstruction or salvage arthrodesis.

References

Almquist EE, Bach AW, Sack JT, Fuhs SE, Newman DM: Four-Bone Ligament Reconstruction for Treatment of Chronic Complete Scapholunate Separation. J Hand Surg Am, 16:322–327, 1991.

Cooney WP, Linscheid RL, Dobyns JH: Carpal Instability: Treatment of Ligament Injuries of the Wrist. Instr Course Lect, 41:33–44, 1992.

56. **a** *Pronator syndrome,* first known as neuralgic amyotrophy, involves the entrapment of the anterior interosseous nerve. Figure 1.4 demonstrates the pinch deformity seen with pronator syndrome. The Phalen test is negative in pronator syndrome. There is a loss of interphalangeal flexion because of flexor pollicis longus loss, as well as a loss of index distal interphalangeal flexion, resulting from flexor digitorum profundus of index loss. It may be the result of traumatic injury, such as a supracondylar fracture. It has also been related to a leash of vessels from a persistent medial artery. The symptoms include forearm pain as well as neuropathy of the anterior interosseous nerve. The muscles supplied by the anterior interosseous nerve are the flexor pollicis longus, the flexor digitorum profundus of the index, and the pronator quadratus. Because pronation is a combination of many muscles, it is more difficult to delineate than flexor pollicis longus or flexor digitorum profundus of index loss. The strength of the pronator quadratus may be differentiated from the pronator teres by flexing the elbow to full flexion and asking the patient to pronate against resistance. Full flexion minimizes the contribution of the pronator teres (normally 75%) to pronation. There may also be sensory changes in the palmar cutaneous nerve, supplying the palm over the thenar eminence. More than 50% of these patients lack electrodiagnostic confirmation of the syndrome. Reduced conduction velocity in the forearm has also been noted with carpal tunnel syndrome, in up to 30% or more.

Reference

Szabo RM: Nerve Compression Syndromes. In Hand Surgery Update. American Society for Surgery of the Hand, pp. 221–231, 1996.

57. **d** It is critical to recognize purulent flexor tenosynovitis at an early stage, to prevent the sequelae that can result in severe disability. The purulence in the tendon sheath will quickly destroy the gliding mechanism by creating adhesions that will limit tendon function and result in severe loss of motion. In addition, the purulence will destroy the blood supply to the tendon, with resulting tendon necrosis. Kanavel described the four classic findings earlier regarding purulent flexor tenosynovitis. Often, the pain on passive extension may be the only finding, especially early in the course of the infection.

Reference

Neviaser RJ. Infections. In Green DP, ed: Operative Hand Surgery, 3rd Ed. New York, Churchill Livingstone, pp. 1021–1038, 1993.

58. **e** The defect in Fig. 1.5 is a radial deficient limb, which has had previous centralization. The thumb that is present is basically nonfunctional, and no attempt should be made to make it more functional. It results in a stiff nonfunctional thumb. The best option for treatment is an excision with index pollicization. A toe-to-thumb transfer is not an appropriate treatment option because the morbidity to the foot is unnecessary. In addition, these children often lack the cortical mapping for a thumb, and a toe transferred to this area may be left unused as well.

References

Gilbert A: Congenital Absence of the Thumb and Digits. J Hand Surg [Br], 14:6–17, 1989.

Light TR (ed): The Pediatric Upper Extremity. Hand Clin, 6(4):551–738, 1990.

59. **c** The Wassel classification of bifid thumb is broken down into I to VII. All the odd numbers represent incomplete separation of the bone distal to proximal: I, the distal phalanx; III, the proximal phalanx; and V, the metacarpal. The even numbers correspond to the previous level with a complete duplication. Type VII is the triphalangeal thumb. The most common bifid thumb is type IV (more than 50%).

References

Flatt AE: The Care of Congenital Hand Anomalies. St Louis, CV Mosby, pp 99–117, 1977.
Wassel HD: The Results of Surgery for Polydactyly of the Thumb: A Review. Clin Orthop 64:175–193, 1969.
Wood VE: Polydactyly and the Triphanlangeal Thumb. J Hand Surg, 3: 436–444. 1978.

60. **d** Boutonniere deformity is the resultant proximal interphalangeal flexion and distal interphalangeal hyperextension positioning of a digit, which results from palmar subluxation of the lateral bands because of a central slip insufficiency or attenuation of the triangular ligament. Volar plate injury, rupture, and extrinsic adhesions all may lead to a swan neck deformity. The dorsal subluxation of the lateral bands yields proximal interphalangeal joint hyperextension with distal interphalangeal flexion. Disruption of the central slip and volar migration of the lateral bands are also associated with decreased flexion of the distal interphalangeal joint. This illustrates the problem of imbalance in the finger, which is a chain of joints with multiple tendon attachments. This chain assumes abnormal positions if the delicate equilibrium is disturbed by the pathologic imbalance of one joint.

References

Carducci AT: Potential Boutonniere Deformity: Its Recognition and Treatment. Orthop Rev, 10:121–123, 1981.
Doyle JR: Extensor Tendons: Acute Injuries. In Green DP, ed: Operative Hand Surgery, 2nd Ed. New York, Churchill Livingstone, pp. 2055–2060, 1988.

61. **a** The treatment of a passively correctable boutonnière deformity is to splint the proximal interphalangeal joint in extension. Active and passive dorsal interphalangeal flexion exercises are permitted to centralize the lateral bands. Only after prolonged conservative treatment has failed should operative treatment be undertaken. All the listed procedures are appropriate surgical treatment of a resistant boutonnière deformity.

References

Carducci AT: Potential Boutonniere Deformity: Its Recognition and Treatment. Orthop Rev, 10:121–123, 1981.
Doyle JR: Extensor Tendons: Acute Injuries. In Green DP, ed: Operative Hand Surgery, 2nd Ed. New York, Churchill Livingstone, pp. 2055–2060, 1988.

62. **b** A persistent median artery contributes to the superficial palmar arch in 10% of cases. A classic complete palmar arch is present less than 35% of the time. The superficial arch is solely supplied by the ulnar artery in approximately 37% of cases.
63. **c** The muscle described is the opponens digiti quinti. Its function is to adduct and flex the fifth metacarpal. The lumbricals flex the metacarpophalangeal joint and extend the proximal interphalangeal joint of the involved digit. The abductor digit quinti abducts the fifth with a stabilized metacarpophalangeal joint, and it originates in the same location as the opponens digiti quinti, but it inserts into the proximal phalanx and the dorsal apparatus. The abductor pollicis brevis abducts and flexes the thumb metacarpal while extending the distal phalanx.
64. **c** High-pressure injection injuries often present as fairly innocuous wounds with a variable examination. The edema present depends on the amount injected, the site, and the time from injury. Palm injections tend to have a better prognosis than digital injuries. It is imperative that the wounds be explored and any necrotic tissue be débrided. This is best done formally in the operating room. In involved digits with severe injuries, especially involving paint, early amputation is a treatment option.

Reference

Thakore HK: Hand Injury with Paint Gun. J Hand Surg [Br], 10(1):124–126, 1985.

65. **e** Berger studied 37 wrists by anatomic dissection and found the scapholunate ligament is consistently divisible into three anatomic regions: dorsal, proximal, and palmar. The dorsal region is thick and composed of transversely oriented collagen fibers. The proximal region is primarily fibrocartilage extending into the scapholunate joint space (resembling knee meniscus). The palmar region is thin and is composed of obliquely oriented collagen fascicles, just dorsal to the long radiolunate ligament. The radioscapholunate ligament separates the proximal and palmar regions.

Reference

Berger R: The Gross and Histologic Anatomy of the Scapholunate Interosseous Ligament. J Hand Surg Am, 21:170–178, 1996.

66. **d** A scapholunate gap of greater than 3 mm is diagnostic of scapholunate dissociation (Fig. 1.14A). This gap has been called the *Terry Thomas sign* after the

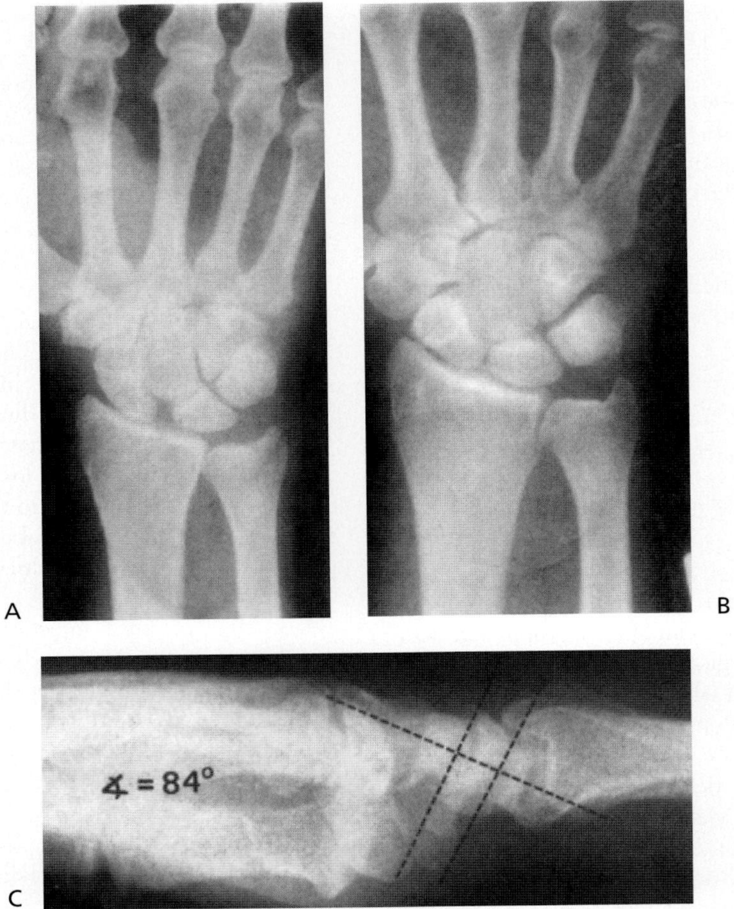

FIGURE 1.14A–C

famous English comedian's dental diastema. The scaphoid assumes a flexed posture from the dissociation and thus appears shortened. An anteroposterior view of the scaphoid on end results in a more prominently visualized cortex appropriately named the *cortical ring sign*. Dorsal intercalated segment instability may occur with scapholunate dissociation as the scaphoid is allowed to rotate into volar flexion, the lunate and triquetrum rotate into dorsiflexion, and the capitate migrates proximally (Fig. 1.14B, C). Volar intercalated segment instability is most commonly associated with lunatotriquetrum laxity.

Reference

Blevens AD, Light TR, Jablonsky WS, Smith DG, Patwardhan AV, Guay ME, Woo TS: Radiocarpal Articular Contact Characteristics with Scaphoid Instability. J Hand Surg Am, 14:781–790, 1989.

67. **c** A carpal instability dissociative lesion is caused by the loss of the interosseous ligaments between the individual bones of the carpal rows and results in dissociative rather than associative motion between the bones of each row (proximal and distal). A carpal instability nondissociative lesion is normal associative motion within each row but dissociation between rows. These include dorsal carpal subluxation, midcarpal instability, volar carpal subluxation, and some ulnar translocations.

References

Taleisnik, J. Current Concepts Review. Carpal Instability. J Bone Joint Surg Am, Sep; 13(5):790–2, 1988.

68. **a** The paradox described by Mayfield et al. for closed reduction states that volar flexion will approximate the volar radioscapholunate ligament; however, this will palmarflex the scaphoid and will separate it from the lunate dorsally. Conversely, if the scaphoid is reduced by dorsiflexing the wrist, the torn ends of the volar ligaments will be distracted. When the ligament is viable and the dissociation is reducible, primary repair may be

attempted. Blatt advocated augmentation such as with the dorsal capsulodesis. The concept of this operation is to create a checkrein to prevent palmarflexion of the scaphoid. Proximal row carpectomy is controversial; however, many large series have reported preservation of wrist motion with decreased pain (and some decreased grip strength). A prerequisite for proximal row carpectomy is good articular cartilage on the proximal pole of the capitate and in the lunate fossa of the radius.

Reference

Wintman BI et al: Dynamic Scapholunate Instability: Results of Operative Treatment with Dorsal Capsulodesis. J Hand Surg Am, 20:971–979, 1995.

69. **a** This is a straightforward anatomic relationship question that is best remembered by realizing that the most sensitive touch is out at the fingers, and therefore, it makes sense that the nerves lie most volar in this region.
70. **b** The most radial structure within the carpal tunnel is the flexor pollicis longus tendon.
71. **d** In 1977, Lanz classified the anatomic variations of the median nerve into four subgroups: (1) variations in the course of the thenar branch of the median nerve, (2) accessory variations of the thenar branch at the distal carpal tunnel, (3) high divisions of the median nerve, and (4) accessory branches proximal to the carpal tunnel. This question addresses the first subgroup. Type C, as described earlier, is the most common variation and is seen approximately half the time. Type B is seen approximately one-third of the time, and type A occurs in approximately one in five cases. Other variations have been described, although they are generally considered extremely rare.

Reference

Eversmann WW Jr: Entrapment and Compression Neuropathies. In Green DP, ed: Operative Hand Surgery, 3rd Ed. New York, Churchill Livingstone, pp. 1341–1385, 1993.

72. **c** Two-point discrimination is a useful clinical adjunct for the evaluation of peripheral nerve function. Sensibility testing is an important part of the workup of a patient with a nerve compression lesion. Four sensory tests are available that test different fiber populations and receptor systems. Touch fibers (groupA β) can be divided into slowly and quickly adapting fiber systems. A quickly adapting fiber signals an onoff event and a slowly adapting fiber continues its pulse response throughout the duration of the stimulus. Static two-point discrimination and SemmesWeinstein monofilament tests evaluate the slowly adapting fibers (Merkle cell receptor), whereas vibration and moving two-point discrimination tests evaluate the quickly adapting fibers (Meissner corpuscle). The normal value for static two-point discrimination is 6 mm. The normal value for moving two-point discrimination is 5 mm.

Reference

Szabo RM: Nerve Compression Syndromes. In Hand Surgery Update. American Society for Surgery of the Hand, pp. 221–231, 1996.

73. **b** The median nerve has many potential sites of compression. This may occur anywhere along the course of this nerve. Four sites are most commonly seen. These sites may comprise an entrapment neuropathy of the median nerve, which is commonly referred to as the *pronator syndrome.* As the nerve courses past the distal third of the humerus, it may be compressed beneath a supracondylar process and the ligament of Struthers. At the level of the elbow joint, the lacertus fibrosus may be the cause of the entrapment. Next, the nerve may be compressed by hypertrophy of the pronator teres, or by the aponeurotic fascia of either its deep or superficial heads. Finally, the arch of the flexor digitorum superficialis muscle may compress the nerve as it passes under it.

Reference

Eversmann, WW: Entrapment and Compression Neuropathies. In Green PD, ed: Operative Hand Surgery, 3rd Ed. New York, Churchill Livingstone, pp. 1341–1385, 1993.

74. **a** Please refer to the combined answer to questions 74 and 75, discussed next.
75. **d** The patient described has *pronator syndrome.* The neuropathy of the median nerve is likely caused by the supracondylar process on the radiographs. This is a small, hookshaped process of bone found approximately 5 cm above the medial epicondyle of the elbow in approximately 10% of the population. The process may form an accessory origin for the pronator teres through the ligament of Struthers. The median nerve can be entrapped by the process or the ligament, and it is generally accompanied by the brachial artery and veins. Early treatment includes avoiding provocative activities, worksite modification, and occasionally splinting or casting. If electrodiagnostic studies are positive, then surgical exploration and decompression are indicated. Surgical treatment includes release of the ligament, with or without resection of the supracondylar process. Care must be taken to follow the course of the nerve, which can be compressed at three other sites distally: the lacertus fibrosis, the pronator teres, and the arch of the flexor digitorum superficialis.

    Anterior interosseous syndrome is caused by compression of the anterior interosseous nerve 4 to 6 cm distal to the elbow. Although the nerve carries no sensory fibers, this syndrome usually presents with forearm pain without sensory findings in the affected hand. Often, the flexor digitorum profundus to the index finger and the flexor pollicis longus are affected, and thus the patient with this syndrome would have a positive Kiloh-Nevin sign.

Carpal tunnel syndrome involves entrapment neuropathy of the median nerve at the wrist. Paresthesias usually follow the distribution of the median nerve in the digits; however, the palm is often spared because the palmar cutaneous branch of the median nerve branches proximal to the tunnel. The Phalen test is positive if paresthesias are elicited in the median distribution of the digits when passively flexing the wrist for 60 seconds. This test is usually negative in the setting of pronator syndrome.

Reference

Eversmann, WW: Entrapment and Compression Neuropathies. In Green DP, ed: Operative Hand Surgery, 3rd Ed. New York, Churchill Livingstone, pp. 1341–1385, 1993.

76. **b** The pronator quadratus is innervated by the median nerve.

Reference

Szabo RM: Nerve Compression Syndromes. In Hand Surgery Update. American Society for Surgery of the Hand, pp. 221–231, 1996.

77. **a** In most dorsal proximal interphalangeal dislocations, the avulsion of the volar occurs from the base of the middle phalanx. In rare instances, the rupture can occur proximally. Three major types of injuries to the ligament system have been described. Type I is a hyperextension injury in which the avulsion of the volar plate occurs from the base of the middle phalanx, and there is often a minor split in the collateral ligaments. The articular surfaces, however, remain in contact. Type 2 injuries are true dorsal dislocations. The avulsion of the volar plate from the base of the middle phalanx is accompanied by a major bilateral split in the collateral ligament system, with no contact between the articular surfaces. Finally, type 3 injuries represent fracturedislocations. In this case, enough compressive force was present to shear away or impact the volar base of the middle phalanx to produce a fracturedislocation.

Reference

Dray GJ, Eaton RG: Dislocations and Ligament Injuries in the Digits. In Green DP, ed: Operative Hand Surgery, pp.767–798, 1996.

78. **c** See the next answer for an explanation.

79. **b** The central tendon is rarely ruptured in closed injuries to the extensor mechanism at zone 5 (at the metacarpophalangeal joint). However, the sagittal bands that hold the central tendon centered over the metacarpophalangeal head are prone to rupture. The long finger is most often affected because it is the most exposed to blunt trauma. Further, its radial sagittal fibers are weaker and more prone to rupture than the ulnar sagittal fibers, although the ulnar sagittal fiber rupture has been reported. This patient's story is typical. Because of the ulnar pull of the flexor and extensor tendons, the extensor tendon usually dislocates into the intermetacarpal valley and prevents extension of the metacarpophalangeal joint. Once extended, however, the extensor tendon is centered over the metacarpophalangeal head and therefore can maintain metacarpophalangeal extension.

Although some authors have advocated conservative splinting, open repair of complete injuries to the sagittal bands is generally recommended because the balance of the extensor mechanism over the metacarpophalangeal joint is delicate. Repair can usually be accomplished by simple reapproximation of the sagittal fibers with 4-0 or 5-0 absorbable sutures in mattress fashion.

Reference

Newport ML: Extensor Tendon Injuries in the Hand. J Am Acad Orthop Surg, 5:59–66, 1997.

80. **b** Although the six-strand repair is the only repair that has been experimentally shown to be safe from rupture during the entire 6-week period of unstrained healing, it is not recommended. The six-strand technique is believed to be technically difficult and may damage the tendon excessively. Although the four-strand technique is not intrinsically strong enough to stand alone, its strength when combined with a running epitendinous stitch should be strong enough to permit even light composite grip during the entire healing period according to experimental evidence. This is further supported by the finding in several studies that gapping at the repair site becomes the weakest part of the tendon, thus unfavorably altering tendon mechanics and attracting adhesions that result in decreased tendon excursion. This gapping is prevented with the epitendinous suture, in addition to providing a 10% to 50% increase in the strength of the repair. Two-stranded repairs are too weak, with or without the epitendinous suture, to be considered safe.

Reference

Strickland JW: Flexor Tendon Injuries: I. Foundations of Treatment. J Am Acad Orthop Surg, 3:44–54, 1995.

81. **d** The most common viral infection in the hand is caused by the herpes simplex virus and results in a cytolytic skin infection known as *herpetic whitlow.* These lesions usually occur on the fingertip (fingers 60%, thumb 40%), but more proximal lesions have been described. The lesions are disseminated by direct contact, and classically health care workers exposed to orotracheal secretions were assumed to be at a greater risk. Some studies have found, however, that only 14% of infections occurred in health care workers. Infections can also be passed by oral or genital lesions. The lesions caused by herpes simplex virus types 1 and 2 are indistinguishable.

The initial signs of infection are the appearance of painful clear vesicles 2 to 14 days after exposure. Pain is out of proportion to the lesions. The vesicles may become turbid, resembling bacterial infections. Over the subsequent 14 days, the vesicles mature, coalesce, and unroof to form an ulcerated base. The ulcer slowly resolves over the ensuing weeks. The virus is believed to reside in the neural ganglia and remains dormant until it is activated by a "stressor." The diagnosis is made by a thorough history and physical examination, which reveals painful, clear vesicles (if early in the course) and a soft pulp space. These infections are often confused with paronychia and felons, and they are treated erroneously with incision and drainage. Incision and drainage are *contraindicated* in these infections because incision may cause local tissue dissemination of the virus with possible bacterial superinfection. Treatment is with oral acyclovir (topical is ineffective), which has been shown to decrease the severity and duration of symptoms and to decrease the number and severity of recurrences.

References

Abrams RA, Botte MJ: Hand Infections: Treatment Recommendations for Specific Types. J Am Acad Orthop Surg, 4:219–230, 1996.
Fowler JR: Viral Infections. Hand Clin, 5(4):599–612, 1989.

82. **a** Most studies of animal bite wounds have focused on the isolation of *Pasteurella multocida* and have disregarded the role of anaerobes. More recent studies of the gingival canine flora and of dog bite wounds, however, point toward an oral flora of multiple organisms, most of which are potential pathogens. Goldstein and associates isolated *P. multocida* from only 26% of dog bite wounds in adults. The most common aerobic isolates were α-hemolytic streptococci (46%) and *Staphylococcus aureus* (13%). Anaerobic pathogens were present in 41% of wounds, including *Bacteroides* and *Fusobacterium* species.

References

Abrams RA, Botte MJ: Hand Infections: Treatment Recommendations for Specific Types. J Am Acad Orthop Surg, 4:219–230, 1996.
Goldstein EJ: Bite Wounds and Infection. Clin Infect Dis, 14(3):633–638, 1992.

83. **b** Immunocompromised patients have a greater susceptibility to infection in general, and many of these represent opportunistic infections. Glickel has published the most extensive series of patients with human immunodeficiency virus and hand infections to date. His work demonstrated that herpes infections were the most common in this population of people.

Reference

Glickel SZ: Hand Infections in Patients with Acquired Immunodeficiency Syndrome. J Hand Surg Am, 13(5):770–775, 1988.

84. **a** This constellation of injuries is referred to as a *floating elbow.* Recommended treatment consists of open reduction and internal fixation of *both* the humerus and the forearm fractures. This permits early range of motion of the wrist, elbow, and shoulder. Nonoperative treatment of the humeral component of this injury is associated with a significantly increased risk of malunion and nonunion. Operative management of these injuries provides more predictably favorable results.

Note: Floating elbows generally stem from high-energy trauma. Thus, many of these fractures are open, and associated injuries are common.

References

Lange RH et al.: Skeletal Management of Humeral Shaft Fractures Associated with Forearm Fractures. Clin Orthop, 195:173–177, 1985.
Rogers JF et al.: Management of Concomitant Ipsilateral Fractures of the Humerus and Forearm. J Bone Joint Surg Am, 66:552–556, 1984.

85. **e** The key landmark in this image is the quadrilateral space (the region of high signal intensity directly inferior to the labeled muscle). The two small *dark circles* within the region of high signal are the axillary nerve and the posterior humeral circumflex artery. Adipose tissue (surrounding this neurovascular bundle) yields the high signal on T1.

The presence of the quadrilateral space localizes the plane of this coronal image to the posterior aspect of the humeral head. The osseous architecture in the image is also consistent with its posterior location. The posterior humeral head can be seen beneath the posterior aspect of the acromion. The remainder of the scapula is not present. If the plane of the image intersected the anterior humeral head, then it would also intersect the coracoid and the acromioclavicular joint. Furthermore, the quadrilateral space would not be evident.

The *teres minor* inserts on the lower aspect of the posterior humeral head directly cephalad to the quadrilateral space. The *infraspinatus* inserts further cephalad. The *teres major* forms the inferior border of the quadrilateral space and inserts on the anterior aspect of the humeral shaft.

86. **d** The *Stryker notch view* is obtained with the ipsilateral hand on the occiput and the ipsilateral elbow pointing straight in the air with the humerus flexed approximately 120 degrees. The patient is supine, and the x-ray beam is angled 10 degrees cephalad and is centered on the coracoid process.

The Stryker notch view is sensitive for detecting *Hill-Sachs lesions.* These lesions are impaction fractures of the posterolateral aspect of the humeral head that are created when this region is compressed against the anterior margin of the glenoid in association with recurrent anterior dislocation.

Note: Reverse Hill-Sachs lesions are impaction fractures of the anterior humeral head. These lesions are associated with recurrent posterior glenohumeral dislocation.

References

Hall, et al.: Dislocations of the Shoulder with Special Reference to Accompanying Small Fractures. J Bone Joint Surg Am, 41:489–494, 1959.

Hill HA, Sachs MD: The Grooved Defect of the Humeral Head: A Frequently Unrecognized Complication of Dislocations of the Shoulder Joint. Radiology, 35:690–700, 1940.

FIGURE CREDITS

Figure 1.1. From Blair WF: Techniques in Hand Surgery. Baltimore, Williams & Wilkins, p. 139, 1996, with permission.

Figure 1.3. From Blair WF: Techniques in Hand Surgery. Baltimore, Williams & Wilkins, p. 123, 1996, with permission.

Figure 1.4. From Chidgey LK, Szabo RM: Anterior Interosseous Nerve Compression Syndrome. In Szabo RM, ed: Nerve Compression Syndromes: Diagnosis and Treatment. Thorofare, NJ, Slack, p. 756, 1989, with permission.

Figure 1.5. From Blair WF: Techniques in Hand Surgery. Baltimore, Williams & Wilkins, p. 1150, 1996;1150, with permission.

Figure 1.6. From Blair WF: Techniques in Hand Surgery. Baltimore, Williams & Wilkins, p. 1118, 1996, with permission.

Figure 1.7. From Blair WF: Techniques in Hand Surgery. Baltimore, Williams & Wilkins, p. 611, 1996, with permission.

Figure 1.8. From Craig EV: Clinical Orthopaedics. Philadelphia, Lippincott, Williams & Wilkins, p. 154, 1999, with permission.

Figure 1.10. From Craig EV: Clinical Orthopaedics. Philadelphia, Lippincott, Williams & Wilkins, p. 100, 1999, with permission.

Figure 1.11. From Strickland JW: Flexor Tendon Injuries: I. Foundations of Treatment. J Am Acad Orthop Surg, 3:47, 1995, with permission.

Figure 1.12. From Blair WF: Techniques in Hand Surgery. Baltimore, Williams & Wilkins, p. 534, 1996, with permission.

Figure 1.13. From Blair WF: Techniques in Hand Surgery. Baltimore, Williams & Wilkins, p. 736, 1996, with permission.

Figure 1.14A–C. From Craig EV: Clinical Orthopaedics. Philadelphia, Lippincott Williams & Wilkins, p. 31, 1999, with permission.

2

SHOULDER AND ELBOW

QUESTIONS

1. During which of the following phases of the overhand pitching motion are the greatest valgus stresses encountered across the medial side of the elbow?
   (a) Windup
   (b) Early cocking
   (c) Acceleration
   (d) Release
   (e) Follow through
2. An unbelted taxi driver is ejected from his vehicle and sustains closed, displaced fractures of the middle third of the clavicle and the ipsilateral glenoid neck. The most appropriate treatment for this combination of injuries would be which of the following?
   (a) Scapulothoracic arthrodesis
   (b) Open reduction and internal fixation of only the glenoid neck
   (c) Open reduction and internal fixation of only the clavicle
   (d) Closed treatment of both fractures with a shoulder immobilizer
   (e) Closed treatment of both fractures with a figure-of-eight brace
3. A 69-year-old croquet enthusiast presents with progressive right shoulder pain. Coronal and axial magnetic resonance images are shown in Fig. 2.1A and B. These images are most consistent with which of the following diagnoses?
   (a) Calcific tendinitis
   (b) Rheumatoid arthritis
   (c) Type IV superior labrum anterior and posterior lesion (SLAP)
   (d) Cuff tear arthropathy
   (e) Neuropathic arthropathy
4. What is the most appropriate position for glenohumeral arthrodesis in a nonparalytic adult shoulder?
   (a) 45 degrees of abduction, 45 degrees of forward flexion, 10 degrees of external rotation
   (b) 30 degrees of abduction, 30 degrees of forward flexion, 30 degrees of internal rotation
   (c) 35 degrees of abduction, 20 degrees of forward flexion, neutral rotation
   (d) 45 degrees of abduction, 50 degrees of forward flexion, neutral rotation
   (e) 60 degrees of abduction, 30 degrees of forward flexion, 20 degrees of internal rotation
5. Which of the following structures is marked by the *thin solid arrow* on the axial T1 magnetic resonance image of the right shoulder shown in Fig. 2.2?
   (a) The anterior humeral circumflex artery
   (b) The tendon of the long head of the biceps
   (c) The ascending branch of the anterior humeral circumflex artery
   (d) The coracohumeral ligament
   (e) The musculocutaneous nerve
6. Which of the following is most commonly encountered when a capitellocondylar total elbow replacement (nonconstrained design) is placed in a patient with rheumatoid arthritis through a lateral approach?
   (a) Transient ulnar nerve dysfunction
   (b) Early loosening of the humeral component
   (c) Anterior dislocation
   (d) Early loosening of the ulnar component
   (e) Infection
7. Which of the following statements is true regarding the Putti-Platt (imbrication of the anterior capsule and subscapularis tendon) procedure for anterior shoulder instability?
   (a) Redislocation has not been reported.
   (b) Glenohumeral arthrosis in the setting of a prior Putti-Platt procedure is associated with minimally compromised range of motion.
   (c) Secondary glenohumeral arthrosis can be successfully relieved by an anterior release technique.
   (d) The objective of the procedure is to rotate large Hill-Sachs lesions posterolaterally by increasing humeral head retroversion.
   (e) Injury to the musculocutaneous nerve is a common complication.

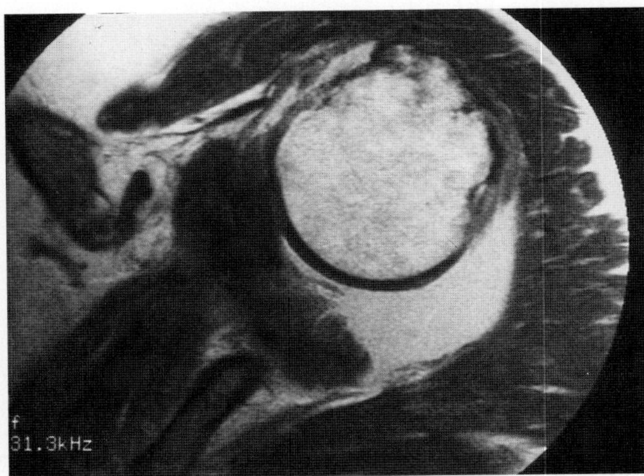

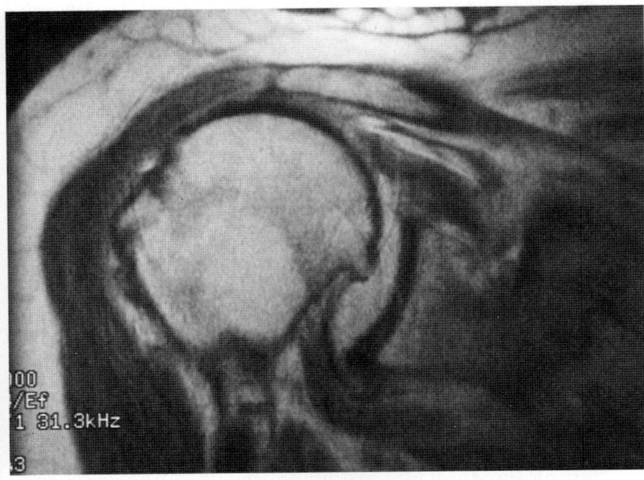

FIGURE 2.1A and B

8. What is the overall ratio of glenohumeral to scapulothoracic motion during abduction of the arm from 0 to 180 degrees?
   (a) 1:1
   (b) 2:1
   (c) 2:3
   (d) 4:1
   (e) 1:2
9. The Judet (posterior) approach to the shoulder reflects a muscular flap on what vascular pedicle?
   (a) The suprascapular artery
   (b) The thoracodorsal artery
   (c) The dorsal scapular artery
   (d) The anterior humeral circumflex artery
   (e) The posterior humeral circumflex artery
10. Figure 2.3 is an axial T1 magnetic resonance image of the right shoulder of a professional wrestler collecting disability insurance. What structure is marked by the *arrow*?
    (a) The thoracodorsal artery
    (b) The circumflex scapular artery
    (c) The acromial branch of the thoracoacromial trunk
    (d) The dorsal scapular artery
    (e) The suprascapular artery
11. What nerve innervates the teres major muscle?
    (a) The lower subscapular nerve
    (b) The axillary nerve
    (c) The upper subscapular nerve
    (d) The thoracodorsal nerve
    (e) The dorsal scapular nerve

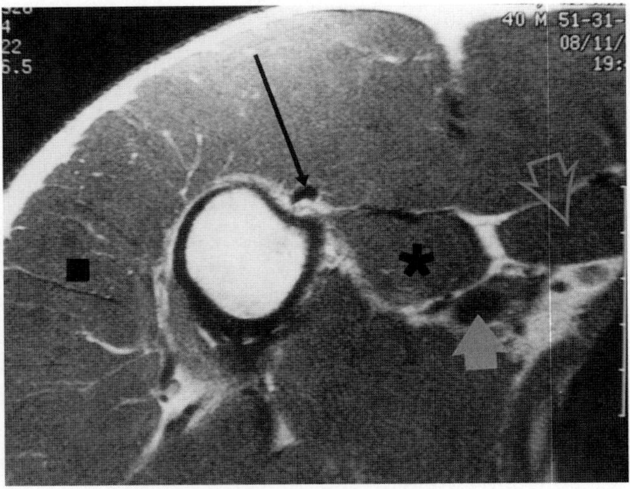

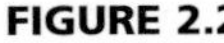

FIGURE 2.2

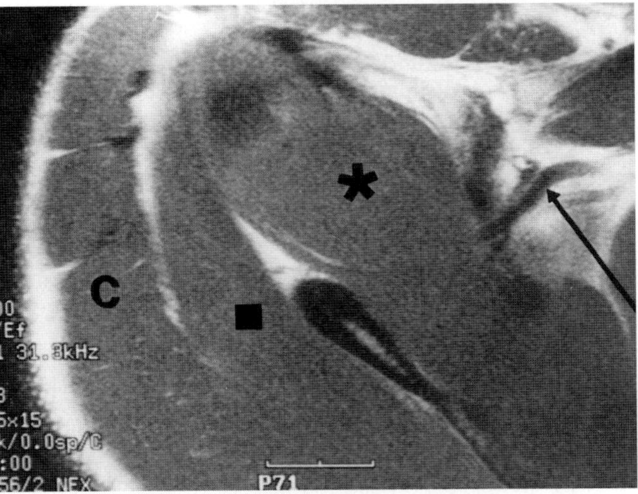

FIGURE 2.3

12. A 34-year-old tennis player presents with burning pain in the posterolateral aspect of his right shoulder that occasionally radiates into his proximal arm. He also complains of "weakness" when he attempts to serve. Examination reveals mild atrophy at the infraspinatus fossa. Examination of the cervical spine is normal. Sensation is normal throughout the upper extremities. Active range of motion of his shoulder is symmetric with the contralateral side. Motor strength is normal throughout the extremity, except for mild weakness with abduction and external rotation. Plain radiographs and a magnetic resonance imaging scan of the shoulder are normal. Electromyograms reveal fibrillations, decreased recruitment, and spontaneous activity in the supraspinatus and infraspinatus. Nerve conduction studies show prolonged motor latencies and decreased amplitude to the same two muscles. What would be the most appropriate course of treatment?
    (a) Anterior decompression and fusion at C4-5
    (b) Surgical exploration and release of the suprascapular ligament
    (c) Arthroscopic subacromial decompression
    (d) Activity modification and physical therapy focusing on strengthening of the rotator cuff and periscapular muscles
    (e) Sural nerve cable grafting to the suprascapular nerve
13. A postal worker presents with chronic pain at his lateral elbow that is aggravated by work activities and recreational softball. Physical examination reveals point tenderness adjacent to his radial head that is exacerbated by resisted wrist extension. A magnetic resonance imaging scan is obtained by the referring primary care physician (Fig. 2.4). Plain radiographs of the elbow are normal. This process predominantly affects what musculotendinous unit?

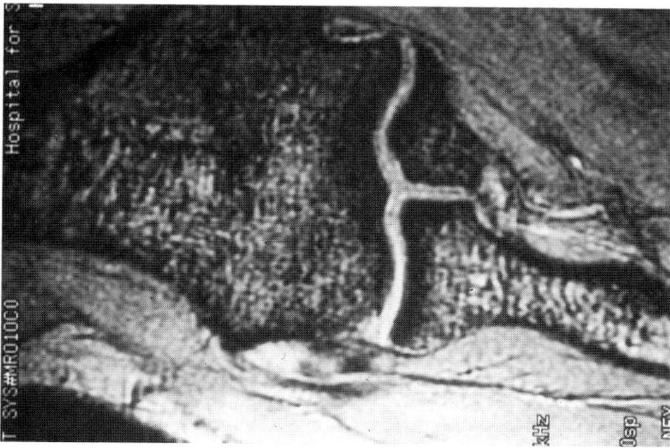

FIGURE 2.4

    (a) The extensor carpi radialis longus
    (b) The brachioradialis
    (c) The extensor pollicis longus
    (d) The extensor carpi ulnaris
    (e) The extensor carpi radialis brevis
14. What would be the anticipated microscopic finding if the lesion in question 13 were to be examined by biopsy?
    (a) Acute inflammation
    (b) Fibrinous necrosis
    (c) Angiofibroblastic hyperplasia
    (d) Fat necrosis
    (e) Granuloma formation
15. What is the average distance proximal to the lateral epicondyle completed by the radial nerve crossing the posterior aspect of the humerus?
    (a) 24 cm
    (b) 19 cm
    (c) 14 cm
    (d) 9 cm
    (e) 6 cm
16. A 50-year-old bowler slips and sustains a transverse fracture of his dominant humeral diaphysis. The injury is closed, and there is no distal neurovascular compromise. However, after reduction and splinting, radial nerve palsy is noted. You recommend surgical exploration of the nerve and internal fixation of the fracture. The patient adamantly refuses surgery, but he asks you to explain the prognosis for his nerve deficit. Which of the following is the most accurate response to his inquiry?
    (a) The nerve was most likely contused during the reduction. Recovery of nerve function is unlikely unless the nerve is surgically decompressed.
    (b) The nerve was most likely contused or stretched during the reduction, but recovery of nerve function is likely even without surgical intervention.
    (c) The nerve was probably lacerated during the reduction. Return of nerve function is unlikely without exploration and microsurgical end-to-end repair.
    (d) The nerve was probably lacerated or entrapped during the reduction. Return of nerve function is unlikely without exploration, decompression, débridement, and interpositional nerve grafting.
    (e) The nerve could have been entrapped or lacerated during the reduction. Early exploration has been proven to improve the overall recovery rate.
17. What is the most common type of clavicle fracture?
    (a) Proximal third
    (b) Middle third
    (c) Distal third (lateral to the coracoclavicular ligaments and extraarticular)

(d) Distal third (lateral to the coracoclavicular ligaments and intraarticular)
(e) Distal third (medial to the coracoclavicular ligaments and extraarticular)

18. Nonunion most commonly occurs after nonoperative management of which of the following types of clavicular fractures?
(a) Intraarticular fracture of the proximal third
(b) Type I fracture of the distal third (lateral to the coracoclavicular ligaments and extraarticular)
(c) Type III fracture of the distal third (lateral to the coracoclavicular ligaments and intraarticular)
(d) Type IIA fracture of the distal third (medial to the coracoclavicular ligaments)
(e) Extraarticular fracture of the proximal third

19. The most common site of developmental nonunion is between which of the following acromial ossification centers?
(a) The basiacromion and the mesoacromion
(b) The mesoacromion and the metaacromion
(c) The basiacromion and the preacromion
(d) The metaacromion and the basiacromion
(e) The preacromion and the metaacromion

20. A 68-year-old man presents with a painful, chronic, locked posterior shoulder dislocation with significant associated wear of the posterior glenoid. A total shoulder arthroplasty is performed. What should be the version of the humeral component?
(a) 60 degrees of anteversion
(b) 30 degrees of anteversion
(c) Neutral version
(d) 30 degrees of retroversion
(e) 60 degrees of retroversion

21. Optimal internal fixation of a C1 (simple bicondylar) fracture of the distal humerus includes which of the following?
(a) A one-third tubular plate placed posteriorly on the lateral column and a 3.5-mm reconstruction plate placed posteriorly on the medial column
(b) Two crossed 4.5-mm cannulated screws
(c) A one-third tubular plate placed posteriorly on the lateral column and a 3.5-mm reconstruction plate placed posteriorly on the medial column
(d) A single Y-plate placed directly posteriorly
(e) A 3.5-mm reconstruction plate placed posteriorly on the lateral column and a one-third tubular plate placed directly medially

22. In which of the following subgroup of patients has early surgical repair (as compared with nonoperative management) of the injury shown in Fig. 2.5 been demonstrated to improve strength and decrease the incidence of late degenerative arthritis?
(a) Football lineman
(b) Swimmers
(c) Patients with generalized ligamentous laxity
(d) Patients with concurrent ipsilateral proximal humerus fractures
(e) None

23. A golfer trips into a sand trap with resultant shoulder pain. The emergency room physician obtains a single radiograph (Fig. 2.6). What does this film demonstrate?
(a) Anterior glenohumeral dislocation
(b) Luxatio erecta
(c) Scapulothoracic dissociation
(d) Posterior glenohumeral dislocation
(e) Scapular body fracture

24. Which of the following is the most appropriate indication for using a short-stemmed humeral component during the performance of a total shoulder arthroplasty?
(a) Paget disease
(b) Rheumatoid arthritis with ipsilateral elbow disease
(c) Rotator cuff incompetence
(d) Prior failed uncemented hemiarthroplasty
(e) Malunion of a prior surgical neck fracture

25. What nerve innervates the trapezius muscle?
(a) The suprascapular nerve
(b) The upper subscapular nerve
(c) The axillary nerve
(d) The dorsal scapular nerve
(e) The spinal accessory nerve

26. A 20-year-old college pitcher undergoes arthroscopic subacromial decompression and acromioplasty for presumed "impingement syndrome." At 12-month follow-up, he has experienced no relief of his preoperative discomfort during the cocking phase. He has been compliant with physical therapy. Examination reveals increased passive external rotation. The most likely diagnosis is
(a) Tendinitis of the long head of the biceps
(b) Internal impingement
(c) Cervical radiculopathy
(d) Inadequate acromioplasty
(e) Posterior subluxation

27. A 27-year-old investment banker presents for follow-up 2 months after an open anterior capsular shift for multidirectional instability. He complains that the operative shoulder has recently become painful. Examination reveals a positive *liftoff test.* The most likely problem is
(a) Axillary nerve injury
(b) Denervation of the subscapularis
(c) Adhesive capsulitis
(d) Subscapularis tendon rupture
(e) Excessive imbrication of the anterior capsule

28. What structures pass through the triangular interval?
(a) The axillary nerve and the posterior humeral circumflex artery
(b) The radial nerve and the profunda brachii artery

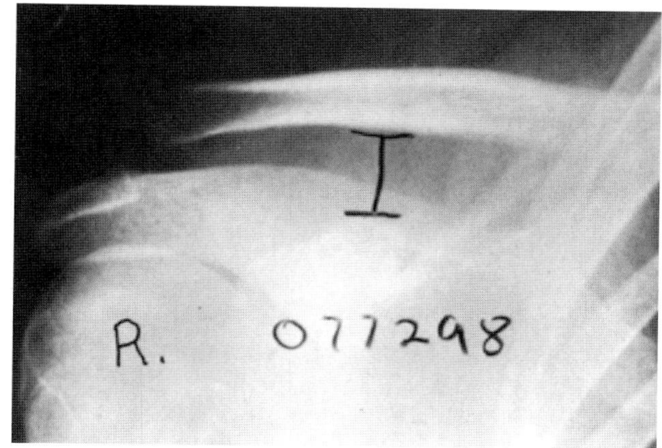

FIGURE 2.5

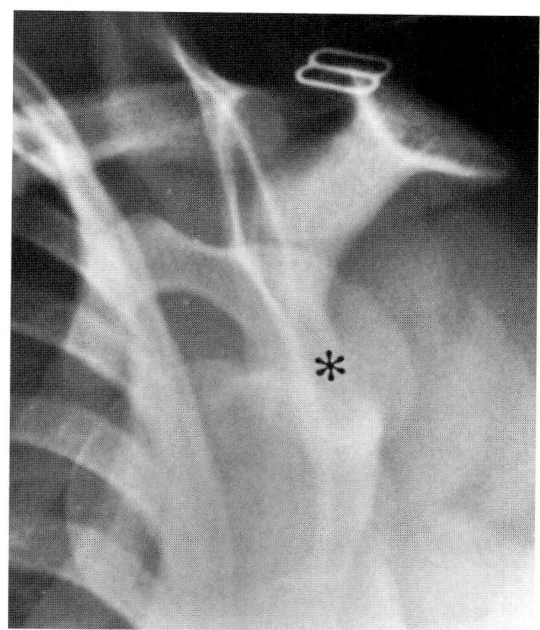

FIGURE 2.6

(c) The circumflex scapular artery and vein
(d) The radial nerve and the posterior humeral circumflex artery
(e) Axillary nerve and the anterior humeral circumflex artery

29. What is the average version of the glenoid relative to the plane of the scapula?
(a) Approximately 27 degrees of retroversion.
(b) Approximately 27 degrees of anteversion.
(c) Approximately 7 degrees of retroversion.
(d) Approximately 7 degrees of anteversion.
(e) Approximately neutral version.

30. A 42-year-old baggage handler presents with right shoulder pain. A coronal magnetic resonance imaging view is shown in Fig. 2.7. What is the most accurate description of the depicted lesion?
(a) Partial (undersurface) rotator cuff tear
(b) Type II SLAP lesion
(c) Partial (outersurface) rotator cuff tear
(d) Type III SLAP lesion
(e) Full-thickness rotator cuff tear

31. Which of the following is not a component of the "superior shoulder suspensory complex"?
(a) The acromioclavicular ligaments
(b) The coracoid process
(c) The superior glenohumeral ligament
(d) The coracoclavicular ligaments
(e) The distal third of the clavicle

32. After a difficult day in the operating room, one of the neurosurgeons at your hospital is involved in a domestic dispute. He is subsequently arrested by the authorities and is placed in handcuffs. During transport to the station, he attempts to free himself by inferiorly displacing his adducted arm. What is the primary static restraint to inferior translation of the humeral head when the arm is in this position?
(a) The posterior glenohumeral ligament
(b) The superior glenohumeral ligament
(c) The middle glenohumeral ligament
(d) The anterior band of the inferior glenohumeral ligament
(e) The anterior and posterior bands of the inferior glenohumeral ligament

33. A 30-year-old helmeted investment banker is thrown off his motorcycle and strikes the pavement with the side of his head. His brachial plexus is completely disrupted at Erb's point. The brachial plexus is otherwise intact. Which of the following functions is most likely to be preserved?
(a) Elbow flexion
(b) Arm abduction
(c) Shoulder external rotation
(d) Metacarpophalangeal extension
(e) Forearm supination

34. Figure 2.8 is a sagittal magnetic resonance image of an elbow. What is the innervation of the muscle marked by the *solid black arrow*?
(a) The radial nerve
(b) The musculocutaneous nerve
(c) The median nerve
(d) The median and musculocutaneous nerves
(e) Musculocutaneous and radial nerves

35. Which of the following patients with anterior shoulder instability would be the best candidate for arthroscopic stabilization with an arthroscopic tack, staple, or suture?
(a) A 20-year-old pitcher who has dislocated his dominant shoulder 15 times. The initial dislocation occurred 1 year ago while he was sliding into second base. A magnetic resonance imaging scan reveals no Bankart lesion.
(b) A 16-year-old gymnast who has dislocated her dominant shoulder twice. Her first dislocation occurred

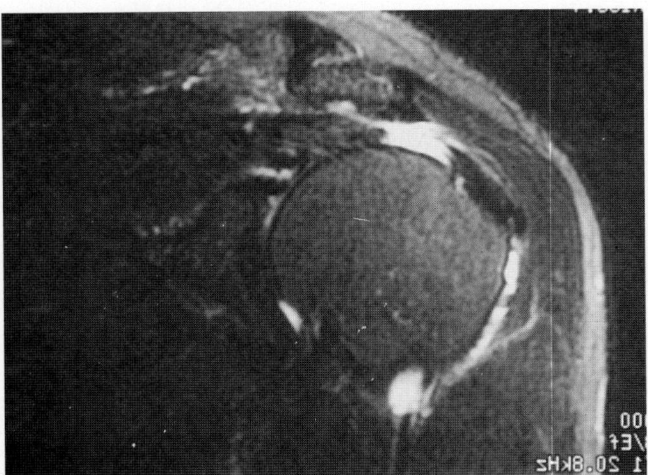

FIGURE 2.7

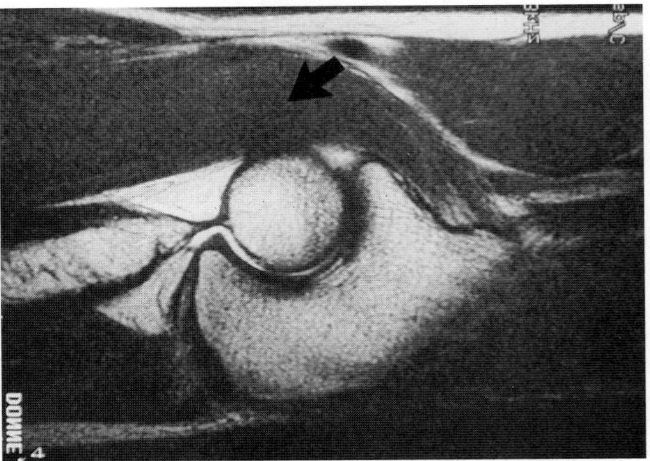

FIGURE 2.8

when she fell off a horse 5 weeks ago. A magnetic resonance imaging scan reveals a Bankart lesion.

(c) A 26-year-old aerobics instructor who has dislocated her dominant shoulder 10 times in her sleep. She has also dislocated her contralateral shoulder twice in the past. Her examination is remarkable for elbow hyperextension.

(d) An 18-year-old quarterback who complains of shoulder pain when cocking his arm to throw. He has never had a dislocation. Examination with the patient under anesthesia reveals moderate anterior shoulder subluxation. His magnetic resonance imaging examination is unremarkable.

(e) A 62-year-old security guard who dislocated his dominant shoulder last week when he fell down a flight of stairs. He has a history of antecedent impingement symptoms, but no history of prior instability.

36. The internervous plane for the Kocher approach to the elbow is between
   (a) The radial and ulnar nerves
   (b) The median and musculocutaneous nerves
   (c) The radial and musculocutaneous nerves
   (d) The posterior interosseous and radial nerves
   (e) The ulnar and musculocutaneous nerves
37. The "safe zone" for placement of hardware in a radial head fracture is 100 degrees centered over the coronal equator, with the forearm held in what position?
   (a) Neutral rotation
   (b) 45 degrees of supination
   (c) Full pronation
   (d) 45 degrees of pronation
   (e) Full supination
38. What is the primary restraint to valgus instability of the elbow?
   (a) The transverse component of the medial collateral ligament
   (b) The ulnar component of the lateral collateral ligament
   (c) The anterior component of the medial collateral ligament
   (d) The radial head
   (e) The posterior component of the medial collateral ligament
39. Which of the following statements accurately describes the electromyographic muscle activity in the elbows of competitive baseball pitchers with medial collateral ligament insufficiency during the late cocking and acceleration phases of throwing a fastball?
   (a) The extensor carpi radialis brevis demonstrates decreased activity versus uninjured pitchers.
   (b) The pronator teres demonstrates increased activity versus uninjured pitchers.
   (c) The extensor carpi radialis longus demonstrates decreased activity versus uninjured pitchers.
   (d) The triceps demonstrates increased activity versus uninjured pitchers.
   (e) The flexor carpi radialis demonstrates decreased activity versus uninjured pitchers.
40. What is the nerve supply to the latissimus dorsi?
   (a) The lateral thoracic nerve
   (b) The long thoracic nerve
   (c) The dorsal scapular nerve
   (d) The thoracodorsal nerve
   (e) The subscapular nerve
41. What is the nerve supply to the rhomboids?
   (a) The axillary nerve
   (b) The long thoracic nerve
   (c) The dorsal scapular nerve
   (d) The thoracodorsal nerve
   (e) The subscapular nerve
42. A patient has a focal contracture of the shoulder capsule in the region of the rotator interval. Which of the following passive motions would most likely be limited?
   (a) Internal rotation with the arm adducted
   (b) Internal rotation with the arm abducted
   (c) External rotation with the arm abducted
   (d) External rotation with the arm adducted
   (e) Internal rotation with the arm forward flexed
43. Which of the following is the most common cause of a Charcot shoulder?
   (a) Tabes dorsalis
   (b) Diabetic neuropathy
   (c) Syringomyelia
   (d) Charcot-Marie-Tooth disease
   (e) Arnold-Chiari malformation
44. A 21-year-old law student sustains a dislocation of his dominant glenohumeral joint when he is tackled in a touch football game against the medical school team. He has never dislocated his shoulder before. He demands a numeric estimation of his risk for redislocation. What would be the most appropriate estimation of the incidence of recurrence in someone his age?
   (a) 1%
   (b) 5%
   (c) 10%
   (d) 25%
   (e) More than 40%
45. Which of the following factors has been shown to be the most significant determinant of a favorable functional outcome after a minimally displaced (one-part) fracture of the proximal humerus?
   (a) Duration of sling use of less than 3 weeks
   (b) Patient age of less than 65 years
   (c) Initiation of physical therapy within 2 weeks of injury
   (d) Fracture of the surgical neck
   (e) Fracture of the greater tuberosity
46. Which of the following structures is the most significant restraint to inferior displacement of the medial clavicle?

(a) The costoclavicular ligament
(b) The first costal cartilage
(c) The sternoclavicular intraarticular disc ligament
(d) The sternoclavicular capsular ligament
(e) The coracoclavicular ligaments

47. Which of the following structures does not attach to the coracoid process?
(a) The pectoralis minor
(b) The trapezoid ligament
(c) The conoid ligament
(d) The conjoined tendon
(e) The long head of the biceps

48. A 29-year-old snowboarder presents with a right tension pneumothorax after colliding with a tree. His dyspnea completely resolves after chest tube placement. Tenderness and deformity at the ipsilateral sternoclavicular joint prompt a computed tomography scan of the chest that confirms a posterior sternoclavicular dislocation. He has no stridor, and neurovascular examination of the upper extremities is normal. What would be the most appropriate management of this injury?
(a) Figure-of-eight strap until the patient's discomfort resolves
(b) Acute closed reduction under general anesthesia followed by figure-of-eight strap for 6 weeks
(c) Acute open reduction and pin fixation of the sternoclavicular joint with Kirschner wires
(d) Initial observation, with delayed open reduction and costoclavicular ligament reconstruction if late symptoms arise
(e) Initial observation, with delayed open reduction and sternoclavicular capsular ligament reconstruction if late symptoms arise

49. What is the prevalence of rotator cuff tears (partial plus complete) detected by magnetic resonance imaging in asymptomatic volunteers between the ages of 40 and 60 years?
(a) Approximately 5%
(b) Approximately 15%
(c) Approximately 30%
(d) Approximately 50%
(e) Approximately 75%

50. During shoulder arthroscopy with interscalene regional anesthesia, supplemental local anesthetic is frequently necessary because of failure of the interscalene block adequately to anesthetize which of the following?
(a) The lateral antebrachial cutaneous nerve distribution
(b) The T2 dermatome
(c) The inferior cord of the brachial plexus
(d) The cutaneous distribution of the axillary nerve
(e) The C4 dermatome

51. The lateral pivot shift test of the elbow includes which of the following maneuvers?
(a) Axial compression and varus stress with the forearm in full supination
(b) Axial distraction and varus stress with the forearm in neutral rotation
(c) Axial compression and valgus stress with the forearm in full supination
(d) Axial distraction and valgus stress with the forearm in full pronation
(e) Axial compression and varus stress with the forearm in full pronation

52. Insufficiency of which of the following structures is primarily responsible for a positive lateral pivot shift test of the elbow?
(a) The lateral ulnar collateral ligament
(b) The annular ligament
(c) The accessory collateral ligament
(d) The radial collateral ligament
(e) The ulnar collateral ligament

53. A Buford complex is encountered during the diagnostic arthoscopy of a 42-year-old recreational squash player with suspected impingement syndrome and a positive preoperative impingement test. How should this patient be managed?
(a) Open stabilization and acromioplasty
(b) Arthroscopic stabilization and acromioplasty
(c) Intraarticular debridement and acromioplasty
(d) Arthroscopic stabilization only
(e) Arthroscopic acromioplasty only

54. Figure 2.9 is an axial T1 magnetic resonance image of the shoulder. Which of the following nerves innervates the structure that is marked by the *solid black box*?
(a) The axillary nerve
(b) The suprascapular nerve
(c) The lateral pectoral nerve

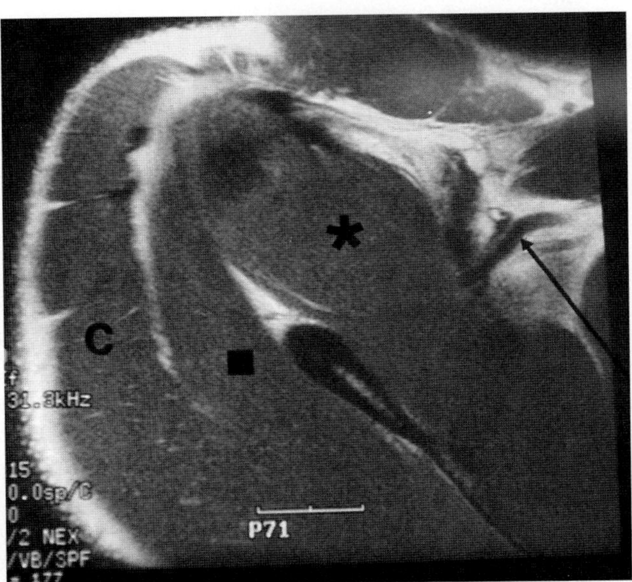

FIGURE 2.9

(d) The upper subscapular nerve
(e) The thoracodorsal nerve

55. The most common elbow disorder among golfers is
(a) Medial epicondylitis in the lead arm
(b) Medial epicondylitis in the trailing arm
(c) Lateral epicondylitis in the lead arm
(d) Lateral epicondylitis in the trailing arm
(e) Posterior impingement

56. Which of the following is false regarding calcific tendinitis of the shoulder?
(a) It may occur in the absence of degenerative joint disease of the glenohumeral joint.
(b) Radiographs during the formative phase characteristically reveal a dense, well-circumscribed, homogeneous mineral deposit.
(c) Radiographs during the resorptive phase characteristically reveal an irregular, fluffy density.
(d) Rupture into the bursa occurs during the resorptive phase.
(e) Pain is most prominent during the formative phase.

57. A 26-year-old windsurfer sustained an anterior shoulder dislocation while crash landing a back flip. Over the ensuing 8 months, he dislocated the shoulder three more times. A preoperative magnetic resonance imaging scan revealed a Bankart lesion and a small Hill-Sachs lesion. Arthroscopically, a lax anterior capsule was encountered. The Bankart lesion was repaired anatomically using a bioabsorbable (polyglyconate) arthroscopic tack. Four months later, the patient sustained a recurrent atraumatic anterior dislocation, and an open anterior shoulder stabilization was performed. What would be the most likely intraoperative findings?
(a) Bankart lesion not healed, patulous capsule
(b) Bankart lesion not healed, reactive synovitis
(c) Bankart lesion not healed, tack impinging on the humeral head
(d) Bankart lesion healed, patulous capsule
(e) Bankart lesion healed, subscapularis rupture

58. What is the most common complication of semiconstrained total elbow replacement for posttraumatic osteoarthrosis at 5-year follow-up?
(a) Aseptic loosening of the humeral component
(b) Aseptic loosening of the ulnar component
(c) Mechanical failure of the prosthesis (other than aseptic loosening)
(d) Infection
(e) Osteolysis

59. A 30-year-old man presents with a 2-week history of left shoulder pain in the region of the acromioclavicular joint. He denies fevers, chills, weight loss, and pain in other joints. He attributes his discomfort to his aggressive use of the nautilus machine that his girlfriend gave him for Christmas. His acromioclavicular joint is tender. An anteroposterior radiograph is shown in Fig. 2.10. A radiograph of the contralateral acromioclavicular joint is normal, and the patient is otherwise healthy. The most appropriate next step in the management of this patient would be
(a) Test parathyroid hormone level
(b) Acromioclavicular joint arthrocentesis for cell count, culture, and sensitivity
(c) Open biopsy of the distal clavicle
(d) Distal clavicular resection (Mumford procedure)
(e) Prescription of a sling for comfort, nonsteroidal antiinflammatory drugs, and activity modification

60. A 30-year-old rollerblader complains of severe left medial clavicle pain and altered phonation after a high-speed collision with a lamppost. The clavicles and sternum are not fractured. However, on a 40-degree cephalic tilt radiograph *(serendipity view),* the left medial clavicle appears to be caudally displaced (relative to the level of the right medial clavicle). What type of injury has she suffered?
(a) Inferior sternoclavicular dislocation
(b) Superior sternoclavicular dislocation
(c) Anterior sternoclavicular dislocation
(d) Posterior sternoclavicular dislocation
(e) Ipsilateral posterior acromioclavicular dislocation

61. What is the main blood supply to the humeral head?
(a) The posterior humeral circumflex artery
(b) The circumflex scapular artery
(c) The arcuate branch of the profunda brachial artery
(d) The acromial branch of the thoracoacromial artery
(e) The anterolateral ascending branch of the anterior humeral circumflex artery

62. What is the most common adverse outcome after antegrade intramedullary nail fixation of a humeral shaft fracture?
(a) Shoulder pain
(b) Ulnar nerve injury
(c) Radial nerve injury
(d) Nonunion
(e) Infection

63. During which phase of the baseball pitch is muscle activity greatest in the pronator teres?
(a) Windup
(b) Early cocking
(c) Late cocking
(d) Acceleration
(e) Follow through

64. The borders of the quadrangular space include
(a) The teres minor, teres major, lateral head of the triceps, and long head of the triceps
(b) The teres minor, teres major, latissimus dorsi, and humerus
(c) The teres major, long head of the triceps, subscapularis, and latissimus dorsi
(d) The teres major, lateral head of the triceps, humerus, and infraspinatus

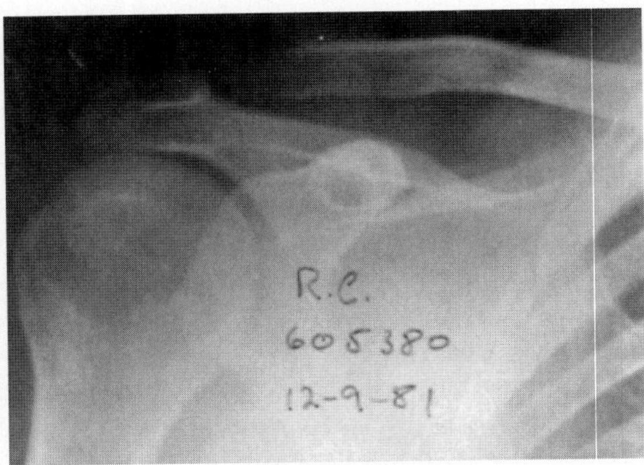

FIGURE 2.10

(e) The teres minor, teres major, long head of the triceps, and humerus

65. When performing an examination of the shoulder under anesthesia, how much posterior translation of the humeral head (in terms of percentage of glenoid diameter) may be considered normal?
    (a) 10%
    (b) 25%
    (c) 50%
    (d) 75%
    (e) 90%
66. A 42-year-old man falls 12 feet from a ladder and sustains a type I Monteggia fracture (anterior radial head dislocation with anterior ulnar angulation). A deficit of which of the following nerves is most commonly associated with this injury?
    (a) The median nerve
    (b) The ulnar nerve
    (c) The anterior interosseous nerve
    (d) The posterior interosseous nerve
    (e) The radial nerve
67. Which of the following statements is *false* regarding the pectoralis major muscle?
    (a) It is innervated by the medial pectoral nerve.
    (b) It is perfused by a branch of the thoracoacromial artery.
    (c) It inserts on the medial aspect of the intertubercular groove caudal to the subscapularis insertion.
    (d) It internally rotates the humerus.
    (e) It is innervated by the lateral pectoral nerve.
68. A 50-year-old patient with rheumatoid arthritis underwent a cemented total shoulder replacement 6 years ago. She presents for routine follow-up. Her shoulder is asymptomatic. Which of the following would be the most likely radiographic finding in this patient?
    (a) Linear radiolucency at the cement-bone interface of the humeral component
    (b) Subsidence of the humeral component
    (c) Linear radiolucency at the cement-bone interface of the glenoid component
    (d) Medial migration of the glenoid component
    (e) Linear radiolucency at the cement-prosthesis interface of the humeral component
69. A 25-year-old snowboarder falls onto his outstretched hand and sustains a complete posterior elbow dislocation. After closed reduction under general anesthesia is performed, range of motion reveals no posterior instability except in terminal extension. The elbow is unstable to valgus stress. Repeat radiographs confirm a concentric reduction and no fracture. The most appropriate management of this patient would be
    (a) Immobilization in 90 degrees of flexion for 5 to 7 days, followed by initiation of range-of-motion exercises.
    (b) Immobilization in 90 degrees of flexion for 4 weeks, followed by initiation of range-of-motion exercises.
    (c) Immobilization in 90 degrees of flexion for 6 weeks, followed by initiation of range-of-motion exercises.
    (d) Acute primary repair of the medial collateral ligament, followed by immediate commencement of range of motion in a hinged, extension block splint
    (e) Acute reconstruction of the medial collateral ligament using a palmaris longus graft, followed by immediate commencement of range of motion in a hinged, extension block splint
70. Which of the following anatomic factors is not a potential direct cause of thoracic outlet syndrome?
    (a) Clavicular malunion
    (b) Cervical rib
    (c) Congenital fibrous bands
    (d) The posterior scalene muscle
    (e) Trapezius weakness
71. Which of the following findings would be least characteristic of chronic valgus extension overload of the elbow in a throwing athlete?
    (a) Traction spurs on the medial aspect of the ulnar notch
    (b) Avulsion of the medial epicondyle through the apophysis
    (c) Hypertrophy of the humerus
    (d) Osteophyte formation on the posterolateral olecranon
    (e) Chondromalacia of the medial olecranon fossa
72. Which of the following types of proximal humerus fractures typically have the most favorable outcome if managed by open reduction and internal fixation rather than immediate hemiarthroplasty?
    (a) Four-part fracture with anterior displacement of the shaft

(b) Four-part fracture with posterior displacement of the shaft
(c) Four-part fracture with varus impaction of the head
(d) Four-part fracture with valgus impaction of the head
(e) Four-part fracture with a massive rotator cuff tear

73. A 39-year-old woman complains of right shoulder pain that is precipitated by overhead activities, particularly during her tennis serve. She notes associated vague shoulder fatigue. She denies numbness or paresthesias. She has a positive Neer impingement sign. Her past medical history is significant for breast cancer that was treated with mastectomy and chemotherapy. Shoulder radiographs are negative. She takes tamoxifen, and she is considered to have no known residual disease. Which of the following is the most appropriate first step in the workup of this patient?
    (a) Electromyograms to rule out brachial plexus damage from the chemotherapy agents
    (b) Referral to physical therapy for infraspinatus and subscapularis strengthening
    (c) Bone scan to rule out occult metastasis
    (d) Magnetic resonance imaging to assess the integrity of the rotator cuff
    (e) Examination for scapular winging
74. Osteoarthritis of the elbow is characterized by all the following except
    (a) Pain at the extremes of range of motion
    (b) Equal sex distribution
    (c) Predilection for the dominant extremity
    (d) Relative sparing of forearm rotation
    (e) Osteophytes of the olecranon and coronoid
75. Fibrosis and tendinitis are the prevailing features of impingement syndrome among patients of what age group?
    (a) Less than 25 years old
    (b) 25 to 40 years old
    (c) 40 to 60 years old
    (d) 60 to 80 years old
    (e) More than 80 years old
76. What is the most common site of compression of the posterior interosseous nerve?
    (a) The fibrous bands at the entrance of the radial tunnel
    (b) The fan-shaped radial recurrent vessels (the leash of Henry)
    (c) The tendinous margin of the extensor carpi radialis brevis muscle
    (d) The proximal border of the superficial belly of the supinator (the arcade of Frohse)
    (e) The distal border of the supinator
77. Which of the following is the least appropriate indication for operative management of midshaft humerus fractures?
    (a) Pathologic humerus fracture
    (b) Segmental humerus fracture
    (c) Ipsilateral humerus and both-bone forearm fractures
    (d) Bilateral humerus fractures
    (e) Closed, transverse fracture with associated complete radial nerve palsy
78. A 23-year-old man presents with a history of recurrent shoulder instability. His shoulder is currently reduced. What is the most appropriate radiographic view to detect a bony Bankart lesion?
    (a) Standard anteroposterior view with internal rotation
    (b) True anteroposterior view
    (c) Axillary view
    (d) West Point view
    (e) Stryker notch view
79. What is the nerve supply to the pectoralis minor?
    (a) The lateral thoracic nerve
    (b) The subscapular nerve
    (c) The lateral pectoral nerve
    (d) The medial pectoral nerve
    (e) Both lateral and medial pectoral nerves
80. A pediatrician slips and falls while attempting to protect an infant from a postnatal hip screening examination by an orthopaedic resident. The pediatrician orders a computed tomography scan, which reveals a type III fracture of the distal third of the clavicle (a minimally displaced fracture that is lateral to the coracoclavicular ligaments with intraarticular acromioclavicular joint extension). The most appropriate treatment of this injury would be
    (a) Closed reduction and percutaneous pin fixation
    (b) Closed reduction and gunslinger cast immobilization
    (c) Open reduction and internal fixation
    (d) Sling immobilization for comfort
    (e) Mumford procedure
81. The radiographs in Fig. 2.11 represent various types of acromial morphology. Which type of acromial morphology is most common in asymptomatic healthy persons?
    (a) I
    (b) II
    (c) III
82. A 60-year-old woman with rheumatoid arthritis presents with progressive elbow pain. She underwent an interpositional arthroplasty on the elbow 8 years ago. Her present discomfort has not improved with bracing, and she states that her medications do not help anymore. Her radiographs reveal severe metaphyseal bone loss. What would be the most appropriate salvage procedure for this patient?
    (a) Revision interpositional arthroplasty using a cutis graft

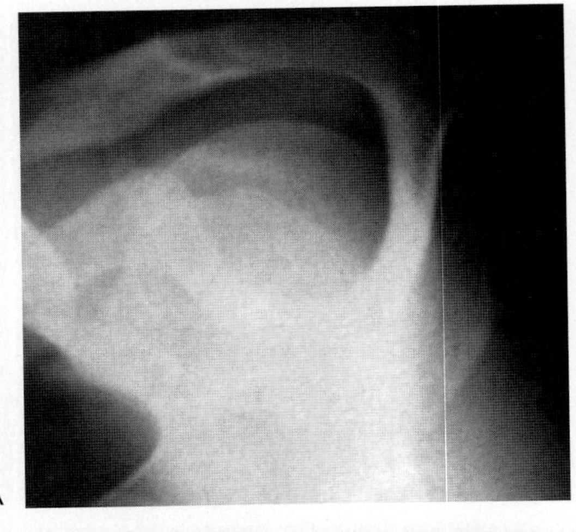
A

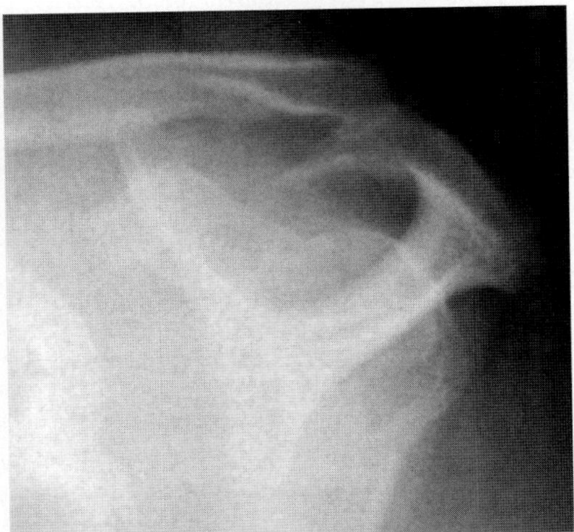
C

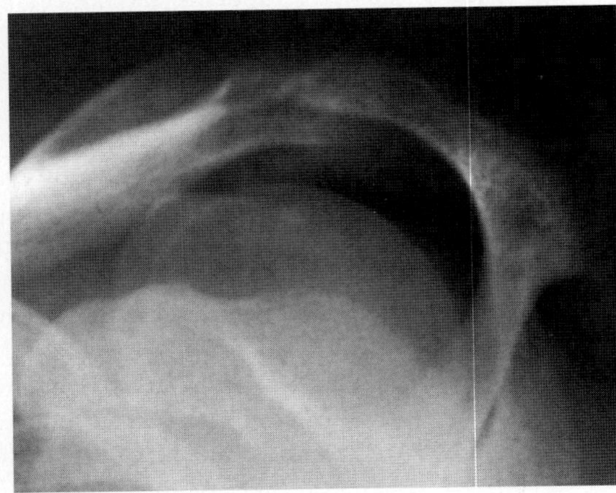
B

FIGURE 2.11A–C

(b) Nonconstrained total elbow arthroplasty
(c) Semiconstrained total elbow arthroplasty
(d) Hinged (constrained) total elbow arthroplasty
(e) Elbow arthrodesis

83. What range of elbow flexion and extension is required to perform most activities of daily living (i.e., what is the functional range of motion of the elbow)?
   (a) 0 to 160 degrees
   (b) 10 to 150 degrees
   (c) 30 to 130 degrees
   (d) 45 to 120 degrees
   (e) 0 to 90 degrees
84. A retained drop of fluid in the Morse taper housing of a modular total shoulder prosthesis will reduce the strength of the assembly linkage by how much?
   (a) No effect, as long as the head is firmly impacted
   (b) 5% compromise
   (c) 10% compromise
   (d) 25% compromise
   (e) More than 50% compromise
85. Which of the following factors has been shown to correlate most favorably with the outcome of patients treated nonoperatively for subacromial impingement syndrome?
   (a) Involvement of the nondominant shoulder
   (b) Tenderness of the acromioclavicular joint
   (c) A type I (flat) acromion
   (d) Age greater than 60 years
   (e) Female gender
86. The anterior approach to the humerus involves which internervous planes?
   (a) The axillary and radial nerves (proximally) and the musculocutaneous and median nerves (distally)
   (b) The radial and musculocutaneous nerves (proximally) and the ulnar and median nerves (distally)
   (c) The musculocutaneous and lateral pectoral nerves (proximally) and the radial and musculocutaneous nerves (distally)
   (d) The suprascapular and axillary nerves (proximally) and the radial and musculocutaneous nerves (distally)
   (e) The axillary and lateral pectoral nerves (proximally) and the radial and musculocutaneous nerves (distally)

87. The axillary artery gives off several branches. Which of the following sequences is the proper order, from proximal to distal?
    (a) The supreme thoracic, lateral thoracic, subscapular, thoracoacromial, posterior humeral circumflex, and anterior humeral circumflex
    (b) The supreme thoracic, lateral thoracic, thoracoacromial, subscapular, posterior humeral circumflex, and anterior humeral circumflex
    (c) The supreme thoracic, thoracoacromial, lateral thoracic, anterior humeral circumflex, subscapular, and posterior humeral circumflex
    (d) The supreme thoracic, lateral thoracic, thoracoacromial, anterior humeral circumflex, subscapular, and posterior humeral circumflex
    (e) The supreme thoracic, thoracoacromial, lateral thoracic, subscapular, anterior humeral circumflex, and posterior humeral circumflex
88. A 57-year-old man with advanced cuff tear arthropathy has not responded to prolonged conservative therapy. Which of the following would be the most appropriate surgical procedure for this patient?
    (a) Arthroscopic débridement of the rotator cuff
    (b) Rotator cuff repair
    (c) Hemiarthroplasty
    (d) Total shoulder replacement
    (e) Arthroscopic subacromial decompression
89. A 76-year-old retired auto racer with Alzheimer's disease is brought for orthopaedic evaluation because his nursing home attendants have noticed unilateral (right) "shoulder stiffness." Active range of motion is painless but limited to 30 degrees of abduction, 30 degrees of external rotation, 50 degrees of elevation, and 5 degrees of internal rotation. The right hand is neurovascularly intact. A radiograph of the shoulder is obtained and demonstrates a posterior glenohumeral dislocation. There is no history of recent trauma. Gentle closed reduction is unsuccessful. The radiographic folder from the nursing home contains only a chest radiograph, obtained 4 months ago because of the patient's history of a positive purified protein derivative test, that shows the dislocation present at that time. What would be the most appropriate form of management for this patient?
    (a) Humeral head resection arthroplasty
    (b) Open reduction, stabilization, and primary hemiarthroplasty
    (c) Open reduction and glenohumeral arthrodesis
    (d) Open reduction and stabilization
    (e) Observation
90. A 60-year-old dancer presents with right shoulder pain after a collision on the dance floor. A radiograph is obtained (Fig. 2.12). What is the most appropriate initial treatment?
    (a) Open reduction and internal fixation
    (b) Closed reduction

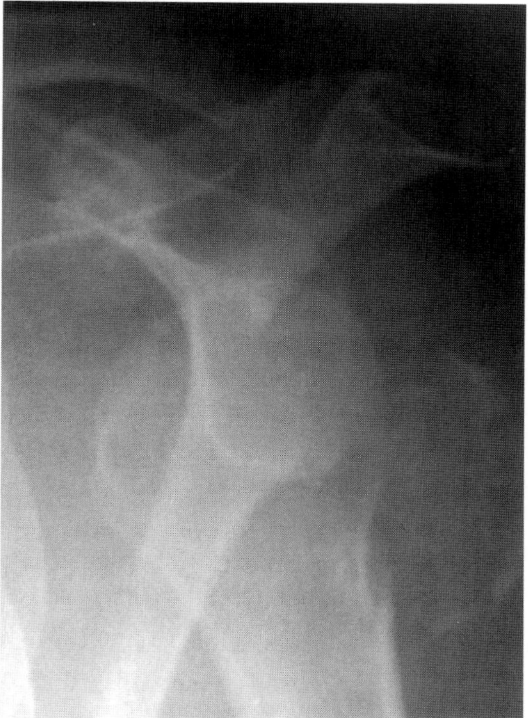

FIGURE 2.12

    (c) Hemiarthroplasty
    (d) Total shoulder arthroplasty
    (e) Open reduction and anterior stabilization
91. The first total shoulder replacement was performed for which of the following conditions?
    (a) Cuff tear arthropathy
    (b) Rheumatoid arthritis
    (c) Tuberculosis
    (d) Chondrosarcoma
    (e) Neuropathic arthropathy

ANSWERS

1. **c** Acceleration. The five classically described stages of overhead throwing are windup, early cocking, late cocking, acceleration, and follow through. Maximal valgus stresses occur across the medial joint line during the late cocking and acceleration phases of overhand throwing. These forces can produce attenuation and tearing of the medial collateral ligament. The resultant syndrome of medial instability and lateral compression can produce significant pain and dysfunction.

References

Jobe FW, et al.: Reconstruction of the Ulnar Collateral Ligament in Athletes. J Bone Joint Surg Am, 68:1158–1163, 1986.

Jobe FW, Nuber G: Throwing Injuries of the Elbow. Clin Sports Med, 5(4):621–636, 1986.

2. **c** Open reduction and internal fixation of only the clavicle. Most midshaft clavicle fractures can be successfully managed nonoperatively with either a sling or a figureofeight brace. However, there are several indications for open reduction and internal fixation of midshaft clavicle fractures. These include (1) concomitant ipsilateral glenoid neck fracture *(floating shoulder);* (2) concomitant scapulothoracic dissociation; (3) open fracture; (4) fracture fragments that tent the overlying skin (impending open fracture); and (5) established nonunion.

   When concomitant clavicular and glenoid neck fractures are both displaced, direct reduction of the clavicle generally provides an acceptable indirect reduction of the glenoid neck. Nonoperative management of the floating shoulder is associated with inferior results.

References

Goss TP: Double Disruptions of the Superior Shoulder Suspensory Complex. J Orthop Trauma, 7:99–106, 1993

Hersovici, et al.: The Floating Shoulder. J Orthop Trauma, 6:499, 1992.

3. **d** Cuff tear arthropathy. The radiographic findings in this patient are consistent with *cuff tear arthropathy,* an entity originally described by Neer in which massive rotator cuff tears lead to glenohumeral arthrosis. Characteristic radiographic findings include superior migration of the humeral head, narrowing of the acromiohumeral interval, and degeneration of the humeral articular surface.

   The magnetic resonance images in Fig. 2.1 manifest all the salient features of cuff tear arthropathy. The coronal image (Fig. 2.1A) reveals marked superior migration of the humeral head in association with a massive, fullthickness supraspinatus tear that is retracted almost to the glenoid. The axial image (Fig. 2.1B) reveals posterior extension of the massive cuff tear into the infraspinatus.

   The osteophyte at the inferior margin of the humeral articular surface is a sign of glenohumeral articular degeneration. Although massive rotator cuff deficiency is often encountered in association with advanced rheumatoid arthritis of the shoulder, osteophyte formation is uncharacteristic of rheumatoid arthritis.

Reference

Neer CS, Craig EV, Fukuda H: Cuff Tear Arthropathy. Orthop Trans, 5:447–448, 1981.

4. **b** 30 degrees of abduction, 30 degrees of forward flexion, 30 degrees of internal rotation. The precise recommendations for glenohumeral arthrodesis have varied slightly in recent literature. Rowe recommended 15 to 25 degrees of abduction, 25 to 30 degrees of forward flexion, and 40 to 50 degrees of internal rotation. Hawkins and Neer recommended 25 to 40 degrees of abduction, 20 to 30 degrees of forward flexion, and 25 to 30 degrees of internal rotation.

   The position of glenohumeral arthrodesis determines the points in space to which the hand will have access after fusion. If the glenohumeral joint is fused in an appropriate position, residual scapulothoracic motion will allow the patient to perform most basic activities of daily living. However, arthrodesis in a suboptimal position can sacrifice residual function. For instance, insufficient internal rotation compromises the ability to bring the hand to the face, head, and the midline of the body for feeding and hygiene.

   Fusion in excessive abduction causes a prominence of the medial scapular border when the arm is adducted. Fusion in excessive forward flexion produces scapular winging when the arm is brought to the side of the torso. These situations not only are cosmetically displeasing, but also they may be associated with discomfort and functional compromise (such as inability to reach one's rear pockets or perform perineal care). For cases of brachial plexopathy, the position of glenohumeral arthrodesis must often be tailored according to which shoulder girdle muscles are nonfunctional.

   Note: Whereas the leading indications for shoulder arthrodesis were formerly poliomyelitis and tuberculosis, the operation is currently performed most commonly as a salvage procedure for arthritic conditions, brachial plexopathies, and multidirectional instability.

References

Hawkins RJ, Neer CS: A Functional Analysis of Shoulder Fusions. Clin Orthop, 223:65–76, 1987.

Rowe CR: Reevaluation of the Position of the Arm in Arthrodesis of the Shoulder in the Adult. J Bone Joint Surg Am, 56A:913–922, 1974.

5. **b** Tendon of the long head of the biceps. The indicated structure is situated along the anteromedial humerus. The crosssectional shape of the humerus localizes this axial image to the proximal shaft. The overlying deltoid muscle is marked by the *black box.*

   The structure in question lies in a groove along the humerus (the bicipital groove). Hence, this structure must be the tendon of the long head of the biceps brachii. The low T1 signal intensity of this structure is consistent with its tendinous composition. Note the pectoralis minor muscle (marked by the *hollow white arrow*) and the axillary artery (marked by the *solid white arrow*). Components of the brachial plexus are evident surrounding the axillary artery. The *asterisk* marks the short head of the biceps brachii and the coracobrachialis (the two appear as a single mass on this cross section). The large muscle mass directly posterior to the short head of the biceps brachii and the axillary artery (between the chest wall and the scapula) is the latissimus dorsi.

Note: The sequence of structures that attach to the coracoid process (from medial to lateral) is as follows: (1) pectoralis minor, (2) coracobrachialis, and (3) short head of the biceps brachii.

6. **a** Transient ulnar nerve dysfunction. The most common complication of nonconstrained total elbow arthroplasty in Ewald and Jacob's series (50 patients with rheumatoid arthritis) was transient ulnar nerve palsy. The incidence of transient ulnar nerve dysfunction was 14%. The operations were performed through a lateral approach (without anterior transposition of the ulnar nerve). Potential explanations for this problem include mechanical trauma (traction or compression), vascular disruption, and underlying peripheral neuropathy. Permanent ulnar nerve dysfunction occurred in 4% of the patients in the same series. The incidence of deep wound infection was 2%.

   The dislocation rate in Ewald and Jacob's series was 7%. Dislocation is relatively common after placement of a nonconstrained prosthesis. However, instability typically occurs in a *posterior* direction. Premature loosening has not been a significant problem in nonconstrained total elbow designs.

Reference

Ewald FC, Jacobs MA: Total Elbow Arthroplasty. Clin Orthop, 182:137–142, 1984.

7. **c** Secondary glenohumeral arthrosis can be successfully relieved by an anterior release technique. The *Putti-Platt procedure* is an imbrication of the anterior capsule and subscapularis tendon. Excessive tightening of these structures during the Putti-Platt procedure has been implicated as a source of subsequent glenohumeral arthrosis.

   The *Weber subcapital osteotomy* was designed to rotate large HillSachs lesions posterolaterally by increasing humeral head retroversion so such defects do not contact the glenoid articular surface during functional range of motion.

   The *Bristow procedure* involves transfer of a portion of the coracoid process to the anterior glenoid rim. The transferred coracobrachialis and short head of the biceps theoretically serve as dynamic stabilizers to hold the humeral head posteriorly, and the transferred portion of coracoid provides a static bone block effect.

   Injury to the musculocutaneous nerve is an infrequent complication of the Putti-Platt procedure. Musculocutaneous nerve damage is more common after the Bristow procedure because of potential tethering of the nerve by the transferred soft tissues. Both the Putti-Platt and the Bristow procedures can produce internal rotation contractures.

   Glenohumeral osteoarthrosis in the setting of a prior Putti-Platt procedure is associated with a substantially compromised range of shoulder motion. Hawkins and Angelo reported successful management of this condition through an anterior release technique.

Reference

Hawkins R, Angelo R: Glenohumeral Osteoarthrosis: A Late Complication of the Putti-Platt Repair. J Bone Joint Surg Am, 72:1193–1197, 1990.

8. **b** 2:1. The overall ratio of glenohumeral to scapulothoracic motion from zero degrees to full abduction is approximately 2:1 (although the precise ratio varies slightly among the various studies).

   Note: During the initial 30 degrees of abduction, scapulothoracic motion is minimal.

Reference

Freedman L, et al.: Abduction of the Arm in the Scapular Plane: Scapular and Glenohumeral Movements. J Bone Joint Surg Am, 48:1503, 1966.
Inman VT et al.: Observations on the Function of the Shoulder Joint. J Bone Joint Surg, 26:1–30, 1944.

9. **a** The suprascapular artery. The *Judet approach* permits broad posterior exposure of the posterior scapula. The infraspinatus, teres minor, and teres major are mobilized from the infraspinatus fossa and are reflected laterally, preserving the suprascapular neurovascular pedicle as well as the circumflex scapular artery. The posteromedial edge of the deltoid is released from the scapular spine to gain adequate visualization of the glenoid neck and lateral scapular margin. The Judet exposure is useful for open reduction and internal fixation of fractures of the scapular body, acromion, glenoid neck, and scapular spine.

Reference

Von Torklus D, Nicola T: Atlas of Orthopaedic Exposures. New York, Urban & Schwarzenburg, 1986.

10. **e** The suprascapular artery. The absence of the humerus and the presence of the scapular spine localize

this axial image to the apical aspect of the scapula. The *asterisk* marks the supraspinatus muscle. The *arrow* marks the suprascapular artery as it passes beneath the supraspinatus with the suprascupular nerve. This artery perfuses the supraspinatus and the infraspinatus muscles. The infraspinatus (marked by the *black box*) can be seen posterior to the scapula and deep to the deltoid (marked by the letter *C*).

The acromial branch of the thoracoacromial trunk would be found in a more anterior and lateral location at the level of this cross section. The dorsal scapular artery runs vertically along the medial border of the scapula. The circumflex scapular artery is a branch of the subscapular artery that loops around the inferolateral margin of the scapula. Neither it nor the thoracodorsal artery is present above the level of the humeral head.

11. **a** The lower subscapular nerve. The teres major is innervated by the lower subscapular nerve. The upper subscapular nerve innervates the subscapularis. The *thoracodorsal nerve* (middle subscapular nerve) innervates the latissimus dorsi. The teres minor is innervated by the *axillary nerve.* The *dorsal scapular nerve* (a branch of the C5 root) innervates the rhomboids.
12. **d** Activity modification and physical therapy focusing on strengthening of the rotator cuff and periscapular muscles. This is a case of suprascapular neuropathy. This entity is sometimes caused by the compressive effects of a specific mass lesion (such as a ganglion). Alternative causes include macrotrauma or repetitive microtrauma. Recurrent overhead shoulder motion can subject the nerve to repetitive traction that can produce suprascapular neuropraxia.

    Focal electromyographic alterations in the suprascapular nerve distribution (supraspinatus and infraspinatus) are diagnostic. Magnetic resonance imaging is useful for detecting specific sources of compression (mass lesions).

    Treatment depends on the underlying problem. If a specific compressive lesion is responsible for the neuropathy, then surgical decompression is indicated. Conversely, if the magnetic resonance imaging scan fails to demonstrate a mass lesion, then nonoperative treatment should be pursued. Most patients will respond favorably to nonoperative treatment. If nonoperative treatment fails in this setting, then surgical release of the suprascapular ligament may be considered.

    In a retrospective study by Martin et al., 12 of the 15 patients who were initially treated nonoperatively had good to excellent results. The remaining three patients experienced persistent symptoms and required operative treatment.

Reference

Martin SD, Warren RF, et al.: Suprascapular Neuropathy: Results of Nonoperative Treatment. J Bone Joint Surg Am, 79:1159–1165, 1997.

13. **e** The extensor carpi radialis brevis. The situation describes a characteristic presentation of chronic lateral humeral epicondylitis. This disease affects the common extensor tendon. Chronic lateral epicondylitis can produce partial discontinuity of the common extensor origin (as depicted in Fig. 2.4). Muscles that originate from the common extensor tendon include the extensor carpi radialis brevis (which is the principal site affected by lateral epicondylitis), the extensor digitorum communis, the extensor indicis, the extensor digiti minimi, and the extensor carpi ulnaris. The extensor carpi ulnaris originates most ulnarly from the common extensor tendon and is not characteristically involved in this disease. The extensor carpi radialis longus and brachioradialis originate proximally to the common extensor tendon (on the lateral supracondylar ridge), and the extensor pollicis longus originates distally to the elbow (from the ulna and the interosseus membrane).

    Although lateral epicondylitis is characteristically associated with tennis *(tennis elbow),* it can be associated with many other activities that apply repetitive stress across the extensor origin (such as golf, throwing, batting, or occupational tasks that require recurrent extreme forearm pronation and wrist flexion).

    Note: The extensor carpi radialis brevis was ruptured in 35% of the surgical specimens reported by Nirschl and Pettrone.

Reference

Nirschl RP, Pettrone FA: Tennis Elbow: The Surgical Treatment of Lateral Epicondylitis. J Bone Joint Surg Am, 61:832–839, 1979.

14. **c** Angiofibroblastic hyperplasia. Nirschl and Pettrone described the characteristic appearance of specimen retrieved from surgically treated cases of lateral epicondylitis. The excised tissue manifests an invasion of fibroblasts and vascular tissue. This granulation-like tissue lacks a significant acute or chronic inflammatory component. Nirschl coined the term *angiofibroblastic hyperplasia* to describe this characteristic finding.

Reference

Nirschl RP, Pettrone FA: Tennis Elbow: The Surgical Treatment of Lateral Epicondylitis. J Bone Joint Surg Am, 61:832–839, 1979.

15. **c** 14 cm. Operative exposure of the posterior humeral diaphysis requires precise understanding of the course of

the radial nerve. This course has been described with specific reference to its position relative to the epicondyles. The radial nerve crosses the posterior aspect of the humerus (from medial to lateral) between the medial and lateral heads of the triceps. This traverse begins 20.7±1.2 cm proximal to the medial epicondyle and ends 14.2±0.6 cm proximal to the lateral epicondyle.

Note: As it crosses the humerus, the radial nerve yields many branches to the lateral head of the triceps. However, the nerve typically gives off no branches to the medial head of the triceps until it has finished crossing the humerus. Thus, the nerve may be safely mobilized proximally and laterally to facilitate exposure of this region of the posterior humeral diaphysis.

Reference

Gerwin M, Hotchkiss R, Weiland A: Alternative operative exposures of the posterior aspect of the humeral diaphysis. J Bone Joint Surg Am, 78:1690–1695, 1996.

16. **b** The nerve was most likely contused or stretched during the reduction, but recovery of nerve function is likely even without surgical intervention. The prognosis for radial nerve palsy that occurs at the time of a humeral shaft fracture is good. If it is treated nonoperatively, the most (approximately 90%) of these deficits will ultimately resolve.

The onset of radial nerve palsy after closed reduction of a humeral shaft fracture has often been considered an indication for nerve exploration and open reudction and internal fixation of the fracture. However, surgical intervention has not definitively been shown to improve the ultimate overall recovery rate in this setting. In fact, Bostman et al. documented that early surgical exploration did not have a favorable effect on the recovery rate for either primary or secondary radial nerve palsies.

Recovery rates do not differ for early exploration versus those lesions that ultimately require delayed exploration. Early exploration may subject a contused nerve to an unnecessary risk of iatrogenic injury.

Note: Radial nerve laceration and entrapment are more commonly associated with spiral fractures of the distal third of the humerus (Holstein-Lewis fractures) than with transverse diaphyseal fractures. Most radial palsies associated with transverse diaphyseal fractures are the result of neuropraxia.

Reference

Bostman O, et al.: Radial Palsy in Shaft Fracture of the Humerus. Acta Orthop Scand, 57:316–319, 1986.

17. **b** Middle third. Fractures of the middle third of the clavicle account for approximately 80% of clavicle fractures.

Reference

Rockwood CA, Green DP, eds: Fractures in Adults, 4th Ed. Philadelphia, Lippincott–Raven, 1996.

18. **d** Type IIA fracture of the distal third (medial to the coracoclavicular ligaments). *Type II* fractures of the distal third of the clavicle are associated with a higher incidence of nonunion than the other types of distal clavicular fractures. This fracture subtype is associated with significant displacement. The proximal segment is displaced cephalad by the deforming action of the sternocleidomastoid, and the weight of the upper extremity is transmitted to the distal segment through the intact coracoclavicular ligaments.

Type I fractures of the distal third are minimally displaced because of the stabilizing effect of the intact acromioclavicular and coracoclavicular ligaments. Likewise, *type III* fractures of the distal third are associated with minimal displacement and no ligamentous disruption.

Regional differences in the cross-sectional anatomy of the clavicle are often invoked to account for the relative infrequency of nonunions of the medial third. This region of the clavicle is relatively broad with abundant cancellous bone. The middle third (which is narrowed and tubular) and the distal third (which is flattened) are more intrinsically prone to nonunion because of the relative paucity of cancellous medullary bone in these regions (Fig. 2.13).

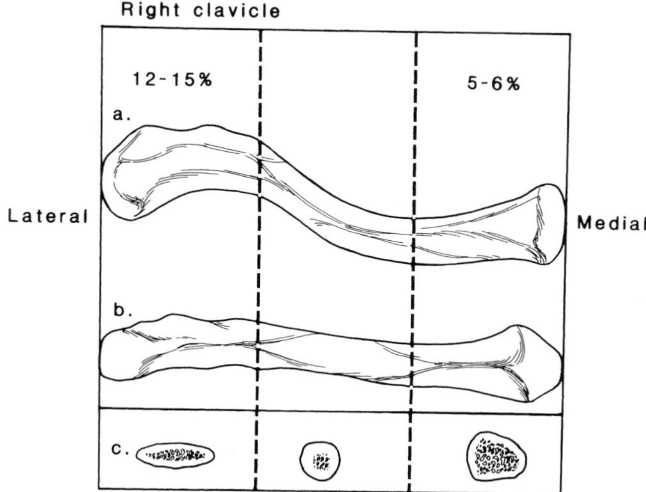

FIGURE 2.13

Note: the coracoclavicular ligaments remain linked to the proximal fragment in type I and type III fractures of the distal third, whereas they remain linked to the distal fragment in type II fractures.

Reference

Neer CS: Nonunion of the Clavicle. JAMA, 172:1006–1011, 1960.
Neer CS: Fractures of the Distal Third of the Clavicle. Clin Orthop, 58:43–50, 1968.
Simpson NS, Jupiter JB: Clavicular Nonunion and Malunion. J Am Acad Orthop Surg, 4:1–8, 1996.

19. **b** The mesoacromion and metaacromion. Four ossification centers contribute to the development of the acromion (Fig. 2.14). Failure of fusion between adjacent ossification centers produces an *os acromiale.* This most often occurs at the junction of the mesoacromion and metaacromion. The best plain radiographic view for demonstrating this unfused apophysis is the axillary view.

Os acromiale is clinically significant for two reasons: (1) the unfused physis may simulate a fracture and (2) it has been associated with rotator cuff disorders. Smooth, rounded contours and bilaterality help to distinguish an incidental os acromiale from a fractured acromion.

Note: The incidence of os acromiale is 2.7% of the general population. The incidence of bilateral os acromiale is 62%.

Reference

Liberson F: Os Acromiale: A Contested Anomaly. J Bone Joint Surg, 19:683–689, 1937.

20. **c** Neutral version. In an uncomplicated total shoulder arthroplasty, the humeral component should be placed in approximately 30 to 40 degrees of retroversion. The corresponds to the anatomic retroversion of the humerus. A useful landmark is the bicipital groove, which should be situated just anterior to the fin on the humeral component.

When there is instability and/or uneven wear of the native glenoid, then the version of the humeral component may be adjusted to increase stability. For cases of chronic posterior dislocation and/or excessive wear of the posterior glenoid, the component should be anteverted approximately 30 degrees more than usual (in other words, approximately neutral version). Conversely, for cases of chronic anterior dislocation (or excessive anterior glenoid wear), the humeral component should be placed in more retroversion than usual.

Reference

Azar FM, Wright PE: Arthroplasty of the Shoulder and Elbow. In Campbell's Operative Orthopaedics, 9th Ed. Mosby, St. Louis, MO, pp. 486–487, 1997.

21. **e** A 3.5-mm reconstruction plate placed posteriorly on the lateral column and a one-third tubular plate placed directly medially. Double plating provides greater rigidity than crossed screws or a single Y plate. The 90-degree offset construct (one plate directly medially and one plate posterolaterally) provides optimal stability. There is no significant difference between the 3.5-mm reconstruction plate and the one-third tubular plate when they are applied in the 90-degree offset configuration.

Reference

Helfet DL, Hotchkiss RN: Internal Fixation of the Distal Humerus: A Biomechanical Comparison of Methods. J Orthop Trauma, 4:260–264, 1990.

22. **e** None. The radiograph demonstrates a type III separation of the acromioclavicular joint (torn acromioclavicular ligaments and coracoclavicular ligaments with inferior acromioclavicular dislocation). Surgical intervention for this type of acromioclavicular separation remains controversial. Early surgical repair of this lesion has yet to be definitively proven to improve ultimate strength or decrease the incidence of acromioclavicular joint arthritis in any patient population.

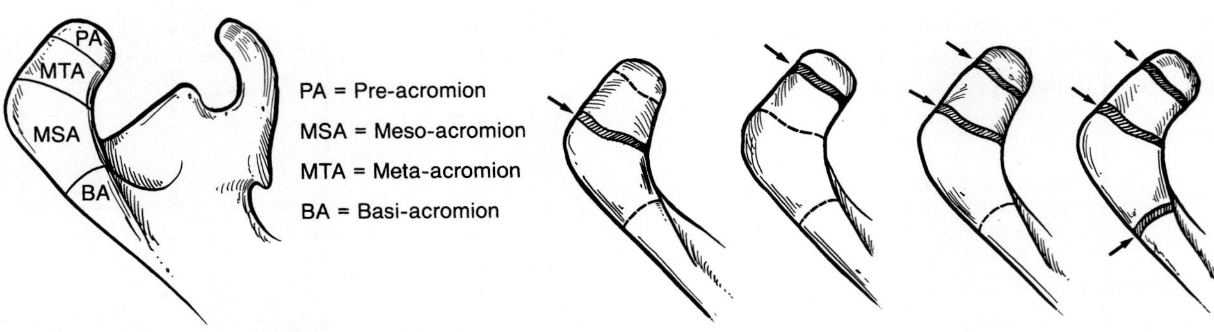

FIGURE 2.14A and B

Recommended treatments for other types of acromioclavicular separations are less controversial. Nonoperative management is recommended for types I and II, and surgical treatment is generally indicated for types IV to VI (Fig. 2.15).

References

Taft TN, et al.: Dislocation of the Acromioclavicular Joint: An End-Result Study. J Bone Joint Surg Am, 69:1045–1051, 1987.

Tibone J, et al.: Strength Testing After Third Degree Acromioclavicular Dislocations. Am J Sports Med, 20:328–331, 1992.

23. **a** Anterior glenohumeral dislocation. Figure 2.6 is a scapular Y view. To obtain this image, the x-ray beam is directed parallel to the plane of the scapular body. The projections of three structures (scapular body, scapular spine, and acromial process) form the Y. The projection of the glenoid is located at the convergence of these three structures. Under normal circumstances, the humeral head should be superimposed on the glenoid on this image. In Fig. 2.6, the humeral head is anterior to the glenoid (closer to the thorax).

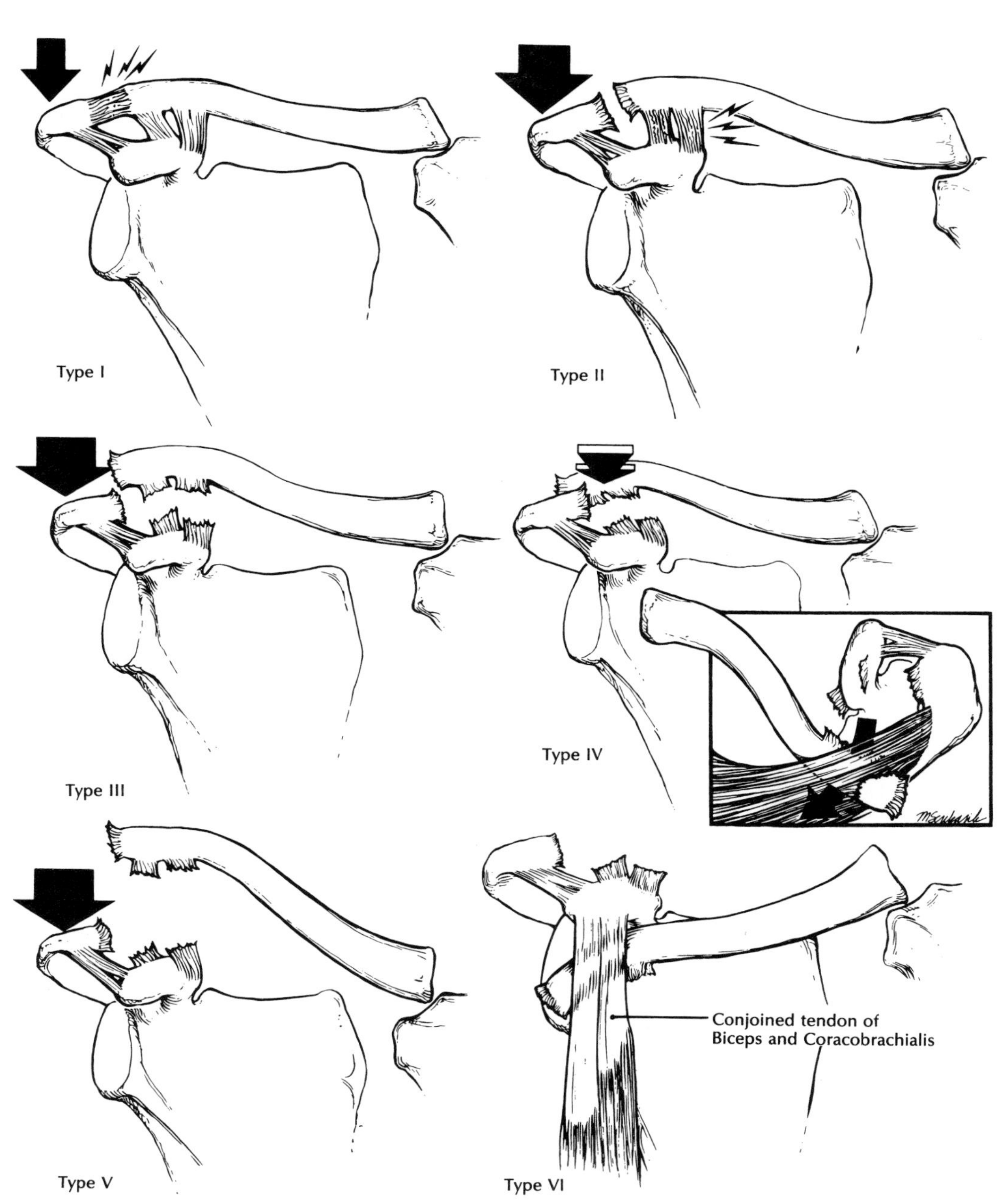

FIGURE 2.15

Luxatio erecta refers to a subglenoid dislocation of the humeral head in which the humerus is locked in extreme abduction with the elbow above the level of the humeral head. The humeral shaft in Fig. 2.6 is not abducted to that extent.

Scapulothoracic dissociation has been referred to as a *closed forequarter amputation.* The precipitating violent trauma produces avulsions of the periscapular muscles and lateral scapular displacement. This condition is associated with a high incidence of injury to the subclavian vessels and the brachial plexus. Although scapulothoracic dissociation may be associated with dislocations of the the glenohumeral joint (as well as the sternoclavicular or acromioclavicular joints), the diagnosis cannot be inferred from this film. Furthermore, the described low-energy mechanism of injury would be incapable of causing scapulothoracic dissociation.

Reference

Ebraheim: Scapulothoracic Dissociation. J Bone Joint Surg Am, 70:428–432, 1988.

24. **b** Rhematoid arthritis with ipsilateral elbow disease. Shortstemmed humeral components are useful in patients with polyarticular disease (e.g., rheumatoid arthritis) that has affected the ipsilateral elbow. If ipsilateral elbow replacement is contemplated for the future, then a short-stemmed humeral component should be employed at the shoulder to prevent abutment with the humeral component of the future elbow prosthesis. Stem tips in close proximity can create a significant stress riser and can lead to periprosthetic fracture.

Reference

Kraay MJ, Figgie MP. In Sculco TP, ed: Surgical Treatment of Rheumatoid Arthritis. St Louis, CV Mosby, p. 133, 1992.

25. **e** The spinal accessory nerve. The trapezius is innervated by the spinal accessory nerve (cranial nerve XI).
26. **b** Internal impingement. Although arthroscopic subacromial decompression is generally efficacious, the procedure is less successful in young throwing athletes who present with signs and symptoms of impingement. In this younger population, impingement symptoms are commonly produced by underlying glenohumeral instability. In young throwing athletes, subtle anterior instability can lead to abutment of the posterior superior undersurface of the rotator cuff on the posterior superior glenoid labrum during abduction and maximal external rotation (i.e., during cocking and early acceleration). This phenomenon is referred to *internal impingement.*

    Internal impingement has been associated with increased passive external rotation and partial tears involving the undersurface of the supraspinatus and infraspinatus. Internal impingement can be misconstrued as simple impingement syndrome.

Reference

Jobe CM, et al.: Theories and Concepts. In Jobe FW, et al., eds: Operative Techniques in Upper Extremity Sports Injuries. St Louis, Mosby-Year Book, 1996.

27. **d** Subscapularis tendon rupture. A positive *liftoff test* (inability to lift one's palm off the small of one's back) is diagnostic of subscapularis insufficiency. In a patient who recently has undergone open anterior capsulorrhaphy, rupture of the subscapularis tendon repair is the probable cause. The upper subscapular nerve is not in close proximity to the subscapularis tendon, and hence denervation of the subscapularis is highly unlikely during the procedure.

Reference

Gerber C, Krushell: Isolated Rupture of the Tendon of the Subscapularis Muscle. J Bone Joint Surg Br, 73:389–394, 1991.

28. **b** Radial nerve and profunda brachii artery. The radial nerve and profunda brachii artery pass through the triangular interval. The boundaries of this interval are the teres major (superiorly), the long head of the triceps (medially), and the humerus (laterally). The triangular *interval* should not be confused with the triangular space, through which passes the circumflex scapular artery (Fig. 2.16).
29. **c** Approximately 7 degrees of retroversion. Although there is marked individual variation, the normal glenoid is retroverted approximately 7 degrees relative to the plane of the scapula. The scapular plane itself is anteverted approximately 30 degrees relative to the coronal plane of the thorax.

    The normal humeral head is retroverted 20 to 30 degrees relative to the transepicondylar axis of the distal humerus. The neckshaft angle of the proximal humerus is approximately 130 to 150 degrees.

References

Pagnani MJ, Warren RF: Sports Med Arthrosc Rev, 1(3):177–189, 1993.
Saha AK: Dynamic Stabilizers of the Glenohumeral Joint. Acta Orthop Scand, 42:491–505, 1971.

30. **e** Full-thickness rotator cuff tear. The image in Fig. 2.7 reveals a fullthickness defect in the supraspinatus tendon. The defect is visible directly cephalad to the humeral head. The proximal tendon is partially retracted. This T2 image clearly demonstrates continuity between the glenohumeral joint and fluid in the subacromial space.

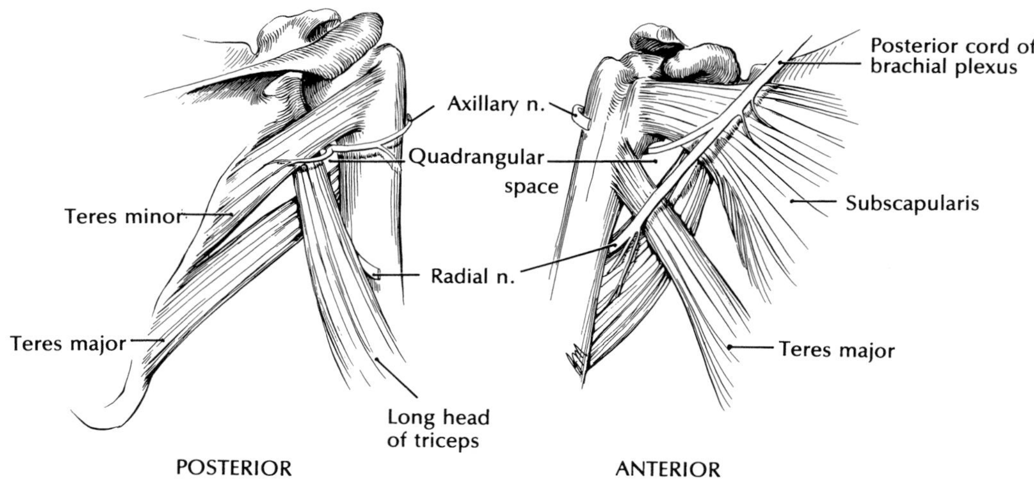

FIGURE 2.16

31. **c** The superior glenohumeral ligament. The superior shoulder suspensory complex consists of a bone–soft tissue ring perched at the end of two bony struts. The ring is composed of the distal clavicle, the acromioclavicular ligaments, the acromion, the superior glenoid, the coracoid, and the coracoclavicular ligaments. The two bony struts are the clavicle and the scapular body.

The concept of the superior shoulder suspensory complex helps to define the linkage between the upper extremity and the torso. The concept also aids in determining stability of injuries of the shoulder girdle. Single disruptions of the superior shoulder suspensory complex are typically stable, whereas double disruptions are generally unstable.

Note: The coracoclavicular ligaments are composed of two principal components: the trapezoid ligament (laterally) and the conoid ligament (medially).

Reference

Goss TP: Double Disruptions of the Superior Shoulder Suspensory Complex. J Orthop Trauma, 7:99–106, 1993.

32. **b** The superior glenohumeral ligament. The capsular ligaments of the shoulder have been well defined. There are three primary glenohumeral ligaments: (1) the superior glenohumeral ligament, (2) the middle glenohumeral ligament, and (3) the inferior glenohumeral ligament complex, which, in turn, is composed of an anterior portion, a posterior portion, and an axillary pouch. The stabilizing role of the individual ligaments depends on the position of the humerus with respect to the glenoid. Sectioning studies have demonstrated that the superior glenohumeral ligament is the principal restraint to inferior translation of the humerus when the arm is adducted. The inferior glenohumeral ligament complex is the principal restraint to anterior, posterior, and inferior translation when the arm is abducted. The middle glenohumeral ligament is a highly variable structure and may be totally absent in certain individuals. The middle glenohumeral ligament limits anterior translation in the midrange of abduction and is regarded as a secondary restraint.

Reference

Warner JJ, Deng, XH, Warren, RF, et al.: Static Capsuloligamentous Restraints to Superior-Inferior Translation of the Glenohumeral Joint. Am J Sports Med, 20:675–685, 1992.

33. **d** Metacarpophalangeal extension. Erb's point describes the site where the C5 and C6 nerve roots merge to form the superior trunk of the brachial plexus. Transection at Erb's point produces a characteristic "waiter's tip" deformity resulting from loss activities mediated by the C5 and C6 roots (shoulder abduction, forearm supination, elbow flexion, shoulder external rotation, and wrist extension). Metacarpophalangeal joint extension is mediated by the C7 root. Although traction injuries to the upper brachial plexus may also affect the C7 root, metacarpophalangeal extension should be preserved if brachial plexus damage does not extend beyond Erb's point.

Note: The suprascapular nerve arises from the superior trunk of the brachial plexus after the C5 and C6 roots merge.

34. **e** Musculocutaneous and radial nerves. The labeled muscle is the brachialis. Its identity is unmistakable based on (1) its course directly anterior to the distal humeral shaft and (2) its insertion on the ulna immediately distal to the

tip of the coronoid process. The brachialis has a dual innervation (musculocutaneous and radial nerves).

35. **b** A 16-year-old gymnast who has dislocated her dominant shoulder twice. Her first dislocation occurred when she fell off a horse 5 weeks ago. A magnetic resonance imaging scan reveals a Bankart lesion.

Open shoulder stabilization is considered the current standard for the treatment of anterior shoulder instability. The utility of arthroscopic shoulder stabilization is controversial because of an associated higher rate of recurrence (approximately 20% versus 5%).

However, arthroscopic stabilization may be considered for selected patients. The optimal patient is one with recurrent, unidirectional instability and a traumatic cause of the disorder in association with a Bankart lesion and a robust anterior band of the inferior glenohumeral ligament.

Patients with multidirectional instability, generalized ligamentous laxity, a history of multiple dislocations, and no Bankart lesion are less amenable to arthroscopic intervention. These factors compromise the quality of tissue available for arthroscopic repair.

Note: Modalities currently under development (i.e., thermal capsular shrinkage) may redefine the indications for arthroscopic stabilization.

Reference

Peterson CA, Altchek DW, Warren RF: Arthroscopic Management of Shoulder Instability. In Rockwood , Matsen FA, eds: The Shoulder, 2nd Ed. Philadelphia, WB Saunders, 1998.

36. **d** The posterior interosseous and radial nerves. The posterolateral (Kocher) approach to the elbow exploits the interval between the extensor carpi ulnaris (posterior interosseous nerve) and the anconeus (radial nerve). Applications of this approach include open reduction and internal fixation and excision of the radial head. During this exposure, the posterior interosseous nerve is vulnerable at the level of the radial neck. Pronation of the forearm will protect the posterior interosseous nerve by mobilizing it medially (away from the incision).

References

Strachan J: Vulnerability of the Posterior Interosseous Nerve During Radial Head Excision. J Bone Joint Surg Br, 53:320, 1971.

37. **a** Neutral rotation. The *safe zone* refers to the region of the radial head that does not impinge on the proximal radioulnar joint during a full arc of pronation and supination. Hardware can be safely positioned within this region without compromising motion. This zone measures approximately 100 degrees and is centered over the coronal equator of the radial head when the forearm is held in neutral rotation.

Reference

Hotchkiss RN: Displaced Fractures of the Radial Head. J Am Acad Orthop Surg, 5(1):1–10, 1997.

38. **c** The anterior component of the medial collateral ligament. The anterior bundle of the medial collateral ligament is the primary restraint to valgus instability of the elbow. The radial head is of secondary significance. Radial head excision alone does not produce pathologic valgus laxity. Replacement of the radial head with an implant will not restore elbow stability in the absence of a functional anterior band of the medial collateral ligament.

Reference

Morrey BF, et al.: Valgus Stability of the Elbow: A Definition of Primary and Secondary Constraints. Clin Orthop, 265:187–195, 1991

39. **e** The flexor carpi radialis demonstrates decreased activity versus uninjured pitchers. Electromyographic investigations of the dynamic stabilizers of the elbow in competitive baseball pitchers have been performed at the Kerlan-Jobe Clinic. These studies have documented an asynchronous pattern of muscle action among patients with dysfunctional medial collateral ligaments. During late cocking and early acceleration, the extensor carpi radialis brevis and extensor carpi radialis longus demonstrated *increased* activity compared with uninjured pitchers; the triceps, flexor carpi radialis, and pronator teres demonstrated *decreased* activity compared with uninjured pitchers.

These findings do not represent an adaptive response. If the flexor carpi radialis and pronator teres were compensating for a deficient medial collateral ligament, then increased activity in these muscles would be anticipated. The presence of decreased activity in these muscles may predispose the insufficient medial collateral ligament to further injury.

Reference

Glousman RE, et al.: An Electromyographic Analysis of the Elbow in Normal and Injured Pitchers with Medial Collateral Ligament Insufficiency. Am J Sports Med, 20(3):311–317, 1992.

40. **d** The nerve supply to the latissimus dorsi is the thoracodorsal nerve.
41. **c** The nerve supply to the rhomboids is the dorsal scapular nerve.
42. **d** External rotation with the arm adducted. Patients with regional shoulder capsule contractures may present with limitation of motion in specific planes depending on which portion of the capsule is involved. Contracture of the anterosuperior capsule (superior and middle glenohumeral ligaments) will result in lim-

itation of external rotation with the arm in adduction. Contracture of the anteroinferior capsule (the anterior band of the inferior glenohumeral ligament) will limit external rotation with the arm in abduction.

Note: The rotator interval is the capsular region defined by the gap between the anterior border of the supraspinatus and the superior border of the subscapularis.

Reference

O'Connell, et al.: The Contribution of the Glenohumeral Ligaments to Anterior Stability of the Shoulder Joint. Am J Sports Med, 8:579, 1991.

43. **c** Syringomyelia. Each of the listed diseases has been associated with neuropathic osteoarthropathy. Diabetes mellitus is the most common cause of neuropathic joints in general (affecting approximately 5% to 10% of patients with diabetes). However, diabetic neuropathy predominantly affects the lower extremities (most commonly the midfoot). Syringomyelia is the most common cause of neuropathic arthropathy of the shoulder and the upper extremity in general.

Note: Approximately 25% of patients with syringomyelia develop neuropathic osteoarthropathy of the upper extremity.

Reference

Alpert et al.: Neuropathic Arthropathy. J Am Acad Orthop Surg, 4(2): 100–108, 1996.

44. **e** More than 40%. Rowe and Sakellarides found that the age of the patient at the time of primary dislocation was the most significant determinant of the incidence of recurrence. They reported a 100% recurrence rate for patients less than 10 years old, a 94% recurrence rate for patients 11 to 20 years old, a 79% recurrence rate for patients 21 to 30 years old, a 50% recurrence rate for patients 31 to 40 years old, and a progressively decreasing incidence with increasing age.

Simonet and Cofield reported a 66% incidence of recurrence in patients less than 20 years old, a 40% incidence of recurrence in patients 20 to 40 years old, and no dislocations in patients older than 40 years.

Hovelius reported a 55% incidence of recurrence in patients less than 22 years old, a 37% incidence of recurrence in patients 23 to 29 years old, and a 12% incidence of recurrence in patients 30 to 40 years old.

References

Hovelius L: Anterior Dislocation of the Shoulder in Teenagers and Young Adults: Five Year Prognosis. J Bone Joint Surg Am, 69:393–396, 1987.
Rowe CR, Sakellarides HT: Factors Related to Recurrences of Anterior Dislocation of the Shoulder. Clin Orthop, 20:40, 1961.
Simonet WT, Cofield RH: Prognosis in Anterior Shoulder Dislocation. Am J Sports Med, 12:19–24, 1984.

45. **c** Initiation of physical therapy within 2 weeks of injury. In a study that evaluated the functional outcome of minimally displaced fractures of the proximal humerus, patients who started supervised physical therapy less than 14 days after the injury had significantly better results than patients who began therapy after 14 days; 42% of the 104 fractures were of the surgical neck, 30% were of the greater tuberosity, and 28% had multiple fracture lines. Results were not influenced by the age of the patient, the location of the fracture, the duration of sling use, dominance of the shoulder, or displacement of the greater tuberosity. Preexisting rotator cuff disease had an adverse effect on outcome.

Reference

Koval, et al.: Functional Outcome After Minimally Displaced Fractures of the Proximal Humerus. J Bone Joint Surg Am, 79:203–207,1997.

46. **d** The sternoclavicular capsular ligament. A cadaveric biomechanical model has demonstrated that the sternoclavicular capsular ligament alone can prevent drooping of the medial clavicle. Secondary stabilizers of the sternoclavicular joint include the intraarticular disc ligament, the costoclavicular ligament, and the first costal cartilage. After sectioning the sternoclavicular capsular ligament, the remaining stabilizers of the sternoclavicular joint were incapable of maintaining suspension of the clavicle. However, division of all the secondary stabilizers did not compromise the ability of the intact sternoclavicular capsular ligament to suspend the lateral clavicle.

Note: The clavicle suspends the scapula through the intact coracoclavicular ligaments. These ligaments do *not* suspend the lateral clavicle.

Reference

Bearn JG: Direct Observations on the Function of the Sternoclavicular Joint in Clavicular Support. J Anat, 101:159–170, 1967.

47. **e** The long head of the biceps. The *short* head of the biceps attaches to the coracoid process, but the long head attaches to the superior glenoid. The conjoined tendon consists of the biceps short head and the coracobrachialis. The pectoralis minor tendon, the coracohumeral ligament, and the coracoclavicular ligaments (trapezoid and conoid) also attach to the coracoid process.
48. **b** Acute closed reduction under general anesthesia followed by a figure-of-eight strap for 6 weeks. Acute posterior sternoclavicular dislocations should uniformly be reduced in skeletally mature patients. Even if an adult manifests no acute signs or symptoms of mediastinal compression, failure to reduce the posteriorly dislocated clavicle is associated with a significant incidence of late complications.

Optimal management consists of closed reduction followed by 4 to 6 weeks of immobilization in a figureofeight strap. Closed reduction becomes increasingly difficult with increased time elapsed from injury. Most posterior dislocations are stable after successful closed reduction. If delayed surgical intervention is required, the most appropriate form of intervention appears to be medial clavicular resection with costoclavicular ligament reconstruction.

Stabilization of the sternoclavicular joint with Steinmann pins or Kirschner wires is fraught with complications related to pin migration (including death).

Note: In contrast to posterior dislocations, most anterior dislocations are unstable. However, aside from minor cosmetic compromise, chronic anterior instability is associated with negligible adverse sequelae. Standard management of anterior dislocations is nonoperative, with "benign neglect" of residual instability if it arises. Operative stabilization should be undertaken with significant trepidation.

Reference

Wirth MA, Rockwood CA: Acute and Chronic Traumatic Injuries of the Sternoclavicular Joint. J Am Acad Orthop Surg, 4(5):268–278, 1996.

49. **c** Approximately 30%. The prevalence of rotator cuff tears (partial plus complete) detected by magnetic resonance imaging in asymptomatic volunteers was reported by Sher et al. The prevalence is highly dependent on age. In patients more than 60 years of age, the prevalence rises to more than 50% (Table 2.1).

Reference

Sher JS, et al.: Abnormal Findings on Magnetic Resonance Images of Asymptomatic Shoulders. J Bone Joint Surg Am, 77:10–15, 1995.

50. **b** The T2 dermatome. An interscalene block anesthetizes the brachial plexus (C5 to T1). However, skin at the standard posterior arthroscopy portal lies within the distribution of the T2 dermatome. Thus, the posterior portal incision site should be infiltrated with supplemental local anesthetic.

Note: Interscalene regional anesthesia is also noted for providing a suboptimal or unpredictable block of the most distal components of the plexus (specifically, the ulnar nerve distribution).

TABLE 2.1. PREVALENCE OF ROTATOR CUFF TEARS

Patient Age	Partial Tears	Complete Tears
<40 yr	4%	0%
40–60 yr	24%	4%
>60 yr	26%	28%

Reference

Ready LB: Anesthesia for Shoulder Procedures. In Rockwood CA, Matsen FA, eds: The Shoulder, 2nd Ed. Philadelphia, WB Saunders, 1998.

51. **c** Axial compression and valgus stress with the forearm in full supination. The lateral pivot shift test was described by O'Driscoll et al. to detect posterolateral rotary instability. The test is performed with the patient supine. A combination of axial load and valgus stress is applied to the elbow with the forearm in full supination. This maneuver attempts to provoke subluxation of the radial head and ulna from their proper alignment with the distal humeral articular surface. Subluxation of the radial head can be visualized as a prominence at the posterolateral elbow. As the forearm is brought from a position of extension to flexion, a palpable or visible spontaneous reduction is typically appreciated at approximately 30 to 60 degrees of flexion.

Note: This test may evoke apprehension rather than subluxation when it is performed on a nonanesthetized patient.

Reference

O'Driscoll SW, Bell DF, Morrey BF: Posterolateral Rotatory Instability of the Elbow. J Bone Joint Surg Am, 73:440–446, 1991.

52. **a** The lateral ulnar collateral ligament. Insufficiency of the lateral ulnar collateral ligament is the essential lesion. An incompetent lateral ulnar collateral ligament allows the radial side of the ulnar articular surface to rotate away from the humerus as the radial head subluxates posterolaterally. Surgical intervention for posterolateral rotary instability focuses upon reconstruction of the lateral ulnar collateral ligament.

Note: The lateral ulnar collateral ligament must be distinguished from the ulnar collateral ligament (also known as medial collateral ligament). Insufficiency of the ulnar collateral ligament produces valgus instability (medial elbow gapping to valgus stress). In posterolateral rotary instability, the ulnar collateral ligament remains intact and serves as a hinge. Posterolateral rotary instability may be misconstrued as ulnar collateral ligament insufficiency by the nonastute clinician. Combined ulnar collateral ligament and lateral ulnar collateral ligament insufficiency is also possible.

Reference

Nestor BJ, O'Driscoll SW, Morrey BF: Ligamentous Reconstruction for Posterolateral Rotatory Instability of the Elbow. J Bone Joint Surg Am, 74:1235–1241, 1992.

53. **e** Arthroscopic acromioplasty only. The *Buford complex* is a normal anatomic variant. It consists of a robust middle glenohumeral ligament in association with a recess adjacent to the anterosuperior labrum. The Buford complex must not be mistaken for a Bankart lesion or a labral tear. No intervention is indicated for this incidental finding.

Reference

Williams MM, Snyder SJ, Buford D: The Buford Complex. J Arthrosc, 10: 241–247, 1994.

54. **b** Suprascapular nerve. The *solid black box* identifies the infraspinatus. This muscle is readily identified on this image by its origin from the *dorsal* surface of the scapula. The *asterisk* indicates the supraspinatus, which is also innervated by the suprascaular nerve. The letter *C* indicates the deltoid, innervated by the axillary nerve.
55. **c** Lateral epicondylitis in the lead arm. Although medial epicondylitis is termed *golfer's elbow,* it is not the most common elbow complaint among golfers. Lateral epicondylitis *(tennis elbow)* is most prevalent. In addition, medial epicondylitis is more common in tennis players than in golfers.

    Note: The golfer's lead arm is most commonly affected by lateral epicondylitis, whereas medial epicondylitis most typically involves the gofer's trailing arm.

References

McCarroll JR, Rettig AC, Shelbourne KD: Injuries in the Amateur Golfer. Phys Sports Med, 18(3):125, 1990.

Vangsness CT, Jobe FW: Surgical Treatment of Medial Epicondylitis: Results in 35 Elbows. J Bone Joint Surg Br, 73:409–411, 1991.

56. **e** Pain is most prominent during the formative phase. Although many authorities believe that calcific tendinitis stems from intratendinous degeneration, this process is not predicated on the presence of intraarticular degeneration.

    Calcific tendinitis is commonly divided into two phases: (1) formative and (2) resorptive. Radiographs during the formative phase characteristically demonstrate a dense, well-circumscribed, homogeneous deposit. Pain is less acute during this phase. The calcific deposit has a chalk-like consistency during this phase.

    Pain is most prominent during the resorptive phase. During this phase, radiographs reveal an ill-defined density with a toothpaste consistency. Rupture into the bursa occurs most often during this phase.

Reference

Uhthoff HK, Loehr JW: Calcific Tendinopathy of the Rotator Cuff: Pathogenesis, Diagnosis, and Management. J Am Acad Orthop Surg, 5(4): 183–191, 1997.

57. **d** Bankart lesion healed, patulous capsule. In one study, 52 consecutive patients treated by a single surgeon for recurrent anterior instability underwent arthroscopic stabilization with a bioabsorbable tack; 50 of the 52 patients had Bankart lesions. The repair failed in 11 patients (21%); seven of the 11 failures occurred atraumatically, and eight of the 11 patients with treatment failures underwent subsequent open capsulorrhaphy. Intraoperative findings at the open procedures revealed that seven of the eight Bankart lesions were completely healed.

    This study illustrates that the degree of capsular laxity is a determinant of the success or failure of arthroscopic stabilization. To restore stability to the shoulder, the Bankart lesion and the patulous capsule (if present) must both be adressed surgically. Anterior capsular laxity is less amenable to arthroscopic tack stabilization than is a Bankart lesion.

Reference

Speer K, Warren R, Pagnani M, Warner J: An Arthroscopic Technique for Anterior Stabilization of the Shoulder with a Bioabsorbable Tack. J Bone Joint Surg Am, 78:1801–1807, 1996.

58. **c** Mechanical failure of the prosthesis (other than aseptic loosening). In a review of semiconstrained total elbow arthroplasties performed for posttraumatic osteoarthritis, the most common complication after an average follow up of 5.6 years was mechanical failure. The ulnar component fractured in 12%, and the polyethylene bushings wore out in 5% of the patients. These complications were attributed principally to the performance of strenuous physical labor (lifting more than 10 kg) on a regular basis, an unstable traumatic injury, and excessive preoperative deformity. The infection rate was 5%, and there was a 0% incidence of aseptic loosening and osteolysis.

Reference

Schneeberger A, Adams R, Morrey B: Semiconstraied Total Elbow Replacement for the Treatment of Posttraumatic Osteoarthritis. J Bone Joint Surg Am, 79:1211–1222, 1997.

59. **e** Prescription of a sling for comfort, nonsteroidal anti-inflammatory drugs, and activity modification. The radiograph reveals osteolysis of the distal clavicle. This disease typically occurs in weightlifters and persons who conduct heavy manual labor. Characteristic radiographic findings include osteopenia and resorption of the distal clavicle with cystic changes. The acromioclavicular joint is widened, but osseous changes are absent on the acromial side of the joint.

    Distal clavicular osteolysis is frequently selflimited, and, thus, initial treatment should be nonoperative. Conservative management includes a sling, nonsteroidal antiinflammatory drugs, and avoidance of aggravating activities. Distal clavicle resection (Mumford procedure) can be performed if the condition is recalcitrant to a reasonable trial of conservative measures or if activity modification is unacceptable to the patient.

Although the exact origin is unknown, distal clavicular osteolysis is hypothesized to be associated with trauma to the acromioclavicular joint and subsequent aseptic necrosis.

Note: Bilateral distal clavicular resorption warrants a workup for hyperparathyroidism.

References

Cahill BR: Osteolysis of the Distal Part of the Clavicle in Male Athletes. J Bone Joint Surg Am, 64:1053, 1982.

Rockwood CA, et al.: Osteolysis of the Distal Clavicle. In Rockwood CA, Matsen FA, eds: The Shoulder, 2nd Ed. Philadelphia, WB Saunders, 1998.

60. **d** Posterior sternoclavicular dislocation. The 40degree cephalic tilt view of the sternoclavicular joint can be used to discern the direction of clavicular displacement. If the projection of the medial clavicle appears superior to the contralateral medial clavicle, it is anteriorly dislocated. If the projection of the medial clavicle appears inferior to the contralateral medial clavicle, it is posteriorly dislocated (Fig. 2.17). Inferior sternoclavicular dislocation is not a described entity.

Note: Computed tomography is the study of choice to evaluate sternoclavicular dislocations. Projectional difficulties are eliminated, and the mediastinal structures can be visualized.

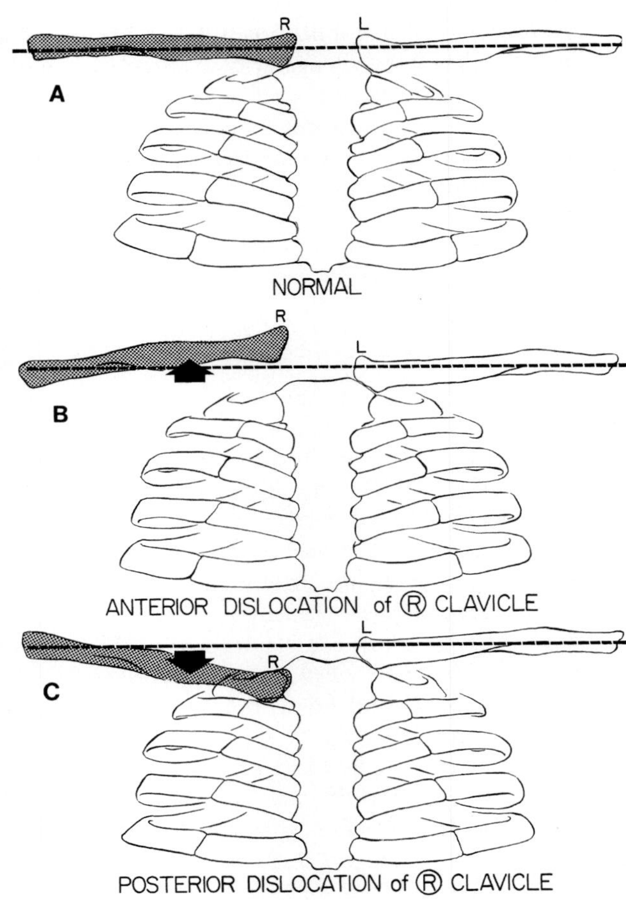

FIGURE 2.17A–C

Reference

Rockwood CA, Green DP, eds: Fractures in Adults, 4th Ed. Philadelphia, Lippincott–Raven, 1996.

61. **e** The anterolateral ascending branch of the anterior humeral circumflex artery. This branch runs parallel to the tendon of the long head of the biceps (on the side of the greater tuberosity) and then enters the humeral head at the end of the intertubercular groove. This vessel perfuses almost the entire humeral epiphysis. The terminal, intraosseous branch of this vessel is referred to as the arcuate artery. The posterior humeral circumflex artery supplies only a small posteroinferior portion of the humeral head.

Reference

Gerber C, et al.: The Arterial Vascularization of the Humeral Head. J Bone Joint Surg Am, 72:1486, 1990.

62. **a** Shoulder pain. The most common complication of antegrade intramedullary nailing of a humeral shaft fracture is residual shoulder pain. In studies by Wagner et al. and Chapman et al., plate fixation was compared with antegrade intrameduallary fixation. The rates of residual shoulder pain were 31% and 42% for the respective nailed cohorts. The reported incidence of nonunion after antegrade humeral nailing ranges from 0% to 8%. Infection and iatrogenic nerve injury occur in approximately 2% to 3% of cases.

Reference

Gregory P, Sanders R: Compression Plating Versus Intramedullary Fixation of Humeral Shaft Fractures. J Am Acad Orthop Surg, 5(4):215–223, 1997.

63. **d** Acceleration. Electromyography has demonstrated that pronator teres activity is greatest during the acceleration phase. Peak activity of this muscle occurs during this phase in both medial collateral ligament–deficient and normal elbows when either a fastball or a curveball is thrown.

Reference

Glousman RE, et al.: An Electromyographic Analysis of the Elbow in Normal and Injured Pitchers with Medial Collateral Ligament Insufficiency. Am J Sports Med, 20(3):311–317, 1992.

64. **e** The teres minor, teres major, long head of the triceps, and humerus. The *quadrilateral space* transmits the posterior humeral circumflex vessels and the axillary nerve. It is bordered by the teres minor (superiorly), the teres major (inferiorly), the long head of the triceps (medially), and the humerus (laterally).

    The *triangular space* lies medialy to the quadrilateral space. It is defined by the long head of the triceps (laterally), the teres minor (superiorly), and the teres major (inferiorly). It transmits the circumflex scapular vessels.

    The triangular interval lies inferiorly to the quadrilateral space. It is bordered by the teres major (superiorly), the long head of the triceps (medially), and the humerus/lateral head of the triceps (laterally). It transmits the profunda brachii artery and the radial nerve (Fig. 2.16).
65. **c** 50%. Normal posterior translation of the humeral head may be as much as 50% of the diameter of the glenoid. In addition, a symptomatic shoulder should always be compared with the contralateral (asymptomatic) side, to determine what degree of laxity is normal for a particular person.

Reference

Hawkins RJ, Neer CS, Pianta RM, Mendoza FX: Recurrent Posterior Instability (Subluxation) of the Shoulder. J Bone Joint Surg Am, 66:169–174, 1984.

66. **d** Posterior interosseous nerve. Monteggia fractures account for fewer than 5% of all forearm fractures. They have been classified by Bado as shown in Table 2.2.

    Most associated neurologic defecits involve the posterior interosseous nerve (regardless of the Bado type). Compression of the posterior interosseus nerve at the arcade of Frohse (the fibrous proximal border of the supinator muscle) is commonly held responsible in these instances.

    Palsies of the entire radial nerve have also been described. The proposed mechanism in these cases is stretch of the nerve by the dislocated radial head. Associated anterior interosseous and ulnar nerve palsies occur very infrequently.

    Monteggia lesions should be managed by closed reduction of the radial head followed by open reduction and internal fixation of the ulna.

References

Engber WE, Keene JS: Anterior Interosseous Nerve Palsy Associated With a Monteggia Fracture. Clin Orthop, 174:133–137, 1983.

Stein F, Deffer P: Nerve Injuries Complicating Monteggia Lesions. J Bone Joint Surg Am, 53(7):1432–1436, 1971.

67. **c** It inserts on the medial aspect of the intertubercular groove caudal to the subscapularis insertion. The pectoralis major is innervated by the medial and lateral pectoral nerves. It is perfused by the pectoral branch of the thoracoacromial artery. It inserts on the *lateral* aspect of the intertubercular groove caudal to the subscapularis insertion. Its principal functions include adduction and internal rotation of the humerus.
68. **c** Linear radiolucency at the cement-bone interface of the glenoid component. Glenoid radiolucencies lines are extremely common after total shoulder arthroplasty. Reports of their incidence range from 30% to 82%. Most of these radiolucencies are nonprogressive and asymptomatic. Radiolucencies at the humeral component are less common.

References

Barret: J Arthroplasty, 4:91, 1989.: J Arthroplasty, 3:123, 1988.

Neer CS: J Bone Joint Surg Am, 64:319, 1982.

69. **a** Immobilization in 90 degrees of flexion for 5 to 7 days, followed by initiation of range-of-motion exercises. After immobilization in a position of stability for 5 to10 days, motion should be initiated within the arc of stability. Immobilization for longer than 3 weeks has been associated with compromised ultimate range of motion.

    Most complete elbow dislocations are associated with rupture of the medial and lateral collateral ligaments. However, acute sugical intervention is rarely appropriate in the absence of associated fractures or intraarticular osteochondral fragments that preclude concentric reduction. A prospective randomized study

TABLE 2.2. MONTEGGIA FRACTURES

Type	Radial Head Dislocation	Ulnar Fracture	Percentage of All Monteggia Fractures
I	Anterior	Diaphyseal with anterior angulation	~65%
II	Posterior	Diaphyseal with posterior angulation	~18%
III	Lateral	Metaphyseal	~16%
IV	Anterior	Radius and ulna both fractured at proximal third	~1%

demonstrated that acute collateral ligament repair provided no advantage over early, protected range of motion for simple dislocations.

Note: In patients less than 18 years old, a longer period of initial immobilization (2 to 3 weeks) is acceptable.

References

Cohen MS, Hastings H: Acute Elbow Dislocation: Evaluation and Management. J Am Acad Orthop Surg, 6:15–23, 1998.

Josefsson PO et al.: Surgical Versus Nonsurgical Treatment of Ligamentous Injuries Following Dislocation of the Elbow Joint: A Prospective, Randomized Study. J Bone Joint Surg Am, 69:605–608, 1987.

Mehlhoff TL et al.: Simple Dislocation of the Elbow in the Adult: Results After Closed Treatment. J Bone Joint Surg Am, 70:244–249, 1988.

70. **d** The posterior scalene muscle. Potential anatomic structures that can cause constriction of the thoracic outlet include adventitious (cervical) ribs, congenital fibrous bands, the *anterior or middle* scalene muscles (particularly when their insertions are anomalous), the clavicle, and the first rib. Obesity cannot, by itself, cause thoracic outlet syndrome, but it may aggravate it.

Reference

Leffert RD: Thoracic outlet syndrome. J Am Acad Orthop Surg, 2(6):317–325, 1994.

71. **d** Osteophyte formation on the posterolateral olecranon. Several characteristic changes can occur around the joint because of the chronic valgus extension loading pattern placed on the elbow. Attenuation of the medial collateral ligament permits a "windshield wiper" pattern of instability. Osteophyte formation is characteristically encountered at the postero*medial* aspect of the olecranon because of impingement against the medial aspect of the olecranon fossa (Fig. 2.18). A reciprocal region of chondromalacia *(kissing lesion)* is often present at the point where the olecranon process contacts the olecranon fossa.

Other associated findings include traction spurs on the medial aspect of the ulnar notch, avulsion of the medial epicondyle through the apophysis (skeletally immature), osteochondral lesions of the capitellum, and hypertrophy of the humerus.

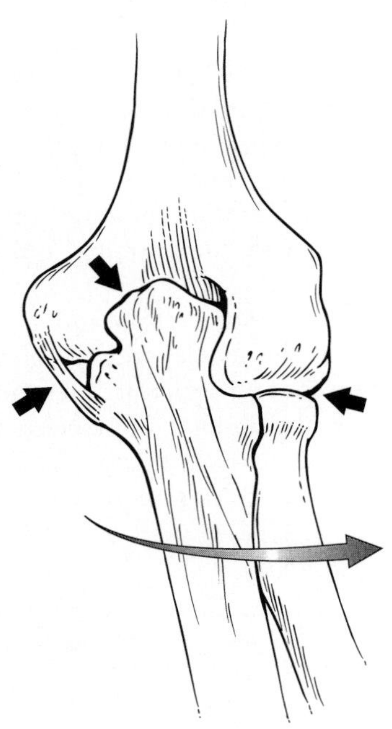

FIGURE 2.18

References

Miller,CD, Savoie FH: Valgus Extension Injuries of the Elbow in the Throwing Athlete. J Am Orthop Surg, 2(5):264, 1994.

Wison FD, Andrews JR, et al.: Valgus Extension Overload in the Pitching Elbow. Am J Sports Med, 11(2):83–87, 1983.

72. **d** Four-part fracture with valgus impaction of the head. Immediate hemiarthroplasty has become the recommended treatment for most fourpart proximal humerus fractures because the incidence of subsequent avascular necrosis has been reported to be as high as 90%. An exception is the fourpart valgus impacted fracture, in which the rate of avascular necrosis is significantly lower (approximately 20%).

Reference

Schlegel TF, Hawkins RJ: Displaced Proximal Humerus Fractures. J Am Acad Orthop Surg, 2(1):54–66, 1994.

73. **e** Examination for scapular winging. The long thoracic nerve is vulnerable to injury along the floor of the axilla during mastectomy axillary node dissection. Iatrogenic long thoracic nerve palsy is a potential cause of scapular winging. Serratus anterior deficit leads to medial scapular translation, medial rotation of the inferior pole of the scapula, and inferior rotation of the acromion (Fig. 2.19). Inability to rotate the glenoid upwardly produces difficulty in achieving full arm elevation. Pain arises from resultant subacromial impingement and fatigue of other periscapular muscles in their efforts to compensate for the serratus anterior deficit.

Concern over potential osseous metastasis is warranted in any patient with a history of cancer. However, an appropriate physical examination should be conducted before considering adjunctive tests (e.g., a bone scan).

Note: The long thoracic nerve arises from the ventral rami of C5, C6, and C7.

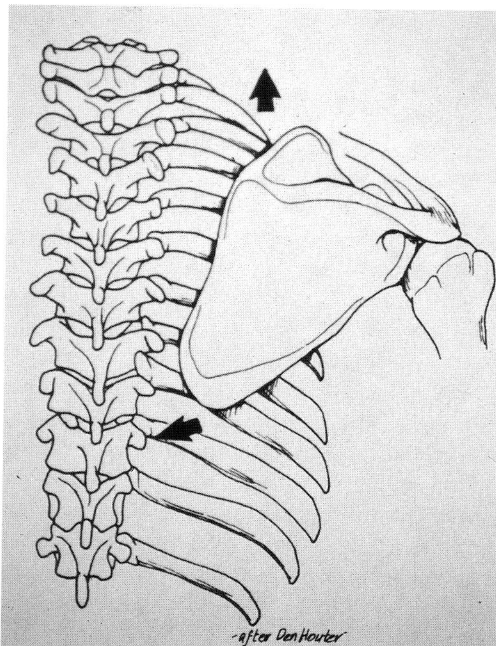

FIGURE 2.19

Reference

Kuhn JE, Plancher KD, Hawkins RJ: Scapular Winging. J Am Acad Orthop Surg, 3:319–325, 1995.

74. **b** Equal sex distribution. Osteoarthritis of the elbow is relatively uncommon, but its presentation and radiographic findings are consistent. Men are affected far more commonly than women. The dominant elbow is predominantly involved. Pain at the extremes of extension and flexion is a characteristic finding.

    The ulnohumeral articulation is the principal focus of disease, with characteristic osteophytes at the olecranon and coronoid. The flexion-extension arc is characteristically compromised. Loss of extension is the most common presenting complaint. The radiocapitellar and radioulnar joints remain relatively spared until the very advanced stages (this accounts for the preserved forearm rotation).

Reference

O'Driscoll SW: Elbow Arthritis: Treatment Options. J Am Acad Orthop Surg, 1(2):106–116, 1993.

75. **b** 25 to 40 years old. Neer classified impingement into three clinicopathologic stages. *Stage I* is characterized by edema and hemorrhage and most commonly affects patients less than 25 years old. *Stage II* affects patients 25 to 40 years old and is characterized by fibrosis and tendinitis. *Stage III* involves partial or complete tearing of the rotator cuff with bony changes and generally affects patients who are more than 40 years old.

Reference

Neer CS: Impingement Lesions. Clin Orthop, 173:70–77, 1983.

76. **d** The proximal border of the superficial belly of the supinator (the arcade of Frohse). Two separate syndromes have been defined for compression of the posterior interosseous nerve: (1) the radial tunnel syndrome (compression of the posterior interosseous nerve in the radial tunnel that results in pain but no motor weakness) and (2) posterior interosseous nerve compression syndrome (compression of the posterior interosseous nerve in the radial tunnel that produces motor weakness but no pain). The mnemonic FREAS is a useful way to recall (in order of appearance during dissection from superficial to deep to expose the posterior interosseous nerve) the structures that have the potential to compress the posterior interosseous nerve in the radial tunnel: *F*ibrous bands (anterior to the radial head at the entrance to the radial tunnel), *R*ecurrent radial vessels (the leash of Henry), *E*xtensor carpi radialis brevis, *A*rcade of Frohse (the fibrous proximal border of the supinator), and the distal border of the *S*upinator. The arcade of Frohse is the most common site of posterior interosseous nerve compression.

Reference

Gelberman RH, Eaton R, Urbaniak JR: Peripheral Nerve Compression. J Bone Joint Surg Am, 75:1854–1878, 1993.

77. **e** Closed, transverse fracture with associated complete radial nerve palsy. Most humeral shaft fractures are amenable to closed treatment with functional bracing. Indications for operative management include (1) pathologic humerus fractures, (2) segmental humerus fractures, (3) ipsilateral humerus and bothbone forearm fractures *(floating elbow),* (4) bilateral humerus fractures, (5) polytrauma patients, (6) failed closed treatment, (7) patients anticipated to be noncompliant or unable to cooperate with closed management, (8) intraarticular extension, (9) open fractures, and (10) fractures with associated vascular injury requiring repair. The management of humeral shaft fractures with associated radial nerve dysfunction is controversial. However, current consensus favors expectant management of most of these injuries. Most associated radial nerve deficits stem from neuropraxia and/or nerve contusion (rather than laceration). Spontaneous recovery occurs in the majority of cases. Early nerve

exploration subjects the nerve to unnecessary risk for iatrogenic damage. Furthermore, the results of delayed nerve decompression and/or repair are comparable to those of early intervention.

References

Bostman O, et al.: Radial Palsy in Shaft Fracture of the Humerus. Acta Orthop Scand, 57:316–319, 1986.

Sarmiento A, et al.: Functional Bracing of Fractures of the Shaft of the Humerus. J Bone Joint Surg Am, 59:596–601, 1977.

78. **d** West Point view. The *West Point* view is a modified axillary view obtained with the patient prone and arm abducted 90 degrees. The x-ray beam is angled 25 degrees from the horizontal and 25 degrees off the long axis of the body (Fig. 2.20). This is the most sensitive view for assessing the integrity of the anteroinferior glenoid rim. The *outlet view* is useful for assessing the degree of compromise of the subacromial space in cases of impingement. The true *anteroposterior view* is best for assessing the extent of joint space narrowing in cases of osteoarthritis. The *Stryker notch view* is the most sensitive view for detecting a HillSachs lesion.
79. **d** The medial pectoral nerve. The nerve supply to the pectoralis minor is the medial pectoral nerve only. The pectoralis major is innervated by both the lateral and medial pectoral nerves.

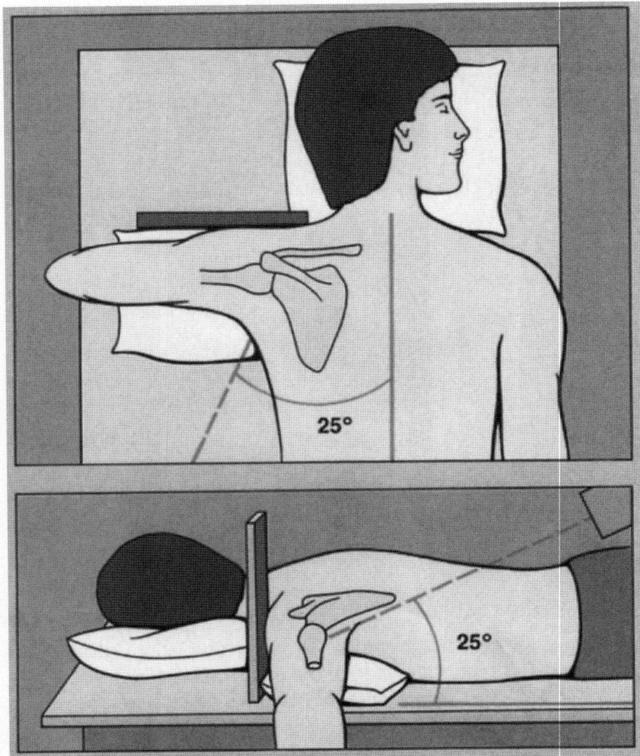

FIGURE 2.20

80. **d** Sling immobilization for comfort. Distal third clavicular fractures are classified into three groups according to Neer. *Type I* injuries occur lateral to the coracoclavicular ligaments and are therefore stable and amenable to sling treatment. *Type II* fractures occur medial to the coracoclavicular ligaments. This disrupts the suspensory mechanism of the scapula, and therefore this injury is typically associated with marked deformity. Type II injuries are unstable and are typically treated operatively. *Type III* fractures occur lateral to the coracoclavicular ligaments with intraarticular (acromioclavicular) extension, no ligamentous disruption, and minimal displacement. They are often missed by plain radiographs and misdiagnosed as grade I acromioclavicular separations. Although posttraumatic acromioclavicular arthritis is a potential sequela, primary management should be conservative, with later surgical management of acromioclavicular symptoms if necessary.

   Note: Some apparent type III fractures are, in fact, type II fractures (fracture medial to the coracoclavicular ligaments) with intraarticular extension. These fractures are unstable and should be treated as type II injuries.

Reference

Rockwood CA, Green DP, eds: Fractures in Adults, 4th Ed. Philadelphia, Lippincott–Raven, 1996.

81. **b** II. Figure 2.11 represent the three types of acromial morphology as described by Bigliani. *Type II* (curved) occurs most commonly in asymptomatic persons (44%). *Type III* (hooked) is the second most common (39%), followed by *type I* (17%). The type III morphology is most common among patients with rotator cuff tears (70%).

Reference

Bigliani L, et al.: Morphology of the Acromion and its Relationship to Rotator Cuff Tears. Orthop Trans, 10:228, 1996.

82. **c** Semiconstrained total elbow arthroplasty. Prerequisites for placement of a nonconstrained prosthesis include preserved metaphyseal bone stock and competent collateral ligaments. Therefore, placement of an nonconstrained prosthesis could not be appropriate in this particular situation. Hinged prostheses are currently not used because of the associated high rates of early loosening. The procedure of choice in this patient would be a semiconstrained elbow prosthesis.
83. **c** 30 to 130 degrees. Normal range of motion of the elbow is approximately 70 degrees of pronation, 85 degrees of supination, and 0 to 140 (±10) degrees of

flexion and extension. The arc of motion needed for most activities of daily living (functional range of motion) is 30 to 130 degrees of flexion and extension and 50 degrees of both pronation and supination.

Reference

Morrey BF, An K: Functional Anatomy of the Ligaments of the Elbow. Clin Orthop, 201:84–89, 1985.

84. **e** More than 50% compromise. Biomechanical testing has revealed that a single drop of fluid or soft tissue debris retained in the Morse taper housing will compromise the strength of the assembly of a modular humeral component by more than 50%. Hence, to maximize the strength of the linkage, the housing should be thoroughly cleaned and dried before impaction of the head.

Reference

Warren RF, et al.: Disassociation of Modular Shoulder Arthroplasty. Presented at the American Shoulder and Elbow Surgeons Annual Meeting, New Orleans, 1994.

85. **c** A type I (flat) acromion. In one study, 636 shoulders with subacromial impingement syndrome were evaluated retrospectively to determine the results of nonoperative treatment; 67% of the patients had a satisfactory outcome. Patients with type I acromial morphology did significantly better (91% successful) than the other patients. Patients who were older than 60 years had the poorest results stratified according to age. Patients with symptom duration of less than 1 month fared significantly better than patients with longer symptom duration. Acromioclavicular joint tenderness did not affect results significantly.

Reference

Morrison, et al.: Nonoperative Treatment of Subacromial Impingement Syndrome. J Bone Joint Surg Am, 79:732–737, 1997.

86. **e** The axillary and lateral pectoral nerves (proximally) and radial and musculocutaneous nerves (distally). The anterior approach to the humerus traverses two internervous planes. Proximally, the approach proceeds between the deltoid (axillary nerve) and the pectoralis major muscle (innervated by the medial and lateral pectoral nerves). Distally, the approach splits the brachialis muscle, which is innervated by the musculocutaneous nerve (medially) and the radial nerve (laterally).
87. **e** The supreme thoracic, thoracoacromial, lateral thoracic, subscapular, anterior humeral circumflex, posterior humeral circumflex. There are three parts to the axillary artery. Each part gives off as many branches as the number of that portion (Table 2.3).

TABLE 2.3. AXILLARY ARTERY

Part	Branches
1	Supreme thoracic
2	Thoracoacromial
	Lateral thoracic
3	Subscapular
	Anterior humeral circumflex
	Posterior humeral circumflex

88. **c** Hemiarthroplasty. The caudally directed vector of a functional rotator cuff ordinarily counters the deltoid's cephalad force on the proximal humerus. Rotator cuff incompetence destabilizes this balance.

    Nonconstrained total shoulder replacement in the setting of cuff tear arthropathy has been associated with premature glenoid loosening. The accelerated rate of glenoid loosening has been attributed to eccentric loading and increased shear forces across the glenoid component *(rocking horse effect)*.

    Hemiarthroplasty has been advocated as a means of avoiding glenoid component failure in the setting of cuff tear arthropathy or osteoarthritis in conjunction with profound, nonreconstructable cuff insufficiency. An oversized humeral head component is recommended to maximize function and stability in these instances.

Reference

Friedman RJ: Glenohumeral Translation After Total Shoulder Arthroplasty. J Shoulder Elbow Surg, 1:312–316, 1992.
Pollack R, et al.: Prosthetic Replacement in Rotator Cuff Deficient Shoulders. J Shoulder Elbow Surg, 1:173–186, 1992.

89. **e** Observation. Benign neglect is a viable treatment option for certain chronic, unreduced glenohumeral dislocations.

    The old chest radiographs reveals that the patient's shoulder has been dislocated for at least 4 months. Closed reduction becomes increasingly difficult and dangerous with increased duration of dislocation. Forceful manipulation carries the risk of fracture as well as neurovascular damage.

    Surgery is not justified when patients have minimal disability (or minimal functional demands), no significant associated pain, and no associated neurovascular deficit. Among the unreduced patients in the study by Schulz et al., 70% of had "good" clinical results, and 90% were subjectively satisfied. In Rowe and Zarins' study, five of eight of the results in the nontreatment group were "good" or "fair."

    Note: In general, the outcomes of untreated posterior dislocations are superior to unreduced anterior dislocations. The position of the arm in an untreated posterior dislocation (adduction and internal rotation) is more functional than in an untreated anterior dislocation (abduction and external rotation).

References

Rowe CR, Zarins B: Chronic Unreduced Dislocations of the Shoulder. J Bone Joint Surg Am, 494–505, 1982.
Schulz TJ, et al.: Unrecognized Dislocations of the Shoulder. J Trauma, 9(12):1009–1023, 1969.

90. **b** Closed reduction. Figure 2.12 reveals a twopart fracture dislocation of the proximal humerus. Initial treatment should be gentle closed reduction. Reduction with the patient under anesthesia should be considered, to avoid further damage to the proximal humerus. Ultimate treatment can be determined only after closed reduction. In this instance, closed reduction produced acceptable reduction of the greater tuberosity fragment. Residual displacement of the greater tuberosity fragment of less than 0.5 cm was correlated with a favorable outcome by McLaughlin. Serial radiographs are necessary during the healing period to rule out late displacement.

Reference

McLaughlin HL: Dislocation of the Shoulder with Tuberosity Fractures. Surg Clin North Am, 43:1615–1620, 1963.

91. **c** Tuberculosis. The first total shoulder arthroplasty was performed in 1893 by Pean for a case of glenohumeral joint destruction secondary to tuberculosis. Pean's implant consisted of a platinum shaft and a rubber humeral head (Fig. 2.21).

Reference

Rowe CR: The Shoulder. New York, Churchill Livingstone, 1988.

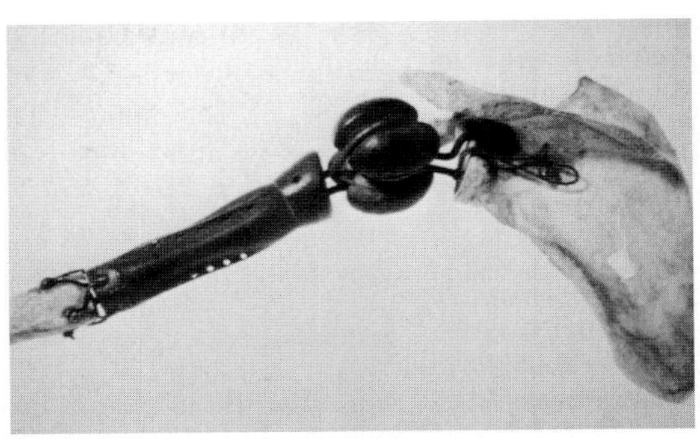

FIGURE 2.21

FIGURE CREDITS

Figure 2.5. From Rockwood CA, Green DP, eds: Fractures in Adults, 3rd Ed. Philadelphia, Lippincott–Raven, p. 1204, 1996, with permission.
Figure 2.6. From Warren R: The Unstable Shoulder. Philadelphia, Lippincott Williams & Wilkins, p. 109, 1999, with permission.
Figure 2.10. From Rockwood CA, Green DP, eds: Fractures in Adults, 3rd Ed. Philadelphia, Lippincott–Raven, p. 1111, 1996, with permission.
Figure 2.11. From Rockwood CA, Matsen FA, eds: The Shoulder. Philadelphia, WB Saunders, p. 45, 1990, with permission.
Figure 2.12. From Rockwood CA, Green DP, eds: Fractures in Adults, 3rd Ed. Philadelphia, Lippincott–Raven, p. 1069, 1996, with permission.
Figure 2.13. From Rockwood CA, Green DP, eds: Fractures in Adults, 3rd Ed. Philadelphia, Lippincott–Raven, p. 1111, 1996, with permission.
Figure 2.14. From Rockwood CA, Green DP, eds: Fractures in Adults, 3rd Ed. Philadelphia, Lippincott–Raven, p. 1171, 1996, with permission.
Figure 2.15. From Rockwood CA, Green DP, eds: Fractures in Adults, 3rd Ed. Philadelphia, Lippincott–Raven, p. 1354, 1996.
Figure 2.16. From Rockwood CA, Green DP, eds: Fractures in Adults, 3rd Ed. Philadelphia, Lippincott–Raven, p. 1201, 1996, with permission.
Figure 2.17. From Rockwood CA, Green DP, eds: Fractures in Adults, 3rd Ed. Philadelphia, Lippincott–Raven, p. 1437, 1996, with permission.
Figure 2.18. From Wilson, et al.: Valgus Extension Overload in the Pitching Elbow. Am J Sports Med, 11:89, 1983, with permission.
Figure 2.19. From Kuhn JE, Plancher KD, Hawkins RJ: Scapular Winging. J Am Acad Orthop Surg, 3:320, 1995, with permission.
Figure 2.20. From Greenspan A.: Orthopaedic Radiology, 2nd Ed. New York, Raven, p. 5.6, 1992, with permission.
Figure 2.21. From Rowe CR: The Shoulder. New York, Churchill Livingstone, p. 14, 1988, with permission.

3

SPINE

QUESTIONS

1. The carotid tubercle is a useful anterior cervical landmark. To what cervical vertebral level does this surface landmark correspond?
   (a) C3
   (b) C5
   (c) C6
   (d) C7
   (e) T1
2. Which of the following statements regarding metastatic disease to the spine in adults is false?
   (a) The spine is the most common site of skeletal metastasis.
   (b) Arterial seeding of the spine is believed to be the most common route of metastasis from the prostate.
   (c) The vertebral body is more commonly involved than the posterior elements.
   (d) Spinal cord compression occurs in fewer than 50% of patients with spinal metastases.
   (e) Pain is the most common presenting symptom.
3. Which of the following statements regarding the epidemiology of degenerative spondylolisthesis is true?
   (a) The incidence among males and females is equivalent.
   (b) L5 to S1 is the most commonly affected level.
   (c) Hemisacralization decreases the risk of this disease.
   (d) The incidence is higher among patients with diabetes mellitus.
   (e) Oophorectomy is not a risk factor.
4. The Brown-Séquard syndrome
   (a) Produces hypesthesia to pain and temperature on the side contralateral to the lesion
   (b) Most commonly results from blunt trauma
   (c) Produces muscle paralysis on the side contralateral to the lesion
   (d) Usually results in permanent loss of bowel and bladder function
   (e) Compromises proprioception on the side contralateral to the lesion
5. A 64-year-old woman presents with 6 weeks of progressive thoracic spine pain, ataxia, and urinary incontinence. Her past medical history is significant for renal cell carcinoma. A computed tomography–guided needle biopsy of the lesion is consistent with metastasis from the renal primary tumor. Her metastatic workup (including bone scan and computed tomography scans of the lung and head) is otherwise negative. The most important step in the preoperative management of this patient would be which of the following?
   (a) Radiation therapy
   (b) Neoadjuvant chemotherapy
   (c) Lumbar puncture for staging purposes
   (d) Arteriography
   (e) Assessment of serum transferrin level
6. A 19-year-old woman crashes her moped into a palm tree. Cervical spine radiographs reveal a C5 burst fracture and an incomplete C5 neurologic level with sacral sparing. Which of the following is the most appropriate treatment?
   (a) Administration of a methylprednisolone bolus (30 mg/kg body weight) within 12 hours of injury
   (b) Administration of a methylprednisolone bolus (30 mg/kg body weight) within 12 hours of injury, followed by a continuous infusion of 5.4 mg/kg per hour for 23 hours
   (c) Administration of a methylprednisolone bolus (30 mg/kg body weight) within 8 hours of injury, followed by a continuous infusion of 5.4 mg/kg per hour for 48 hours
   (d) Administration of a methylprednisolone bolus (30 mg/kg body weight) within 8 hours of injury, followed by a continuous infusion of 5.4 mg/kg per hour for 23 hours
   (e) No steroid protocol in this situation because the lesion is incomplete
7. A 70-year-old sports broadcaster presents with a 3-week history of progressive thoracic spine pain. He denies radicular symptoms, fevers, and weight loss. Examination reveals midthoracic tenderness with paraspinal muscle spasm. He is neurologically intact.

Workup has included negative blood cultures, a white blood cell count of 11, and an erythrocyte sedimentation rate of 75 mm per hour. Plain films were unremarkable. Magnetic resonance images are shown in Fig. 3.1. A culture from a computed tomography–guided aspiration grew Staphylococcus aureus. What would be the most appropriate next step in treatment?

(a) Open biopsy to confirm the diagnosis and to obtain accurate antibiotic sensitivities
(b) Open biopsy with thorough débridement
(c) Six weeks of parenteral antibiotics guided by the culture sensitivities from the aspiration
(d) Vertebral body resection and primary anterior reconstruction with tricortical autograft
(e) Vertebral body resection and staged anterior reconstruction with tricortical autograft

8. A patient sustains a C7-T1 disc herniation. Which of the following reflexes will most likely be affected?
(a) The biceps reflex
(b) The triceps reflex
(c) The brachioradialis reflex
(d) The Moro reflex
(e) None of the above

9. Which of the following incomplete spinal cord injuries generally has the worst prognosis?
(a) The posterior cord syndrome
(b) The anterior cord syndrome
(c) Tabes dorsalis

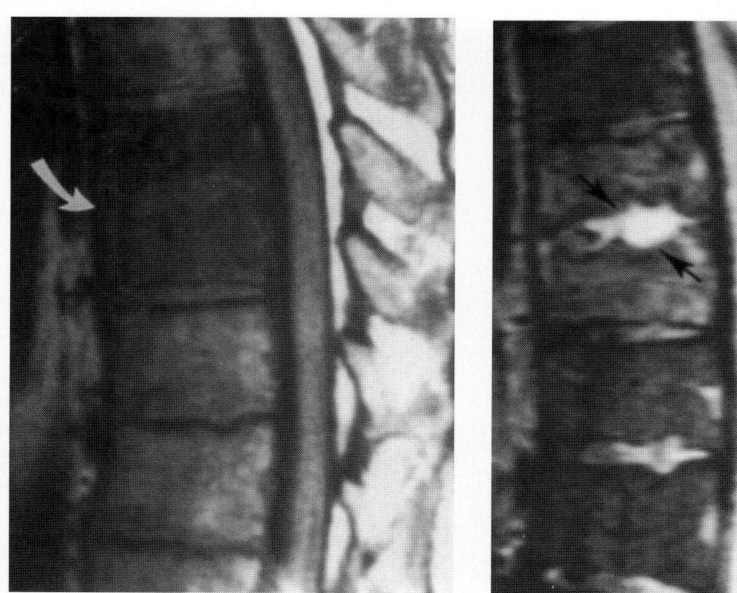

A

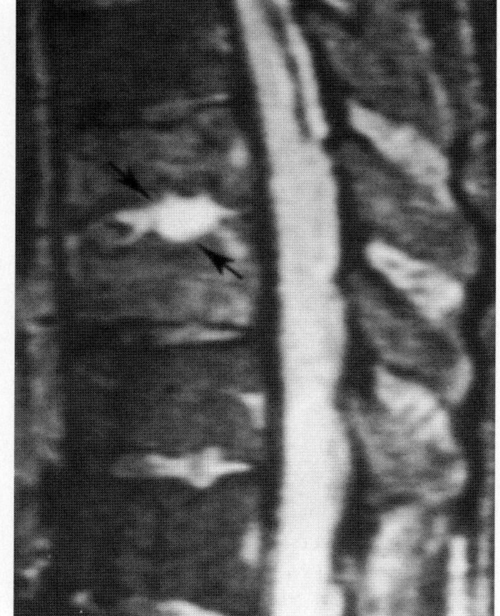

B

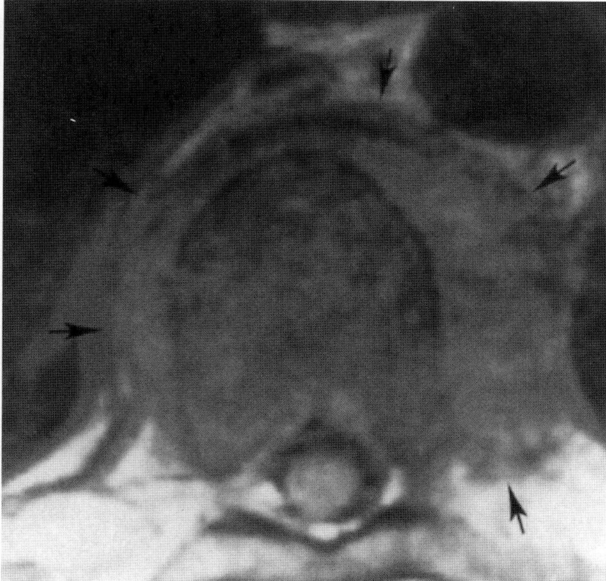

C

FIGURE 3.1A–C

(d) The central cord syndrome
(e) Brown-Séquard syndrome

10. All the following statements regarding central cord syndrome are true except
    (a) It typically results from an extension mechanism.
    (b) It typically occurs in patients older than 50 years.
    (c) It produces greater loss of function in the lower extremities than in the upper extremities.
    (d) Perianal sensation is typically preserved.
    (e) It is the most common incomplete spinal cord injury syndrome.
11. A 24-year-old motorcycle enthusiast presents to the trauma room with a T4 fracture-dislocation (with complete absence of motor and sensory function caudal to T4), a hemopneumothorax, a grossly positive diagnostic peritoneal lavage (DPL), and an L1 burst fracture with 90% canal compromise. Operative stabilization (with complete decompression) of the thoracic spine and lumbar spine injuries is accomplished within the first 24 hours. Forty-eight hours after the injury, there has been no change in the patient's neurologic examination. The bulbocavernosus reflex has not yet returned. What is the most accurate statement regarding this patient's prognosis?
    (a) The patient will remain a T4 paraplegic with a possible one to two level improvement in motor and/or sensory function.
    (b) The patient has a 25% chance of recovering both motor and sensory function caudal to the L1 level.
    (c) The patient has a 75% chance of recovering both motor and sensory function caudal to the L1 level.
    (d) The patient has a 50% chance of recovering full sensory function caudal to the level of L1, but no statement regarding the chances of return of motor function can be made until the bulbocavernosus reflex has returned.
    (e) No prognostic statement can be made until the bulbocavernosus reflex has returned.
12. At the level of the atlas, approximately what percentage of the total spinal canal diameter does the spinal cord occupy?
    (a) 25%
    (b) 35%
    (c) 50%
    (d) 75%
    (e) 90%
13. Which of the following statements regarding assessment of the rheumatoid spine is true?
    (a) Under normal circumstances, the tip of the odontoid will never be above the McGregor line.
    (b) Atlantoaxial impaction is a source of occipital headaches, but it does not produce neurologic deficit.
    (c) The Ranawat index is a measurement of atlantoaxial subluxation.
    (d) Under normal circumstances, the tip of the odontoid will never be above the McRae line.
    (e) Atlantoaxial impaction is the most common form of instability associated with rheumatoid disease of the cervical spine.
14. Waddell signs include all the following except
    (a) Nonorganic tenderness
    (b) Simulation tests
    (c) Neuroanatomic motor and/or sensory compromise
    (d) Distraction tests
    (e) Overreaction
15. A United States senator sustains a complete spinal cord transection through a stab wound from a renegade special interest group member with an osteotome. The senator subsequently wishes to pierce his umbilicus; however, he is extremely concerned about how painful the procedure may be. Medicare will not cover local anesthesia for this procedure. He seeks your advice. Which of the following levels of cord transection would be the most cephalad level at which the patient would still experience pain during the piercing procedure?
    (a) T7
    (b) T9
    (c) T11
    (d) T12
    (e) L1
16. A man complains of neck pain after driving his car into a wall. A lateral cervical spine film is shown in Fig. 3.2. What is the most appropriate description of this injury based on the radiograph?
    (a) Bilateral facet dislocations
    (b) Wedge compression fracture
    (c) Unilateral facet dislocation
    (d) Teardrop fracture
    (e) Lateral mass fracture
17. What is the most appropriate treatment for the patient in question 16?
    (a) Closed reduction with skeletal traction followed by posterior stabilization and fusion
    (b) Closed reduction followed by Philadelphia collar for 8 weeks
    (c) Closed reduction and halo vest immobilization for 2 to 3 months
    (d) Open reduction followed by posterior fusion
    (e) Anterior discectomy followed by reduction and anterior fusion with plate stabilization
18. In the anterior approach to the cervical spine, which of the following structures is retracted medially?
    (a) The vagus nerve
    (b) The internal jugular vein
    (c) The sternocleidomastoid muscle
    (d) The omohyoid muscle
    (e) The common carotid artery
19. Which of the following pathologic reflexes could NOT be produced by a central cervical disc herniation?

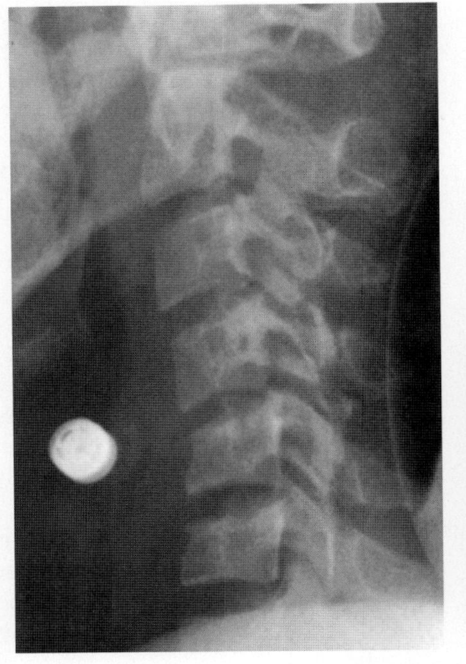

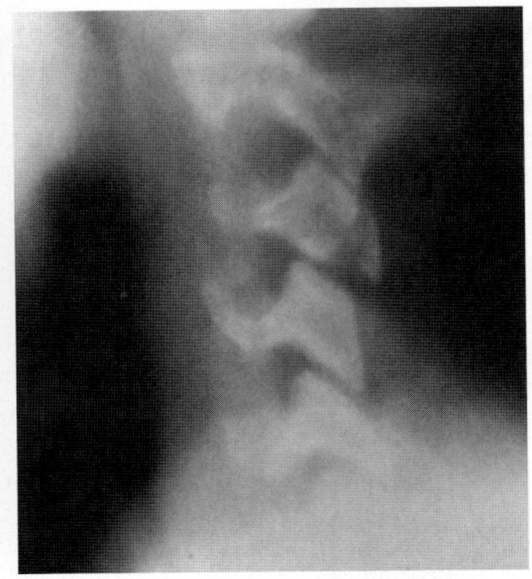

FIGURE 3.2A and B

(a) An inverted radial reflex
(b) Oppenheim sign
(c) Babinski sign
(d) A hyperactive jaw jerk reflex
(e) Hoffman sign

20. A 50-year-old woman is involved in a rollover motor vehicle accident. She is resuscitated and transported to the emergency room, where cervical radiographs and a computed tomography scan reveal a severely angulated traumatic spondylolisthesis of C2. There is minimal translation and no facet dislocation. What is the most appropriate treatment?
(a) Philadelphia collar for 8 to 12 weeks
(b) Halo vest immobilization in extension for 3 months
(c) Minerva vest (cervicothoracic orthosis) immobilization for 3 months
(d) Traction for 3 weeks followed by conversion to halo vest
(e) Posterior spinal fusion

21. In the evaluation of a patient suspected of having a cervical disc herniation, which of the following studies has the greatest diagnostic value?
(a) Magnetic resonance imaging scan
(b) Plain radiographs
(c) Computed tomography scan
(d) Discogram
(e) Bone scan

22. The highest lumbar disc pressure is generated in which of the following positions?
(a) Sitting with lumbar support
(b) Sitting without support
(c) Standing at ease
(d) Lying supine
(e) Lying prone

23. A 58-year-old woman presents with progressive back pain, deformity, and right leg pain. A radiograph of her spine demonstrates 74-degree degenerative thoracolumbar scoliosis. She chooses to undergo operative intervention. During the instrumentation of her spine, increased latencies are noted by somatosensory evoked potential monitoring. What is the most appropriate next step in management?
(a) Finish the instrumentation promptly and close the wound.
(b) Remove all the instrumentation promptly and close the wound.
(c) Remove all the instrumentation promptly and recheck the somatosensory evoked potentials.
(d) Obtain immediate intraoperative radiographs to confirm appropriate hardware placement.
(e) Perform a Stagnara wake-up test.

24. Which of the following types of disc herniations is most likely to produce myelopathic symptoms?
(a) Intraforaminal
(b) Anterocentral
(c) Posterolateral
(d) Posterocentral
(e) Intravertebral

25. Which of the following is the most frequent cause of a "flat back" deformity?

(a) The crankshaft phenomenon
(b) Posterior spinal fusion from T3 to L2 for idiopathic scoliosis with Harrington rod instrumentation
(c) Degenerative changes below the level of a previous posterior spinal fusion
(d) Posterior spine fusion with distraction instrumentation spanning the lumbar spine that ends at the L5 or S1 level
(e) Pseudarthrosis

26. Which of the following statements is most accurate regarding a patient with a Pavlov ratio of 0.76?
(a) The patient has a normal cervical canal.
(b) The patient has atlantooccipital instability.
(c) The patient will salivate in response to the Spurling test.
(d) The patient has atlantoaxial instability.
(e) The patient has an abnormally narrow cervical canal.

27. A 34-year-old heavy-metal singer presents with neck pain and radicular complaints along the radial side of his left forearm and thumb. He had difficulty playing guitar on their latest tour. His left brachioradialis reflex is diminished, and his left wrist extension strength is decreased. Plain films of the cervical spine are normal. Magnetic resonance imaging reveals a left C5-6 posterolateral disc herniation. After failure of nonsurgical treatment, what is the preferred form of intervention for this condition?
(a) Anterior cervical discectomy and fusion
(b) Laminectomy and posterior discectomy
(c) Anterior cervical discectomy without fusion
(d) Anterior cervical corpectomy, discectomy, and strut grafting
(e) Laminectomy and lateral mass plating

28. A patient undergoes a posterior cervical decompression with multilevel laminectomies for cervical spondylosis and stenosis. Which of the following maneuvers is associated with the greatest risk of late cervical spine deformity?
(a) Removal of more than 75% of each lamina
(b) Complete removal of the discs
(c) Resection of over 50% of each facet
(d) Removal of the ligamentum flavum
(e) Removal of the interspinous ligament

29. What percentage of patients with thoracolumbar fractures presents with a neurologic deficit?
(a) 5% to 10%
(b) 15% to 20%
(c) 30% to 40%
(d) 50% to 60%
(e) More than 60%

30. Which of the following is the most common sequela of injury to the sympathetic plexus during an anterior approach to the lumbar spine?
(a) Impaired penile erection
(b) Retrograde ejaculation
(c) Urinary incontinence
(d) Urinary retention
(e) Fecal incontinence

31. Which of the following components of the lumbar spine have sensory innervation?
(a) The annulus fibrosus only
(b) The nucleus pulposus only
(c) The vertebral periosteum
(d) The annulus fibrosus and nucleus pulposus
(e) The annulus fibrosus and vertebral periosteum

32. Which of the following statements is most accurate regarding the addition of spinal fusion at the time of spinal decompression?
(a) Arthrodesis is not indicated when spinal decompression is performed for degenerative spondylolisthesis.
(b) The literature supports decompression and arthrodesis for patients with spinal stenosis associated with progressive degenerative scoliosis.
(c) When arthrodesis is performed at the time of decompression for degenerative spondylolisthesis, there is a tendency for greater bone regrowth (versus when decompression is performed without arthrodesis).
(d) It is inappropriate to perform concomitant arthrodesis on a patient who requires a second decompressive laminectomy at L4-5 unless translational instability is present on preoperative flexion-extension radiographs.
(e) All patients who develop stenosis above a previous posterior fusion should undergo arthrodesis at the time of decompression.

33. Which of the following results constitutes a "positive" computed tomography discogram?
(a) Dye extravasation into or beyond the annulus with concordant pain
(b) Dye extravasation into or beyond the annulus and discordant pain
(c) Concordant pain only
(d) Discordant pain only
(e) Dye extravasation into or beyond the annulus without regard to pain

34. A 62-year-old woman undergoes an L3-4 and L4-5 laminectomy and discectomy for a herniated disc. Postoperatively, she experiences complete relief of her presenting back pain and sciatica. After a 4-month pain-free interval, she experiences a gradual onset of recurrent low back pain without associated neurologic deficit. Myelography and computed tomography images are shown in Fig. 3.3. Which of the following is the most appropriate treatment at this point?
(a) Needle aspiration followed by bed rest and intravenous antibiotic treatment

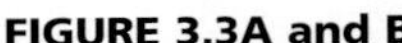
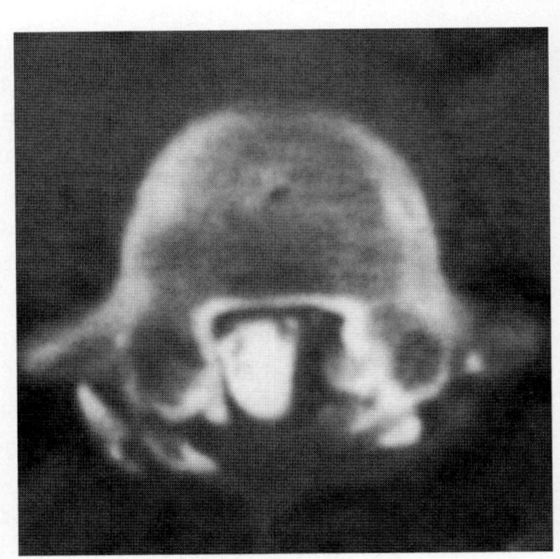
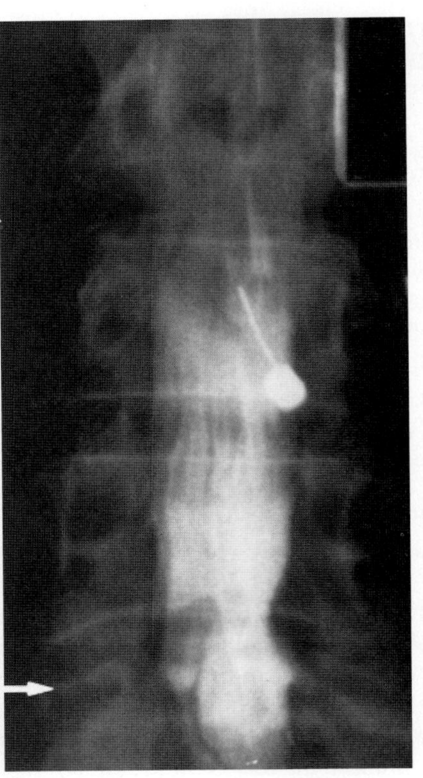
FIGURE 3.3A and B

(b) Epidural steroid injection and physical therapy
(c) Surgical revision with excision of scar tissue
(d) Surgical revision with excision of recurrent disc herniation
(e) Disc excision with concomitant posterolateral fusion

35. A 34-year-old man presents with weakness of his right extensor hallucis longus and decreased sensation over the dorsal aspect of his right foot. Deep tendon reflexes are normal. Which of the following types of lumbar disc herniation would best explain this patient's symptoms?
(a) Posterolateral L5-S1 disc herniation
(b) Extraforaminal L5-S1 disc herniation
(c) Posterolateral L3-4 disc herniation
(d) Extraforaminal L4-5 disc herniation
(e) Lateral L3-4 disc herniation

36. A 25-year-old man sustains a fracture dislocation at the thoracolumbar junction and splenic rupture when he collides with a flagpole after he is ejected from a roller coaster. On arrival at the scene, the emergency medical technicians find the patient alert but hypotensive. He has no lower extremity sensory or motor function. Which of the following would be the most likely associated finding?
(a) A positive Babinski sign
(b) Lower extremity vasoconstriction
(c) An intact bulbocavernosus reflex
(d) Tachycardia
(e) A unilaterally absent cremasteric reflex

37. Which of the following conditions or groups is least likely to be associated with spondylolysis?
(a) Butterfly swimmers
(b) Scheuermann kyphosis
(c) Nonambulators with cerebral palsy
(d) Wrestlers
(e) Football linemen

38. A 21-year-old college football player is injured in a high-energy collision with another player during a game. He relates that he has burning pain and tingling in both arms, and he is unable to move either upper extremity. His symptoms gradually resolve, and recovery is complete within 36 hours. Which of the following statements is most accurate?
(a) This player is at high risk of a permanent neurologic injury if he continues to play football.
(b) This clinical picture does not constitute transient neuropraxia because the symptoms lasted for more than 24 hours.
(c) Patients with a permanent neurologic deficit from a football injury usually have a history of another previous incident like the one described here.
(d) A lateral radiograph of this player's cervical spine is likely to show a spinal canal diameter to vertebral body diameter of less than 0.8.
(e) A finding of developmental narrowing of the cervical canal in an athlete should preclude participation in contact sports.

39. Which of the following forms of venous thromboembolism prophylaxis is most appropriate for patients after major reconstructive spinal surgery?
    (a) Low-molecular-weight heparin
    (b) Compression stockings
    (c) Heparin
    (d) Warfarin (Coumadin)
    (e) Aspirin
40. What is the most appropriate initial management for a competitive high school gymnast who has a symptomatic L5 spondylolysis with a grade 1 spondylolisthesis and no neurologic deficit?
    (a) Open reduction and instrumented fusion
    (b) Posterolateral fusion *in situ*
    (c) Exercise and brace treatment
    (d) Gill procedure
    (e) Instrumented fusion *in situ*
41. Which of the following statements is most accurate with regard to thoracolumbar fractures?
    (a) A wedge compression fracture implies failure of the anterior and middle columns of the spine.
    (b) A wedge compression fracture is a stable fracture and therefore never requires internal fixation.
    (c) In a stable burst fracture, the middle column is not disrupted.
    (d) In a translational shear injury, all three spinal columns are usually injured, and the alignment of the neural canal is typically disrupted.
    (e) A Chance fracture results from distraction forces of the anterior and middle columns and classically occurs in the upper thoracic spine.
42. What is believed to be responsible for the abnormal translation in degenerative lumbar spondylolisthesis?
    (a) A congenital pars defect with superimposed arthrosis
    (b) Fatigue fracture of the pars
    (c) Facet deterioration and incompetence
    (d) Excessive surgical facet resection
    (e) Dysplasia of the superior facets
43. Which of the following situations is the most appropriate indication for posterior surgical management of a lumbar burst fracture?
    (a) A patient who was injured 14 days ago has an incomplete neurologic deficit with 50% canal compromise.
    (b) A patient without neurologic deficit demonstrates a 10-degree sagittal plane deformity with 10% canal compromise and no loss of vertebral height.
    (c) The posterior longitudinal ligament is disrupted in a patient with 50% canal compromise and an incomplete neurologic deficit.
    (d) A large fragment from the posterior wall of the vertebral body is turned, the cancellous portion is facing backward and produces 50% canal compromise in a patient with an incomplete neurologic deficit.
    (e) A patient has an incomplete neurologic deficit, a 20-degree kyphotic deformity, and 35% canal compromise; the computed tomography scan shows a minimally displaced laminar fracture.
44. The preferred treatment for a 60-year-old woman with grade 2 L4-5 spondylolisthesis and evidence of symptomatic, dynamic spinal stenosis is which of the following?
    (a) *In situ* posterolateral fusion
    (b) In situ posterolateral fusion with decompression and instrumentation
    (c) Posterior decompression alone
    (d) *In situ* posterolateral fusion, decompression, and anterior vertebral body fusion with fibular strut grafting
    (e) Epidural steroids
45. A 45-year-old exercise video celebrity sustains a dens fracture and undergoes a posterior C1 to C2 fusion. How much rotation of the cervical spine will he lose?
    (a) 10%
    (b) 30%
    (c) 50%
    (d) 75%
    (e) 100%
46. A 65-year-old patient presents with a history of progressive low back pain and lower extremity fatigue, which increases with activity and is relieved by rest. Which of the following statements is most accurate?
    (a) Weakness of the extensor hallucis longus would be the most common associated motor deficit.
    (b) Degenerative spondylolisthesis at the L5-S1 level is the most likely anatomic abnormality to be associated with her condition.
    (c) A positive straight leg raise test is likely to be present.
    (d) Her symptoms are likely to improve in an extended posture.
    (e) Loss of sensation of light touch is a likely finding on clinical examination.
47. Which of the following statements is most accurate regarding immobilization of a patient with a potentially injured cervical spine in the field?
    (a) A soft collar is the method of choice for immobilizing the cervical spine during the extraction of a victim from a motor vehicle accident.
    (b) Ideally, a patient who has been injured by diving into the shallow end of a pool should be removed from the pool promptly and transferred directly onto a spine board at poolside.
    (c) All patients with significant head injuries should have their cervical spines immobilized before transportation (including conscious patients without neck pain).
    (d) An infant with a suspected cervical injury should be immobilized on a spine board with supplementary support behind the head.

(e) A football player with a potential cervical spine injury should be transported to the emergency room with his helmet and facemask in place to avoid harm to the spine during helmet removal.

48. Which of the following statements is true regarding osteoblastoma in the spine?
 (a) It typically occurs in the thoracic and lumbar pedicles.
 (b) It usually presents as painless scoliosis.
 (c) It rarely causes neurologic deficit.
 (d) Malignant transformation never occurs.
 (e) The best initial treatment is radiotherapy.

49. During which phase of the reduction and fixation of high-grade L5-S1 spondylolisthesis is the L5 nerve at greatest risk of injury?
 (a) During the instrumentation
 (b) During the first 50% of reduction
 (c) During the last 50% of reduction
 (d) During the application of bone graft
 (e) During the correction of the slip angle

50. Which of the following statements is most accurate regarding herniated cervical discs in athletes?
 (a) The condition is usually associated with bilateral symptoms.
 (b) Participation in sports activities has no protective effect against disc herniation.
 (c) It commonly occurs in sports such as football and rugby because of neck rotation and hyperextension.
 (d) It is commonly associated with myelopathy in younger athletes.
 (e) It has no definite association with the recreational use of weight-lifting equipment.

51. Which of the following fixation techniques provides the weakest rotatory stability for C1 to C2 fixation?
 (a) Bilateral posterior clamps (Halifax)
 (b) Wire fixation with a single midline graft (Gallie)
 (c) Wire fixation with bilateral grafts (Brooks)
 (d) Anterior odontoid screw placement
 (e) Transarticular screw fixation (Magerl technique)

52. Which of the following statements is most accurate with regard to the treatment of lumbar spinal stenosis?
 (a) Spinal decompression should be uniformly avoided when a patient is older than 80 years.
 (b) The incidence of complications after spinal decompression is not increased in patients who are older than 75 to 80 years of age.
 (c) Patients with spinal stenosis will experience a definite, predictable progression in their symptoms and/or neurologic deficit if they opt not to undergo surgical decompression.
 (d) The mainstay of the surgical approach to lumbar spinal stenosis is laminectomy.
 (e) If nonoperative management fails, surgical decompression is indicated for persistent back pain that interferes with the patient's quality of life.

53. A 34-year-old actor (who plays the role of a lifeguard on TV) falls from his lifeguard stand and lands directly on his head. In the emergency room, he complains of neck pain, but he is found to have no neurologic deficit. His thought process is noted to be fragmented and tangential, but his friends assure you that this is no change from his baseline. A computed tomography scan of the head is normal. A plain cervical spine film is shown in Fig. 3.4A. A cervical computed tomography scan reveals no abnormality, except at the level of the image that is shown in Fig. 3.4B. The most appropriate management would be
 (a) Immobilization for 6 weeks in a Minerva cervicothoracic orthosis
 (b) Initial traction (3 to 6 weeks) followed by halo vest immobilization for 3 months
 (c) Posterior spinal fusion (C1 to C2) with posterior wiring
 (d) Posterior spinal fusion (occiput to C2)
 (e) Posterior spinal fusion (C1 to C2) with transarticular screw fixation

54. Which of the following factors is not considered to be a clinical or radiographic sign of subaxial instability?
 (a) Relative sagittal plane intersegmental translation greater than 3.5 mm
 (b) Relative sagittal plane intersegmental angulation greater than 7 degrees
 (c) A positive stretch test
 (d) Cervical cord damage
 (e) Structural or functional destruction of the posterior elements

55. In an anterior approach to C5, what structure is less vulnerable from the left side than from the right?
 (a) The superior laryngeal nerve
 (b) The recurrent laryngeal nerve
 (c) The sympathetic chain
 (d) The carotid sheath
 (e) The thoracic duct

56. Which of the following statements is true regarding the surgical management of spinal stenosis?
 (a) The decision to fuse the spine should always be made before surgery is performed for spinal stenosis.
 (b) When performing a laminectomy, it is technically easier and safer to enter the canal distally and to proceed proximally.
 (c) Lateral stenosis is usually produced by osteophyte formation on the inferior articular facet of the superior vertebral body.
 (d) Most patients with spinal stenosis have compression at the L5-S1 level with involvement of the S1 nerve root.
 (e) The neuroforamina should not be probed with a metal instrument because this may traumatize the nerve roots.

A

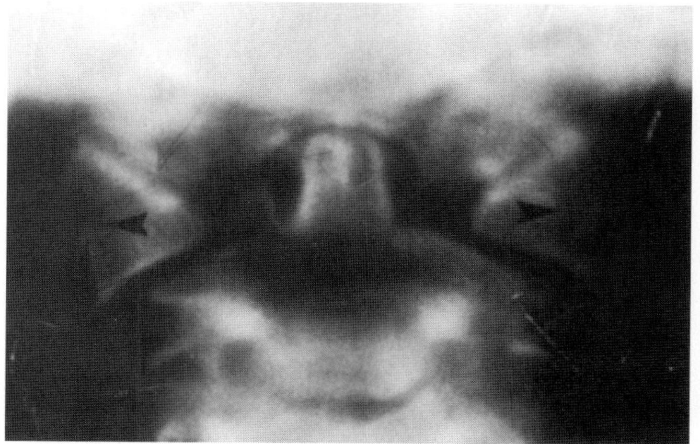

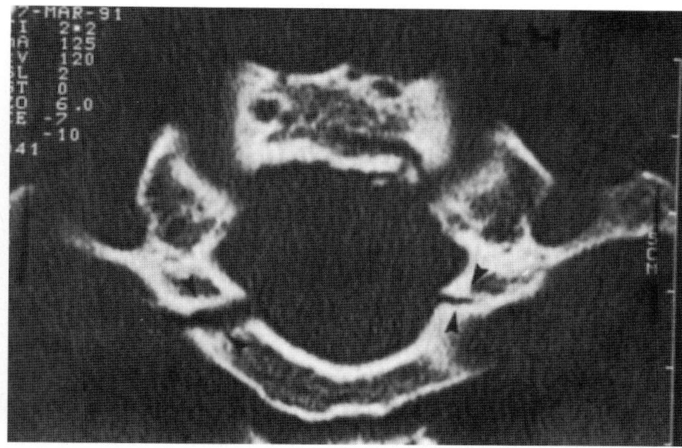

B

C

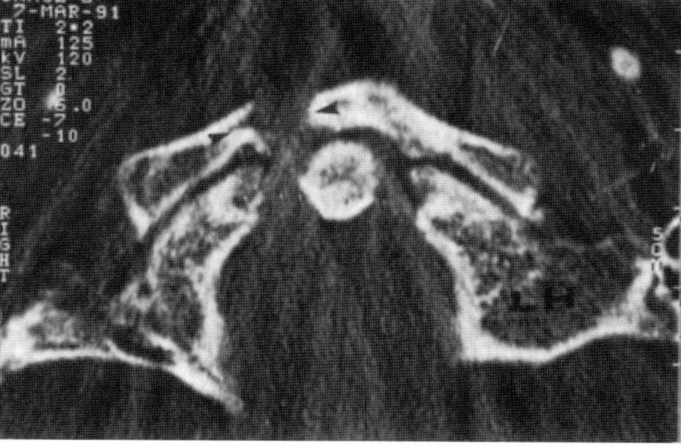

FIGURE 3.4A–C

57. Most cases of quadriplegia that occur during football stem from which of the following mechanisms of injury to the cervical spine?
    (a) Hyperflexion
    (b) Extension-compression
    (c) Flexion-distraction
    (d) Extension-distraction
    (e) Vertical compression
58. Which of the following statements is false regarding traumatic failure of the transverse ligament of the atlas?
    (a) An anterior atlantodens interval of 3.5 mm is the upper limit of normal in adults.
    (b) An anterior atlantodens interval of 1.0 mm does not exclude the diagnosis.
    (c) An anterior atlantodens interval of 4.5 mm is the upper limit of normal in children.
    (d) Initial management should consist of 6 to 8 weeks in a halo vest followed by repeat flexion extension views to confirm adequate ligament healing.
    (e) Isolated traumatic failure of the transverse ligament is less common than the combination of ligament rupture with atlas fracture.
59. A 20-year-old fast-food restaurant drive-through window clerk is seen with complaints of persistent neck pain after a motor vehicle accident 7 months earlier. He was told that he had "strained" his neck, and he was treated with a soft collar for 10 days. His present lateral radiograph is shown in Fig. 3.5A, and a tomographic image is shown in Fig. 3.5B. The best treatment at this moment is
    (a) Soft collar and activity modification (relocation at work from the window to a position requiring less neck rotation)
    (b) Posterior fusion from C1 to C2
    (c) Posterior fusion from the occiput to C2
    (d) Anterior screw fixation
    (e) Halo vest immobilization for 3 months
60. Which of the following points is true regarding surgical decompression for spinal stenosis?
    (a) Even in appropriately selected patients, surgical management rarely yields success rates of greater than 60% to 70% with regard to the relief of leg symptoms.
    (b) The literature contains several reports of poor results, many of which can be attributed to multilevel decompression and the development of postoperative instability.
    (c) No correlation exists between preoperative myelographic findings and outcome.

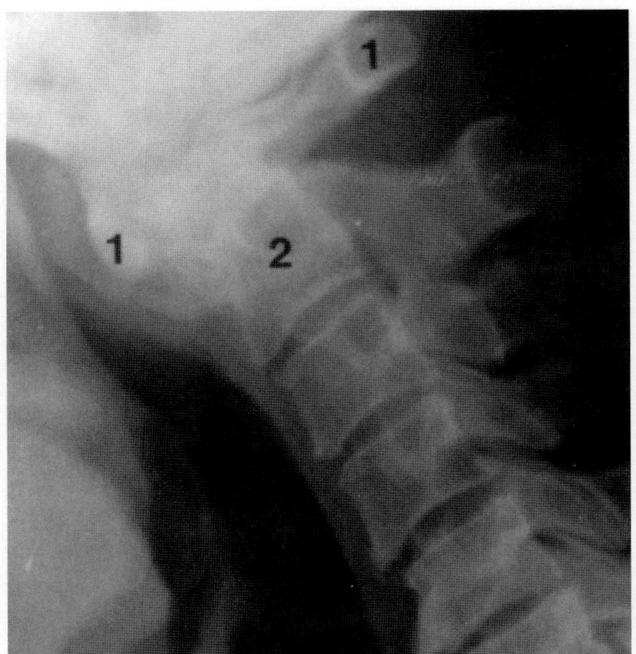

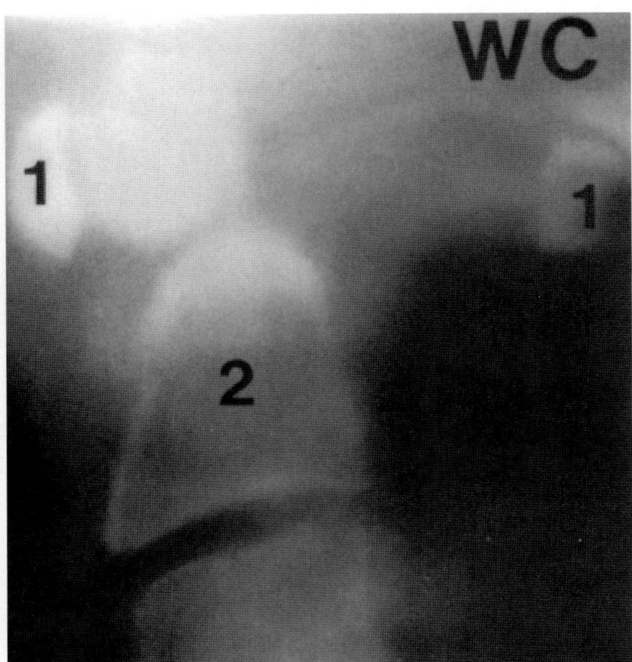

FIGURE 3.5A and B

(d) Postoperative results are independent of the duration of preoperative symptoms.
(e) Low back pain after decompression is less likely when multiple levels are decompressed than when only one or two levels are decompressed.

61. Which of the following statements regarding lumbar burst fractures is true?
    (a) Dural lacerations are commonly encountered, even in the setting of burst fractures without associated laminar fractures.
    (b) Posterior spinal decompression and fusion are contraindicated when there is an associated laminar fracture because of the potential for a concomitant dural laceration and iatrogenic nerve damage.
    (c) Retropulsed bone fragments have been shown to resorb from the canal over time.
    (d) Anterior spinal decompression and fusion are preferable in the setting of an associated laminar fracture because laminar hooks cannot obtain adequate purchase on the fractured lamina.
    (e) L2 is the most commonly affected level.
62. A 13-year-old boy scout presents with neck pain and no neurologic deficit. A radiograph and bone scan are obtained (Fig. 3.6A–C). A biopsy is shown in Fig. 3.6D. The most appropriate treatment for this lesion would be which of the following:
    (a) Observation with careful follow-up at regular intervals
    (b) Chemotherapy followed by radiotherapy and surgical excision
    (c) Resection of the lesion through a posterior approach after an initial course of radiotherapy
    (d) Resection of the tumor and stabilization of the spine through a combined anterior and posterior approach
    (e) Embolization of the tumor followed by excision through a posterior approach
63. Which of the following statements is a correct description of the normal alignment of the spine?
    (a) A curve of less than 20 degrees in the frontal plane is considered normal.
    (b) The normal apex of thoracic kyphosis is at T4.
    (c) The majority of lumbar lordosis exists below L3.
    (d) The normal sagittal vertical axis from the center of the C7 vertebral body should fall 7 cm posterior to the sacral promontory.
    (e) The normal range of thoracic kyphosis is 40 to 50 degrees.
64. Which of the following is the best example of a structural curve?
    (a) A lumbar curve secondary to leg length inequality
    (b) The lumbar component of a King-Moe type III curve
    (c) A thoracic curve without vertebral rotation
    (d) A lumbar curve that does not manifest vertebral wedging
    (e) A thoracic curve that fails to correct on bending films
65. Which of the following statements regarding the natural history of adolescent idiopathic scoliosis is false?

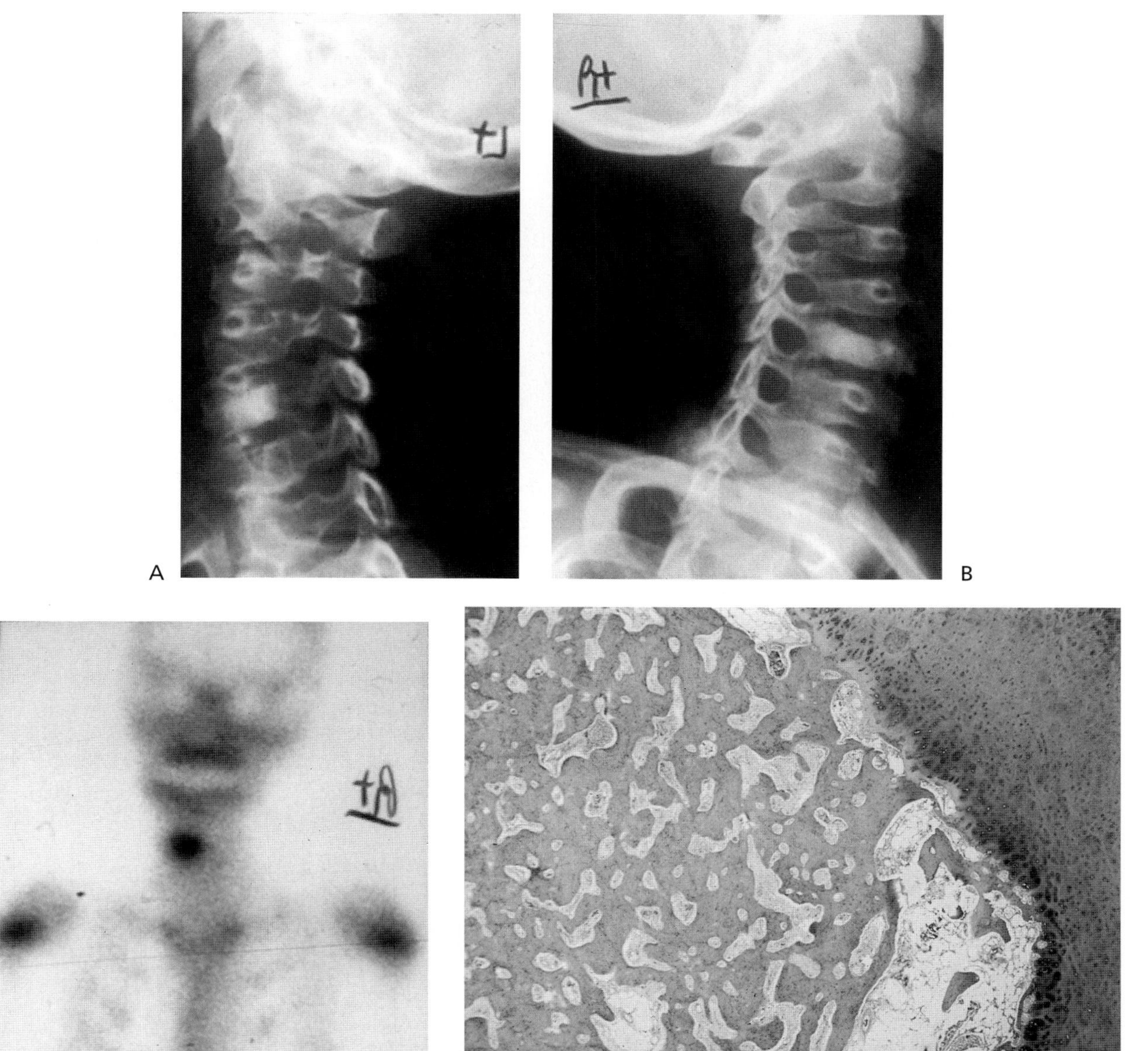

FIGURE 3.6A–D

(a) Some 40-degree curves may continue to progress after skeletal maturity.
(b) Pregnancy and delivery can cause curve progression.
(c) Curves greater than 100 degrees are associated with an increased mortality rate compared with the general population.
(d) The incidence of curve progression is significantly lower in single lumbar and single thoracolumbar curves than in other patterns.
(e) Lumbar curves greater than 60 degrees are associated with increased incidence of low back pain compared with the general population.

66. Which of the following statements about tuberculosis of the spine is false?
    (a) Most patients with spinal tuberculosis do not have neurologic deficit.
    (b) Only 10% of all patients with tuberculosis have skeletal involvement.
    (c) The disc spaces are spared early in the process.

(d) The thoracic spine is the most frequently involved portion of the spine.
(e) Age does not affect the risk of paralysis in instances of cervical involvement.

67. Which of the following statements regarding the treatment of adolescent idiopathic scoliosis is false?
(a) Thoracoplasty is indicated when the thoracic prominence is greater than 6 cm.
(b) Anterior instrumentation has powerful corrective capability and may save fusion levels compared with posterior instrumentation.
(c) King-Moe type I curves should not be treated with selective thoracic fusion.
(d) Fusion of a King-Moe type III or IV pattern short of the neutral and stable vertebra may produce decompensation to the right.
(e) Overcorrection of a King-Moe type II curve may produce decompensation to the left.

68. A 45-year-old x-ray technician presents with complaints of fatigue in her lumbar spine, buttocks, and thighs. Her past orthopaedic history is significant for posterior spinal fusion from L3 to S1 for degenerative disc disease 3 years earlier. The hardware was removed, but she has persistent pain. Standing anteroposterior and lateral radiographs are shown in Fig. 3.7. What is the best explanation for her symptoms?
(a) Malingering
(b) Thoracic hypokyphosis
(c) Sagittal decompensation
(d) Pseudarthrosis
(e) Junctional kyphosis

69. Which of the following congenital spine abnormalities has the worst prognosis?
(a) A unilateral unsegmented bar with a contralateral hemivertebra
(b) A unilateral unsegmented bar
(c) A double convex hemivertebra
(d) An incarcerated single hemivertebra
(e) A block vertebra

70. A 58-year-old woman with long-standing rheumatoid arthritis presents with complaints of occipital headaches and intermittent "electric shocks" into her arms and legs. Physical examination reveals no myelopathic findings. Flexion and extension views of her cervical spine are shown in Fig. 3.8A and B. A magnetic resonance imaging view is shown in Fig. 3.8C. The Ranawat index measures 10 mm. What is the most appropriate management for this patient?

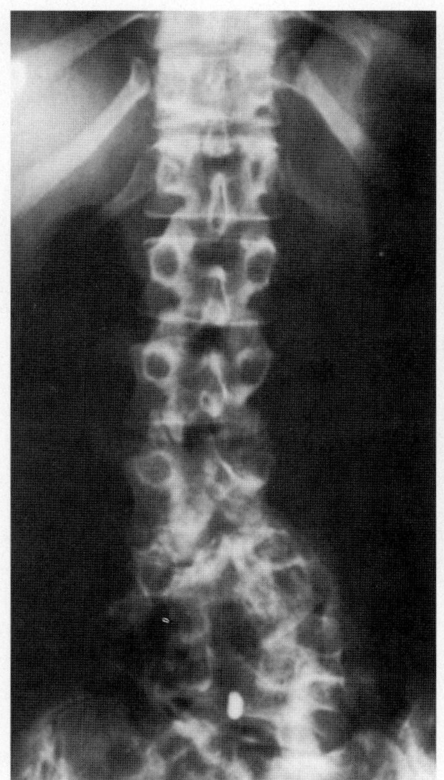
A

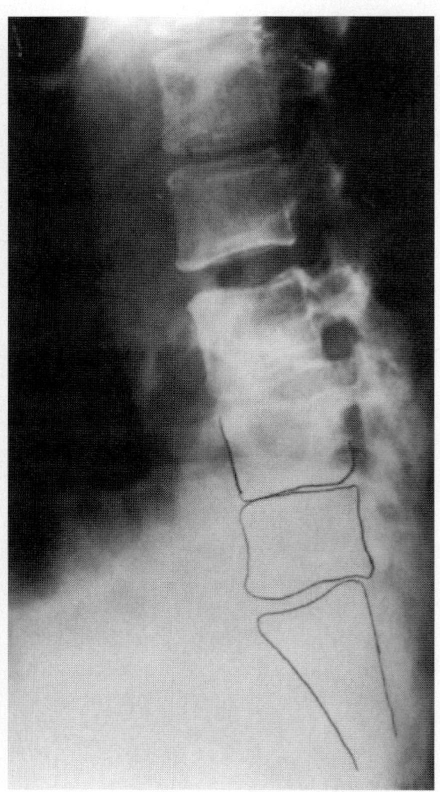
B

FIGURE 3.7A and B

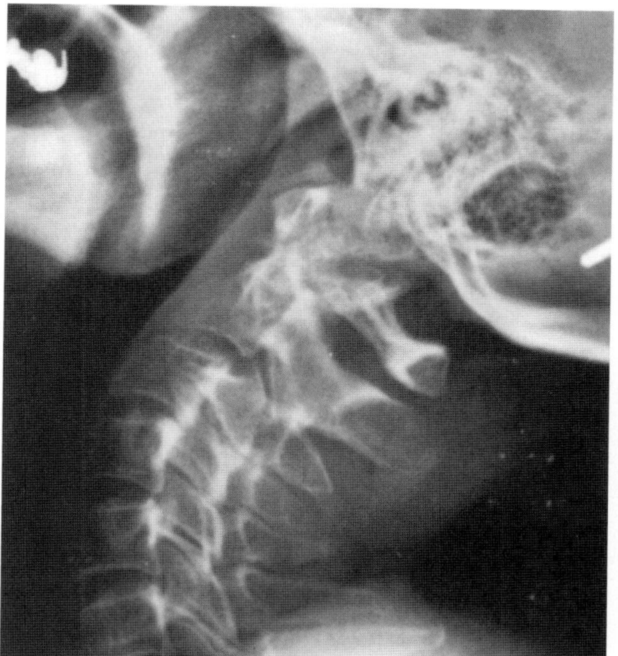

A

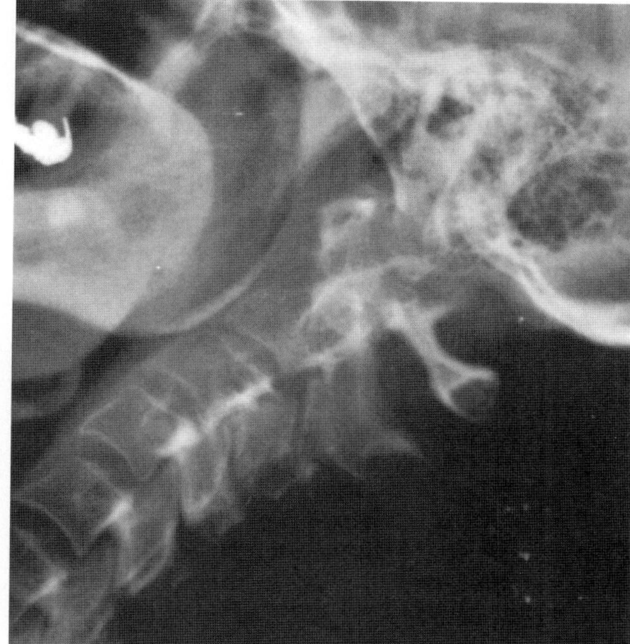

B

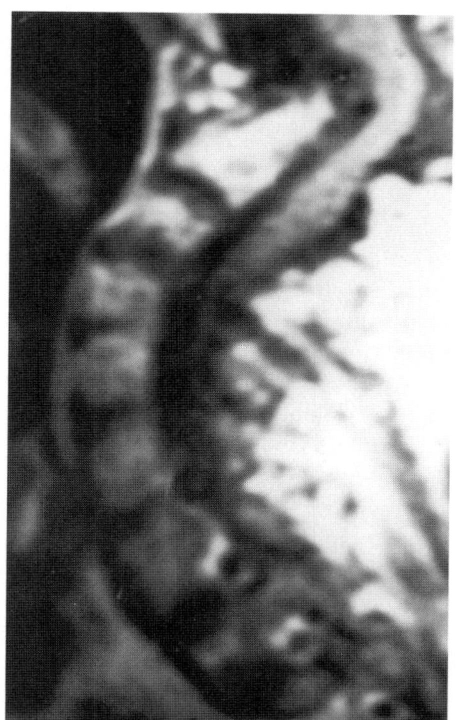

C

FIGURE 3.8A–C

(a) Two months of full-time Philadelphia collar use followed by clinical reassessment
(b) Atlantooccipital fusion
(c) Atlantoaxial fusion
(d) Axis to occiput fusion
(e) Transoral resection of the dens

71. All the following statements regarding congenital spine deformity are true except
   (a) Associated genitourinary system anomalies occur in approximately 20% of affected persons.
   (b) Congenital kyphosis is the most common of the three major patterns of congenital spine deformity.

(c) Kyphosis resulting from a defect of segmentation tends to have a better prognosis than kyphosis produced by a defect of formation.
(d) All forms of nonoperative treatment of congenital kyphosis are useless.
(e) Bracing has no proven efficacy for short, stiff congenital scoliosis curves.

72. An 11-year-old girl presents with a right thoracic idiopathic scoliosis. She is premenarchal and neurologically intact. Radiographic examination reveals a 45-degree right thoracic curve (T5 to T10) and a 20-degree left compensatory curve (T12 to L4). The lateral film shows 5 degrees of thoracic kyphosis and 30 degrees of lumbar lordosis. Bending films show that the right thoracic curve corrects to 15 degrees, and the left lumbar corrects to 0 degrees. She is Risser stage 1. What would be the most appropriate management of this patient?
(a) Repeat radiographs in 3 months
(b) Bracing with follow-up radiographs in 3 months
(c) Anteroposterior fusion
(d) Posterior spinal fusion
(e) Electric stimulation, melatonin supplementation, and follow-up in 3 months

73. A 10-year-old girl and her 15-year-old brother present for scoliosis evaluation. She is Risser stage 1 with a 17-degree right thoracic curve. Her brother is Risser stage 4 with a 22-degree right thoracic curve. Which of the following statements is most accurate?
(a) If untreated, she has a significantly higher chance of curve progression than her brother.
(b) If untreated, he has a significantly higher chance of curve progression than his sister.
(c) If untreated, they have similar chances of curve progression.
(d) They both should be braced on initial evaluation because they are affected siblings.
(e) He has a "twisted sister."

74. A 14-year-old boy is brought to you because his family is concerned about his progressive, painful, "hunchedback" deformity. Physical examination confirms a kyphotic deformity that does not correct with attempted hyperextension. Muscle tightness of the hamstrings and anterior shoulder girdle is noted. He is neurologically intact. Radiographs reveal 12 degrees of wedging at T7, T8, and T9 with an 80-degree thoracic kyphosis that corrects to 45 degrees on lateral cross-table hyperextension radiography. What is the most appropriate treatment at this stage?
(a) Milwaukee bracing and reevaluation in 3 months
(b) Thoracolumbosacral orthosis bracing and reevaluation in 3 months
(c) Postural hyperextension exercises
(d) Anterior discectomy and fusion plus instrumented posterior spinal fusion
(e) Instrumented posterior spinal fusion

75. A 20-year-old hospital cafeteria cashier presents for scoliosis evaluation. She is otherwise perfectly healthy and is Risser 5. The right thoracic and left lumbar curves measure 78 and 72 degrees, respectively. She has no pain. Bending films show correction of the thoracic curve to 40 degrees and the lumbar curve to 40 degrees. The curve is classified as a King-Moe double major curve. Which of the following statements is true?
(a) She needs operative spinal stabilization.
(b) The most appropriate treatment is bracing.
(c) This curve necessitates a magnetic resonance imaging scan.
(d) The most appropriate treatment is selective thoracic fusion.
(e) No treatment is necessary because the patient is skeletally mature and has no pain.

76. An 11-year-old cheerleader presents for scoliosis evaluation. Her past medical history is unremarkable. She is Risser stage 1. Radiographs reveal a 20-degree single left thoracic curve. She is neurologically intact and denies back pain. What is the most appropriate initial management?
(a) Anteroposterior spinal fusion
(b) Observation with follow-up radiographs in 3 to 6 months
(c) Initiate bracing with follow-up radiographs in 3 to 6 months
(d) Observation with follow-up radiographs in 1 year
(e) Magnetic resonance imaging of the entire spine

77. A 74-year-old woman presents with a 3-month history of progressive midthoracic back pain. She complains of leg weakness and intermittent fevers. She denies bowel and bladder dysfunction. Laboratory studies include a white blood cell count of 6,000 and an erythrocyte sedimentation rate of 90 mm per hour. Examination shows a significant kyphotic deformity at the midthoracic area, grade 3/5 motor strength in the lower extremities, and lower extremity hyperreflexia. A sagittal magnetic resonance image is shown in Fig. 3.9. A computed tomography–guided biopsy and multiple blood cultures reveal *Staphylococcus aureus*. Culture-specific intravenous antibiotics are initiated. The most appropriate additional treatment at this time would be
(a) Supine bed rest with observation for signs of sepsis
(b) Casting in extension
(c) Decompressive laminectomy
(d) Anterior débridement, decompression, and anterior fusion
(e) Decompressive laminectomy and posterior spinal fusion

78. A 60-year-old woman with lumbar stenosis and instability undergoes an instrumented posterior spinal fusion with laminectomy and decompression from L3 to S1. Pedicle screws are used at multiple levels. She is unable to void when the Foley catheter is removed on

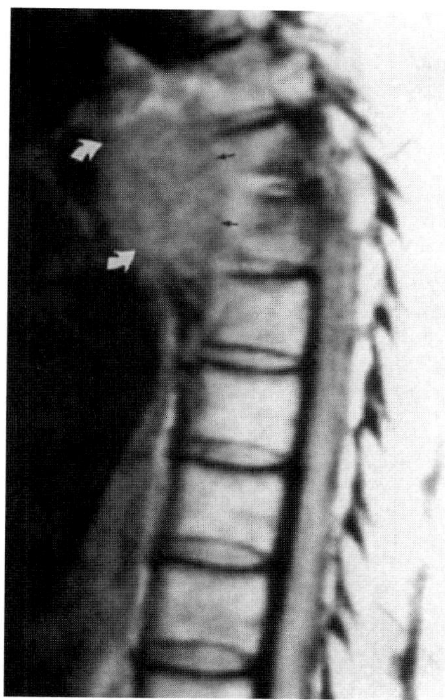

FIGURE 3.9

postoperative day 2. Physical examination reveals normal motor strength, sensation, and deep tendon reflexes in both lower extremities. What is the most appropriate next step to elucidate the source of her urinary dysfunction?

(a) Urology consultation for urodynamic testing
(b) Magnetic resonance imaging scan to rule out epidural hematoma
(c) Computed tomography scan to rule out neural compromise from pedicle screw malposition
(d) Urinalysis and culture to rule out urinary tract infection
(e) Digital rectal examination and assessment of perianal sensation

79. A 45-year-old man presents with a 6-month history of midthoracic pain. In the past month, he has experienced paresthesias and a feeling of heaviness in both legs. His past medical history is unremarkable, and he denies fevers and weight loss. His motor examination is grade 4/5 in all lower limb muscle groups, and his sensory examination is normal. Plain radiographs of his thoracic spine are normal. Which of the following would be the most appropriate next diagnostic test in this situation?
(a) Flexion extension radiographs
(b) Thoracic spine computed tomography scan
(c) Nerve conduction studies
(d) Thoracic myelography
(e) Thoracic computed tomography myelography

80. What is the incidence of lumbar herniated nucleus pulposus in asymptomatic patients less than 60 years of age?
(a) 0%
(b) 2%
(c) 10%
(d) 20%
(e) 30%

81. Which of the following statements about posterior lumbar interbody fusion (PLIF) is false?
(a) Wide posterior decompression is necessary.
(b) It has been proven to result in a lower rate of pseudarthrosis compared with standard posterolateral intertransverse process fusion.
(c) There is a theoretical biomechanical advantage to having the site of arthrodesis anteriorly.
(d) Adequate nerve root decompression can be achieved.
(e) It permits complete disc excision and restoration of disc height.

82. A 13-year-old boy is referred from his primary care physician for scoliosis evaluation. He states that he was not aware that he had scoliosis until now, but he has recently experienced difficulty sleeping because of back pain. His curve is 26 degrees and does not correct with side bending. Plain films and computed tomography images are shown in Fig. 3.10 A and B, respectively. Based on this information, which of the following statements is most accurate?
(a) He should be treated with nonsteroidal antiinflammatory drugs immediately.
(b) He will require a posterior spinal fusion to correct his curvature regardless of the duration of his symptoms.
(c) If complete excision of the lesion is accomplished within 15 months of the onset of his symptoms, then significant curve regression and/or complete resolution can be anticipated.
(d) His curve has a high likelihood of regressing spontaneously regardless of the duration of his symptoms.
(e) Primary spinal fusion (at the time of excision of the lesion) is never indicated in the management of this disorder.

83. A 33-year-old podiatrist presents with a 5-month history of midthoracic back pain. He has been under the care of his roommate (who is a chiropractor), but his pain has worsened despite multiple manipulations. His roommate has referred him for orthopaedic evaluation because of a 24-hour history of ataxia. Review of systems reveals a recent 20-pound weight loss, intermittent fevers, and occasional night sweats. Physical examination is significant for lower extremity hyperreflexia and a positive Babinski reflex (upgoing hallux). A magnetic resonance imaging scan of the thoracic spine is

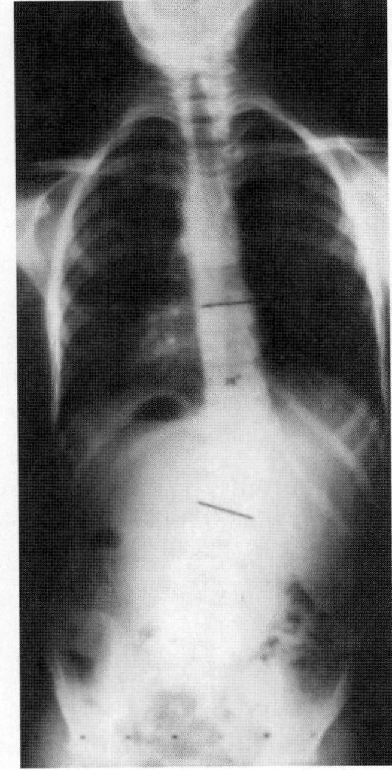

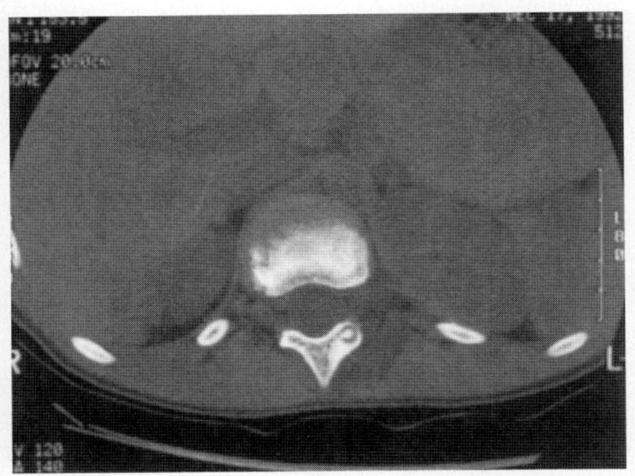

FIGURE 3.10A and B

shown in Fig. 3.11. A computed tomography–guided biopsy is performed. What will be the most likely findings of the biopsy?
(a) Gram-positive cocci in pairs
(b) Gram-negative rods
(c) Gram-positive cocci in clusters
(d) Acid-fast, nonmotile rods
(e) Gram-negative intracellular cocci

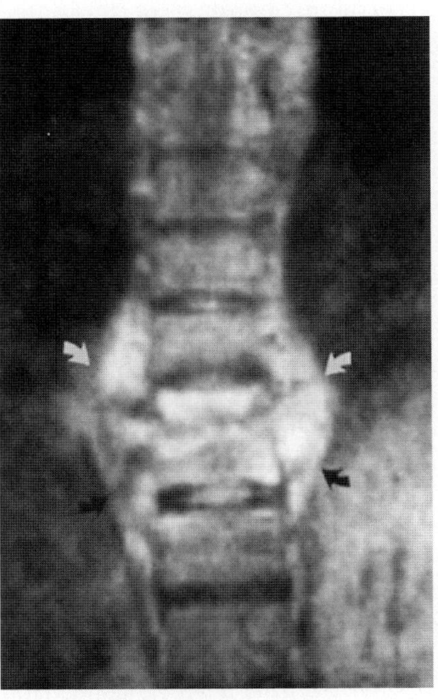

FIGURE 3.11

84. Which of the following would be the most appropriate treatment for the patient described in question 83?
    (a) 3 to 6 months of bed rest and culture-directed chemotherapy
    (b) Cast application followed by 3 to 6 months of culture-directed, outpatient chemotherapy
    (c) Anterior débridement and decompression followed by 3 to 6 months of culture-directed, outpatient chemotherapy
    (d) Posterior decompression (laminectomy) followed by 3 to 6 months of culture-directed, outpatient chemotherapy
    (e) Anterior débridement and decompression with strut grafting followed by 3 to 6 months of culture-directed, outpatient chemotherapy
85. Which of the following statements is false regarding the artery of Adamkiewicz?
    (a) It is also known as the great anterior radicular artery.
    (b) It arises most commonly from an anterior intercostal artery on the right side.
    (c) It sometimes arises from a superior lumbar artery.
    (d) It most commonly enters the vertebral canal through an intervertebral foramen at the T9-12 level.
    (e) It is the main arterial supply for the inferior two-thirds of the anterior spinal cord.

86. An 11-year-old male football player presents to your office with grade 1 spondylolisthesis (20% slippage) and back pain. No treatment is prescribed. At 6-month follow-up, the spondylolisthesis has progressed to 45% with worsened back pain. The most appropriate treatment at this time would be which of the following?
    (a) Restriction from contact sports and a hyperextension cast with thigh extension
    (b) Restriction from contact sports and a lumbosacral orthosis
    (c) A one-level bilateral posterior fusion *in situ*
    (d) Laminectomy and posterior fusion *in situ*
    (e) Combined anteroposterior fusion *in situ*
87. The predominant collagen composition of the lumbar disc is
    (a) Annulus, type 1; nucleus, type 2
    (b) Annulus, type 2; nucleus, type 1
    (c) Annulus, type 1; nucleus, type 1
    (d) Annulus, type 2; nucleus, type 2
    (e) Annulus, type 1; nucleus, type 3
88. What is the recommended target depth for pedicle screw insertion in the lumbar spine?
    (a) 25% through the vertebral body
    (b) 40% through the vertebral body
    (c) 80% through the vertebral body
    (d) Slight penetration of the anterior cortex of the vertebral body
    (e) To the anterior cortex of the vertebral body without penetrating it
89. A 50-year-old man with diffuse idiopathic skeletal hyperostosis presents with cervical stiffness and weakness of his triceps. What disc level and nerve root are most likely affected?
    (a) C5-6 level, C6 root
    (b) C6-7 level, C6 root
    (c) C 6-7 level, C7 root
    (d) C7-T1 level, C7 root
    (e) C7-T1 level, C8 root
90. A 55-year-old woman presents for follow-up 1 year after anteroposterior spinal fusion for lumbar scoliosis. She states that she has experienced progressive thoracolumbar pain over the preceding 4 months. She denies fever or chills. She is neurologically intact. Anteroposterior and lateral standing films demonstrate junctional kyphosis at the superior end of the hardware (T10-11). What is the most appropriate management for this situation?
    (a) Thoracolumbosacral orthosis until fusion matures
    (b) Conversion of the superior pedicle screws to hooks
    (c) Extension of the instrumentation and fusion to T3
    (d) Technetium scan
    (e) Removal of all the hardware and bracing of the patient
91. A 30-year-old dancer presents to your office for the evaluation of acute low back pain. All the following factors would persuade you to obtain plain lumbar radiographs within the first month of this patient's symptoms except
    (a) Radiation of the pain to the right posterior thigh
    (b) Saddle anesthesia
    (c) History of recent urinary tract infection
    (d) History of malignant disease
    (e) Recent onset of overflow incontinence
92. A 3-year-old boy presents with a left thoracic scoliosis. Plain radiographs reveal no evidence of a congenital deformity. Magnetic resonance imaging of the head and spine reveal no intraspinal or intracranial lesions. The apical vertebra is phase 1, and the rib-vertebral angle difference is 25 degrees. What is the most appropriate treatment for this patient?
    (a) Anteroposterior spinal fusion
    (b) Observation with follow-up radiographs in 4 to 6 months
    (c) Posterior instrumentation without fusion
    (d) Posterior spinal fusion without instrumentation
    (e) Serial casting followed by full-time bracing
93. A 40-year-old woman with a 1-month history of thoracic back pain presents with acute bilateral leg weakness and a partial sensory deficit at the L1 level. A sagittal magnetic resonance imaging scan is shown in Fig. 3.12. The most appropriate next step in management is which of the following?
    (a) A short trial of bed rest with gradual mobilization and limitation of activities
    (b) Thoracolumbosacral orthosis
    (c) Posterior thoracic laminectomy and excision
    (d) Transthoracic transpleural exposure and excision
    (e) Computed tomography–guided biopsy

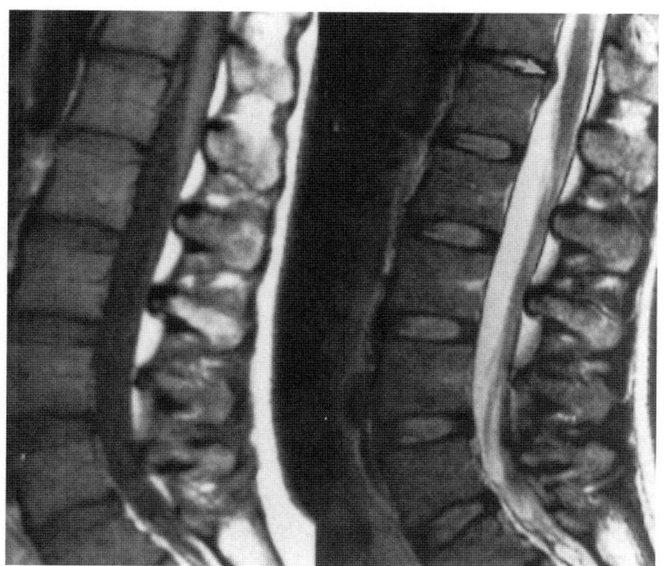

FIGURE 3.12

94. A 52-year-old hairdresser with rheumatoid arthritis presents with lower extremity weakness and recalcitrant neck pain. Cervical spine flexion and extension films show pronounced C1-2 subluxation and mild C2-3 subluxation (Fig. 3.13A). The posterior alantodens interval measures 12 mm in extension. A sagittal magnetic resonance image is shown in Fig. 3.13B. The Ranawat index measures 16 mm. Which of the following would be the most appropriate form of intervention?
    (a) Anterior odontoid resection
    (b) Posterior fusion of C1 to C2 with Gallie wiring
    (c) Posterior C1 decompression and fusion of C1 to C5 with transarticular C1 to C2 screw fixation
    (d) Occiput to C3 fusion
    (e) Posterior occiput to C2 fusion
95. The patient in question 94 undergoes a posterior occiput to C5 fusion with occipitocervical plating. At 1-year follow-up, she complains of urinary incontinence, ataxia, and progressive lower extremity weakness. Radiographs, flexion-extension views, and tomograms reveal a solid fusion at all levels. The C2-3 subluxation has been reduced. However, C1 and C2 have been fused in a subluxated position with a posterior alantodens interval of 10-mm. What is the most appropriate form of intervention at this time?
    (a) Takedown of the C1 to C2 fusion and revision of the fusion in a more lordotic position
    (b) Application of a halo vest
    (c) Cervical traction until symptoms resolve, then conversion to a halo vest
    (d) Anterior odontoid resection
    (e) Takedown of the posterior fusion and revision of the fusion in a more flexed position
96. During scoliosis screening, which of the following scoliometer measurements is the cutoff for referral to an orthopaedist?
    (a) 5 degrees
    (b) 7 degrees
    (c) 9 degrees
    (d) 10 degrees
    (e) 12 degrees
97. A 40-year-old man presents with insidious, progressive low back pain. Sagittal reformatted computed tomography images are shown in Fig. 3.14. Which of the following diagnosis does the computed tomography scan suggest?

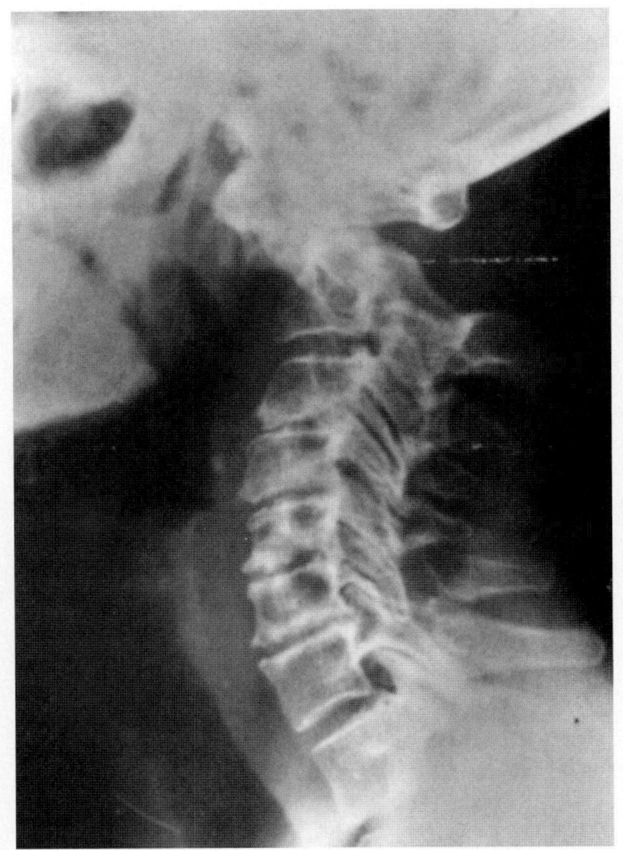
A

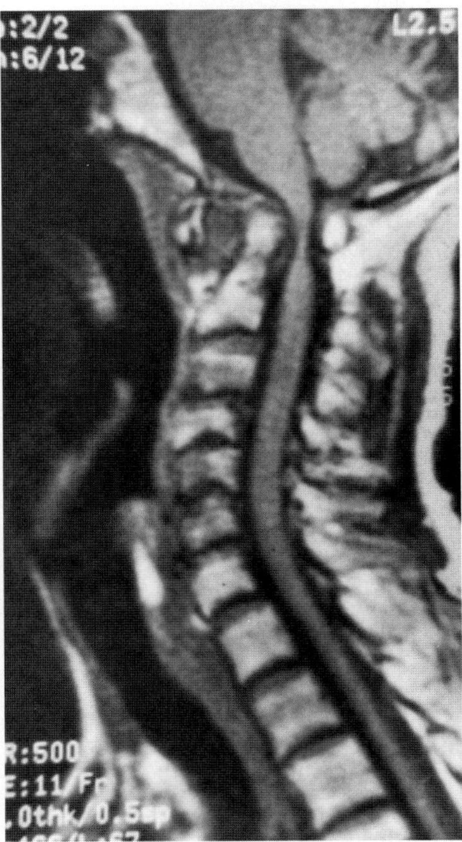

B

FIGURE 3.13 A and B

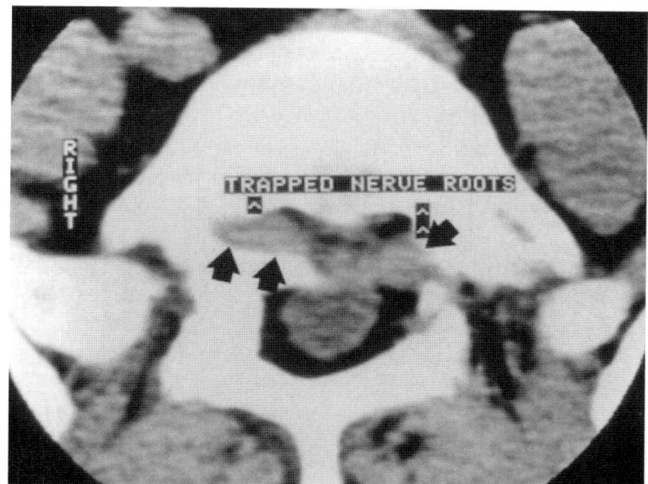

A

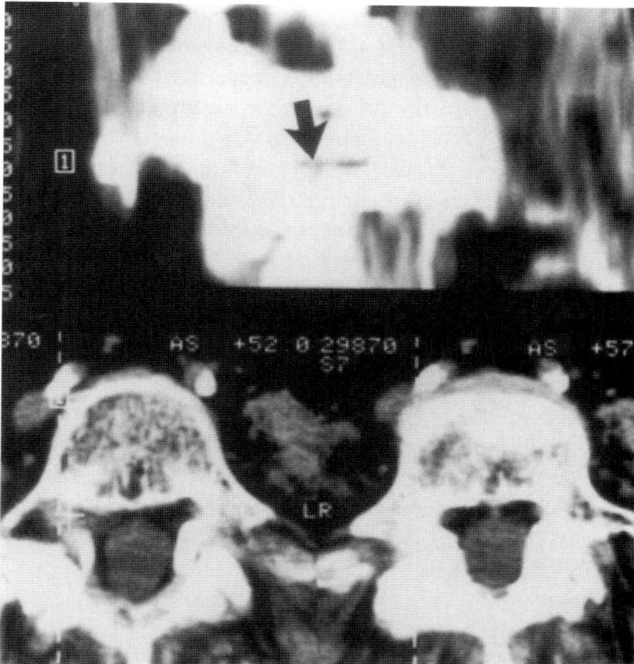

B

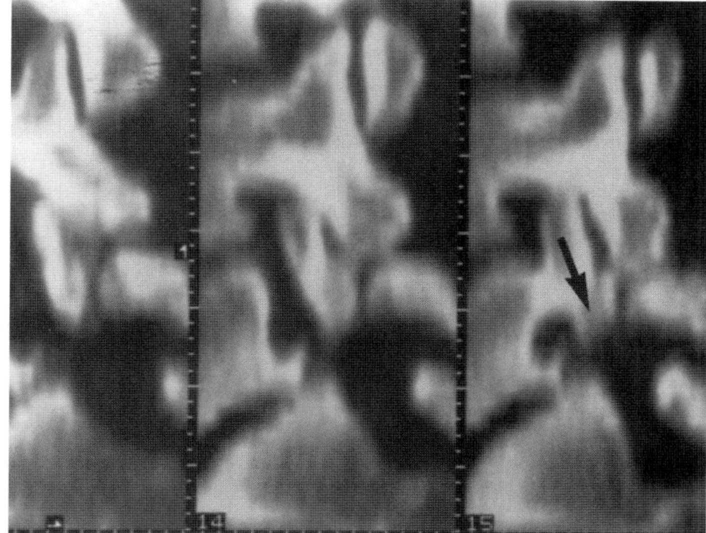

C

FIGURE 3.14A–C

(a) L4-L5 facet osteoarthritis
(b) L5 spondylolysis
(c) L5-S1 facet osteoarthritis
(d) Lumbar scoliosis
(e) L3-L4 facet osteoarthritis

98. What structure (or structures) passes (or pass) through the foramen transversarium of C7?
(a) The vertebral artery and vein
(b) An accessory vertebral vein
(c) The vertebral artery and the greater occipital nerve
(d) The vertebral artery
(e) The vertebral artery and the long thoracic nerve

99. The primary arterial blood supply to the spinal cord in the cervical spine is derived from
(a) Branches from the thyrocervical trunks
(b) Segmental branches from the aorta
(c) Branches from the first segments of the subclavian arteries
(d) Branches from the common carotid arteries
(e) The basilar artery

ANSWERS

1. **c** C6. The carotid tubercle (Chassaignac tubercle) is an enlargement of the anterior tubercle of the transverse process of C6. It is a useful surface landmark that can be used to determine the appropriate level for incision in an anterior approach to the cervical spine. The cricoid cartilage is another palpable surface landmark that corresponds to the C6 vertebral level. Other useful anterior cervical surface landmarks and their corresponding vertebral levels are as follows: hard palate (C1), angle of mandible (C2), hyoid bone (C3), and thyroid cartilage (C4 to C5). Posteriorly, the spinous processes of C2, C7, and T1 are the most prominent palpable landmarks.

   Note: The spinous processes of C2 to C6 are bifid; the spinous process C7 is not.

Reference

Hoppenfeld S: Surgical Exposures in Orthopaedics, 2nd Ed. Philadelphia, JB Lippincott, pp. 264–275, 1994.

2. **b** Arterial seeding of the spine is believed to be the most common route of metastasis from the prostate. Statement b is false. Hematogenous seeding is *not* believed to represent the most common vehicle of metastasis to the spine. The Batson venous plexus is commonly believed to be the route for prostatic metastases. This low-pressure system is valveless and has been proven capable of draining the pelvic and abdominal viscera when intraabdominal pressure increases. Tumors of the prostate, breast, lung, and kidney are the most common primary tumors for vertebral metastases in adults. The most common primary tumors for spinal metastases in children include Ewing sarcoma, osteosarcoma, rhabdomyosarcoma, lymphoma, and neuroblastoma. Myeloma is, in fact, the most common tumor involving the spine, but, technically, it represents a primary tumor of the marrow elements rather than a metastatic lesion.

   The spine is the most common site of skeletal metastasis. Approximately 85% of spinal metastases occur in the vertebral body. Spinal metastases have been detected in up to 80% of patients who die of cancer. However, most metastases to the spine are clinically insignificant, and fewer than 25% of them produce spinal stenosis. Cadaveric studies suggest that most spinal metastases are asymptomatic. Pain (not neural compromise) is the most common presenting symptom.

3. **d** The incidence is higher among patients with diabetes mellitus. Patients with diabetes mellitus are at increased risk of developing degenerative spondylolisthesis. A defect in collagen cross-linking has been invoked to account for this observed phenomenon. The incidence increases with advancing age. Females are more commonly affected than males. Oophorectomy is also a risk factor. The most common level of involvement is L4 to L5. Relative immobility of the more caudal vertebral segment predisposes to degenerative spondylolisthesis. Thus, hemisacralization of L5 predisposes to degenerative spondylolisthesis at L4 to L5. Other sources of L5 immobility (e.g., advanced L5-S1 spondylosis or L5-S1 fusion) also focus stress at L4 and L5 and increase susceptibility to degenerative L4-L5 spondylolisthesis.

Reference

Frymoyer JW: Degenerative Spondylolisthesis. J Am Acad Orthop Surg, 2(1):9–15, 1994.

4. **a** Produces hypesthesia to pain and temperature on the side contralateral to the lesion. The Brown-Séquard syndrome is caused by unilateral transection of the spinal cord. Classically, it is produced by penetrating trauma (i.e., a projectile or stab wound). Consequently, ipsilateral motor function is lost distal to the level of the lesion because the pyramidal decussation (the crossing of the upper motor neurons of the corticospinal tracts) occurs cephalad to the spinal cord (in the caudal medulla oblongata). Similarly, ipsilateral proprioception is lost caudal to the level of a Brown-Séquard lesion because the ascending fibers of the posterior column (fasciculus gracilis and fasciculus cuneatus) cross the midline cephalad to the spinal cord (also in the medulla). Contralateral sensation of pain and temperature is lost caudal to the level of the lesion because pain and temperature afferent fibers cross the midline at the level of their dorsal root ganglia immediately on entering the spinal cord (before ascending in the lateral spinothalamic tracts). Most patients with Brown-Séquard syndrome recover bowel and bladder function.

Reference

Benson DR, Keenan TL: Evaluation and Treatment of Trauma to the Vertebral Column. Instr Course Lect, 71:577–589, 1990.

5. **d** Arteriography. The history and magnetic resonance imaging findings are consistent with renal metastasis to the thoracic spine with vertebral body destruction. The tumor and bone debris have caused spinal cord compression with resultant myelopathy. Prompt decompression is warranted and could not be accomplished by either radiation or chemotherapy. Renal metastases are notable for their relative resistance to radiotherapy. A spinal tap would not be appropriate because the dura is resistant to direct invasion from local tumor expansion, and intrathecal metastasis is rare. Furthermore,

the presence or absence of intrathecal metastasis would not affect the decision to decompress and stabilize this spine (given the patient's neurologic status).

Renal metastases tend to be extremely vascular. Thus, preoperative diagnostic angiography is an integral part of managing such lesions. Concomitant embolization can be conducted to minimize intraoperative blood loss and should be performed within 48 hours preoperatively. With thoracic lesions, the artery of Adamkiewicz should be located to ensure that it is preserved during embolization (as well as during surgery), to avoid spinal cord infarction. Serum transferrin is a useful baseline nutritional parameter, but it is less important than preventing intraoperative exsanguination.

6. **d** Administration of a methylprednisolone bolus (30 mg/kg body weight) within 8 hours of injury, followed by a continuous infusion of 5.4 mg/kg per hour for 23 hours. According to Bracken's multicenter, randomized, prospective trial, the recommended methylprednisolone protocol is a loading dose of 30 mg/kg given within the 8 hours after injury, followed by 5.4 mg/kg per hour for the next 23 hours. This pharmacologic approach provided significant improvement in neurologic recovery after acute spinal cord injury. The rationale behind high-dose steroid administration is to minimize secondary injury to the cord by curtailing local edema and free radical formation.

   Sacral sparing (intact perianal sensation, with preserved motor function to the anal sphincter and flexor hallucis longus) is a good prognostic sign because it signifies that at least some of the spinal tracts remain in continuity. The presence of sacral sparing implies that there has not been a complete cord transection and, therefore, that there is potential for recovery of additional function. In such a setting, optimizing the milieu for recovery and minimizing secondary injury (by immobilization and control of local swelling) are crucial.

References

Bracken MB: A Randomized, Controlled Trial of Methylprednisolone or Naloxone in the Treatment of Acute Spinal Cord Injury. N Engl J Med, 322:1406–1461, 1990.

Bracken MB: Pharmacological Treatment of Acute Spinal Cord Injury: Current Status and Future Projects. J Emerg Med, 11:43–48, 1993.

7. **c** Six weeks of parenteral antibiotics guided by the culture sensitivities from the aspiration. This situation is a typical presentation of subacute pyogenic vertebral osteomyelitis. Many affected persons do not present with constitutional symptoms. The magnetic resonance images reveal involvement of the disc space and the vertebral bodies. The process is believed to begin in the disc space with secondary spread into the adjacent vertebral bodies. Other pertinent features of the magnetic resonance images include the absence of bony collapse, canal compromise, or abscess formation.

   Precise identification of the inciting organism is mandatory. More than 50% of cases of pyogenic vertebral osteomyelitis are caused by *Staphylococcus aureus*. *Pseudomonas* species are commonly associated with vertebral infection in intravenous drug abusers. Cases associated with genitourinary instrumentation of infection are commonly associated with gram-negative organisms such as *Escherichia coli* and *Proteus*.

   In cases of putative vertebral osteomyelitis, positive blood cultures can be used to guide antibiotic therapy. However, blood cultures are negative in more than 75% of cases. In all other cases, biopsy is required to confirm the diagnosis and identify the organism and its antibiotic sensitivities (computed tomography–guided closed needle biopsy is the preferred technique). Recommended treatment is 6 weeks of culture-specific parenteral antibiotics. Immobilization and brace use should be incorporated into the treatment regimen for analgesia as well as to prevent deformity and neurologic deterioration.

   Surgical intervention is warranted in the following specific situations: (1) for open biopsy to identify the inciting organism (when computed tomography–guided biopsy is nondiagnostic), (2) in cases of prolonged, unsuccessful nonoperative treatment, (3) in the presence of an abscess with clinical sepsis, (4) in spinal cord compression from abscess formation or from collapsed vertebral elements, or (5) in significant spinal deformity from vertebral destruction.

8. **e** None of the above. In the cervical spine, nerve roots exit over the disc that lies above their numerically corresponding vertebrae (i.e., the C4 nerve root exits over the C3-4 disc). The C8 nerve root is the one exception to this rule (the C8 root has no numerically corresponding vertebra; it exits above the C7-T1 disc). In contradistinction to the cervical spine, nerve roots in the thoracolumbar spine exit below the pedicles of their numerically corresponding vertebrae.

   A cervical disc herniation affects the nerve root that exits above the affected disc. Thus, a C6-7 disc herniation would impinge on the C7 root. Likewise, a C7-T1 disc herniation would impinge on the C8 nerve root. The C8 root does not have a testable reflex arc. The biceps reflex arc is primarily mediated by the C5 nerve root. The brachioradialis reflex tests the function of the C6 nerve root. The triceps reflex arc is primarily mediated by the C7 nerve root. The Moro reflex is the startle reflex in infants; it is irrelevant to a discussion of cervical radiculopathy. Manifestations of C8 nerve root compromise include (1) loss of finger flexion motor strength and (2) decreased sensation in the ring and small fingers.

9. **b** Anterior cord syndrome. The anterior cord syndrome results from a flexion or compression mechanism that produces a total loss of motor function distal to the level of the lesion. Sensation of deep pressure, vibration, and proprioception (dorsal columns) is preserved. This syndrome carries the worst prognosis of all partial cord injuries (no recovery in approximately 90% of affected patients). The Brown-Séquard syndrome and the central cord syndrome are associated with better prognoses because of their partial sparing of motor function and their greater potential for recovery (functional recovery in approximately 90% of patients with Brown-Séquard syndrome and functional recovery in approximately 75% of patients with central cord syndrome). Posterior cord syndrome is extremely rare. Full motor function is preserved, but posterior column function is lost caudal to the level of the lesion. Tabes dorsalis (a manifestation of syphilis) produces symptoms similar to those of the posterior cord syndrome. However, unlike the other listed answers, tabes dorsalis is atraumatic in origin.

Reference

Garfin SR, Vaccaro AR: Orthopaedic Knowledge Update: Spine. Rosemont, IL, American Academy of Orthopedic Surgeons, p. 38, 1997.

10. **c** It produces greater loss of function in the lower extremities than in the upper extremities. The central cord syndrome is the most common incomplete spinal cord injury syndrome. The syndrome typically occurs in elderly persons in whom the hypertrophied ligamentum flavum predisposes the cord to contusion (with or without associated fracture) from a hyperextension mechanism. Cord contusion produces central hemorrhage and edema. Motor function in the upper extremities is more severely affected than in the lower extremities because of the somatotopic organization of the lateral corticospinal tracts wherein the upper motor neurons to the upper extremity are located most centrally (Fig. 3.15). Perianal sensation is typically spared (sacral-sparing) because of the more peripheral position of the more caudal afferent fibers in the spinothalamic tracts.
11. **a** The patient will remain a T4 paraplegic with a possible one to two level improvement in motor and/or sensory function. In general, a statement regarding the prognosis for neurologic recovery cannot be made until spinal shock is over. The return of the bulbocavernosus reflex (Fig. 3.16) is typically a reliable indicator of the termination of spinal shock. Spinal shock represents physiologic rather than structural disruption of the reflex arc. However, in the setting of a conus lesion, the bulbocavernosus reflex (S3 and S4) arc may be anatomically disrupted, and, thus, this reflex will not be elicited regardless of the presence or absence of spinal shock. Thus, in the situation described in this question (in which the severe L1 burst fracture would certainly have inflicted great structural damage to the adjacent conus), the bulbocavernosus cannot be used as an indicator of the presence or absence of spinal shock. Under

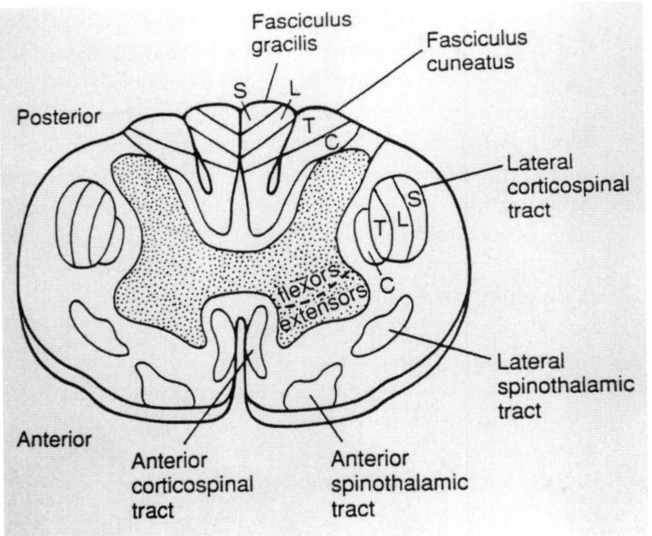

FIGURE 3.15

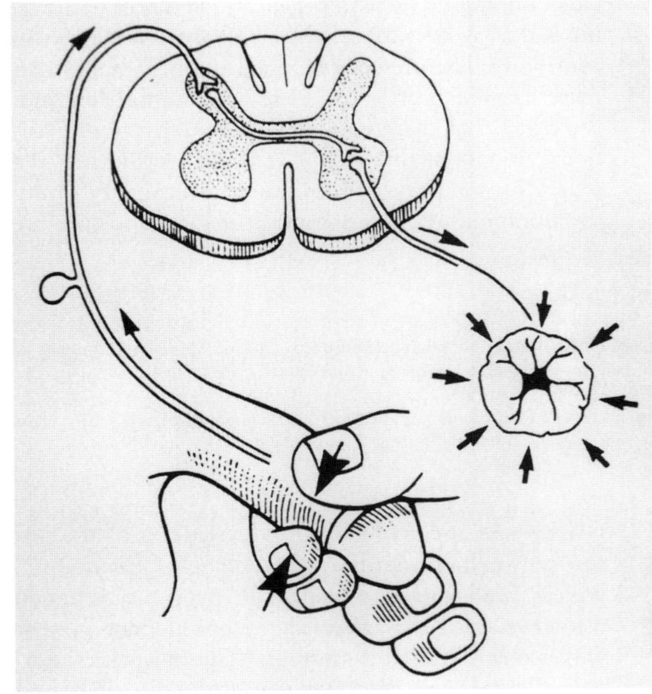

FIGURE 3.16

virtually all circumstances, spinal shock lasts no more than 48 hours. After termination of spinal shock, total absence of motor and sensory function caudal to the level of injury signifies a complete spinal cord lesion. The prognosis for significant further neurologic improvement is dismal in this setting, with maximal potential recovery of one to two levels of motor and/or sensory function.

Reference

Garfin SR, Vaccaro AR: Orthopaedic Knowledge Update: Spine. Rosemont, IL, American Academy of Orthopedic Surgeons, p. 37, 1997.

12. **b** 35%. At the level of the atlas, the cervical spinal cord occupies approximately one-third of the canal diameter. The diameters of both the canal and the cord vary considerably along the course of the spine. There is bulbous enlargement of the cord in the cervical and lumbar regions owing to the volume of anterior horn cells giving rise to motor axons to the extremities at these levels. In the subaxial cervical spine and thoracolumbar segments, the cord occupies approximately 50% of the canal diameter. The cervical canal widens considerably at the C1 level because of the absence of a vertebral body and the specialized (condensed) structure of the dens.

    Note: Steel's rule of thirds describes the cross-sectional anatomy at the level of the axis: approximately one-third of the space is occupied by the dens; approximately one-third of the space is occupied by the cord; and approximately one-third of the space is "empty." In reality, "empty" is cerebrospinal fluid plus epidural fat plus dura.

Reference

Steel HH: Anatomic and Mechanical Considerations of the Atlanto-Axial Articulations. J Bone Joint Surg Am, 50:1481–1482, 1968.

13. **d** Under normal circumstances, the tip of the odontoid will never be above the McRae line. There are three basic types of cervical instability in rheumatoid spondylitis: (1) atlantoaxial subluxation, (2) atlantoaxial impaction, and (3) subaxial subluxation. All three of these phenomena are capable of producing a neurologic deficit. Atlantoaxial subluxation is the most common.

There are multiple reference lines for quantifying atlantoaxial impaction (Fig. 3.17). The McGregor line is a reference line drawn from the hard palate to the base of the occiput. Under normal circumstances, the tip of the odontoid should not protrude more than 4.5 mm above this line. The McRae line is a reference line drawn from the anterior foramen magnum (clivus) to the posterior foramen magnum. Under normal circumstances, the tip of the odontoid should never protrude above the McRae line. The Ranawat index is another method of quantifying atlantoaxial impaction. (It is not a measurement of atlantoaxial instability.) The Ranawat index is the perpendicular distance from a line connecting the anterior and posterior arches of C1 to the midpoint of the pedicles of C2. The lower limit of normal is 13 mm.

References

Lipson SJ: Rheumatoid Arthritis of the Cervical Spine. Clin Orthop, 239:121–127, 1989.

Ranawat CS, et al.: Cervical Spine Fusion in Rheumatoid Arthritis. J Bone Joint Surg Am, 61:1003–1010, 1979.

14. **c** Neuroanatomic motor and/or sensory compromise. Waddell signs are clinical findings that are typically elicited from patients who are experiencing pain of nonphysical (supratentorial) origin. The five classic signs of Waddell are as follows: (1) nonorganic tenderness (such as

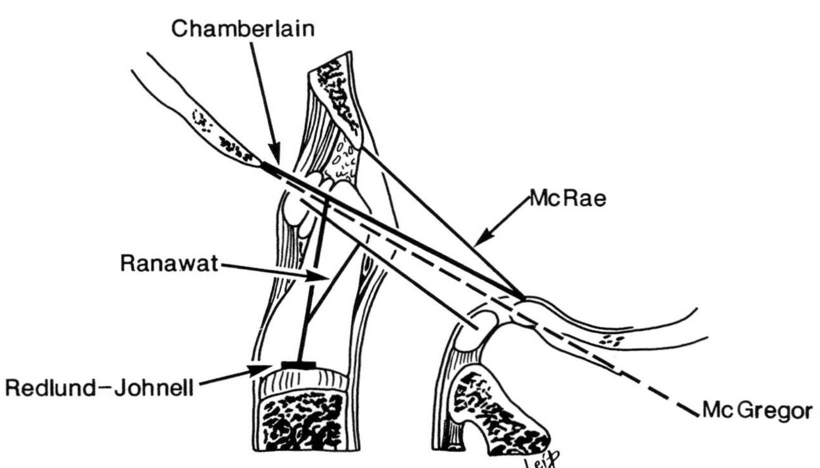

FIGURE 3.17

superficial tenderness to light touch), (2) simulation tests (designed to suggest to the patient that a specific provocative maneuver is being performed when, in fact, it is not), (3) overreaction to nonnoxious stimuli, (4) regional (non-neuroanatomic) motor and/or sensory compromise, and (5) distraction tests (e.g., performing a seated straight leg raise while seemingly focusing on the knee).

Reference

Waddell G, et al.: Nonorganic Physical Signs in Low Back Pain. Spine, 5:117–125, 1980.

15. **c** T11. The umbilicus is characteristically innervated by the T10 dermatome (Fig. 3.18). Classic anterior thoracic dermatomal landmarks include the nipple line (T4), the xiphoid process (T7), the umbilicus (T10), and the inguinal crease (T12).
16. **c** Unilateral facet dislocation. The radiograph in Fig. 3.2 reveals a unilateral facet dislocation at C4 to C5. The mechanism of this injury is flexion-distraction with a component of rotation. The injury is purely ligamentous with disruption of the supraspinous ligament, interspinous ligament, ligamentum flavum and facet capsule. On the side of the dislocated facet, the neural foramen is narrowed, giving rise to a high incidence of ipsilateral radiculopathy. Lateral radiographs demonstrate approximately 25% anterior displacement of the vertebral body and a typical "bow-tie" appearance of the laminae. Bilateral facet dislocations produce approximately 50% anterior displacement of the vertebral body.

Oblique radiographs demonstrate the dislocation (or, in cases of subluxation, a "perched" facet) and narrowing of the foramen. Deviation of the spinous process toward the side of the dislocation will be seen on the anteroposterior radiographs. A computed tomography scan can assist in defining the anatomy and detecting associated fractures. An empty or "naked" superior articulating facet of the lower vertebra is seen because the inferior articulating facet of the upper vertebra has dislocated anteriorly.

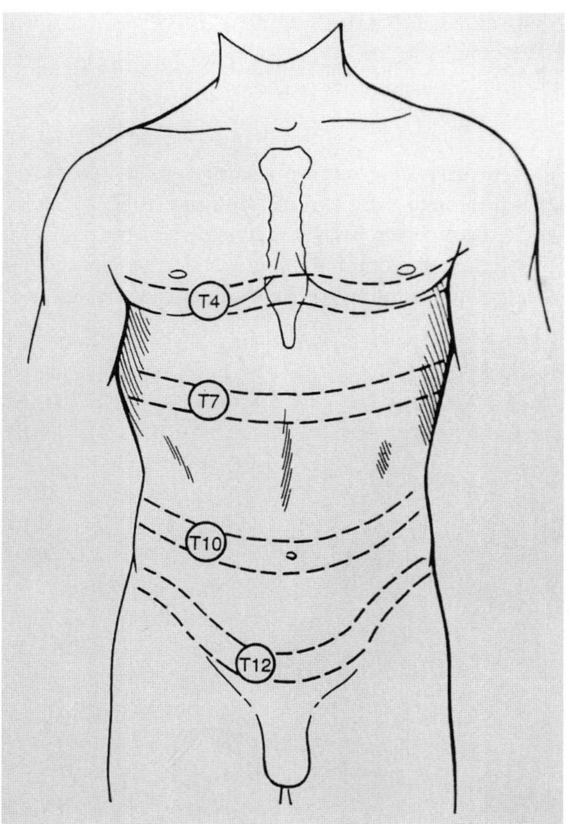

FIGURE 3.18

Reference

Penning L: Obtaining and Interpreting Plain Films in Cervical Spine Injury. The Cervical Spine, 2nd Ed. Philadelphia, JB Lippincott, 1989.

17. **a** Closed reduction with skeletal traction followed by posterior stabilization and fusion. Unilateral facet dislocation is best treated by closed reduction (by skeletal traction) and subsequent posterior stabilization and fusion. Closed reduction followed by halo immobilization is a potential alternative. However, the risk of recurrent instability and chronic pain is lower after posterior stabilization and fusion.

   In cases of bilateral facet dislocation, controversy exists regarding whether a magnetic resonance imaging scan should be obtained before closed reduction. Potential associated disc herniation can lead to neurologic damage during closed reduction. Therefore, if the magnetic resonance imaging scan demonstrates a significant disc herniation, the appropriate treatment will consist of anterior discectomy followed by reduction, anterior fusion, and anterior plate stabilization. If no disc herniation is present, then treatment should be closed reduction followed by posterior fusion.

References

Bohlman HH: Acute Fractures and Dislocations of the Cervical Spine. J Bone Joint Surg Am, 67:1340–1348, 1979.
Garfin SR, Vaccaro AR: Orthopaedic Knowledge Update: Spine. Rosemont, IL, American Academy of Orthopedic Surgeons, p. 206, 1997.

18. **d** Omohyoid muscle. After division of the platysma during the superficial dissection in the anterior approach to the cervical spine, the carotid sheath (common carotid artery, internal jugular vein, and vagus nerve) is retracted laterally with the sternocleidomastoid muscle. The strap muscles (including the omohy-

oid) are retracted toward the midline with the trachea and the esophagus. The pretracheal fascia (connecting the carotid sheath to the strap muscles) is divided just medial to the sheath (Fig. 3.19).

The anterior approach to the cervical spine provides access to vertebral bodies C3 to T1 as well as to the regional discs and uncinate processes. The superior thyroid artery diverges from the carotid artery in a medial direction and (unless sacrificed) may compromise proximal extension of this exposure. The inferior thyroid artery arises from the thyrocervical trunk (not from the carotid).

Reference

Hoppenfeld S: Surgical Exposures in Orthopaedics, 2nd Ed. Philadelphia, JB Lippincott, pp. 263–274, 1994.

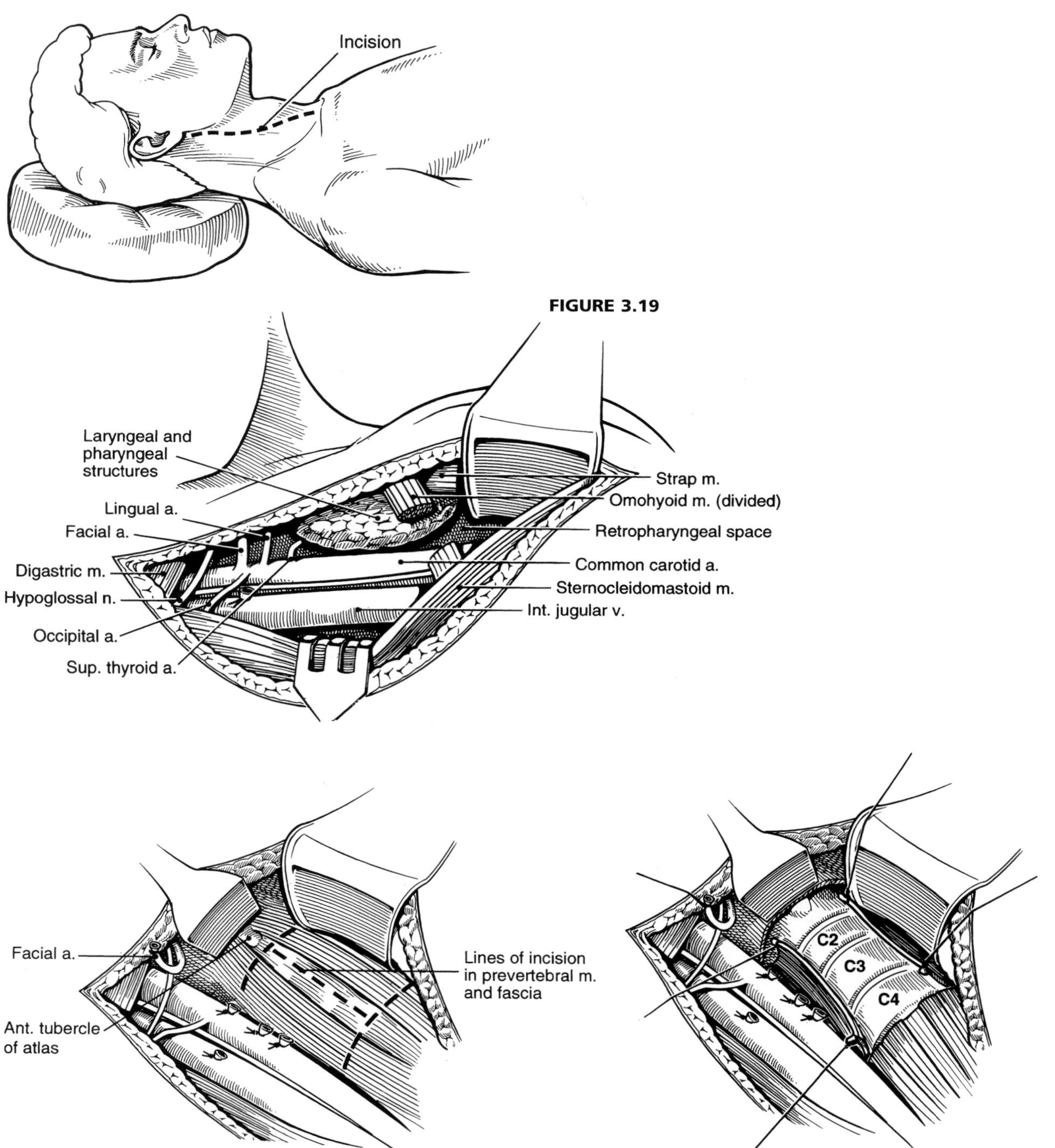

FIGURE 3.19

19. **d** Hyperactive jaw jerk reflex. A hyperactive jaw jerk reflex indicates disease above the foramen magnum. The inverted radial reflex, Oppenheim sign, Babinski sign, and Hoffman sign are all signs of upper motor neuron lesions that could be produced by a central cervical disc herniation.

The jaw jerk reflex is protrusion of the mandible in response to a tap on the chin. The Babinski sign is great toe extension and fanning of the lesser toes in response to stroking of the plantar surface of the heel proximally along the lateral border of the foot and across the forefoot. The Hoffman sign is flexion of the distal phalanx of the thumb and index finger in response to flicking the nail of the long finger. A positive Oppenheim sign is great toe extension and fanning of the lesser toes in response to firm stroking of the tibial crest. The inverted radial reflex is finger flexion in response to attempted elicitation of the brachioradialis reflex.

20. **b** Halo vest immobilization in extension for 3 months. There are four types of traumatic spondylolisthesis of the axis (C2). Type 1 injuries are nondisplaced (less than 3 mm) and show no angulation. A type 2 injury shows significant anterior translation of C2 on C3 (more than 3 mm) and may demonstrate mild angulation. Type 2A injuries (such as the injury described in the question) have severe angulation with less anterior translation. Type 3 fractures demonstrate considerable anterior translation with either unilateral or bilateral facet dislocation.

Management of the four types of "hangman's" fractures is as follows:

Type 1: Philadelphia collar
Type 2: Longitudinal traction in extension for several weeks with conversion to a halo vest
Type 2A: Halo vest immobilization in extension *(no traction)*
Type 3: Open reduction and posterior spinal fusion

Although traction plays an integral role in establishing and maintaining initial alignment for type 2 injuries, it is imperative that traction be avoided in type 2A injuries because traction has the potential to increase the deformity and compromise the neurologic status of these patients.

Although a cervicothoracic orthosis may be acceptable in certain forms of cervical spine trauma, there is a general consensus that the halo vest should be used in truly unstable cervical spine fractures.

Reference

Levine AM, Edwards CC: The Management of Traumatic Spondylolisthesis of the Axis. J Bone Joint Surg Am, 67:217–226, 1985.

21. **a** Magnetic resonance imaging. This technique provides excellent visualization of cervical disc herniations and excellent resolution of the neural elements. However, the clinician must bear in mind that 10% of all asymptomatic patients younger than age 40 years and 5% of asymptomatic persons older than age 40 years manifest disc herniation on magnetic resonance imaging scans. Therefore, magnetic resonance imaging results must be correlated with the history and clinical examination. The value of the history and physical examination cannot be overemphasized. Approximately 25% of asymptomatic persons younger than 40 years of age and approximately 60% of asymptomatic patients older than 40 years show disc degeneration or narrowing on magnetic resonance imaging scans.

Computed tomography is good for bony disease but is not as sensitive for detecting soft tissue changes. Likewise, plain films and bone scans do not provide resolution of either the intervertebral disc tissue or the neural elements. The utility of discograms remains a subject of controversy.

Reference

Boden SD, et al.: Abnormal Magnetic-Resonance Scans of the Cervical Spine in Asymptomatic Subjects. J Bone Joint Surg Am, 72:1178–1184, 1990.

22. **b** Sitting without support. In Nachemson and Morris' *in vivo* investigations, sitting without a support produced greater intradiscal pressures than the other listed options. Even greater pressures were generated when study subjects sat flexed forward with weights in their hands.

In general, sitting produces greater intradiscal pressure than standing. A useful guideline is that positions that place a greater flexion moment across the lumbar spine will produce greater intradiscal pressure. The supine position produces the lowest lumbar intradiscal pressures.

References

Andersson BJ, et al.: The Sitting Posture: An Electromyographic and Discometric Study. Orthop Clin North Am, 6(1):105–120, 1975.
Nachemson A, Morris JM: *In vivo* Measurements of Intradiscal Pressure: Discometry, a Method for the Determination of Pressure in the Lower Lumbar Discs. J Bone Joint Surg Am, 46:1077–1092, 1964.

23. **e** Perform a Stagnara wake-up test. Patients with advanced scoliosis are at increased risk of neurologic injury because of the severity of their deformity and by virtue of the complexity of the surgical procedures that they often require. The risk of intraoperative spinal cord injury is increased if the amount of intraoperative correction exceeds the amount of correction that can be obtained on preoperative bending films. Maintaining adequate intraoperative perfusion to the spinal cord is

also important. Hypotension may compromise spinal cord circulation, and excessive blood loss should be avoided.

Some form of intraoperative spinal cord monitoring is imperative in all deformity-correcting spinal surgery. The wake-up test was first described by Vauzzelle, Stagnara, and Jounvinroux in 1973. With this test, the patient is awakened from anesthesia after final curve correction has been achieved and is asked to move his or her feet. The desired response may sometimes be difficult to elicit from a young child or from patients with mental retardation. Despite isolated reports of false-negative tests, the Stagnara test remains the most reliable and commonly used method of assessing spinal cord function.

Somatosensory evoked potential monitoring provides the advantage of being capable of providing a continuous reading of spinal cord function during surgery. False-negative and false-positive somatosensory evoked potential recordings may result from to the effects of anesthetic agents, changes in operating room temperature, spinal cord irrigation, and monitor dysfunction.

When significant somatosensory evoked potential waveform changes occur during a procedure, a wake-up test should be performed to rule out spinal cord injury. If movement of the feet cannot be elicited during the Stagnara test, then the instrumentation should be removed immediately. In most cases, the tracing will return to baseline within 15 to 30 minutes, and the spine may be reinstrumented (attempting to obtain less correction) with no adverse sequelae.

Reference

Bieber E, Tolo V, Uematsu S: Spinal cord monitoring during posterior spinal instrumentation and fusion. Clin Orthop, 229:173–178, 1973.

24. **d** Posterocentral. The most common type of intervertebral disc herniation is posterolateral. A posterolateral herniation is typically associated with radicular signs and symptoms only. Posterocentral (midline) disc herniation, conversely, can compress the spinal cord and produce myelopathy. Cervical myelopathy can produce a variety of symptoms including ataxia, weakness, hyperreflexia, upper extremity radicular symptoms, and bowel or bladder dysfunction. Loss of vibratory sense and proprioception are late findings and confer a poor prognosis. The relative strength of the anterior longitudinal ligament makes anterior disc herniation extremely unlikely, and an anterior extrusion would obviously not compromise the spinal cord.

Reference

Levine MJ, et al.: Cervical Radiculopathy: Diagnosis and Non-operative Management. J Am Acad Orthop Surg, 4:305–316, 1996.

25. **d** Posterior spinal fusion with distraction instrumentation spanning the lumbar spine that ends at the L5 or S1 level. Flat back is characterized by a loss of lumbar lordosis with associated back pain, forward inclination of the trunk, and inability to stand erect. The use of Harrington distraction instrumentation across the lumbosacral junction is the most frequent cause of this syndrome. Less common causes of flat back include tumor, infection, ankylosing spondylitis, and posttraumatic lumbar kyphosis.

The majority of lumbar lordosis occurs below L3. Posterior distraction instrumentation that extends to L5 or the sacrum can significantly compromise spinal lordosis. When a posterior spinal fusion terminates proximal to L3, flat back is less likely because of the preserved lordosis at the remaining motion segments.

Surgical correction of this deformity is challenging and consists of posterior closing wedge osteotomies through the fusion mass to restore appropriate sagittal contour (with or without anterior release and fusion). Prevention is a preferable form of management. With contemporary segmental instrumentation systems, proper sagittal alignment is more easily preserved than with simple distraction rods.

Reference

La Grone MO, Bradford DS, Moe JH, et al.: Treatment of Symptomatic Flatback after Spinal Fusion. J Bone Joint Surg Am, 70:569–580, 1988.

26. **e** The patient has an abnormally narrow cervical canal. The Pavlov ratio is the ratio of the spinal canal diameter to the diameter of the vertebral body (measured on the lateral radiograph). A normal ratio is 1.0. A ratio of less than 0.82 indicates significant cervical canal stenosis and implies an increased risk of the development of cervical myelopathy. The cited study compared a control population with 23 athletes who had experienced cervical neuropraxia.

The Spurling test is an attempt to reproduce upper extremity radicular symptoms (not salivation) by axial compression while the cervical spine is extended and is ipsilaterally rotated.

Reference

Pavlov H, Torg J, et al.: Cervical Spine Stenosis: Determination with Vertebral Body Ratio Method. Radiology, 164:771–775, 1987.

27. **a** Anterior cervical discectomy and fusion. Although some controversy persists, most surgeons prefer anterior discectomy with fusion for a single level soft disc herniation. Discectomy followed by fusion preserves stability at the operative level and therefore avoids late deformity. Discectomy without fusion is associated with a high rate of postoperative neck pain. Laminec-

tomy may be considered in the presence of normal cervical lordosis, but it is still not the procedure of choice because access to the cervical disc is limited from a posterior approach.

Reference

Bohlman H, et al.: Robinson Anterior Discectomy and Arthrodesis for Cervical Radiculopathy: Long-Term Follow-up of 122 patients. J Bone Joint Surg Am, 75:1298–1307, 1993.

28. **c** Resection of more than 50% of each facet. Although cervical laminectomy is not the preferred treatment for a single-level cervical disc herniation, it is often appropriate for cases of multilevel cervical spondylosis. Reservations regarding cervical laminectomy center on the potential for postoperative cervical instability and kyphosis. Instability and deformity depend on the amount of facet joint resected. Zdeblick documented that resection of more than 50% of the facet can produce segmental hypermobility. Resection of more than 50% of the facet also significantly compromises facet strength. Thus, when posterior cervical decompression is performed, care should be taken to ensure that less than 50% of the facet is resected. If greater than 50% of the facet is resected, then some form of concomitant posterior stabilization should be performed.

References

Raynor R, et al.: Cervical Facetectomy and its Effect on Spine Strength. J Neurosurg, 63:278–282, 1985.
Zdeblick TA: Cervical Stabilization after Sequential Capsule Resection. Spine, 18:2005–2008, 1993.

29. **b** 15% to 20%. The number of patients with thoracolumbar fractures who present with a neurologic deficit is approximately 15% to 20%. This is considerably less than for cervical spine fractures (approximately 40%). Most patients with spinal cord injuries are male, and their mean age is in the middle 20s. The survival rate for patients with spinal cord fractures decreases dramatically after the age of 50 years.

References

Geisler WO, Jousse AT, Wynne-Jones M: Survival in Traumatic Spinal Cord Injury. Paraplegia, 21:364–373, 1983.
Riggins RS, Kraus JF: The Risk of Neurologic Damage with Fractures of the Vertebrae. J. Trauma, 17:126–133, 1977.

30. **b** Retrograde ejaculation. Anterior exposure of the lumbar spine may be complicated by injury to the sympathetic plexus with resultant sexual dysfunction. Penile erection is a parasympathetically controlled function that is mediated by the pelvic splanchnic nerves (nervi erigentes). Ejaculation, conversely, is controlled by the sympathetic nervous system. Sympathetic fibers typically coordinate closure of the bladder neck with sperm expulsion. Damage to the sympathetic fibers in the superior hypogastric plexus can compromise coordinated bladder neck function and can produce retrograde ejaculation. The incidence of this complication is approximately 1%, and it is usually related to the anterior approach to the L5-S1 disc space.

Note: If the lumbar sympathetic chain (as opposed to the superior hypogastric plexus) is injured, vasodilatation occurs and causes warmth of the ipsilateral foot, with a feeling of coolness in the contralateral foot.

Reference

Watkins RG: Complications of Lumbar Spine Surgery. In Bell GR, ed: The Lumbar Spine, 2nd Ed. Philadelphia, WB Saunders, p. 1270, 1996.

31. **e** The annulus fibrosus and vertebral periosteum. The annulus fibrosus is innervated by the sinuvertebral nerves. Both encapsulated and free nerve endings have been documented in the annulus. The vertebral periosteum is also innervated (free nerve endings). The nucleus pulposus is aneural. The cartilage end plates contain perivascular nerves but no other nerve endings.

Reference

Bogduk N: The Innervation of the Lumbar Spine. Spine, 8:286–293, 1983.

32. **b** The literature supports decompression and arthrodesis for patients with spinal stenosis associated with progressive degenerative scoliosis. Not all patients with degenerative scoliosis and associated spinal stenosis require arthrodesis at the time of decompression. However, associated curve progression is an indication for concomitant fusion. Decompression without fusion in this situation is associated with an increased tendency for postoperative curve progression.

There is considerable evidence to support the addition of an arthrodesis at the time of decompression of a stenotic segment that is associated with degenerative spondylolisthesis. In the prospective study by Herkowitz and Sidhu, 96% of patients who underwent simultaneous fusion and decompression had "satisfactory" outcomes (in comparison with 44% of patients who underwent decompression without concomitant fusion).

Progressive instability and listhesis are far more common in patients with degenerative spondylolisthesis who undergo decompression without fusion. Furthermore, this population experiences more bone regrowth at the decompression site than those who undergo a concomitant arthrodesis.

Patients who require a second decompressive laminectomy at the same segment are generally considered candidates for a concomitant arthrodesis (even when translational instability is not demonstrated on preoperative flexion-extension radiographs). Revision decompression often requires additional facet resection to ensure adequate decompression. This can precipitate iatrogenic spondylolisthesis, particularly if more than 50% of the facet is resected. Patients who develop a stenotic segment above a previous posterior fusion require only decompression (unless an excessive facetectomy is performed).

References

Herkowitz HN, Kurz LT: Degenerative Lumbar Spondylolisthesis with Spinal Stenosis: A Prospective Study Comparing Decompression with Decompression and Intertransverse Process Arthrodesis. J Bone Joint Surg Am, 73:802–808, 1991.

Herkowitz HN, Sidhu KS: Lumbar Spinal Fusion in the Treatment of Degenerative Conditions: Current Indications and Recommendations. J Am Acad Orthop Surg, 3(3)123–135, 1995.

Postacchini F, Cinotti G: Bone Regrowth After Surgical Decompression for Lumbar Spinal Stenosis. J Bone Joint Surg Br, 74:862–869, 1992.

33. **a** Dye extravasation into or beyond the annulus with concordant pain. Reproduction of concordant pain (pain similar to patient's presenting pain) is required for a positive discogram. The addition of a computed tomography scan allows one to evaluate the condition of the annulus during the discography. Dye leakage into the annulus or beyond is considered positive. Therefore, a positive computed tomography discogram requires both (1) concordant pain and (2) dye leakage into or beyond the annulus.

References

Guyer RD, et al.: Contemporary Concepts in Spine Care: Lumbar Discography. Spine, 20:2048–2059, 1995.

Walsh TR, et al.: Lumbar Discography in Normal Subjects. J Bone Joint Surg Am, 72:1081–1088, 1990.

34. **b** Epidural steroid injection and physical therapy. This is a case of arachnoiditis. Arachnoiditis is defined as inflammation of the pia-arachnoid membrane. Although several cases of congenital or familial forms have been described, most cases are attributed to the use of myelographic contrast or lumbar spine surgery. Postoperative infections may also play an etiologic role. A 1- to 6-month postsurgical pain-free interval, followed by gradual recurrent back pain and sciatica, is typical of the clinical presentation of this phenomenon. The sciatica tends to be constant and aggravated by activity; it may be unilateral or bilateral. Neurologic deficits are characteristically absent, although positive tension signs may be evident.

    Recurrent disc herniation must also be considered in this clinical situation. However, the radiographic findings in this case are not consistent with recurrent herniated nucleus pulposus. Either gadolinium-enhanced magnetic resonance imaging or computed tomography myelography may be used to make the diagnosis of arachnoiditis. The characteristic finding is diffuse abundant epidural scar tissue.

    Surgery is futile for these patients, and no definitive treatment exists. Epidural steroid injections, electrostimulation, and physical therapy have been tried with variable results. None of these modalities leads to a cure, but they may provide symptomatic relief.

Reference

Burton CV: Lumbosacral Arachnoiditis. Spine, 3:24–30, 1978.

35. **b** Extraforaminal L5-S1 disc herniation. Posterolateral disc herniation in the lumbar spine typically affects the root, which traverses the affected disc space to exit below the pedicle of the vertebra below the affected disc (Fig. 3.20A). (Hence, the number of the affected root corresponds to the number of the lumbar vertebra below the affected disc space). The nerve root that numerically corresponds to the vertebra above the affected disc space is typically not disturbed by the protruding disc because this root exits the canal below the pedicle of the superior vertebral body, which is markedly cephalad to the involved disc.

    Note: A lateral (or extraforaminal) disc herniation is a caveat to this rule. This type of disc herniation can affect the nerve root that exits at the level of the affected disc. As it herniates laterally, the disc contacts the nerve root as it continues distally after having exited the canal through the foramen (Fig. 3.20B).

    This patient presents with typical signs of an L5 radiculopathy (Fig. 3.20C). This could be caused by either a posterolateral L4-5 herniation or by an extraforaminal L5-S1 disc herniation. The posterolateral L4-5 herniation would be a more common cause, but it is not a listed option.
36. **d** Tachycardia. Neurogenic shock after cervical or high thoracic spinal cord injury is associated with low blood pressure and bradycardia. The bradycardia stems from loss of sympathetic innervation to the heart. (The sympathetic fibers to the cardiac plexus originate from the cervical and high thoracic regions of the spinal cord.) The hypotension in neurogenic shock stems from both (1) vasodilation from a loss of vascular sympathetic tone and (2) a loss of reflexive tachycardia.

    A transection of the spinal cord at the level of the thoracolumbar junction would disrupt sympathetic tone to the lower extremities, but it would not disrupt the sympathetic innervation of the heart. Thus, reflexive tachycardia would be preserved. Tachycardia would be expected in the described situation because of the

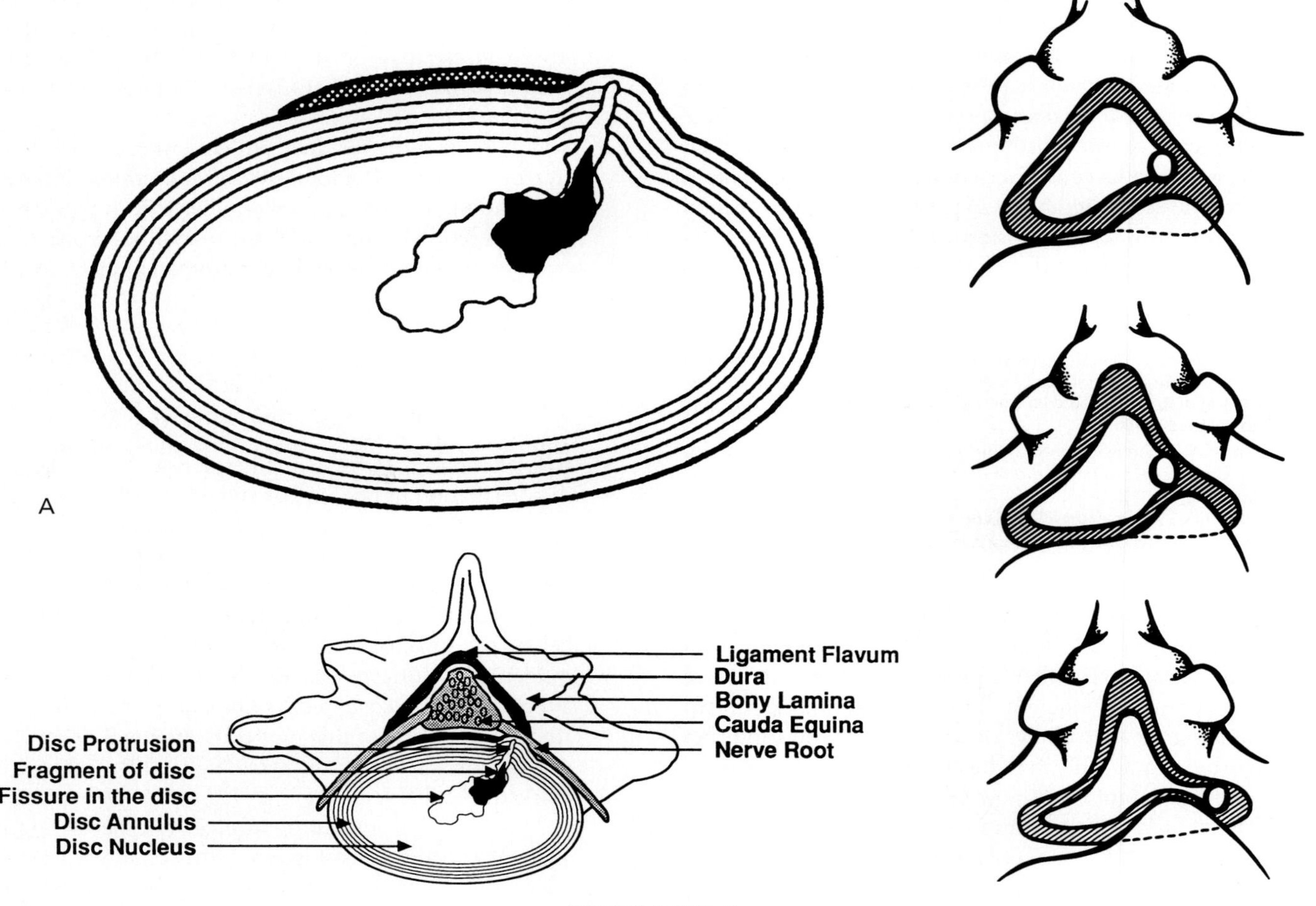

FIGURE 3.20A–C

splenic hemorrhage and the lower extremity vasodilatation.

The cremasteric reflex may be unilaterally disrupted with an isolated L1 lower motor neuron lesion. However, acute cord transection (as in this case) would produce a state of spinal shock. Hence, all reflexes distal to the level of transection would be absent.

Although most patients with a complete spinal cord injury ultimately develop lower extremity hyperreflexia and a positive Babinski sign, this pathologic reflex would not be present in the acute setting. In fact, spinal shock would be present, and, thus, there would be no reflexes present distal to the level of transection.

37. **c** Nonambulators with cerebral palsy. A study of nonambulators with cerebral palsy revealed a 0% incidence of spondylolysis. The apparent protective effect of a nonambulatory state supports the hypothesis that isthmic spondylolisthesis stems from repetitive microtrauma.

Athletes who participate in sports that require repetitive lumbar hyperextension (e.g., football linesmen, gymnasts, weight lifters, and butterfly swimmers) have a considerably higher incidence of spondylolysis and spondylolisthesis than age-matched controls.

Patients with Scheuermann kyphosis also have a high incidence of spondylolysis. This putatively results from the lumbar hyperlordosis that these patients develop in compensation for their exaggerated thoracic kyphosis.

Reference

Rosenberg NJ, et al.: The Incidence of Spondylolysis and Spondylolisthesis in Nonambulatory Patients. Spine, 6:5, 1981.

38. **d** A lateral radiograph of this player's cervical spine is likely to show a spinal canal diameter to vertebral body diameter of less than 0.8. This clinical picture is typical of transient neuropraxia. The symptoms of transient neuropraxia may persist for up to 36 hours. A history of transient neuropraxia does not predispose a player to a subsequent permanent neurologic injury. Patients

with a permanent neurologic injury usually have no previous history of a transient neuropraxia. In fact, none of the quadriplegic patients in the study by Torg et al. had experienced a transient neuropraxia before their catastrophic spine injuries. Persons who have had an episode of transient neuropraxia usually have a cervical canal to vertebral body ratio of less than 0.8. A ratio less than 0.8 constitutes narrowing of the cervical canal, but (if the spine is stable) this finding should not preclude participation in contact sports.

Reference

Torg JS, Naranja JR, Pavlov H, et al.: The Relationship of Developmental Narrowing of the Cervical Spinal Canal to Reversible and Irreversible Injury of the Cervical Spinal Cord in Football Players. J Bone Joint Surg Am, 78:1308–1314, 1996.

39. **b** Compression stockings. Given the very low prevalence of deep venous thrombosis in patients who undergo spine operations and the potentially catastrophic consequences of bleeding complications (e.g., epidural hematoma) in this population, routine pharmacologic anticoagulation is not warranted. Likewise, routine screening for asymptomatic deep venous thrombosis is not indicated. Mechanical modalities (i.e., compression stockings or boots) are the recommended form of deep venous thrombosis prophylaxis in the setting of spine surgery.

References

Rokito SE: Deep Venous Thrombosis After Major Reconstructive Spinal Surgery. Spine, 21(7):853–859, 1996.
Smith MD: Deep Venous Thrombosis and Pulmonary Embolism After Major Reconstructive Operations on the Spine. J Bone Joint Surg Am, 76:980–985, 1994.

40. **c** Exercise and brace treatment. The preferred initial treatment for spondylolysis with a low-grade spondylolisthesis is nonsurgical. Brace treatment, activity modification, and exercise are indicated for this patient. Return to full activities (including contact sports) is permitted in this setting once the patient is entirely asymptomatic. Surgical treatment should be considered only after failure of nonsurgical treatment (intractable pain and/or progressive slippage).

Risk factors for progression include female sex, recurrent symptoms, a high-grade slip (more than 50%), and young age at presentation (less than 10 to 15 years old).

The Gill procedure (removal of the loose arch) is rarely indicated (particularly in children) because of its destabilizing consequences. Posterolateral fusion *in situ* is the procedure of choice for most children who require surgery. Instrumented fusion in the setting of spondylolisthesis is indicated (1) if a decompression is performed (e.g., a Gill procedure) or (2) if a reduction is performed. Decompression is contraindicated unless a preoperative neurologic deficit is present.

41. **d** In a translational shear injury, all three spinal columns are usually injured, and the alignment of the neural canal is typically disrupted. In a translational injury, all three spinal columns are usually injured, and the alignment of the neural canal is typically disrupted.

A wedge compression fracture implies failure of only the anterior column. There is no posterior ligamentous injury and no failure of the middle osteoligamentous column. These injuries rarely require internal fixation. However, such intervention may sometimes be required when the degree of compression exceeds 50%. All burst fractures, by definition, involve failure of the anterior and middle columns secondary to an axial load. A Chance fracture results from distraction forces of the posterior and middle columns and characteristically occurs in the lower thoracic and lumbar areas (usually secondary to a seat belt injury).

Reference

McAfee PC, Yuan HA, Fredrickson BE, et al.: The Value of Computed Tomography in Thoracolumbar Fracture: An Analysis of One Hundred Consecutive Cases and a New Classification. J Bone Joint Surg Am, 65: 461–473, 1983.

42. **c** Facet deterioration and incompetence. Degenerative spondylolisthesis is believed to stem from arthritic deterioration of the facets and intervertebral disc with resultant facet incompetence. There is no discontinuity of the pars in degenerative spondylolisthesis. Degenerative slips rarely progress past a grade 2 status.

Other types of spondylolisthesis include the following:

Congenital: Congenital dysplasia of a superior facet (usually S1)
Isthmic: Pars defect
Traumatic: Acute pars and/or facet fracture
Postsurgical: Excessive surgical resection of facets
Pathologic: Compromise of pars and/or facet by tumor

43. **e** A patient has an incomplete neurologic deficit, a 20-degree kyphotic deformity, and 35% canal compromise. The computed tomography scan shows a minimally displaced laminar fracture.

Posterior decompression is strongly indicated when a laminar fracture occurs in association with a burst fracture. Dural lacerations are common in this setting, and elements of the cauda equina can become entrapped in the lamina fracture. Even when there is minimal residual displacement of the laminar fracture, significant opening of the fracture site can occur at the moment of injury. Subsequent recoil can entrap nerve roots. A posterior approach is the best way to ensure that the roots are clear, to maximize the chance for neurologic recovery.

For most other circumstances, significant controversy persists regarding the optimal form of intervention (anterior versus posterior). A posterior approach relies on ligamentotaxis to accomplish an indirect reduction of the retropulsed vertebral body fragments when distraction is applied. Thus, the posterior approach is not optimal when ligamentotaxis is unlikely to clear the canal sufficiently. Such instances would include (1) a disrupted posterior longitudinal ligament (reduction by ligamentotaxis requires an intact ligament to serve as a restraint to distraction), (2) patients who were injured more than 10 days earlier (callous formation has commenced), and (3) patients in whom the posterior cortical fragment is rotated 180 degrees (this is an indicator that the posterior longitudinal ligament is disrupted).

Many authorities advise an anterior approach in the setting of neurologic deficit because they believe that it affords a more complete decompression and optimizes the milieu for neurologic recovery. This concept remains controversial.

Patients who are neurologically intact with minimal sagittal deformity and minimal canal compromise (e.g., the patient described in option b) should be managed nonoperatively with an extension cast or brace.

Reference

Denis F, Burkus JK: Diagnosis and Treatment of Cauda Equina Entrapment in the Vertical Lamina Fracture of Lumbar Burst Fractures. Spine, 16:S433–S439, 1991.

44. **b** *In situ* posterolateral fusion with decompression, and instrumentation.

Decompression is indicated because of the symptomatic stenosis. Although *in situ* fusion alone would stabilize the listhesis, it would not adequately address the stenosis. Fusion not only stabilizes the listhesis but also prevents iatrogenic exacerbation of the instability by the decompression. Anterior fusion is not indicated in this case because of the low grade of the slip, but it may be used for grade 4 slips or vertebral optosis. The efficacy of epidural steroids is variable in the management of spinal stenosis.

Reference

Bridwell KM, et al.: The Role of Fusion and Instrumentation in the Treatment of Degenerative Spondylolisthesis with Spinal Stenosis. J Spinal Disord, 6:461–472, 1993.

45. **c** 50%. Rotation between C1 and C2 accounts for 50% of the total rotation of the cervical spine.

Reference

Hohl M, Baker HR: The Atlanto-Axial Joint: Roentgenographic and Anatomical Study of Normal and Abnormal Motion. J Bone Joint Surg Am, 46:1739–1752, 1964.

46. **a** Weakness of the extensor hallucis longus would be the most common associated motor deficit. The question describes stereotypical symptoms of spinal stenosis. These symptoms are characteristically exacerbated with extension and improved with flexion because the capacity of the spinal canal and neural foramen decreases in extension. Degenerative spondylolisthesis is often seen in association with spinal stenosis, but it typically occurs at the L4-5 level. Straight leg raise testing is typically negative in spinal stenosis because the associated nerve root entrapment occurs slowly and circumferentially, unlike the sudden asymmetric compression produced by a disc herniation. Weakness of the extensor hallucis longus is the most common motor deficit associated with spinal stenosis. Loss of sensation of light touch is unusual and, if present, should raise the possibility of an associated peripheral neuropathy.

Reference

Lipson S: Clinical Diagnosis of Spinal Stenosis. Semin Spine Surg, 1:143–144, 1989.

47. **c** All patients with significant head injuries, including conscious patients without neck pain, should have their cervical spines immobilized before transportation. The Philadelphia collar is the method of choice for immobilizing the cervical spine during the extraction of a victim from a motor vehicle accident. It can be applied before patient mobilization (whether the patient is found in a prone or supine position), and it will not interfere with the remainder of the extraction, resuscitation, or radiographs. It provides stabilization superior to that of a soft collar.

Ideally, a patient who has been injured by diving into shallow water should initially be supported supine at the surface of the water (making use of the support provided by the water). He or she should be transferred onto a spine board while still in the water.

Because of the large head-to-body ratio in an infant, placing the infant on a standard spine board will force the neck into a flexed posture and potentially damage an unstable spine (additional support behind the head will worsen this situation). The head of an infant needs to be immobilized in a recessed position relative to the torso so normal alignment is maintained.

A football player with a potential cervical spine injury should not be transported to the emergency room with his facemask in place. Although concern exists regarding the potential for exacerbation of cervical damage during helmet removal, the facemask must be removed from the helmet in order to provide airway access.

All patients with significant head trauma have cervical spine damage until proven otherwise. Injuries to the head and elsewhere can distract a patient's attention from neck discomfort.

48. **a** It typically occurs in the thoracic and lumbar pedicles. Osteoblastoma in the spine typically arises in the thoracic and lumbar pedicles. Patients present with painful scoliosis in approximately two-thirds of cases, and there is neurologic involvement in more than 50% of cases. Malignant transformation can occur in osteoblastoma. Radiotherapy is not effective in the management of osteoblastoma.

49. **c** During the last 50% of reduction. During reduction of an L5-S1 spondylolisthesis, the L5 nerve root is at risk for a traction neuropraxia because of its course under the L5 pedicle. The risk of stretch injury to the L5 root during reduction of a high-grade slip is not linear. Petraco et al. showed that the L5 nerve is at greatest risk during the last 50% of reduction. In fact, 71% of L5 root strain occurs during the second half of the reduction. In this study, the correction of the slip angle did not jeopardize the L5 nerve root, and there was minimal strain during the first 50% of translation. The reported potential for recovery from such an injury is variable.

Reference

Petraco DM, et al.: An Anatomic Evaluation of L5 Nerve Stretch in Spondylolisthesis. Spine, 21(10):1133–1139, 1996.

50. **e** It has no definite association with the recreational use of weight-lifting equipment. Herniated nucleus pulposus has a weak association with certain sports, but most literature suggests a protective effect of sports activity against disc herniation. When this condition occurs in football or rugby it is most likely caused by repetitive cervical loading. This is in contrast to swimming or tennis, in which it is the result of neck hyperextension and rotation. The condition has not been definitively associated with the recreational use of weight-lifting equipment, although a possible association has been noted with the use of free weights. Symptoms tend to be unilateral, and myelopathy is more likely to occur as a clinical finding in an older patient than in a younger athlete.

Reference

Northeast Collaborative Group on Low Back Pain: An Epidemiologic Study of Sports and Weight Lifting as Possible Risk Factors for Herniated Lumbar and Cervical Discs. Am J Sports Med, 21:854–860, 1993.

51. **b** Wire fixation with a single midline graft (Gallie). Posterior clamps and wiring techniques resist flexion, but they do not provide optimal restraint against rotation. In the study by Grob et al., Gallie wiring provided the least rotational stability. The Magerl transarticular screw technique with posterior wiring allowed the least rotation. This technique provides true three-point fixation and optimal multidirectional stability.

Reference

Grob D, Crisco JJ III, Panjabi MM, et al.: Biomechanical Evaluation of Four Different Posterior Atlantoaxial Fixation Techniques. Spine, 17:480–490, 1992.

52. **d** The mainstay of the surgical approach to lumbar spinal stenosis is laminectomy. Complications of decompressive surgery for spinal stenosis have been shown to be increased in patients who are more than 75 to 80 years of age. However, chronologic age, by itself, should not be used as an exclusion criteria for surgery. Many chronologically old patients are physiologically young and healthy enough to undergo operative intervention. Such patients should not be deprived of potential surgical benefit. There is no evidence that patients with spinal stenosis who opt to forgo surgery will definitely experience progressive symptoms and/or neurologic deterioration. Surgical decompression is recommended for persistent leg pain (not back pain). The mainstay of the surgical approach to spinal stenosis is lumbar laminectomy.

Reference

Deyo RA, et al.: Morbidity and Mortality in Association with Operations on the Lumbar Spine: The Influence of Age, Diagnosis and Procedure. J Bone Joint Surg Am, 74:536–543, 1992.

53. **b** Initial traction (3 to 6 weeks) followed by halo vest immobilization for 3 months. The imaging studies in Fig. 3.4 reveal a burst fracture of the atlas with failure of the anterior and posterior arches of the C1 ring (Jefferson fracture). Salient features of this injury include (1) lateral subluxation of the lateral articular masses of C1 (seen on the odontoid view), (2) characteristic absence of neurologic deficit, and (3) favorable outcome with nonoperative treatment.

With significant displacement, a period of initial traction is usually recommended before halo vest application, although this is a matter of debate. This is particularly true if there is lateral mass separation of more than 7 mm (which implies greater ring instability because of associated transverse ligament failure). A halo vest does not provide sufficient axial distraction to achieve a reduction.

Primary surgical intervention may be indicated if other fractures in the cervical spine require operative intervention or if trauma to the chest and/or skull precludes the use of a halo. Late surgical intervention may be indicated if (after halo removal) flexion-extension views manifest C1-C2 instability. This may be treated with standard posterior C1-C2 wiring techniques if the posterior arch of C1 has healed. Otherwise, the atlantoaxial instability should be addressed with either Magerl screws or occiput-C2 fusion.

Note: Up to 50% of patients with Jefferson fractures have associated fractures elsewhere in the spine.

References

Garfin SR, Vaccaro AR: Orthopaedic Knowledge Update: Spine. Rosemont, IL, American Academy of Orthopedic Surgeons, p. 203, 1997.

Pierce DS, Barr JS: Fractures and Dislocations at the Base of the Skull and Upper Cervical Spine. The Cervical Spine, 2nd Ed. Philadelphia, JB Lippincott, 1989.

54. **b** Relative sagittal plane intersegmental angulation greater than 7 degrees. White and co-authors described a point-weighted checklist of criteria for establishing the diagnosis of traumatic subaxial instability. These criteria include (1) anterior elements destroyed or unable to function, (2) posterior elements destroyed or unable to function, (3) relative sagittal plane translation of more than 3.5 mm; (4) relative sagittal plane rotation of more than 11 degrees, (5) positive stretch test (progressive segmental distraction with longitudinal traction), (6) spinal cord damage, (7) root damage, (8) abnormal disc narrowing, and (9) dangerous loading anticipated.

    This is a useful list. However, the absence of all these factors does not rule out an unstable cervical spine. In particular, the clinician needs to employ flexion-extension views to rule out occult ligamentous instability when clinically indicated.

References

McAfee PC: Cervical Spine Trauma. In Frymoyer FW, ed: The Adult Spine. Philadelphia, JB Lippincott, 1991.

White A, Southwick W, Panjabi M: Clinical Instability in the Lower Cervical Spine. Spine, 1:15, 1976.

55. **b** Recurrent laryngeal nerve. The recurrent laryngeal nerve is less vulnerable on the left side, where it is better protected ascending in the tracheoesophageal groove after looping around the aortic arch. On the right, the nerve ascends alongside the trachea after looping around the subclavian artery. Injury to the recurrent laryngeal nerve may result in hoarseness or vocal fatigability.

    One should be conscious of the thoracic duct in a low left-sided anterior approach to the cervical spine. This structure ascends along the esophagus in the left thorax and enters the left cervical region, where it crosses posterior to the internal jugular vein to empty into the subclavian vein. If the duct is violated, it should be ligated both proximally and distally.

56. **b** When performing a laminectomy, it is technically easier and safer to enter the canal distally and to proceed proximally. Most patients with spinal stenosis have compression at the L4-5 level with involvement of the L5 nerve root. Lateral stenosis usually stems from impingement on the nerve root by osteophyte formation on the superior articular facet of the inferior vertebral body (Fig. 3.21). The superior facet is the principal component of the posterior wall of the foramen. It is important to evaluate the adequacy of foraminal decompression by passing a small nerve probe out the neuroforamen. The decision to fuse the spine may be made preoperatively or decided on intraoperatively, based on the degree of instability present after decompression.

    During a laminectomy, it is technically easier and safer to enter the canal distally and then to proceed proximally with the decompression. The insertion of the ligamentum flavum on the ventral surface of the superior lamina and the oblique orientation of the facets (proximal anterior to distal posterior) renders the distal edge of the facet more accessible.

57. **e** Vertical compression. Most cases of quadriplegia in football occur in association with burst fractures, which stem from an axial compression mechanism. Historically, this phenomenon has occurred as the result of spear tackling (making contact with the opponent with one's head down, leading with the crown of one's helmet). This position eliminates normal cervical lordosis. As a result, all the compressive force (between the

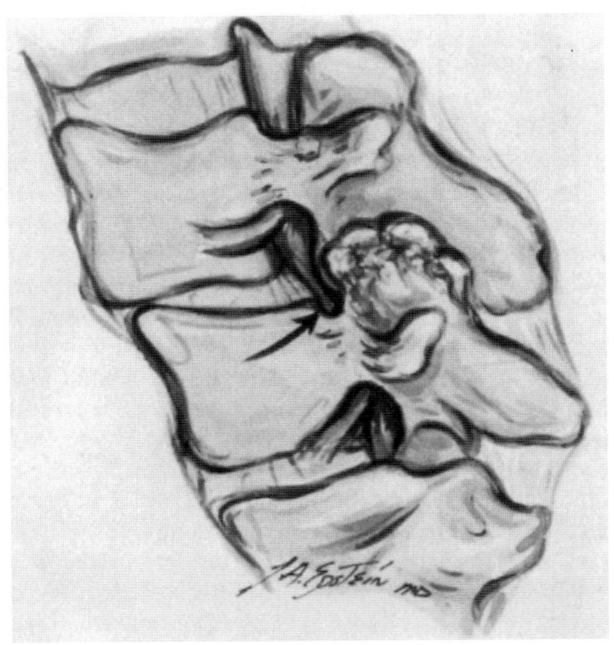

FIGURE 3.21

rapidly decelerating head and continued body momentum) is translated along the vertical axis of the cervical spine. When the cervical spine is in its normal lordotic posture, forces can be dissipated to adjacent soft tissues by controlled motion. Slight cervical flexion obliterates the natural lordosis and precludes the ability to dissipate axial compressive energy by controlled motion. Rules against spear tackling have led to a significant reduction in the incidence of quadriplegia in football.

Reference

Torg J: The Epidemiology, Pathomechanics, and Prevention of Athletic Injuries to the Cervical Spine. The Cervical Spine, 2nd Ed. Philadelphia, JB Lippincott, pp. 442–463, 1989.

58. **d** Initial management should consist of 6 to 8 weeks in a halo vest followed by repeat flexion views to confirm adequate ligament healing. Isolated traumatic failure of the transverse ligament is a rare phenomenon. It usually occurs in association with fracture of the atlas. The injury may not be detected on a single lateral cervical spine film. Once bony injuries have been ruled out, active flexion-extension views may be obtained. The diagnosis is made based on these studies if the anterior atlantodens interval is greater than 3.5 mm in adults (or greater than 4.5 mm in children). Management should consist of primary C1-C2 arthrodesis because ligament healing does not reliably occur.

Reference

Levine A: Orthopaedic Knowledge Update: Trauma. Rosemont, IL, American Academy of Orthopedic Surgeons, 1996.

59. **b** Posterior C1-C2 fusion. This patient has a type 2 odontoid fracture nonunion with marked associated C1-C2 instability. Given the time elapsed between injury and diagnosis, a halo vest would have an extremely poor chance of establishing union. The atlantoaxial instability requires surgical stabilization. Anterior odontoid screw fixation has a low success rate in the setting of an established nonunion, in contrast to its approximately 92% efficacy in acute fractures.

Posterior C1-C2 fusion would be the most appropriate option in this situation. In the absence of associated occiput-C1 instability or discontinuity of the C1 ring, extension of the fusion to the occiput would not be indicated.

References

Aebi M, et al.: Fractures of the Odontoid Process Treated with Anterior Screw Fixation. Spine, 14:1065–1069,1989.
Anderson LD, Clark CR: Fractures of the Odontoid Process of the Axis. The Cervical Spine, 2nd Ed. Philadelphia, JB Lippincott, pp. 325–343, 1989.
Clark CR, White AA: Fractures of the Dens. J Bone Joint Surg Am, 67:1340–1348, 1985.

60. **b** The literature contains several reports of poor results, many of which can be attributed to multilevel decompression and the development of postoperative instability. In properly selected patients (who receive adequate surgical decompression with fusion if necessary), success rates of 85% to 90% can be anticipated. Preoperative symptom duration of less than 2 years is associated with superior results. When preoperative myelograms document high-grade stenosis, outcomes are superior than when preoperative myelograms show minimal or no stenosis. Low back complaints are more common after multiple level decompression than after one- to two-level decompressions. The primary reason for poor results in most series is related to multilevel decompression and the development of postoperative instability.

References

Herkowitz HN: Lumbar Stenosis: Indications for Arthrodesis and Spinal Instrumentation. Instr Course Lect, 43:425–433, 1994.
Herkowitz HN, Kurz LT: Degenerative Lumbar Spondylolisthesis with Spinal Stenosis: A Prospective Study Comparing Decompression with Decompression and Intertransverse Process Arthrodesis. J Bone Joint Surg Am, 73:802–808, 1991.
Johnsson KE, Willner S, Petersson H: Analysis of Operated Cases with Lumbar Spinal Stenosis. Acta Orthop Scand, 52;427- —433, 1981.

61. **c** Retropulsed bone fragments have been shown to resorb from the canal over time. The optimal indications and approach (anterior versus posterior) for operative management of burst fractures remain a subject of controversy. Radiographic criteria for surgical management of these injuries (in the absence of neurologic deficit) are inconsistent in the literature. The degree of canal compromise is particularly debatable in light of the finding that numerous studies have documented that retropulsed bone will resorb over time.

Cammisa et al. showed that a laminar fracture in association with a burst fracture predicts the possibility of a dural laceration. Among 30 patients with burst fractures and associated laminar fractures, 11 were found to have dural lacerations at the time of operation. Each of these eleven had a preoperative neurologic deficit, and four of the 11 were found to have neural elements entrapped in the laminar fracture. Failure to recognize and relieve the neural entrapment in this setting may preclude neurologic recovery. Thus, a posterior procedure may be preferable to an anterior procedure in the setting of a laminar fracture and neurologic deficit. Modern segmental posterior instrumentation techniques can bypass the level of injury and do not require fixation to the fractured lamina. Complications related to posterior procedures for burst fractures in the setting of dural lacerations (i.e., dural-cutaneous fistulas or pseudomeningoceles) have not been documented to occur with increased frequency. None of the patients with burst fractures in the series reported by Cammisa et al. who did not have laminar fractures had dural lacerations.

L1 is the most common site for burst fractures because of its transitional position between the inflexible thoracic spine and the more mobile lumbar spine. Furthermore, its neutral (horizontal) orientation between the kyphosis of the thoracic spine and the lordosis of the lumbar spine renders it less resistant to axial loads.

References

Cammisa F, et al.: Dural Laceration Occurring with Burst Fractures and Associated Laminar Fractures. J Bone Joint Surg Am, 71:1044–1052, 1989.
Cantor JB, et al.: Nonoperative Management of Stable Thoracolumbar Burst Fractures with Early Ambulation and Bracing. Spine, 18:971–976, 1993.

62. **d** Resection of the tumor and stabilization of the spine through a combined anterior and posterior approach. Given the patient's age, this well-circumscribed, expansile lesion of the cervical spine is most likely to be an osteoblastoma. The histologic features are indicative of an osteoblastoma with sclerotic bony trabeculae.

Osteoblastoma is a benign yet aggressive tumor with a high chance of local recurrence. Radiotherapy is not an effective treatment for this tumor. Complete surgical excision (preferably with wide margins) is required to minimize the chance of recurrence. However, wide excision is often not possible in the spine, as in this case. Complete excision would be most effectively accomplished in this instance through a combined anterior and posterior approach. Given the extent of involvement, a stabilization procedure would be required after resection of this lesion. Radiotherapy does not significantly alter the natural history of this tumor.

Note: The three most common primary tumors that involve the posterior elements of the spine are osteoblastoma, osteoid osteoma, and aneurysmal bone cyst.

Reference

Marsh BW, et al.: Benign Osteoblastoma: Range of Manifestations. J Bone Joint Surg Am, 57:1–9, 1975.

63. **c** The majority of lumbar lordosis exists below L3. A normal spine is straight in the frontal projection (more than 10 degrees of curvature is considered scoliosis). The amount of thoracic kyphosis and lumbar lordosis is variable, with normal ranges of 20 to 50 and 20 to 60 degrees, respectively. These curves compensate for one another, so the sagittal vertical axis (from the center of the C7 vertebral body) should normally fall 3.2 ± 3.2 cm behind the sacral promontory. The thoracic apex is usually located between T5 and T8. Most lumbar lordosis exists within the last two segments.

References

Bernhardt M, Bridwell KH: Segmental Analysis of the Sagittal Plane Alignment of the Normal Thoracic and Lumbar Spine and Thoracolumbar Junction. Spine, 14:717–721, 1989.
Gelb D, et al.: An Analysis of Sagittal Spinal Alignment in 100 Asymptomatic Middle and Older Aged Volunteers. Spine, 20:1351–1358, 1995.

64. **e** A thoracic curve that fails to correct on bending films. A structural scoliotic curve is characterized by its lack of flexibility. By definition, structural curves do not correct on bending films. Associated characteristics of structural curves include vertebral wedging and vertebral rotation.

Lumbar curves that exist secondary to leg length inequality are not structural. Likewise, the lumbar component of a King-Moe type III curve is highly flexible by definition.

The primary (or major) curve is the most structural component of a scoliotic deformity in an idiopathic scoliosis deformity. However compensatory curves may secondarily acquire structural characteristics.

Reference

Lonstein JE, et al.: Moe's Textbook of Scoliosis and Other Spinal Deformities, 3rd Ed. Philadelphia, WB Saunders, 1995.

65. **b** Pregnancy and delivery can cause curve progression. Pregnancy and delivery do not affect scoliosis progression. Curves greater than 100 degrees restrict pulmonary function and confer an increased mortality rate compared with the general population. Lumbar curves greater than 60 degrees are associated with an increased incidence of low back pain compared with the general population. Lonstein and Carlson documented that the incidence of curve progression is significantly lower in single lumbar and single thoracolumbar curves than in other patterns.

References

Betz RR, Bunnel WP, Lamrecht-Mullier, MacEen GD: Scoliosis and Pregnancy. J Bone Joint Surg Am, 69:90–96, 1987.
Lonstein JE and Carlson JM: The Prediction of Curve Progression in Untreated Idiopathic Scoliosis During Growth. J Bone Joint Surg Am, 66:1061–1071, 1984.
Lonstein JE, et al.: Moe's Textbook of Scoliosis and Other Spinal Deformities, 3rd Ed. Philadelphia, WB Saunders, 1995.
Weinstein SL, Ponseti IV: Curve Progression in Idiopathic Scoliosis. J Bone Joint Surg Am, 65:447–455, 1983.

66. **e** Age does not affect the risk of paralysis in instances of cervical involvement. Approximately 10% of all patients with tuberculosis have skeletal involvement. Half of those with skeletal involvement have spinal lesions, and 10% to 45% of patients with spinal involvement will manifest neurologic deficit. The disc spaces are spared early in the process.

Cervical tuberculosis in children younger than 10 years of age carries a relatively low risk of spinal cord compromise (17%) as compared with patients who are older than 10 years, in whom the risk of spinal cord compromise rises to 81%.

References

Ho EKW, Leong JC: Tuberculosis of the Spine. In Weinstein SL, ed: The Pediatric Spine: Principles and Practice. New York, Raven Press, pp. 837–850, 1994.

Hsu LC, Leong JC: Tuberculosis of the Lower Cervical Spine (C2 to C7): A Report on 40 Cases. J Bone Joint Surg Br, 66:1–5, 1984.

67. **e** Overcorrection of a King-Moe type II curve may produce decompensation to the left. King-Moe type I curves are double major curves in which the magnitude and stiffness of the lumbar curve exceed the thoracic curve. Selective thoracic fusion is not an option in this context. Selective thoracic fusion is reserved for King-Moe type II (double major curve with lumbar smaller than thoracic) and King-Moe type III (single thoracic curve) patterns.

When selective thoracic fusion is applied to a King-Moe type II curve, overcorrection must be avoided. The thoracic curve should be corrected only as much as the left lumbar curve is able to compensate. Overcorrection will produce decompensation to the right.

After correction, the most caudal fused segment should be neutral and stable. Fusion of a King-Moe type III or IV pattern short of the neutral and stable vertebra may produce decompensation to the right.

Thoracoplasty is indicated in patients with significant rib prominence (more than 6 cm of elevation). The thoracoplasty not only yields cosmetic improvement, but also the resected rib serves as a good source of bone graft.

Anterior instrumentation has powerful corrective capability and may save fusion levels compared with posterior instrumentation. This is most applicable to single lumbar and thoracolumbar curves.

References

Hall JE: Anterior Surgery in the Treatment of Idiopathic Scoliosis. J Bone Joint Surg Br, 76:3–6, 1994.

King HA, Moe JH, Bradford DS, et al.: The Selection of Fusion Levels in Thoracic Idiopathic Scoliosis. J Bone Joint Surg Am, 65:1302–1313, 1983.

Lonstein JE, et al.: Moe's Textbook of Scoliosis and Other Spinal Deformities, 3rd Ed. Philadelphia, WB Saunders, 1995.

68. **c** Sagittal decompensation. The lateral radiograph demonstrates sagittal decompensation. The patient has lost her normal lumbar lordosis. This case demonstrates the significance of preserving normal lumbar lordosis, most of which typically exists below L3. Failure to contour the rods appropriately when using segmental instrumentation renders the instrumentation functionally equivalent to simple posterior distraction instrumentation. The result is a form of flat back. This was a common problem seen with Harrington-type instrumentation. The severe loss of lordosis has exceeded the capacity of adjacent spinal segments to compensate.

Thoracic hypokyphosis will develop as an attempt to compensate sagittally. Hip hyperextension also occurs as a compensatory measure to achieve appropriate sagittal balance. Increased demand on the hip extensors accounts for the thigh and buttock pain that is commonly observed in patients with flat back. Compromised hip extension will exacerbate clinical decompensation in these patients.

69. **a** Unilateral unsegmented bar with a contralateral hemivertebra. Congenital spinal anomalies are classified into two basic groups: defects of formation (i.e., hemivertebra) and defects of segmentation (i.e., unsegmented bar). The anomaly with the greatest potential for progressive curvature is the combination of a unilateral unsegmented bar on the concavity with a contralateral hemivertebra. Such curves have been documented to progress at rates as high as 12 degrees per year.

The unilateral bar is the second most severe defect, followed by double convex hemivertebrae. A single hemivertebra may or may not cause a progressive curvature.

Curves progress because of growth imbalance. Block vertebrae have no growth potential, and therefore they usually do not produce growth imbalance. Progression occurs more rapidly during periods of rapid growth (i.e., between 0 and 3 years and at the pubertal growth spurt).

Reference

Winter RB, Lonstein JE, Boachie-Adjei O: Congenital Spinal Deformity. J Bone Joint Surg Am, 78:300–311, 1996.

70. **d** Axis to occiput fusion. This patient manifests advanced atlantoaxial subluxation and atlantoaxial impaction (the lower limit of normal Ranawat index is 13 mm). The presence of these two conditions in conjunction with the neurologic symptoms mandates surgical intervention. Despite the absence of a neurologic deficit, her spinal cord is at risk.

Theoretically, resection of the dens alone (option e) would provide additional space for the spinal cord. However, this case appears to be anterior cord compression from the dens. This is best seen on the magnetic resonance imaging scan. Her intermittent symptoms suggest that her principal problem stems from dynamic instability. Dens resection (by itself) would do nothing to address the C1-C2 instability; in fact, it would further destabilize the C1-C2 articulation. Furthermore, the transoral approach to the dens is associated with an extremely high complication rate.

An atlantooccipital fusion would not address the atlantoaxial instability. An atlantoaxial fusion would not treat the associated atlantoaxial impaction. An axis to occiput fusion would treat both levels of instability.

Note: This patient should be fiberoptically intubated with the cervical spine rigidly immobilized.

Reference

Monsey RD: Rheumatoid Arthritis of the Cervical Spine. J Am Acad Orthop Surg, 5:240–248, 1997.

71. **b** Congenital kyphosis is the most common of the three major patterns of congenital spine deformity. Congenital spinal deformity is associated with multiple other anomalies. Approximately 40% of patients with a congenital spinal deformity have some form of spinal dysraphism. Genitourinary and cardiac malformations are present in 20% and 12%, respectively, of patients with congenital spinal deformity. Congenital lordosis is the least common of the three major patterns of congenital deformity (scoliosis, kyphosis and lordosis), and scoliosis is the most common.

Kyphosis from a defect of segmentation tends to have a better prognosis than kyphosis produced by a defect of formation. Segmentation defects tend to cause gradual, round curves, whereas defects of formation show a tendency for causing sharp angular deformities and paraplegia.

Congenital kyphosis (of all types) is a surgical disease. No form of nonoperative management is useful in this population. Treatment goals include early recognition, prompt posterior fusion to halt progression, and prevention of paraplegia.

Although bracing does have limited utility in the management of congenital scoliosis (specifically, for long flexible curves), it has no efficacy for short, stiff congenital curves.

Reference

Winter RB, Lonstein JE, Boachie-Adjei O: Congenital Spinal Deformity. Instructional Course Lecture. J Bone Joint Surg Am, 78:300–311, 1996.

72. **d** Posterior spinal fusion. The two most important factors in determining treatment in idiopathic scoliosis are the magnitude of the curve and the remaining growth potential of the child. When the deformity reaches 40 to 45 degrees in a skeletally immature patient, surgery is indicated.

General guidelines for treatment of adolescent idiopathic scoliosis are given in Table 3.1.

TABLE 3.1. GUIDELINES FOR TREATMENT OF ADOLESCENT IDIOPATHIC SCOLIOSIS

Curve Magnitude (Degrees)	Risser Stage	Treatment
0–25	Immature	Observation (serial radiograph)
25–30	Immature	Brace (if progressive)
30–40	Immature	Brace (+/– progression)
>40	Immature	Fusion
0–50	Mature	No brace; no fusion
>50–60	Mature	Fusion

The two principal indications for a combined anterior-posterior procedure in idiopathic scoliosis are (1) a large stiff curve and (2) young skeletal age and concern over potential for the "crankshaft" phenomenon with continued growth of the vertebral bodies. There may be some postoperative loss of correction (from the "crankshaft" phenomenon) in this adolescent patient, but not enough to warrant a combined anteroposterior fusion.

Reference

Lonstein JE, et al.: Moe's Textbook of Scoliosis and Other Spinal Deformities, 3rd Ed. Philadelphia, WB Saunders, 1995.

73. **c** If untreated, they have similar chances of curve progression. Lonstein and Carlson provided cross-correlated data that is useful for predicting the chance of idiopathic curve progression during skeletal growth. These authors focused on two factors: curve magnitude and Risser sign. In their study, the incidence of progression was significantly less in patients whose initial curve magnitude was less than 19 degrees (versus those whose initial curve magnitude was 20 to 29 degrees). They found that the chance of progression was approximately the same for a large curve (20 to 29 degrees) in a mature child (Risser 2 to 4) as it was for a small curve (less than 19 degrees) in an immature child (Risser 0 to 1).

One can see from Table 3.2 that the sister and brother described in this question have quite similar chances of progression (22% and 23% respectively).

Reference

Lonstein JE, Carlson JM: The Prediction of Curve Progression in Untreated Idiopathic Scoliosis During Growth. J Bone Joint Surg Am, 66:1061–1071, 1984.

TABLE 3.2. CHANCE OF IDIOPATHIC CURVE PROGRESSION DURING SKELETAL GROWTH

Riser Sign	<19 Degrees	20–29 Degrees
0–1	22%	68%
2–4	1.6%	23%

TABLE 3.3. TREATMENT GUIDELINES FOR SCHEUERMANN KYPHOSIS

Amount of Kyphosis (Degrees)	Treatment
<50	Observation, serial radiographs, extension exercise program
50–74	Milwaukee brace
>75	Consider surgery if symptomatic
>75 (corrects to <50)	Single-staged posterior procedure
>75 (corrects to >50)	Anterior and posterior spinal fusion

74. **e** Instrumented posterior spinal fusion. Scheuermann kyphosis is diagnosed based on the following radiographic features: (1) kyphosis exceeding 45 degrees, (2) 5 degrees or more of wedging at least three adjacent vertebrae, and (3) end plate changes.

Treatment depends on the severity of the deformity. General guidelines are given in Table 3.3.

Most cases recognized during adolescence are treated successfully with a brace. Severe kyphosis (more than 75 degrees), skeletal maturity, and increased vertebral wedging (averaging greater than 10 degrees) are factors that limit the success of bracing. Surgery should be considered in these uncommon instances.

If the deformity is flexible, then posterior fusion is adequate. However, staged anterior and posterior fusion with instrumentation is recommended for patients with kyphosis that does not correct to less than 50 degrees on a hyperextension lateral radiograph.

References

Boachie-Adjei O, Lonner B: Spinal Deformity. Pediatr Clin North Am, 43:885–897, 1996.

Murray PM, Weinstein SL, Spratt KF: The Natural History and Long-Term Follow-up of Scheuermann's Kyphosis. J Bone Joint Surg Am, 77:236–248, 1993.

75. **a** She needs operative spinal stabilization. Even though she is Risser stage 5, several studies have demonstrated that curves greater than 50 degrees continue to progress after skeletal maturity. Her curve requires stabilization to prevent further deterioration. Correction at a later time will be more difficult and more dangerous. Brace use has no utility in this context, given her skeletal maturity and lack of pain.

Because both the thoracic and the lumbar curves cross the midline, this patient has a double major curve. Selective thoracic fusion is not indicated for a double major curve. The King-Moe type V pattern is a double thoracic curve (with T1 tilted into the concavity of the upper curve).

References

King HA, Moe JH, Bradford DS, et al.: The Selection of Fusion Levels in Thoracic Idiopathic Scoliosis. J Bone Joint Surg Am, 65:1302–1313, 1983.

Weinstein SL, Ponseti IV: Curve Progression in Idiopathic Scoliosis. J Bone Joint Surg Am, 65:447–455, 1983.

76. **e** Magnetic resonance imaging of the entire spine. Most adolescent idiopathic scoliosis curves are right thoracic curves. Left thoracic idiopathic curves are extremely atypical. This finding warrants consideration of the diagnosis of nonidiopathic scoliosis. A left thoracic curve pattern is associated with a 20% incidence of intraspinal disease.

Reference

Winter RB, et al.: The Prevalence of Spinal Canal or Cord Abnormalities in Idiopathic, Congenital, or Neuromuscular Scoliosis. Orthop Trans, 16:135, 1992.

77. **d** Anterior débridement, decompression, and anterior fusion. This patient has pyogenic vertebral osteomyelitis with significant deformity and neurologic compromise. Surgical intervention is indicated because of the neurologic deficit, associated bony deformity, and compression of the dura. An anterior procedure is preferred in this situation for multiple reasons: (1) a posterior approach could not effectively débride the infected tissue; (2) a posterior approach could not mechanically reconstitute the destroyed anterior and middle columns; and (3) the source of cord compression is anterior. A posterior approach could not decompress the spinal cord as effectively as an anterior procedure.

Optimal intervention would consist of anterior débridement, decompression, and fusion with strut grafting. Supplementary posterior instrumentation may be necessary as well. Laminectomy would not only provide suboptimal decompression, but it would also destabilize the posterior column. Posterior instrumentation would be destined to fail in the absence of anterior-middle column reconstitution.

Reference

Malawski SK, Lukawski S: Pyogenic Infection of the Spine. Clin Orthop, 272:58–66, 1991.

78. **e** Digital rectal examination and assessment of perianal sensation. Of the multiple potential causes of urinary retention in the early postoperative period, cauda equina syndrome is one of the least frequent. However, it is crucial not to overlook this possible source in

patients who have had lumbar surgery. Potential reversible causes (epidural hematoma or pedicle screw malposition) must be detected and corrected as soon as possible to ensure maximal recovery. Thus, in such a setting, perianal sensation and rectal sphincter function should be assessed promptly. If an abnormality is detected, then it will be necessary to proceed with magnetic resonance imaging and/or computed tomography scanning to rule out epidural hematoma and/or pedicle screw malposition. These studies should be performed urgently because cauda equina syndrome is a surgical emergency.

79. **e** Thoracic computed tomography myelography. The most likely diagnosis in this case is thoracic disc herniation. Thoracic myelography (without computed tomography) is less than 70% sensitive for thoracic disc herniation. Thoracic computed tomography myelography is diagnostic for thoracic disc herniation in 95% of cases. Computed tomography myelography can accurately demonstrate canal compromise and the presence of lateral disc herniations.

The relative utility of magnetic resonance imaging versus computed tomography myelography remains controversial in the setting of thoracic disc herniation. Advantages of computed tomography myelography include the following: (1) computed tomography is superior to magnetic resonance imaging in demonstrating disc calcifications; (2) there is a high incidence of asymptomatic thoracic disc herniation; (3) magnetic resonance imaging may be overly sensitive; and (4) cardiac motion may produce artifact on magnetic resonance imaging scans.

Advantages of magnetic resonance imaging include (1) the capacity to yield both sagittal and axial images, (2) noninvasiveness, (3) its superior ability to detect disc degeneration, and (4) its greater sensitivity in detecting other forms of disease that may mimic thoracic disc herniation (i.e., multiple sclerosis, spinal cord tumors, aneurysms, transverse myelitis, and retroperitoneal neoplasms). Nerve conduction studies have not been found to be helpful for the diagnosis of herniated thoracic discs.

References

Garfin SR, Vaccaro AR: Orthopaedic Knowledge Update: Spine. Rosemont, IL, American Academy of Orthopedic Surgeons, p. 88, 1997.

Wood KB, et al.: MRI of the Thoracic Spine: Evaluation of Asymptomatic Individuals. J Bone Joint Surg Am, 77:1631–1638, 1995.

80. **d** 20%. The study by Boden et al. prospectively evaluated the incidence of abnormalities noted on magnetic resonance imaging scans of asymptomatic persons who had no history of back pain, sciatica, or neurogenic claudication. Twenty percent of asymptomatic persons who were less than 60 years old demonstrated a herniated nucleus pulposus on magnetic resonance imaging scans; 35% of asymptomatic persons less than 60 years old demonstrated degeneration or bulging of a disc on magnetic resonance imaging scans.

Among asymptomatic persons who were more than 60 years old, 36% demonstrated a herniated nucleus pulposus on magnetic resonance imaging scans; 21% of this older cohort manifested spinal stenosis on magnetic resonance imaging scans. All but one demonstrated degeneration or bulging of a disc on magnetic resonance imaging scans.

Although these findings were all subclinical, it would not be correct to categorize them as "false-positive." However, because of the prevalence of abnormal magnetic resonance imaging findings in asymptomatic persons, Boden et al. emphasized the requirement for strict correlation of magnetic resonance imaging findings with clinical symptoms and findings before contemplating surgical intervention.

Reference

Boden S, et al.: Abnormal Magnetic-Resonance Scans of the Lumbar Spine in Asymptomatic Subjects. J Bone Joint Surg Am, 72:403–408, 1990.

81. **b** It has been proven to result in a lower rate of pseudarthrosis compared with standard posterolateral intertransverse process fusion. By providing an anterior fusion through a posterior approach, posterior lumbar interbody fusion offers many potential advantages. Complete discectomy and disc height restitution can be achieved through the same incision used for a thorough decompression of both the cord and nerve roots. Posterior lumbar interbody fusion also allows an extraperitoneal approach to the L5-S1 disc space. In addition, it is biomechanically advantageous to have the site of arthrodesis anteriorly (where it is under compression rather than tension). However, this theoretic advantage has not yet translated into a lower rate of pseudarthrosis compared with standard posterolateral intertransverse process fusion. Supplementary posterior instrumentation may lower the pseudarthrosis rate.

Critics of posterior lumbar interbody fusion invoke concerns over the potential for (1) nerve root irritation from excessive retraction for exposure, (2) posterior graft extrusion, and (3) iatrogenic spine destabilization from the combination of a thorough discectomy and the wide posterior decompression that is required for exposure.

Reference

Herkowitz HN, Sidhu KS: Lumbar Spine Fusion in Degenerative Conditions. J Am Acad Orthop Surg, 3(3):123–135, 1995.

82. **c** If complete excision of the lesion is accomplished within 15 months of the onset of his symptoms, then

significant curve regression and/or complete resolution can be anticipated. This is a stereotypical presentation of scoliosis secondary to osteoid osteoma. Note the radiolucent nidus and surrounding sclerosis at the pedicle. (Although this lesion has been reported in the vertebral body, involvement of the posterior elements is the rule).

Adolescent idiopathic scoliosis is characteristically painless. The diagnosis of osteoid osteoma should be entertained whenever an adolescent with scoliosis complains of significant associated back pain. In the setting of an osteoid osteoma, the concavity of the curve almost invariably faces the side of the osteoid osteoma.

Scoliosis secondary to osteoid osteoma is typically clinically inflexible. Curves that are present for a significant amount of time during growth have a tendency to become structural. However, when the lesion is completely excised within the first 15 months of symptoms, curves tend to resolve spontaneously. Conversely, patients rarely improve when excision is accomplished after symptoms have been present for longer than 15 months. Limited primary fusion of the spine may be indicated if the surgical approach for excision of the lesion significantly destabilizes the posterior elements.

Reference

Pettine KA, et al.: Osteoid Osteoma and Osteoblastoma of the Spine. J Bone Joint Surg Am, 68:354–361, 1986.

83. **d** Acid-fast, nonmotile rods. This clinical history and radiographic findings are most consistent with a diagnosis of granulomatous vertebral osteomyelitis (tuberculosis). *Mycobacterium tuberculosis* is an acid-fast, nonmotile rod.

Characteristic radiographic features of tuberculous spondylitis include (1) involvement of multiple adjacent vertebral bodies, (2) paravertebral shadow (representing paravertebral abscess), and (3) relative sparing of the intervertebral disc. The magnetic resonance imaging scan usually demonstrates multiple adjacent vertebral involvement with relative sparing of the disc.

Note: Unlike pyogenic vertebral osteomyelitis, which initially involves the disc space, tuberculous vertebral osteomyelitis initially spares the disc space.

Reference

Boachie-Adjei O, Squillante RG: Tuberculosis of the Spine. Orthop Clin North Am, 27:95–103, 1996.

84. **e** Anterior débridement and decompression with strut grafting followed by 3 to 6 months of culture-directed, outpatient chemotherapy. Medical treatment would be the treatment of choice in the absence of neurologic deficit. However, based on this patient's magnetic resonance imaging and neurologic examination, surgical decompression of the spinal cord is warranted.

An anterior procedure would be preferable to posterior decompression in this case because it would (1) permit débridement of the large paraspinal abscess, (2) allow thorough débridement of the infected material in the two adjacent involved vertebral bodies, (3) provide optimal decompression of the cord, and (4) permit reconstitution of the compromised anterior and middle columns (strut grafting) to decrease the chance of late progressive collapse and deformity. Radical anterior débridement with fusion has been proven to yield results superior to those of simple anterior fusion and medical treatment, particularly with regard to the incidence and progression of kyphotic deformity.

Laminectomy (alone) is contraindicated in this case. Infectious destruction and neurologic compromise have occurred anterior to the cord. Posterior decompression would further destabilize the spine and would create a diathesis for progressive kyphotic deformity.

Requirements for successful nonoperative management of tuberculous spondylitis include (1) the absence of a neurologic deficit, (2) the presence of a chemotherapy-sensitive organism, and (3) the absence of a significant gibbous deformity.

References

Boachie-Adjei O, Squillante RG: Tuberculosis of the Spine. Orthop Clin North Am, 27:95–103, 1996.
Medical Research Council Working Party on Tuberculosis of the Spine: A Ten-Year Assessment of Anterior Spinal Fusion in the Management of Tuberculosis of the Spine in Patients on Standard Chemotherapy in Hong Kong. J Bone Joint Surg Br, 64:393–398, 1982.

85. **b** It arises most commonly from an anterior intercostal artery on the right side. The artery of Adamkiewicz is also known as the great anterior radicular artery. It is the main tributary to the anterior spinal artery in the lumbar and the lower thoracic regions of the spine. Thus, the artery of Adamkiewicz is the main arterial supply for the inferior two-thirds of the anterior spinal cord. Interruption of this vessel can produce a regional spinal cord infarction.

The artery of Adamkiewicz arises most commonly from a posterior intercostal artery on the left side. However, it sometimes originates from a superior lumbar artery. It most commonly enters the vertebral canal through an intervertebral foramen at the T9-T12 level.

Reference

Garfin SR, Vaccaro AR: Orthopaedic Knowledge Update: Spine. Rosemont, IL, American Academy of Orthopedic Surgeons, p. 15, 1997.

86. **c** A one-level bilateral posterior fusion *in situ*. Spondylolisthesis was graded by Meyerding according to the

amount of slippage of the superior vertebra on the inferior vertebra: grade I, 0% to 25%; grade II, 25% to 50%; grade III, 50% to 75%; and grade IV, 75% to 100%.

The recommended treatment for a child with an asymptomatic grade I slip includes full activity with no restrictions. A grade II slip necessitates restriction from contact sports and serial radiographs until maturity. A grade III slip is treated with a posterior fusion *in situ*. A grade IV slip is also treated with a posterior fusion *in situ*.

Exceptions to these generalizations are as follows. Operative treatment is indicated for low-grade slips with mechanical or neurologic symptoms recalcitrant to appropriate attempts at nonsurgical management. Surgery is also indicated for presentation with more than 50% slippage and for documented progression of slips beyond 25% to 33% (in a growing child).

References

Bradford DS. In Lonstein JE, et al., eds: Moe's Textbook of Scoliosis and Other Spinal Deformities, 3rd Ed. Philadelphia, WB Saunders, 1994.

Garfin SR, Vaccaro AR: Orthopaedic Knowledge Update: Spine. Rosemont, IL, American Academy of Orthopedic Surgeons, p. 158, 1997.

Saraste H: Long-Term Clinical and Radiological Follow-up of Spondylolysis and Spondylolisthesis. J Pediatr Orthop, 7:631–638, 1987.

87. **a** Annulus, type 1; nucleus, type 2. Intervertebral discs are composed of water, proteoglycans, collagen, elastic fibers, and various noncollagenous proteins. The collagen in the nucleus is synthesized by chondrocytes and is predominantly type II. The collagen in the annulus is synthesized by chondrocytes and fibrocytes and is predominantly type I. Water is a major component of both the nucleus (70% to 90%) and the annulus (60% to 70%).

88. **c** 80% through the vertebral body. Biomechanical studies have proven that pedicle screw pullout strength is increased with greater depth of insertion into the vertebral body. Maximum pullout strength is attained when screw threads actually cross the anterior cortex. However, vascular injury from anterior cortex penetration can be catastrophic. Furthermore, screw pullout is not the principal mode of pedicle screw failure, except in extremely osteopenic bone. Rather, under most circumstances, the principal mode of screw failure is bending fatigue.

The risk of vascular injury outweighs the potential for greater resistance to screw pull out with screw insertion across the anterior cortex. Thus, to ensure that the anterior vertebral body cortex is not violated, the recommended depth of screw insertion is 50% to 80% across the anteroposterior diameter of the vertebral body.

References

Vaccaro AR, Garfin SR: Pedicle Screw Fixation in the Lumbar Spine. J Am Acad Orthop Surg, 3(5):263–274, 1995.

Weinstein JN, et al.: Anatomic and Technical Considerations of Pedicle Screw Fixation. Clin Orthop, 284:34–46, 1992.

89. **d** C7-T1 level, C7 root. C7 innervates the triceps and cervical roots exit below the level of the disc space. Therefore, the lower nerve root at any given level is usually affected in the cervical spine.

Diffuse idiopathic skeletal hyperostosis is an idiopathic condition characterized by proliferative ossification along the ventral spine. It typically produces flowing anterior ankylosis of multiple contiguous vertebrae with relative sparing of the apophyseal joints and the intervertebral discs. Diffuse idiopathic skeletal hyperostosis most commonly affects the thoracic spine, but involvement of the cervical and/or lumbar spine is not unusual. The lower segments are more commonly involved than the upper segments.

Ankylosing spondylitis typically produces more severe symptoms and affects young adults, whereas diffuse idiopathic skeletal hyperostosis produces relatively mild symptoms in middle-aged and elderly persons. The syndesmophytes in ankylosing spondylitis are relatively thin compared with the broad excrescences in diffuse idiopathic skeletal hyperostosis. Furthermore, the syndesmophytes in ankylosing spondylitis occur circumferentially around the involved disc spaces (producing the characteristic "bamboo spine" appearance on anteroposterior radiographs). This distribution differs from the strict anterior distribution of ankylosis seen in diffuse idiopathic skeletal hyperostosis.

Likewise, the paravertebral outgrowths in psoriatic arthritis and Reiter syndrome do not demonstrate a predilection for the ventral surface of the spine. In fact, the marginal syndesmophytes in these two conditions are generally best visualized on anteroposterior spine films. Psoriatic arthritis and Reiter syndrome can also be distinguished from diffuse idiopathic skeletal hyperostosis based on their tendency for sacroiliitis and apophyseal joint involvement.

Acromegaly can produce bridging spinal osteophytes that resemble diffuse idiopathic skeletal hyperostosis. However, distinguishing features of acromegaly include posterior vertebral scalloping, peripheral soft tissue hypertrophy, and joint space enlargement.

Hypertrophic osteoarthropathy produces periostitis and digital clubbing. It does not typically affect the spine. It is generally associated with underlying pulmonary disease.

90. **c** Extension of the instrumentation and fusion to T3. This patient has developed a junctional kyphosis at T10 to T11 above the fusion and instrumentation.

Appropriate management for this condition is extension of the posterior fusion to the high thoracic spine. Termination of the extended fusion at the midthoracic or low thoracic spine would leave too long a lever arm at the new junction and would predispose the patient to recurrence of the junctional breakdown.

Technical factors that predispose to this phenomenon include (1) excessive dissection and disruption of the interspinous ligament above the termination of the fusion and (2) placement of excessive lordosis into the lumbar construct.

91. **a** Radiation of the pain to the right posterior thigh. Routine spinal imaging tests are generally not recommended in the first month of low back symptoms except in the presence of specific "red flags" that may portend a more serious underlying condition. These "red flags," as set forth by the Agency for Health Care Policy Research, include the following:

Potential fracture:
Recent significant trauma (any age)
Recent mild trauma (in patients older than 50 years)
Prolonged steroid use
Osteoporosis
Age greater than 70 years
Potential tumor or infection:
Unexplained weight loss
History of malignant disease
Recent infection (including urinary tract infection)
Immunosuppression
Intravenous drug use
Pain increased by rest
Fever
Possible cauda equina syndrome:
Saddle anesthesia
Bladder dysfunction
Severe or progressive lower extremity neurologic deficit
Anal sphincter laxity
Major limb motor weakness

Note: sciatica is not a "red flag."

References

Bigos SJ, et al.: Acute Low Back Problems in Adults. AHCPR Publication No. 95-0643. Washington, DC, United States Department of Health and Human Services, 1994.
Garfin SR, Vaccaro AR: Orthopaedic Knowledge Update: Spine. Rosemont, IL, American Academy of Orthopedic Surgeons, pp. A16-A22, 1997.

92. **e** Serial casting followed by full time bracing. This is a case of infantile idiopathic scoliosis. By definition, the onset of an infantile idiopathic curve is 0 to 3 years of age. Boys are affected more commonly than girls, and left thoracic curves are more common than right thoracic curves. (Note that these characteristics are opposite those of adolescent idiopathic scoliosis.)

Observation is appropriate for phase I curves with a rib-vertebral angle difference of less than 20 degrees. However, active treatment is mandated for (1) phase I curves with an rib-vertebral angle difference of more than 20 degrees and (2) all phase II curves. Initial therapy should consist of serial corrective body casting followed by full-time bracing until adolescence, with close radiographic follow-up.

If casting or bracing fails to control the curve, then surgical stabilization is indicated. Instrumentation without fusion (subcutaneous rodding with serial rod lengthening procedures) would be the most appropriate treatment in such a setting. Instrumentation without fusion has the theoretic advantage of maximizing residual potential growth (height and chest volume).

Posterior spinal fusion alone would be inappropriate for such a young patient because of the likelihood of the crankshaft phenomenon. Combined anteroposterior fusion would prevent the crankshaft phenomenon, but fusion is generally delayed until the late juvenile or early adolescent years in an effort to maximize potential growth.

Note: Each spine segment contributes approximately 0.07 cm to longitudinal growth of the axial skeleton per year.

References

Dubousset J, et al.: The Crankshaft Phenomenon. J Pediatr Orthop, 9:541–550, 1989.
McMaster MJ: The Management of Progressive Infantile Idiopathic Scoliosis. J Bone Joint Surg Br, 61:36–42, 1979.
Mehta MH: The Rib-Vertebra Angle in the Early Diagnosis Between Resolving and Progressive Infantile Idiopathic Scoliosis. J Bone Joint Surg Br, 54:230–243, 1972.

93. **d** Transthoracic transpleural exposure and excision. Thoracic disc herniation is most common in the fourth decade of life. The male-to-female incidence is approximately equal. Seventy five percent of cases occur below the level of T8, and the most common site is the level of the T11-12 interspace. The mode of presentation is highly variable.

Surgical intervention is indicated for patients who present with myelopathy or for those with intractable pain who do not respond to nonsurgical management. The transthoracic transpleural route is the most versatile and is especially suitable for central and centrolateral discs from T4 to the thoracolumbar junction. The transsternal approach is only suitable for access to the upper thoracic spine (T2 to T4). Conventional posterior laminectomy is suboptimal because it requires retraction of the spinal cord and provides inadequate exposure of the disc. A transthoracic approach does not require manipulation of the cord and therefore carries a lower risk of paraplegia.

Reference

Bohlman H, Zdeblick T: Anterior Excision of Herniated Thoracic Discs. J Bone Joint Surg Am, 70:1038–1047, 1988.

94. **c** Posterior C1 decompression and C1-C5 fusion with transarticular C1-C2 screw fixation. The imaging studies reveal two regions of significant spinal cord compromise: (1) atlantoaxial instability and (2) subaxial subluxation at C2 to C3. Either one (or both) could be contributing to the patient's presenting symptoms. Thus, both must be addressed surgically.

   There is no significant cranial settling (as manifested by a Ranawat index of less than 13). Given the absence of significant cranial settling, fusion to the occiput is not indicated.

   Failure of C1 to reduce when the posterior atlanto-dens interval is less than 14 mm mandates posterior decompression. After posterior decompression of the C1 ring, the optimal means of achieving C1-C2 fixation is with transarticular screws. The fusion should be extended caudally to include all significantly subluxated segments. Termination of the fusion mass at C2 (above the unstable C2-3 articulation) would be inappropriate.

Reference

Monsey RD: Rheumatoid Arthritis of the Cervical Spine. J Am Acad Orthop Surg, 5:240–248, 1997.

95. **d** Anterior odontoid resection. Because of its high complication rate, anterior decompression is appropriate in select cases only. Patients with a solid posterior fusion who have persistent, symptomatic anterior cord compression with significant neurologic symptoms are candidates for an anterior odontoid resection. This procedure may lead to increased deformity and should not be performed in the absence of a posterior fusion.

   Traction and/or halo vest application would not be appropriate in this setting because there is no evidence of instability.

   Surgical treatment of the symptomatic rheumatoid spine has been very successful for pain relief (85% to 100%), but it has not proven to be as reliable for improving neurologic function. The degree of neurologic improvement depends on the preoperative impairment level. For Ranawat class II patients (subjective weakness with hyperreflexia and dysesthesia), the recovery rate is 60% to 100%. For Ranawat class III patients (objective weakness and long-tract signs), the rate of recovery is 20% to 60%.

Reference

Monsey RD: Rheumatoid Arthritis of the Cervical Spine. J Am Acad Orthop Surg, 5:240–248, 1997.

96. **b** 7 degrees. The scoliometer provides a means of clinically quantifying the angle of trunk rotation with forward bending. The screening examination is considered positive if the angle of trunk rotation reading is 7 degrees or more. An interval change of 3 degrees or more suggests curve progression. Smaller changes can be produced by variations in posture.

Reference

Scoliosis Research Society, Park Ridge, IL.

97. **b** L5 spondylolysis. This sagittal reformatted computed tomography image clearly demonstrates a disruption of the pars interarticularis. The best answer, therefore, is L5 spondylolysis.
98. **b** An accessory vertebral vein. The vertebral artery does not pass through the foramen transversarium of C7. It enters the C6 foramen transversarium and ascends through all cephalad foramen transversarium. On exiting the C1 foramen transversarium, the artery abruptly turns medially and passes along the superior border of C1 before it pierces the atlantooccipital membrane 1 to 2 cm from the midline. Due respect should be granted to the vertebral artery during a posterior approach to the cervical spine at the C1-occiput level.

   The only structure that passes through the C7 foramen transversarium is an accessory vein. The greater occipital nerve is formed by the posterior ramus of C2. It emerges beneath the obliquus capitis inferior muscle. The long thoracic nerve receives contributions from the C5, C6, and C7 nerve roots; it does not pass through the C7 foramen transversarium.

Reference

Hoppenfeld S: Surgical Exposures in Orthopaedics, 2nd Ed. Philadelphia, JB Lippincott, pp. 252–275, 1994.

99. **c** Branches from the first segments of the subclavian arteries. The paired vertebral arteries provide the primary blood supply to the cervical spinal cord. They originate as direct branches from the first segment of each subclavian artery. The vertebral arteries then ascend within the transverse foramen of the cervical vertebral bodies from C6 to C1. After exiting the transverse foramen of the atlas, the arteries pass posteromedially along the arch of C1, where they penetrate the posterior atlantooccipital membrane approximately 2 cm from the midline. Finally, they ascend through the foramen magnum and fuse to form the basilar artery, which subsequently ascends along the ventral pons. The cervical cord is perfused directly from a single anterior spinal artery and paired posterior spinal arteries. The anterior spinal artery is fed from anterior radicular branches from the vertebral arteries. The posterior

spinal artery is fed from posterior radicular branches form the vertebral arteries.

FIGURE CREDITS

Figure 3.1A–C. From Frymoyer FW: The Adult Spine. Philadelphia, JB Lippincott, p. 493, 1991, with permission.
Figure 3.2. From Rockwood CA, Green D, eds: Fractures in Adults, 3rd ed. Philadelphia, Lippincott–Raven, p. 1500, 1996, with permission.
Figure 3.3A and B. From Frymoyer FW: The Adult Spine. Philadelphia, JB Lippincott, pp. 2125–2126, 1991, with permission.
Figure 3.4A and B. From Levine AM: Orthopaedic Knowledge Update: Trauma. Rosemont, IL, American Academy of Orthopaedic Surgeons, pp. 318–319, 1996, with permission.
Figure 3.5A and B. From Frymoyer FW: The Adult Spine. Philadelphia, JB Lippincott, p. 1112, 1991, with permission.
Figure 3.7A and B. From Frymoyer FW: The Adult Spine. Philadelphia, JB Lippincott, p. 1557, 1991, with permission.
Figure 3.8A–C. From Frymoyer FW: The Adult Spine. Philadelphia, JB Lippincott, pp. 709–710, 1991, with permission.
Figure 3.9. From Stoller: Magnetic Resonance Imaging in Orthopaedics and Sports Medicine. Philadelphia, Lippincott Williams & Wilkins, p. 1140, with permission.
Figure 3.10A and B. From Weinstein JN: Essentials of the Spine. Philadelphia, Lippincott–Raven, p. 890, 1995, with permission.
Figure 3.11. From Stoller: Magnetic Resonance Imaging in Orthopaedics and Sports Medicine. Philadelphia, Lippincott Williams & Wilkins, p. 1140, with permission.
Figure 3.12. From Stoller: Magnetic Resonance Imaging in Orthopaedics and Sports Medicine. Philadelphia, Lippincott Williams & Wilkins, p. 1086, with permission.
Figure 3.13A and B. From Craig EV: Clinical Orthopaedics. Philadelphia, Lippincott Williams & Wilkins, pp. 429–431, 1999, with permission.
Figure 3. 14. From Frymoyer FW: The Adult Spine. Philadelphia, JB Lippincott, p. 357, 1991, with permission.
Figure 3.15. From Weinstein JN: Essentials of the Spine. Philadelphia, Lippincott–Raven, p. 38, 1995, with permission.
Figure 3.16. From Weinstein JN: Essentials of the Spine. Philadelphia, Lippincott–Raven, p. 78, 1995, with permission.
Figure 3.17. From Frymoyer FW: The Adult Spine. Philadelphia, JB Lippincott, p. 750, 1991.
Figure 3.18. From Weinstein JN: Essentials of the Spine. Philadelphia, Lippincott–Raven, p. 34, 1995, with permission.
Figure 3.19. From Crenshaw AH, ed: Campbell's Operative Orthopaedics, 8th Ed. St. Louis, CV Mosby, p. 3503, 1992, with permission.
Figure 3.20A–C. From Weinstein JN, Essentials of the Spine. Philadelphia, Lippincott–Raven, pp. 32–36, 1996, with permission.
Figure 3.21. From Rothman, Simeone: The Spine, 3rd Ed. Philadelphia, WB Saunders; 831, with permission.

4

HIP

QUESTIONS

1. Which of the following statements correctly describes the calcar femorale?
   (a) Its cephalad end merges with the posteromedial aspect of the femoral neck.
   (b) It is thicker laterally than medially.
   (c) It reinforces the superior femoral neck.
   (d) It is less dense than adjacent bone.
   (e) It reinforces the anterior femoral neck.
2. After total hip arthroplasty, what is the magnitude of the compressive force across the hip joint during unsupported ipsilateral single leg stance?
   (a) Approximately 2.5 times body weight
   (b) Approximately 1 times body weight
   (c) Approximately 1.25 times body weight
   (d) Approximately 5 times body weight
   (e) Approximately 0.5 times body weight
3. What is the most appropriate position for hip arthrodesis?
   (a) Neutral rotation, 15 degrees of abduction, 10 degrees of flexion
   (b) 10 degrees external rotation, 15 degrees of abduction, 45 degrees of flexion
   (c) Neutral rotation, 5 degrees of adduction, 30 degrees of flexion
   (d) 5 degrees of external rotation, 5 degrees of adduction, 10 degrees of flexion
   (e) 10 degrees of external rotation, 25 degrees of abduction, 5 degrees of flexion
4. Which of the following statements is true regarding reamed antegrade intramedullary femoral nailing?
   (a) Heterotopic ossification is a common phenomenon after femoral nailing, with a reported incidence of approximately 25%.
   (b) When heterotopic ossification occurs after femoral nailing, it is commonly associated with significant pain and compromised hip function.
   (c) Wound irrigation with pulsatile lavage has been shown to decrease the incidence and severity of heterotopic ossification in this setting.
   (d) Heterotopic ossification is rarely seen after femoral nailing except in association with concomitant intracranial injury.
   (e) Prophylaxis against heterotopic ossification with indomethacin is routinely indicated.
5. Which of the following best sequences the materials according to decreasing order of elastic moduli (stiffest to most elastic)?
   (a) (1) cobalt-chromium, (2) stainless steel, (3) titanium, (4) cortical bone, (5) polyethylene
   (b) (1) stainless steel, (2) titanium, (3) cobalt-chromium, (4) polyethylene, (5) cortical bone
   (c) (1) polyethylene, (2) cortical bone, (3) titanium, (4) stainless steel, (5) cobalt- chromium
   (d) (1) polyethylene, (2) cortical bone, (3) cobalt-chromium, (4) stainless steel, (5) titanium
   (e) (1) titanium, (2) stainless steel, (3) cobalt-chromium,(4) polyethylene, (5) cortical bone
6. A 29-year-old business school student has recently been fitted with an above-knee prosthesis after recovering from a boating (propeller) accident. Analysis of his gait demonstrates exaggerated lumbar lordosis during stance phase. Which of the following is not a potential explanation for this abnormality?
   (a) Weak abdominal muscles
   (b) Hip flexion contracture
   (c) Insufficient support from the anterior socket brim
   (d) Weak hip flexors
7. Displaced femoral neck fractures that are anatomically reduced and fixed with cannulated screws have an osteonecrosis rate of approximately
   (a) 5%
   (b) 15%
   (c) 50%
   (d) 75%
   (e) 90%
8. What structure is labeled by the *curved arrow* in Fig. 4.1?
   (a) The gracilis
   (b) The adductor longus
   (c) The semitendinosus

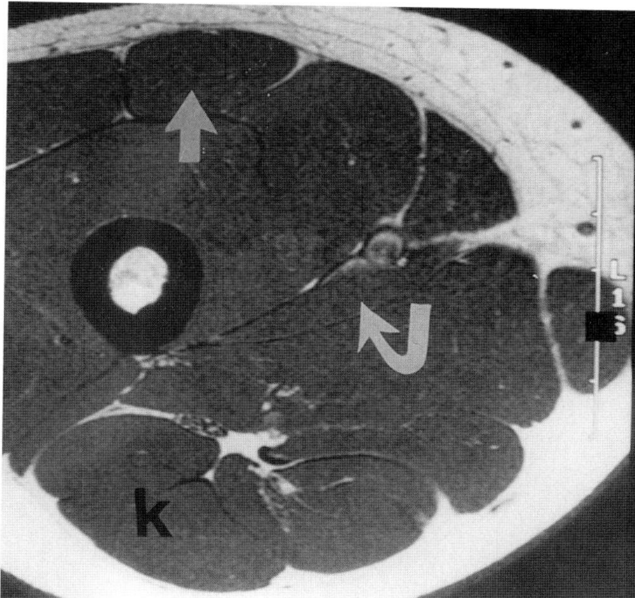

FIGURE 4.1

(d) The sartorius
(e) The vastus medialis

9. Which of the following is least commonly associated with acetabular protrusio?
   (a) Ochronosis
   (b) Paget disease
   (c) Ankylosing spondylitis
   (d) Arthrokatadysis
   (e) Marfan syndrome
10. Compared with cemented all-polyethylene acetabular components, cemented metal-backed acetabular components
    (a) Are associated with a higher rate of dislocation because of impingement of the femoral neck with the metal backing
    (b) Have a higher rate of septic failure
    (c) Are associated with higher peak cement mantle stresses
    (d) Are associated with increased polyethylene cold flow
    (e) Have a higher rate of aseptic loosening
11. In preparing the femoral canal during total hip arthroplasty, "third-generation" cement technique includes which of the following additions to "second-generation" technique?
    (a) Use of an intramedullary canal plug
    (b) Cement porosity reduction with centrifugation or vacuum mixing
    (c) Pulsatile lavage of the canal
    (d) Use of pressurized gas to dry the intramedullary canal
    (e) Use of preheated cement
12. An uncemented acetabular component is implanted with line-to-line reaming and supplemental screw fixation. A 35-mm screw is placed in the anterior superior quadrant of the acetabulum. Which of the following structures is at the greatest risk of being damaged during the drilling and insertion of this screw?
    (a) The obturator vein
    (b) The femoral nerve
    (c) The sciatic nerve
    (d) The internal iliac vein
    (e) The external iliac vein
13. The surgeon in question 12 feels an irresistible urge for more secure fixation, and he elects to place a 70-mm screw into the posterosuperior quadrant. Which of the following structures is at the greatest risk of being damaged by this maneuver?
    (a) This is a "safe zone" and no structures are at risk.
    (b) The pudendal nerve
    (c) The superior gluteal artery
    (d) The inferior gluteal artery
    (e) The external iliac artery
14. The location of the Ward triangle is
    (a) Medial to the principal compressive trabeculae
    (b) Between the principal and secondary compressive trabeculae
    (c) At the apex formed above the convergence of the principal tensile trabeculae and the secondary compressive trabeculae
    (d) Lateral to the secondary compressive trabeculae
    (e) At the apex formed below the convergence of the secondary tensile trabeculae and the secondary compressive trabeculae

Questions 15 to 17 are based on the following situation:

A 69-year-old retired nurse returns for routine follow-up 2 years after a femoral neck fracture that had been treated with an uncemented hemiarthroplasty. She complains of intermittent thigh pain that is worst during her first several steps after a period of inactivity. She has also noted moderate groin discomfort after prolonged walking. A radiograph is shown in Fig. 4.2A. One week later, she trips and falls while shopping, and she is unable to get up. A radiograph in the emergency room is shown in Fig. 4.2B.

15. What is the most likely explanation for her groin pain before her fall?
    (a) Undersizing of the head of the prosthesis
    (b) Wear of the acetabular articular cartilage
    (c) Osteolysis
    (d) Disjunction of the prosthetic head from the shaft
    (e) Oversizing of the head of the prosthesis
16. What is the most likely explanation for her thigh pain before her fall?

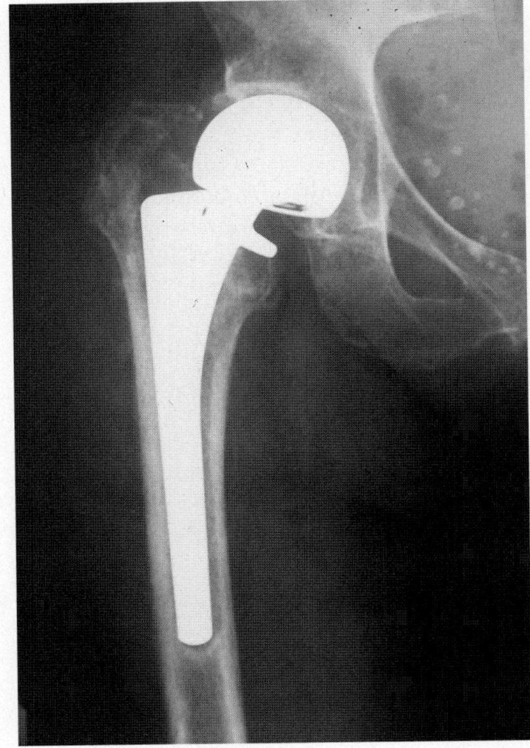

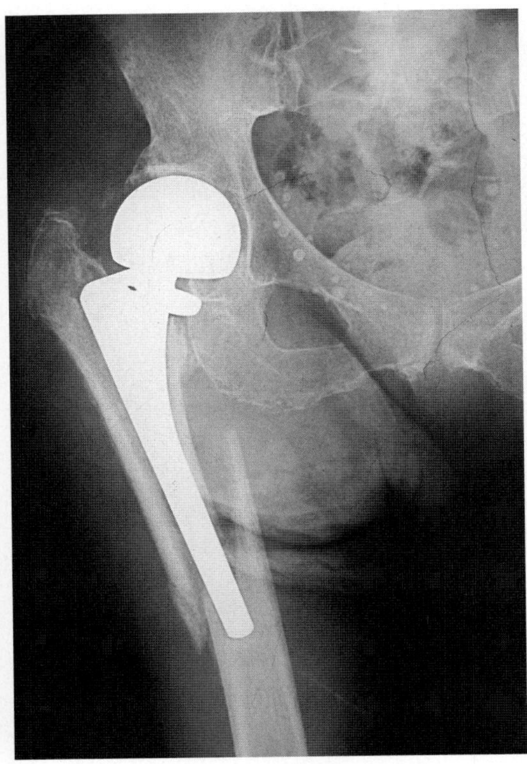

FIGURE 4.2A and B

(a) Stress fracture
(b) Mismatch between the moduli of elasticity of the stem and her cortical bone
(c) Meralgia paresthetica
(d) Aseptic loosening
(e) Iatrogenic shaft fracture at the time of stem implantation

17. How should you treat the patient at this point?
(a) Skeletal traction and bed rest for 6 weeks
(b) Open reduction and internal fixation with cerclage wires
(c) Open reduction and internal fixation with a spanning plate fixed proximally with cerclage wires and distally with screws
(d) Open reduction and internal fixation with conversion to a long-stem prosthesis
(e) Open reduction and internal fixation with conversion to a total hip arthroplasty with a long-stem prosthesis

18. An intertrochanteric osteotomy is contemplated for a 31-year-old investment banker with grade III osteonecrosis. Magnetic resonance imaging demonstrates focal involvement of the anterolateral portion of his femoral head. What would be the most appropriate procedure?
(a) Varus-extension osteotomy
(b) Valgus-flexion osteotomy
(c) Pure varus osteotomy
(d) Varus-flexion osteotomy
(e) Valgus-extension osteotomy

19. Which of the following statements regarding polymethylmethacrylate is correct?
(a) Polymethylmethacrylate is stronger under compression than under tension.
(b) Neither mixing the monomer and polymer in a vacuum nor centrifuging after mixing can improve the strength of polymethylmethacrylate.
(c) Polymethylmethacrylate is radiopaque.
(d) The elastic modulus of polymethylmethacrylate is more than cortical bone.
(e) Polymethylmethacrylate functions primarily as an adhesive.

20. Which of the following statements is most accurate regarding the effect of active movement of the foot and ankle on venous blood flow after total hip arthroplasty?
(a) No published evidence supports the widely accepted concept that active foot and ankle motion has a beneficial hemodynamic effect.
(b) The beneficial hemodynamic effect of active foot and ankle motion has been shown to decrease the incidence of proximal deep venous thrombosis by 50%.

(c) Active foot and ankle motion has been shown to produce a 22% mean increase in lower extremity venous outflow.
(d) Active foot and ankle motion has an unpredictable effect on lower extremity hemodynamics. It increases venous outflow in some persons but decreases venous outflow in others.
(e) The increase in lower extremity venous outflow peaks immediately after foot and ankle exercise and returns to baseline within the first 5 minutes after exercise.

21. A 16-year-old soccer player complains of persistent thigh pain 2 days after he was kicked in the same location by an opponent. His primary care physician orders a magnetic resonance imaging scan, to rule out an occult neoplasm (Fig. 4.3). What structure is labeled by the *O*?
(a) The adductor magnus
(b) The semitendinosus
(c) The gracilis
(d) The biceps femoris
(e) The semimembranosus

22. Which of the following patients has the least risk for developing heterotopic ossification after total hip arthroplasty?
(a) A 44-year-old man with ankylosing spondylitis
(b) A 22-year-old woman with rheumatoid arthritis
(c) A 62-year-old man with hypertrophic osteoarthritis
(d) A 50-year-old man with diffuse idiopathic skeletal hyperostosis
(e) A 72-year-old woman with osteoarthritis who developed heterotopic ossification in the contralateral hip after open reduction and internal fixation of a femoral neck fracture

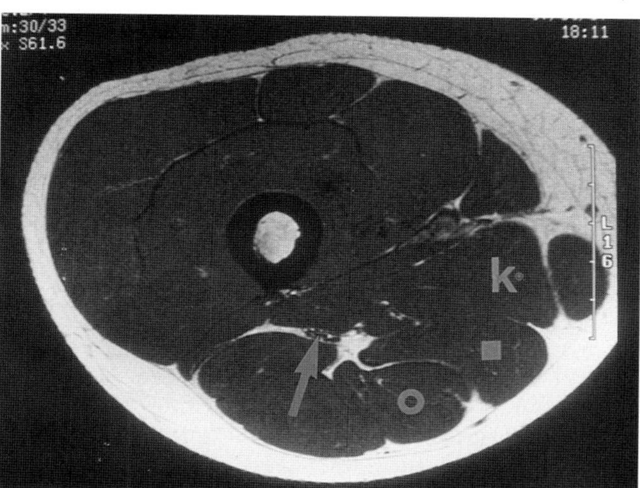

FIGURE 4.3

23. What percentage of DeLee and Charnley's low friction arthroplasty acetabular components demonstrated bone-cement interface radiolucencies at 10-year follow-up?
(a) Approximately 10%
(b) Approximately 30%
(c) Approximately 50%
(d) Approximately 70%
(e) Approximately 95%

24. Increased femoral component offset is associated with which of the following?
(a) Decreased bending stresses on the femoral component
(b) Decreased joint compressive forces
(c) Increased likelihood of impingement
(d) Increased rate of acetabular component mechanical loosening
(e) Increased abductor muscle contraction force during single leg stance

25. An internal medicine resident skis off a cliff and sustains an unstable pelvic fracture with sacroiliac joint disruption. Significant vertical migration and outward rotation of the hemipelvis are noted. Which of the following neurologic injuries is most likely to be encountered?
(a) L5 nerve root laceration
(b) Obturator nerve laceration by disrupted pubic rami
(c) Contusion of the anterior primary rami of the S1-S3 roots
(d) Lumbosacral trunk traction injury
(e) Avulsion of cauda equina nerve roots from the spinal cord

26. The material property that refers to the ability of a material to absorb relatively large amounts of plastic deformation before failing is
(a) Toughness
(b) Ductility
(c) Stress relaxation
(d) Fatigue strength
(e) Brittleness

27. After femoral component removal during a revision total hip arthroplasty, an oblong defect with rounded edges is noted. It involves 50% of the circumference of the cortex of the shaft. What is the residual torsional strength of the femur (expressed as a percentage of the strength of an intact femur)?
(a) Approximately 12%
(b) Approximately 25%
(c) Approximately 50%
(d) Approximately 75%
(e) Approximately 90%

28. Which of the following is a disadvantage of the Bernese (Ganz) periacetabular osteotomy?
(a) It requires two simultaneous surgical approaches.

(b) The shape of the true pelvis is narrowed so the potential for vaginal child delivery is jeopardized.
(c) Rotational corrections can produce undesirable linear translations of the center of rotation of the hip joint.
(d) It sacrifices the continuity of the posterior column of the pelvis.
(e) Subsequent total hip arthroplasty is contraindicated.

29. Which of the following muscles functions as an internal rotator of the hip?
(a) The iliopsoas
(b) The sartorius
(c) The gluteus medius
(d) The obturator internus
(e) The gluteus maximus

30. Which of the following statements is correct regarding the assessment of acute pelvic trauma by plain radiographs?
(a) The obturator oblique view is the best view for assessing the integrity of the anterior column.
(b) The pelvic inlet view is the best view for detecting vertical instability at a sacroiliac joint.
(c) The iliac oblique view is the best view for assessing the integrity of the posterior wall of the acetabulum.
(d) The pelvic outlet view is the best view for detecting rotational instability at a sacroiliac joint.
(e) The pelvic inlet view is the best view for assessing the integrity of the posterior column.

31. Which of the following statements regarding hip arthrodesis is most accurate?
(a) Two decades after fusion, the incidence of low back pain is approximately 60%.
(b) Two decades after fusion, the incidence of ipsilateral knee pain is approximately 15%.
(c) Conversion to a total hip arthroplasty carries the same prognosis as a primary total hip arthroplasty of a nonfused hip.
(d) Conversion to a total hip arthroplasty 2 decades after fusion would be expected to be more effective at relieving ipsilateral knee pain than relieving low back pain.
(e) Optimal management of a malaligned arthrodesis consists of takedown of the arthrodesis and repeat fusion in an improved position.

32. The greatest amount of proximal femoral bone loss resulting from stress shielding would be anticipated with which of the following types of femoral components?
(a) Cemented cobalt-chromium stem
(b) Uncemented, proximally porous-coated titanium alloy stem
(c) Cemented titanium alloy stem
(d) Uncemented, fully porous-coated cobalt-chromium stem
(e) Uncemented, proximally porous-coated cobalt-chromium stem

33. The anterior (Smith-Petersen) approach to the hip uses which internervous plane?
(a) The femoral nerve–inferior gluteal nerve plane
(b) The inferior gluteal nerve–superior gluteal nerve plane
(c) The femoral nerve–superior gluteal nerve plane
(d) The superior gluteal nerve–sciatic nerve plane
(e) No true internervous plane

34. A 28-year-old woman experienced the insidious onset of right groin pain approximately 16 months earlier. She continues to experience progressive pain with activity and an associated intermittent "catching" sensation. A plain radiograph is shown in Fig. 4.4A. Coronal T1 and T2-weighted magnetic resonance images are shown in Fig. 4.4B and C, respectively. Gross and histologic specimens reveal hyaline cartilage in nodules. The most likely diagnosis is
(a) Pigmented villonodular synovitis
(b) Multiple synovial ganglion cysts
(c) Synovial chondromatosis
(d) Synovial sarcoma
(e) Chondrosarcoma

35. Accelerated wear, cracking, and delamination in ultra-high-molecular-weight polyethylene components have been associated with subsurface white bands. To which of the following factors has this band been attributed?
(a) Compression molding
(b) Machining of ram-extruded polyethylene bars
(c) Sterilization with ethylene oxide
(d) Sterilization with γ irradiation and shelf aging in the presence of air
(e) The addition of calcium stearate to the polymer

36. A 67-year-old man undergoes hybrid total hip arthroplasty for posttraumatic coxarthrosis. The acetabular component is inserted with press fitting (2-mm under-reaming) and without supplemental screw fixation. A lucency of 1 mm located centrally in the dome (zone II) is noted on the postoperative radiograph. Which of the following statements is most accurate regarding this lucency at the bone-prosthesis interface?
(a) It is the result of intraoperative acetabular fracture
(b) Press-fit fixation is associated with an increased incidence of gaps in this location (compared with screw fixation with line-to-line reaming)
(c) It is associated with an increased incidence of component loosening at 5-year follow-up (compared with screw fixation with line-to-line reaming)
(d) Most isolated radiolucencies that are present in this location on initial postoperative radiographs will have progressed at 2-year follow-up
(e) It is associated with a approximately 20% incidence of profound focal cavitary osteolysis in the adjacent pelvis within the first 5 years

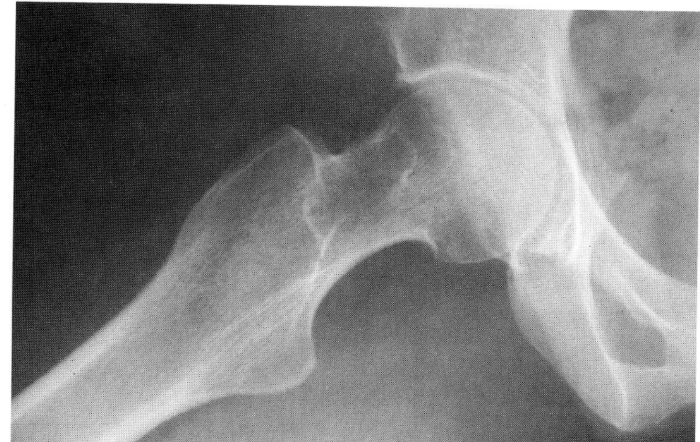

A

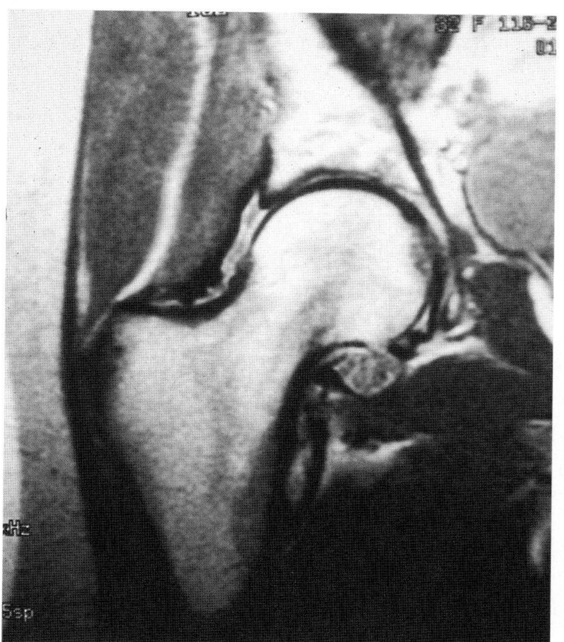

B

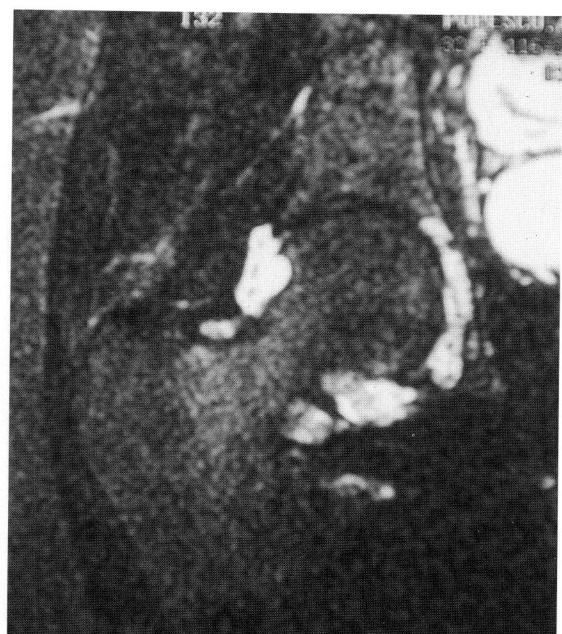

C

FIGURE 4.4A–C

37. What was the most common mechanism for aseptic loosening of the femoral component in primary cemented total hip arthroplasty using first-generation cement technique?
    (a) Pistoning (stem within cement) (type IA)
    (b) Pistoning (cement within bone) (type IB)
    (c) Medial midstem pivot (type II)
    (d) Calcar pivot (type III)
    (e) Bending, cantilever (fatigue) (type IV)
38. Which of the following statements is most accurate regarding the effect of micromotion on bone ingrowth into porous-coated implants?
    (a) Motion of any detectable quantity precludes bone ingrowth.
    (b) Motion of up to 28 μm is compatible with bone ingrowth, but motion greater than 150 μm produces fibrous ingrowth.
    (c) Motion of up to 150 μm is compatible with bone ingrowth, but motion greater than 150 μm produces fibrous ingrowth.
    (d) Motion of up to 10 μm is compatible with bone ingrowth, motion between 10 and 150 μm is compatible with fibrous ingrowth, and motion greater than 150 μm precludes ingrowth of any sort.
    (e) Motion of up to 300 μm is compatible with bone ingrowth.
39. A 33-year-old investment banker has recovered from a traumatic knee disarticulation (bungee-jumping mis-

hap) and has been fitted with an above-knee prosthesis. In observing his gait, you note a circumduction pattern. The *least* likely explanation for this abnormality is
(a) Excessive plantarflexion of the prosthetic ankle
(b) Inadequate overall length of the prosthesis
(c) Incomplete seating of the residual limb in the socket
(d) Inadequate prosthesis suspension
(e) Excessively deep seating of the residual limb in the socket

40. A 65-year-old man is knocked over and sustains a periprosthetic fracture below a loose total hip replacement. He is otherwise healthy and has no history of prosthetic infection. Which of the following would be the most appropriate treatment?
(a) Skeletal traction
(b) Bone stimulation
(c) Above-knee amputation
(d) Total femoral replacement
(e) Open reduction and internal fixation with revision of the femoral component of the total hip arthroplasty using a longer stem

41. While performing a hybrid total hip arthroplasty, a surgeon implants a modular uncemented acetabular component. She subsequently inserts an elevated liner with the elevation positioned directly posteriorly. What is the most significant potential benefit of this construct?
(a) Decreased volumetric wear rate
(b) Compensation for excessive retroversion of the acetabular shell
(c) Decreased incidence of anterior dislocation
(d) Increased range of motion
(e) Decreased impingement

42. What structure is labeled by the tip of the *curved white arrow* on the thigh magnetic resonance image in Fig. 4.5?
(a) The adductor magnus
(b) The vastus medialis
(c) The adductor brevis
(d) The sartorius
(e) The adductor longus

43. Which of the following anatomic alterations is least likely to be encountered during a total hip arthroplasty on a patient with developmental hip dysplasia?
(a) Increased femoral retroversion
(b) A deficient anterior acetabular wall
(c) Narrow (anterior-to-posterior) acetabular dimensions
(d) A false acetabulum
(e) A narrow proximal femoral intramedullary canal

44. Figure 4.6 is an axial T1 magnetic resonance image of the pelvis. The nerve that innervates the muscle marked by the *arrow* also innervates which of the following muscles?
(a) The quadratus femoris
(b) The inferior gemellus
(c) The obturator externus
(d) The superior gemellus
(e) The piriformis

45. All the following are commonly believed to be risk factors for avascular necrosis of the femoral head except
(a) Caisson disease
(b) Sickle cell anemia
(c) Gaucher disease
(d) Intraarticular glucocorticoid injection
(e) Pancreatitis

46. The design of the femoral prosthesis shown in Fig. 4.7 is intended to
(a) Provide increased offset
(b) Increase leg length
(c) Decrease the bending moment on the prosthesis
(d) Decrease the amount of torque transmitted from the prosthesis to the cement mantle

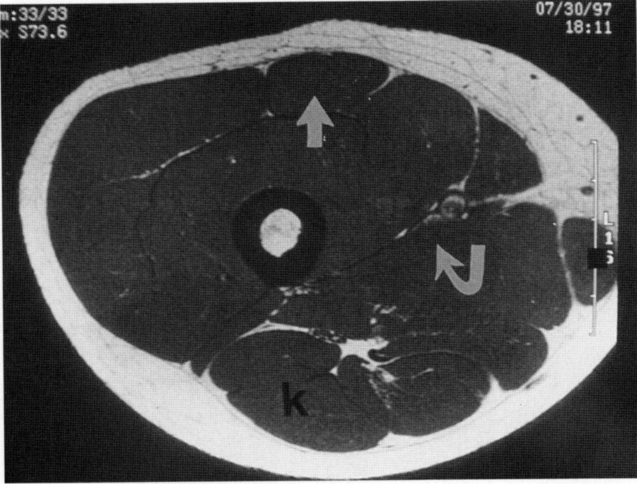

FIGURE 4.5

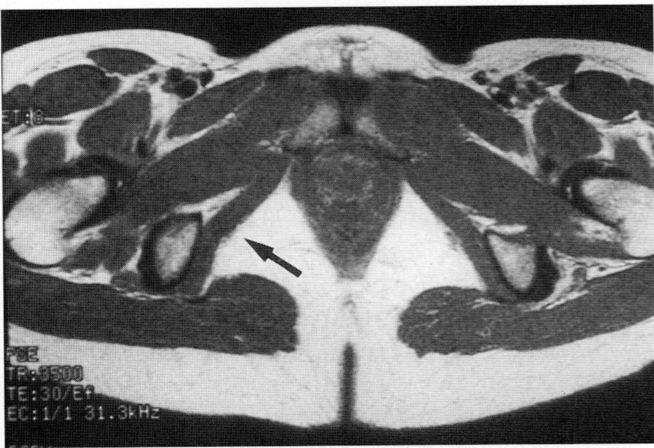

FIGURE 4.6

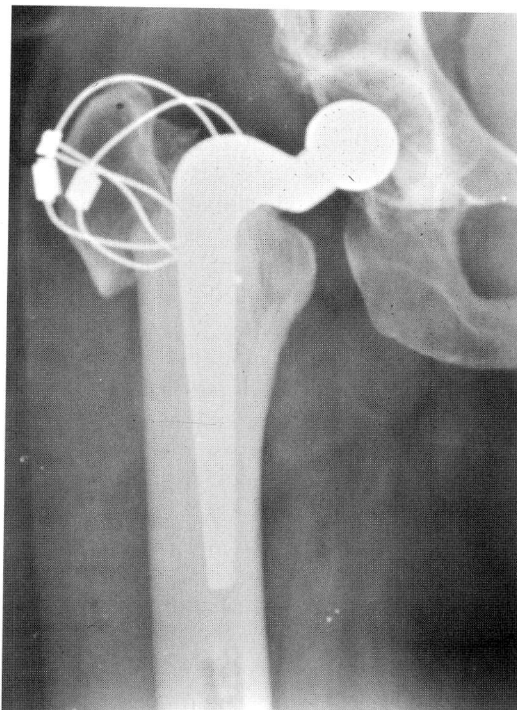

FIGURE 4.7

(e) Decrease the strain in the medial cement mantle

47. Which of the following factors is the most significant prophylactic measure against acute deep infection after large joint arthroplasty?
   (a) Preoperative antibiotics
   (b) Horizontal laminar flow operating theatres
   (c) Body exhaust suits
   (d) Use of double gloves
   (e) Vertical laminar flow operating theatres
48. Which of the following statements is correct regarding the biomechanics of the peritrochanteric region?
   (a) Valgus reductions of intertrochanteric fractures produce increased bending moments on sliding hip screws.
   (b) Bending moments on implants are increased by translating the implant closer to the weight-bearing axis.
   (c) Subtrochanteric fractures are characteristically associated with flexion of the proximal fragment, external rotation of the proximal fragment, and lateral translation of the distal fragment.
   (d) Decreasing the angle of inclination of a sliding hip screw is associated with decreased internal resistance to compression.
   (e) If an intertrochanteric fracture is associated with comminution of the medial cortex, then medial translation of the shaft fragment will decrease the bending moment on the implant.
49. A patient with an above-knee amputation has painful irritation of the skin over the distal lateral aspect of his residual femur. Which of the following gait abnormalities is he most likely to demonstrate as a result of this discomfort?
   (a) Circumduction
   (b) Foot rotation at heel strike
   (c) Vaulting gait
   (d) Lateral trunk bending (to the ipsilateral side)
   (e) Swing-phase whip
50. A 28-year-old man is involved in a head-on motor vehicle accident. A pelvic computed tomography scan in the emergency room reveals a posterior dislocation of his femoral head with no associated fracture. The least common complication of this injury is
   (a) Avascular necrosis of the femoral head
   (b) Recurrent dislocation
   (c) Sciatic nerve palsy
   (d) Posttraumatic arthritis
   (e) Irreducibility
51. All the following structures exit the greater sciatic notch distally to the piriformis except
   (a) The inferior gluteal nerve
   (b) The obturator nerve
   (c) The posterior femoral cutaneous nerve
   (d) The sciatic nerve
   (e) The pudendal nerve
52. A 65-year-old retired postal worker presents with left hip pain 15 years after cemented primary total hip arthroplasty for avascular necrosis. A radiograph is shown in Fig. 4.8. Comparison with a radiograph from

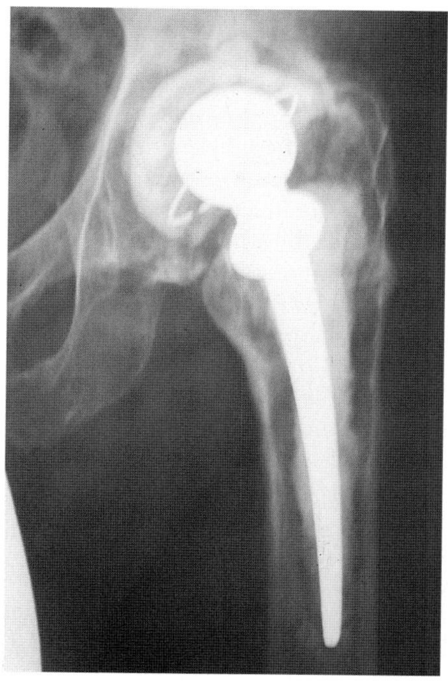

FIGURE 4.8

8 years ago reveals 5 mm of stem subsidence and no migration of the acetabular component. Based on these data, the surgeon should conclude that the (1) femoral and (1) acetabular components are
(a) (1) possibly loose and (2) stable
(b) (1) definitely loose and (2) definitely loose
(c) (1) definitely loose and (2) probably loose
(d) (1) probably loose and (2) possibly loose
(e) (1) infected and (2) infected

53. A revision of both components in Fig. 4.8 is planned. Provided that all defects are contained, what would be the most appropriate method for revising (1) the femur and (2) the acetabulum?
(a) (1) cemented long stem and (2) cemented all-polyethylene cup
(b) (1) uncemented standard length stem and (2) uncemented cup
(c) (1) fully coated uncemented long stem and (2) uncemented cup
(d) (1) cemented standard-lengthened stem and (2) cemented metal-backed cup
(e) (1) uncemented standard length stem and (2) cemented all-polyethylene cup

54. Which two nerves enter the pelvis through the lesser sciatic foramen?
(a) The nerve to the obturator externus and the pudendal nerve
(b) The nerve to the obturator externus and the genitofemoral nerve
(c) The pudendal nerve and the genitofemoral nerve
(d) The nerve to the obturator internus and the genitofemoral nerve
(e) The nerve to the obturator internus and the pudendal nerve

55. All the following steps act to decrease wear debris production after total hip arthroplasty except
(a) Use of thicker polyethylene (greater than 6 mm)
(b) Use of 28-mm heads (as opposed to 32-mm heads)
(c) Use of titanium femoral heads
(d) Avoidance of third-body contamination
(e) Avoidance of modularity

56. A 27-year-old power lifter complains of dysesthesias at the anterolateral aspect of his left thigh. The remainder of his peripheral neurologic examination is unremarkable. Which of the following would be the most appropriate initial clinical step?
(a) Lumbar myelography
(b) Lumbar magnetic resonance imaging
(c) Digital rectal examination
(d) Electromyography
(e) Adjustment of the fit of his weight belt

57. Patients with ankylosing spondylitis function with which of the following forms of acetabular malposition?
(a) Excessive retroversion
(b) Excessive extension
(c) Insufficient abduction
(d) Excessive abduction
(e) Excessive flexion

58. Which of the following statements is incorrect regarding corrosion of metal orthopaedic implants?
(a) The presence of a metal-oxide coating on the surface of an implant will prevent fretting.
(b) Titanium and stainless steel implants may undergo galvanic corrosion when they are inserted in close proximity to one another.
(c) Elevated levels of titanium have been documented in the serum of patients with failed titanium-containing total joint replacements.
(d) Galvanic corrosion can increase polyethylene debris production.
(e) Elevated serum levels of chromium have been detected in patients with well-functioning total hip prostheses composed of cobalt-chromium.

59. A 24-year-old professional squash player presents with persistent right inguinal pain and clicking after an episode of lunging for a backhand. A plain anteroposterior radiograph is unremarkable. Magnetic resonance imaging reveals a labral tear. He has failed to respond to a 3-month course of rest, stretching, and nonsteroidal antiinflammatory therapy. Which of the following would be the most appropriate treatment plan?
(a) 2 more months of relative rest and nonsteroidal antiinflammatory agents with an aggressive, supervised hip-strengthening protocol
(b) Hip arthroscopy and débridement
(c) Arthrotomy and repair
(d) Right inguinal herniorrhaphy
(e) Computed tomography–guided needle biopsy

60. During a direct lateral (Hardinge) approach to the hip, which neurovascular structure may be injured by excessive retraction of the gluteus medius muscle?
(a) The femoral nerve
(b) The superior gluteal nerve
(c) The sciatic nerve
(d) The inferior gluteal nerve
(e) The medial femoral circumflex artery

61. A 23-year-old woman commences training to run a marathon. Eight weeks later, she complains of right groin pain that is aggravated by running and relieved by rest. Physical examination reveals a slight antalgic gait with mildly limited hip flexion and internal rotation. Plain radiographs are unremarkable. A bone scan reveals increased activity in the right inferior femoral neck. T1 magnetic resonance images reveal a linear region of decreased signal intensity at the inferomedial femoral neck that extends 25% across its diameter. T2-weighted images manifest linear increased signal at the same location. How should she be treated?
(a) Urgent percutaneous pinning

(b) Valgus osteotomy and fixation with a 95-degree blade plate
(c) Non–weight bearing, crutches, and close observation
(d) Weight bearing as tolerated but with encouragement to stop running until the pain subsides and the bone scan normalizes
(e) Allowing the patient to continue running with modifications in her training schedule

62. A 70-year-old man presents with debilitating right hip pain. His complete blood count is normal, and his serum alkaline phosphatase level is 202 IU/L. A plain radiograph is shown in Fig. 4.9. What is the most likely diagnosis?
(a) Multiple myeloma
(b) Neurofibromatosis
(c) Paget disease
(d) Myelodysplasia
(e) Vitamin D–deficient rickets

63. Which of the following couples is most susceptible to galvanic corrosion?

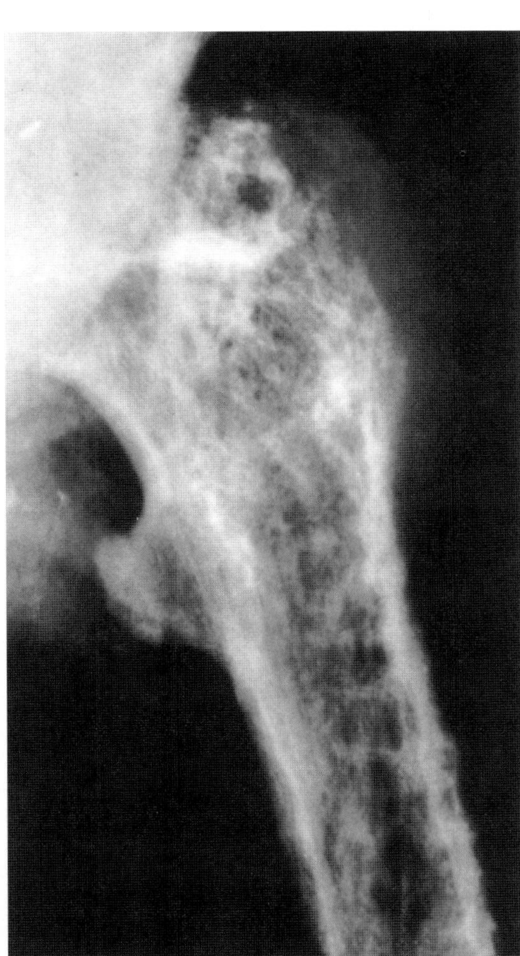

FIGURE 4.9

(a) Cobalt alloy and zirconium
(b) Stainless steel and cobalt alloy
(c) Titanium alloy and zirconium
(d) Cobalt alloy and titanium alloy
(e) Stainless steel and zirconium

64. When a posterior capsulotomy is performed during a posterior approach to the hip for total hip arthroplasty, which of the following structures is divided?
(a) The Y ligament of Bigelow
(b) The iliofemoral ligament
(c) The ischiofemoral ligament
(d) The ligamentum teres
(e) The indirect head of the rectus femoris

65. Low-molecular-weight heparin has as its primary inhibitory effect on which of the following?
(a) Factor II
(b) Factor IXa
(c) Antithrombin III
(d) Factor Xa
(e) Factor XIIa

66. Problems associated with total hip arthroplasty in patients with Paget disease of the hip include all the following except
(a) An increased incidence of heterotopic ossification
(b) Excessive intraoperative hemorrhage
(c) Protrusio acetabuli
(d) An increased incidence of deep venous thrombosis
(e) Varus malalignment of the femoral component

67. Which of the following structures are innervated by the *anterior* branch of the obturator nerve?
(a) The semitendinosus
(b) The gracilis
(c) The rectus femori
(d) The adductor magnus
(e) The adductor brevis

68. A 66-year-old woman falls and sustains a displaced right femoral neck fracture. Her health is otherwise excellent, and she takes no medications. She is independent in all activities of daily living. She denies antecedent hip pain of any sort. She walks 2 miles a day and plays occasional recreational tennis. Which of the following options would provide the most predictably favorable long-term outcome?
(a) Primary total hip arthroplasty
(b) Reduction and pinning with three partially threaded cannulated screws
(c) Bed rest and traction for 6 weeks
(d) Reduction and fixation with a sliding hip screw and side-plate device
(e) Primary hemiarthroplasty

69. If the patient in question 68 is acutely treated with a total hip arthroplasty, which of the following statements most accurately describes her risk of dislocation?
(a) Equivalent to a primary total hip arthroplasty performed for osteoarthritis

(b) Equivalent to a primary total hip arthroplasty performed for rheumatoid arthritis
(c) Equivalent to a primary total hip arthroplasty performed for osteoarthritis for the first 4 months and, thereafter, greater than the risk of dislocation after total hip arthroplasty performed for osteoarthritis
(d) Greater than a primary total hip arthroplasty performed for osteoarthritis for the first 4 months and, thereafter, approximately equivalent to the risk of dislocation after total hip arthroplasty performed for osteoarthritis
(e) Significantly less than hemiarthroplasty performed for acute femoral neck fracture

70. Particulate wear debris from total joint replacements can result in osteolysis and catastrophic implant failure. The particle size that is believed to be most osteolytic is
(a) Greater than 200 μm
(b) 100 to 200 μm
(c) 50 to 100 μm
(d) 20 to 50 μm
(e) 10 μm and smaller

71. The apprehension test for subluxation of a symptomatic dysplastic hip is performed by which of the following maneuvers?
(a) External rotation and hyperextension
(b) Internal rotation and hyperflexion
(c) External rotation and hyperflexion
(d) Internal rotation and hyperextension
(e) Neutral rotation and hyperflexion

72. Which of the following is an accurate description of the Nelaton line?
(a) A radiographic line along the superior femoral neck
(b) A clinical line between the anterior superior iliac spine and the ipsilateral ischial tuberosity
(c) A horizontal radiographic line through the two triradiate cartilages
(d) A curvilinear radiographic line along the inferior femoral neck that continues along the superior obturator foramen
(e) A clinical line from the anterior superior iliac spine to the umbilicus

73. A 72-year-old nun is to undergo total hip arthroplasty for end-stage osteoarthritis. She has a single unicortical screw in the lateral femoral cortex from an unspecified prior procedure. The screw is removed before the femur is reamed. How far must the femoral stem extend to minimize strain in the lateral femoral cortex?
(a) One femoral diameter distal to the screw hole
(b) Just distal to the screw hole
(c) Three femoral diameters distal to the screw hole
(d) One femoral diameter proximal to the screw hole
(e) 1.5 femoral diameters past the screw hole

Questions 74 and 75 are based on the following situation:

A 64-year-old neurosurgeon presents for routine follow-up 15 years after right total hip replacement. The arthroplasty has functioned flawlessly, and the patient is asymptomatic. An anteroposterior radiograph is shown in Fig. 4.10.

74. Based on the radiograph, which of the following statements is most accurate?
(a) The acetabular shell is probably loose.
(b) Both components are infected.
(c) The femoral component is probably loose.
(d) The femoral component and acetabular shell are both well fixed.
(e) The acetabular shell is probably loose and the femoral component is definitely loose.

75. What is the most appropriate next step in management of this patient?
(a) Revise both the acetabular shell and the femoral stem.
(b) Débride the joint and exchange the polyethylene liner and the femoral component.
(c) Observe.
(d) Revise the acetabular component only.

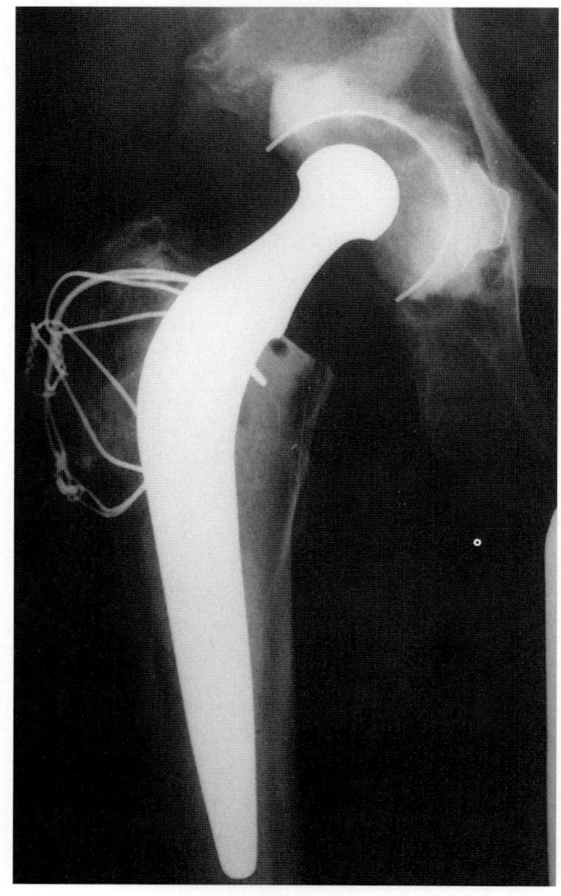

FIGURE 4.10

(e) Débride the joint and exchange the polyethylene liner and the femoral head.

76. Which of the following is not a cause of ipsilateral trunk lean during right-sided stance phase?
 (a) Weak right hip abductors
 (b) Leg length discrepancy (right leg longer)
 (c) Right hip adduction contracture
 (d) Right hip osteoarthritis
 (e) Scoliosis with decompensation to the left

77. Figure 4.11 is a magnetic resonance image of a left hip. What structure is marked by the tip of the *arrow?*
 (a) The gluteus medius
 (b) The pectineus
 (c) The gluteus minimus
 (d) The reflected head of the rectus femoris
 (e) The tensor fasciae latae

78. Which of the following statements is correct regarding polymerization of polymethylmethacrylate?
 (a) The volume contraction during early polymerization is produced by thermal changes.
 (b) Increases in temperature during polymerization produce volume contraction.
 (c) The final stage of cement volume contraction is caused by polymerization.
 (d) Porosity reduction decreases volume expansion during polymerization.
 (e) Polymerization increases cement volume independently of thermally induced volume expansion.

79. You are asked to consult on a patient with an altered gait pattern that has been attributed to "right hip spasm." Analysis of his gait demonstrates limited extension of the right hip during ipsilateral stance phase. Examination of the hip with the patient supine and the leg in 5 degrees of adduction reveals a 10-degree flexion contracture. However, full passive extension is achieved when the hip is abducted to 15 degrees. What is the most likely explanation for these findings?
 (a) Iliopsoas contracture
 (b) Pectinius contracture
 (c) Iliotibial band contracture
 (d) Contracture of the iliofemoral ligament
 (e) Adductor magnus contracture

80. A 76-year-old woman presents with progressive bilateral hip pain. Her past medical history is significant for colon carcinoma. A plain radiograph is shown in Fig. 4.12. A bone scan reveals no increased signal at the hip. A biopsy is performed and reveals multiple small cells with minimal intervening stroma. The cells in this lesion are bland sheets of homogeneous plasma cells. Bence Jones proteins are detected in her urine. What is the most likely diagnosis?
 (a) Multiple myeloma
 (b) Metastatic carcinoma
 (c) Chondrosarcoma
 (d) Osteomyelitis
 (e) Lymphoma

81. Which of the following external-beam radiation protocols is currently recommended for heterotopic ossification prophylaxis?
 (a) 2,000 cumulative cGy in ten divided fractions
 (b) 10,000 cumulative cGy in ten divided fractions
 (c) 800 cGy in a single dose
 (d) 300 cGy in a single dose
 (e) 10,000 cumulative cGy in three divided fractions

82. Which of the following is the most likely source of significant intrapelvic hemorrhage after pelvic fracture?
 (a) The obturator artery
 (b) The superior gluteal artery
 (c) The smaller (unnamed) vessels and fractured cancellous osseous surfaces

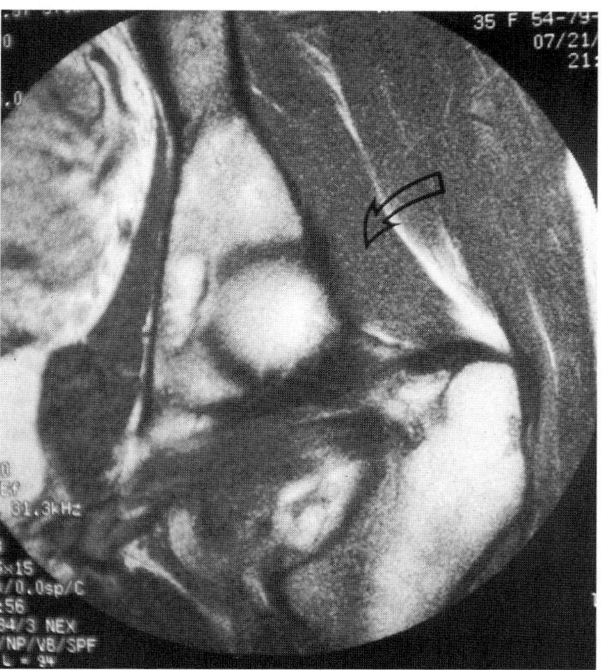

FIGURE 4.11

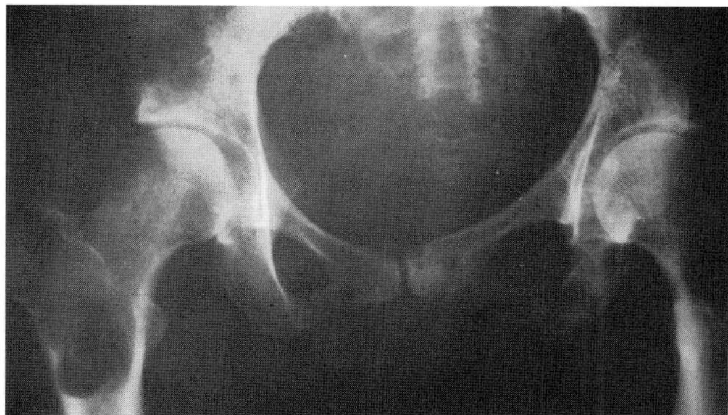

FIGURE 4.12

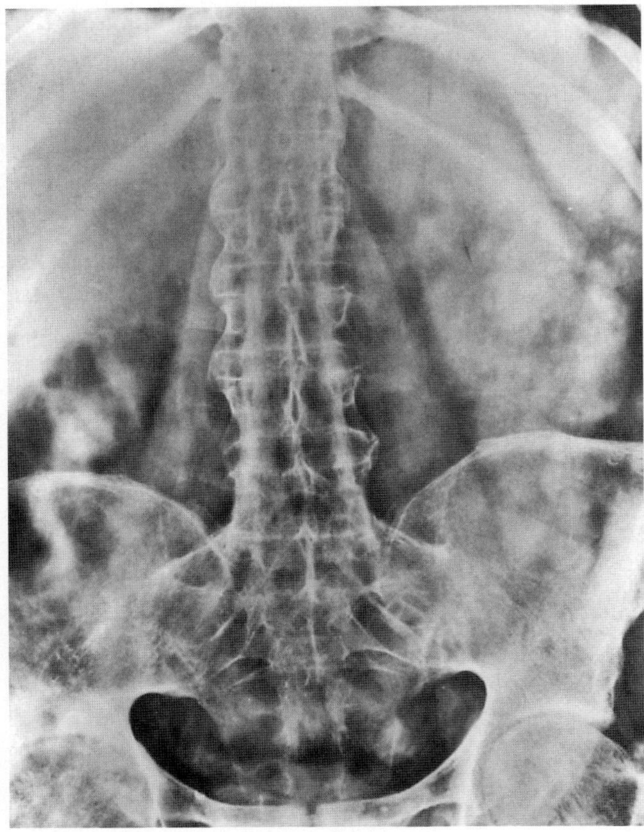

FIGURE 4.13

(d) The pudendal artery
(e) The hypogastric artery

83. A 44-year-old man presents with normal stature and progressive bilateral hip pain and an unspecified past medical history. He denies prior hip surgery. An anteroposterior pelvis film is shown in Fig. 4.13. What is the most likely diagnosis?
    (a) Multiple epiphyseal dysplasia
    (b) Ankylosing spondylitis
    (c) Spondyloepiphyseal dysplasia
    (d) Avascular necrosis
    (e) Hemochromatosis
84. A 44-year-old lawyer presents with right hip pain. He has moderate discomfort that is exacerbated by activity. He recently had to cease playing tennis because of the pain. He takes 30 mg of prednisone a day for inflammatory bowel disease. A radiograph of his affected hip is shown in Fig. 4.14A. A magnetic resonance image is shown in Fig. 4.14B. The most appropriate form of treatment for this patient would be
    (a) Nonoperative management
    (b) Total hip arthroplasty
    (c) Hip arthrodesis
    (d) Core decompression
    (e) Vascularized free fibular autograft
85. The foveal artery is a branch of what vessel?
    (a) The deep femoral artery
    (b) The ascending cervical arteries

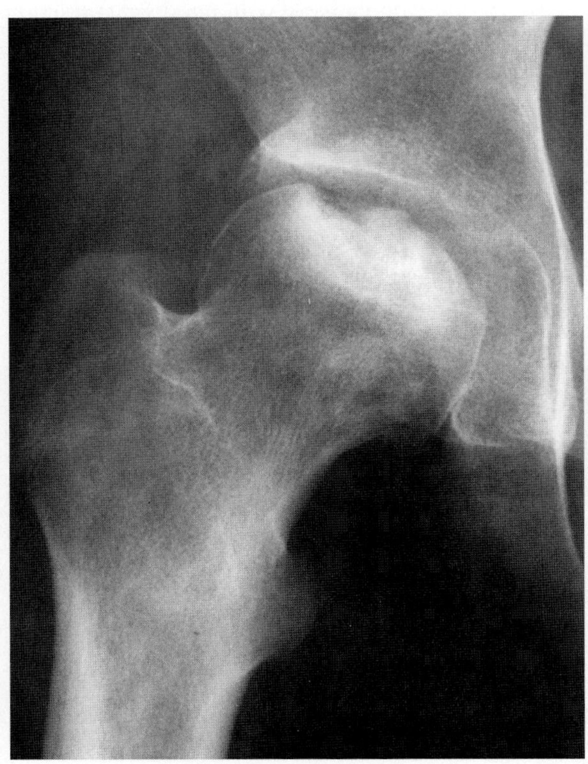

A

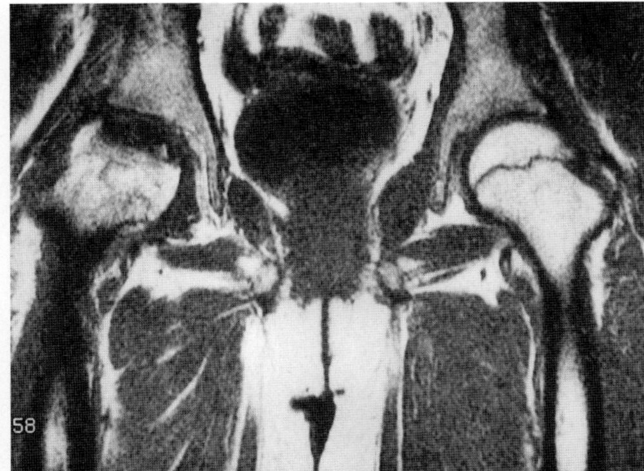

B

FIGURE 4.14 A and B

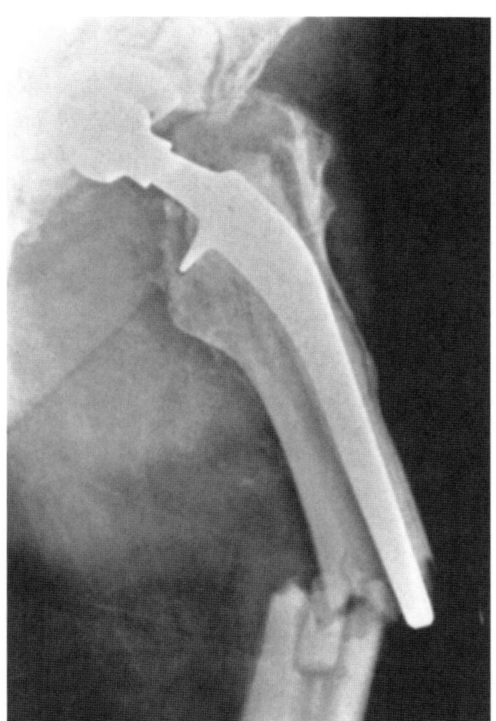

FIGURE 4.15

(c) The inferior gluteal artery
(d) The obturator artery
(e) The lateral femoral circumflex artery

86. Which of the following pore sizes is optimal for promoting biologic fixation of porous-coated components?
(a) Less than 10 μm
(b) 20 to 40 μm
(c) 100 to 300 μm
(d) 500 to 800 μm
(e) More than 900 μm

87. A 56-year-old woman is a restrained passenger in the front seat of a car that is struck from the right by an armored car. The patient presents with acute right hip pain. She underwent a right total hip arthroplasty 2 months earlier. An anteroposterior pelvis radiograph is shown in Fig. 4.15. Which of the following is the best way to describe this situation?
(a) This is bad.
(b) This is a problem.
(c) This is very bad.
(d) This is a serious problem.
(e) This is the resident's fault.

ANSWERS

1. **a** Its cephalad end merges with the posteromedial aspect of the femoral neck. The calcar femorale is a vertically oriented condensation of trabecular bone that extends from the posteromedial cortex of the femoral shaft (below the lesser trochanter) to the posterior femoral neck. This internal buttress reinforces the posteroinferior femoral neck. The density of the trabeculae that form the calcar is greatest medially. The trabeculae attenuate as they radiate laterally toward the posterior aspect of the greater trochanter (Fig. 4.16).

Reference

Harty M: The Calcar Femorale and the Femoral Neck. J Bone Joint Surg Am, 39:625–630, 1957.

2. **a** Approximately 2.5 times body weight. Experiments with a prosthetic strain gauge have demonstrated compressive forces of approximately 2.5 to three times body weight across the hip during static, *unsupported single leg stance.* Simplified frontal plane static mechanical analysis also predicts a joint reactive force of approximately three times body weight. The joint reactive

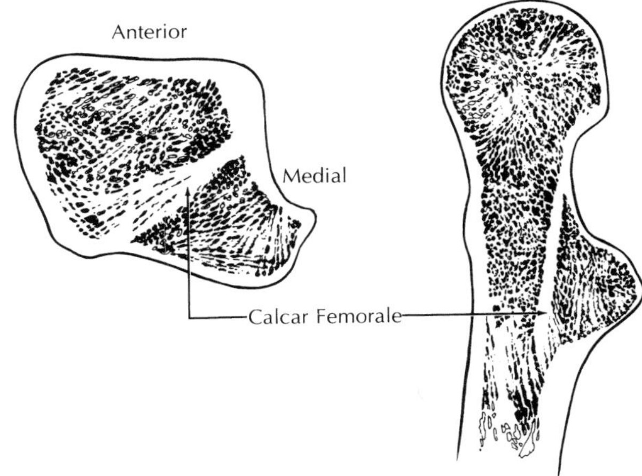

FIGURE 4.16

force is greater than body weight because of the compressive force generated by the hip abductors to prevent pelvic tilt during single leg stance. In preventing rotation around the hip joint (fulcrum), the abductor muscles operate at a mechanical disadvantage because the distance (lever arm) between the abductor insertion and the hip is shorter than the distance (lever arm) between the body's center of gravity and the hip center of rotation.

During static double leg stance, the joint reaction force is equal to approximately 0.5 times body weight across each hip because the abductor force is eliminated. *Supine straight leg raising* generates a compressive force of approximately 1.5 times body weight across the ipsilateral hip. *Running* produces compressive forces of approximately five times body weight.

References

Brand RA, et al.: Comparison of Hip Force Calculations and Measurements in the Same Patient. J Arthroplasty, 9:45–51, 1994.

Davy DT, et al.: Telemetric Force Measurements Across the Hip After Total Hip Arthroplasty. J Bone Joint Surg Am, 70:45–50, 1988.

Rydell N: Biomechanics of the Hip Joint. Clin Orthop, 92:6–15, 1973.

3. **c** Neutral rotation, 5 degrees of adduction, 30 degrees of flexion. Fusion in *abduction* results in a higher incidence of low back pain and ipsilateral knee pain than fusion in neutral to slight *adduction*. Arthrodesis in abduction is also associated with a worse limp (increased ipsilateral sway). Optimizing position in the sagittal plane involves a conflict between the need for adequate flexion (to permit sitting) and adequate extension (to avoid functional limb shortening and resultant gait disturbance). This balance is best achieved at 30 to 40 degrees of flexion; 5 to 10 degrees of flexion would make sitting too difficult. Internal rotation should be avoided in favor of neutral to slight external rotation.

References

Callaghan JJ, et al.: Hip Arthrodesis: J Bone Joint Surg Am, 67:1328–1335, 1985.

Sponseller PD, et al.: Hip Arthrodesis in Young Patients. J Bone Joint Surg Am, 66:853–859, 1984.

4. **a** Heterotopic ossification is a common phenomenon after femoral nailing with a reported incidence of approximately 25%. In the series of Brumback et al., the incidence of moderate to severe heterotopic ossification about the hip after antegrade, reamed intramedullary nailing of the femur was 26%. One of the putative stimuli for the generation of heterotopic ossification in this context is the osseous debris that is deposited in the abductor musculature during reaming. However, in the randomized, prospective study of Brumback et al., copious pulsatile wound irrigation had no effect on the incidence or severity of heterotopic ossification. This series also demonstrated no statistically significant correlation between the presence of a closed head injury and the incidence or severity of heterotopic ossification. Despite the high incidence of heterotopic ossification detected after antegrade intramedullary femoral nailing, this phenomenon is not associated with a clinically significant compromise in hip function.

Reference

Brumback RJ, et al.: Heterotopic Ossification About the Hip After Intramedullary Nailing for Fractures of the Femur. J Bone Joint Surg Am, 72:1067–1073, 1990.

5. **a** (1) cobalt-chromium, (2) stainless steel, (3) titanium, (4) cortical bone, (5) polyethylene. The Young modulus of elasticity equals stress divided by strain. Thus, it is defined by the slope of the stress-strain curve. The more stiff (less elastic) a material is, the higher its Young modulus will be. By definition, a material with a higher Young modulus will have a steeper stress-strain curve. The following sequence of materials is arranged according to decreasing elastic modulus magnitude: Cobalt-chromium > stainless steel > titanium > cortical bone > methyl methacrylate > cancellous bone > polyethylene.

Reference

Berry DJ, Chao EYS: In Morrey BF, ed: Reconstructive Surgery of the Joints, 2nd Ed. Churchill Livingston, p. 946, 1996.

6. **d** Weak hip flexors. There are multiple potential explanations for exaggerated lordosis during stance phase after an above-knee amputation. Lumbar hyperlordosis is a compensatory mechanism for processes that cause the center of gravity of the torso to translate anteriorly to the hips and feet. In this setting, hyperlordosis is an adaptive postural response that brings the center of gravity of the torso back into appropriate sagittal alignment.

   Under normal circumstances, the abdominal muscles pull up on the anterior pelvis, and, thus, they resist forward tilt of the pelvis. Weak abdominal musculature permits forward tilt of the pelvis. Lumbar hyperlordosis compensates for the resultant anterior tilt of the lumbosacral junction. Forward tilt of the pelvis may also be produced by weak hip extensors, insufficient support from the anterior brim of an above-knee prosthetic socket, or a flexion contracture of the hip.

References

Lower Extremity Prosthetics Syllabus. New York, Prosthetic-Orthotic Publications, p. 168, 1996.

Perry J: Gait Analysis: Normal and Pathological Function. Thorofare, NJ, Slack, p. 245, 1992.

7. **b** 15%. Lu-Yao et al. performed a meta-analysis of 106 studies that reported the outcome of displaced femoral neck fractures. The two most common complications that precipitated reoperation after primary open reduction and internal fixation were osteonecrosis and nonunion. The osteonecrosis rate was 16% (95% confidence interval, 11% to 19%). The incidence of nonunion was 33% (95% confidence interval, 23% to 37%).

Reference

Lu-Yao GL, et al.: Outcomes After Displaced Fractures of the Femoral Neck: A Meta-Analysis of One Hundred and Six Published Reports. J Bone Joint Surg Am, 76(1):15–25, 1994.

8. **b** The adductor longus. The key landmark in this image is the superficial femoral artery. The superficial femoral artery travels immediately deep to the sartorius and superficial to the adductor longus *(curved arrow)* in the midthigh. In Fig. 4.1, the *short arrow* marks the rectus femoris. The *k* marks the biceps femoris. The *box at the extreme right* marks the gracilis.
9. **a** Ochronosis. Many conditions are capable of producing acetabular protrusio. This condition is defined in terms of protrusion of the femoral head medial to the Kohler line *(the ilioischial line)* (Fig. 4.17).

   Acetabular protrusio is a characteristic feature of rheumatoid arthritis and the inflammatory arthropathies in general (i.e., ankylosing spondylitis). It is also seen in association with Paget disease, Marfan syndrome, trauma, or component loosening with periprosthetic bone loss after total hip arthroplasty.

   Note: Bilateral, idiopathic acetabular protrusio is called *arthrokatadysis.* This condition has also been referred to as *Otto pelvis.* It is associated with coxa vara and premature degenerative joint disease.

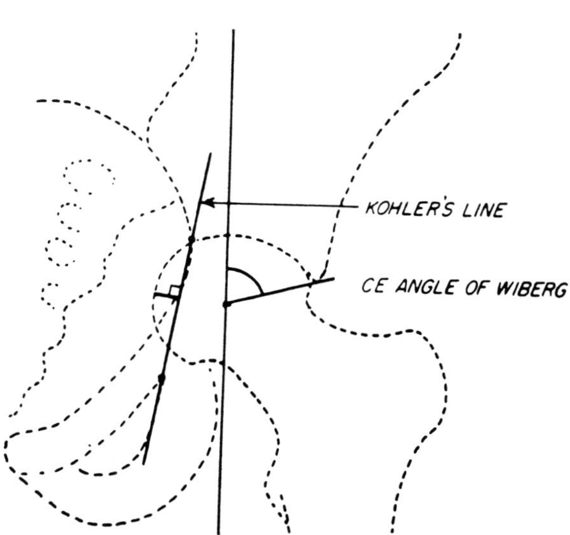

FIGURE 4.17

Reference

Pomeranz MM: Intrapelvic Protrusion of the Acetabulum (Otto Pelvis). J Bone Joint Surg, 14:663–686, 1932.

10. **e** Have a higher rate of aseptic loosening. The notion of adding a metal backing to cemented acetabular components had several potential biomechanical advantages: (1) the stiff shell would theoretically distribute stresses to the cement mantle and cancellous bone more evenly and thus would reduce peak stresses and forestall loosening; (2) worn polyethylene liners could be exchanged without revising the entire component; and (3) the severity of polyethylene cold flow would be reduced. However, despite these advantages, the *in vivo* performance of cemented metal-backed acetabular components has manifested a markedly increased rate of aseptic loosening.

Reference

Ritter MA, et al.: Metal-Backed Acetabular Cups in Total Hip Arthroplasty. J Bone Joint Surg Am, 72:672–677, 1990.

11. **b** Cement porosity reduction with centrifugation or vacuum mixing (Table 4.1).
12. **e** The external iliac vein. Wasielewski et al. delineated four clinically useful acetabular quadrants. The quadrants are defined by a vertical bisector from the anterior superior iliac spine to the ischium (through the posterior aspect of the fovea) and a second line (perpendicular to the first) at the level of the acetabular equator (Fig. 4.18). Screws placed too deeply in the anterior superior quadrant endanger the external iliac artery and vein. Screws placed too deeply in the anterior inferior quadrant endanger the obturator artery and vein. The depth of available bone in the two anterior quadrants is relatively shallow. Hence, screw placement in these regions is undesirable.

TABLE 4.1. CEMENT POROSITY REDUCTION

First generation	Antegrade finger packing of doughy cement
Second generation	Canal plugging; pulsatile lavage; retrograde canal filling with cement gun (components made of superalloys)
Third generation	Porosity reduction (centrifugation or vacuum mixing; implant surface modifications)

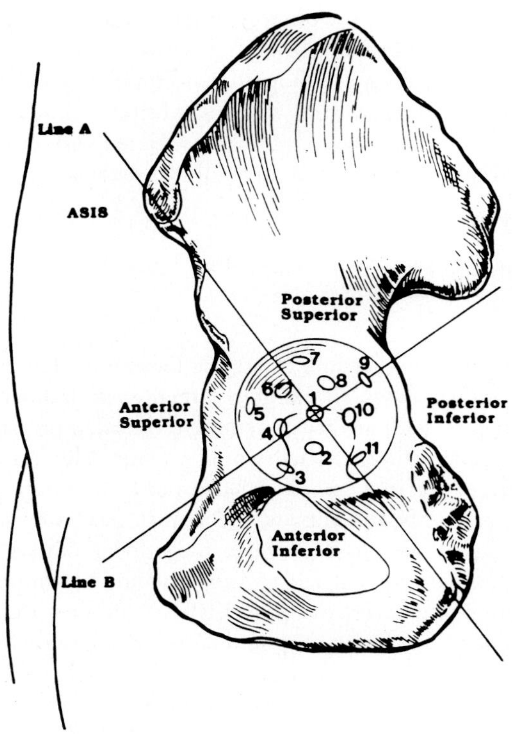

FIGURE 4.18

Reference

Wasielewski RC, et al.: Acetabular Anatomy and the Transacetabular Fixation of Screws in Total Hip Arthroplasty. J Bone Joint Surg Am, 72:501–508, 1990.

13. **c** The superior gluteal artery. The posterior quadrants are typically considered "safe zones." In contrast to the shallow bone in the anterior quadrants, the bone in the two posterior quadrants is relatively thick and can accommodate deeper screw placement. Screws as long as 85 mm may be placed *centrally* in the posterosuperior quadrant (toward the sacroiliac joint) without perforating either the inner or outer cortex of the ilium. However, screw placement in this quadrant is *not* fail-safe. An excessively long posterosuperior screw that is not directed perfectly centrally between the inner and outer tables of the ilium could conceivably perforate the cortex and could damage the sciatic nerve or the superior gluteal neurovascular structures. The sciatic nerve is less susceptible to injury because it is usually palpable and mobile. The superior gluteal neurovascular structures are not palpable and are therefore at increased risk.

    The pudendal and inferior gluteal neurovascular structures may be damaged by an overzealous, plunging drill bit or by an excessively long screw in the postero*inferior* quadrant.

Reference

Wasielewski RC, et al.: Acetabular Anatomy and the Transacetabular Fixation of Screws in Total Hip Arthroplasty. J Bone Joint Surg Am, 72:501–508, 1990.

14. **b** Between the principal and secondary compressive trabeculae. The trabecular framework within the femoral head and neck has been divided into five groups (Fig. 4.19). The Ward triangle is a region of relatively sparse trabeculae in the center of the femoral neck that is defined by the principal tensile trabeculae (superiorly), the principal compressive trabeculae (medially), and the secondary compressive trabeculae (laterally).

    Singh et al. defined a system for grading osteoporosis that is based on deterioration of the normal trabecular pattern of the proximal femur. The calcar femorale is a component of the principal compressive trabeculae.

    Note: The decussation of the principal tensile trabeculae and of the principal compressive trabeculae forms the most dense region of cancellous bone in the femoral head. To maximize purchase within the femoral head, internal fixation devices should target this region.

Reference

Singh M, et al.: Changes in the Trabecular Pattern of the Upper End of the Femur as an Index of Osteoporosis. J Bone Joint Surg Am, 52:457–467, 1970.

15. **b** Wear of the acetabular cartilage. Acetabular erosion is a common source of groin pain after hemiarthroplasty. Figure 4.2A reveals an uncemented bipolar hemiarthroplasty. There is no evidence of head disjunction, and the size of the outer diameter head appears to conform appropriately to the size of the native acetabulum. However, there is evidence of asymmetric joint space narrowing (greatest at the dome). This radiographic finding (in association with the nature of the patient's pain) suggests that acetabular wear is the most likely cause of her groin discomfort.

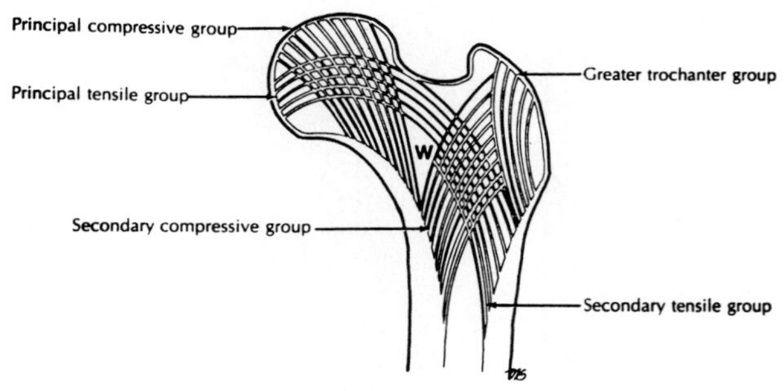

FIGURE 4.19

References

Kofoed H, Kofod J: Moore Prosthesis in the Treatment of Fresh Femoral Neck Fractures: A Critical Review with Specific Attention to Acetabular Degeneration. Injury, 14:531–540, 1983.

Lu-Yao GL, et al.: Outcomes After Displaced Fractures of the Femoral Neck: A Meta-Analysis of One Hundred and Six Published Reports. J Bone Joint Surg Am, 76(1):15–25, 1994.

16. **d** Aseptic loosening. Thigh pain is a frequent complaint after noncemented femoral fixation, and it is not necessarily a sign of loosening. However, the radiograph and the quality of the thigh pain in this question *(startup pain)* are indicative of loosening.

Figure 4.2A reveals pedestal formation at the tip of the stem. Serial radiographs are required to prove the presence of stem subsidence. However, subsidence is implied in this case by the endosteal contour cephalad to the proximal lateral corner of the stem. Additional signs of loosening include radiolucency along the medial side of the stem (suggesting varus rotatory migration of the stem) and the absence of cortical hypertrophy or *spot-welds.*

Pain on initiating weight-bearing (startup pain) is indicative of stem loosening. The quality of thigh pain associated with radiographically stable components characteristically occurs after prolonged weight bearing. One of the commonly invoked explanations for the later variety of thigh pain is the mismatch in stiffness between the metallic stem and the cortical bone.

17. **e** Open reduction and internal fixation with conversion to a total hip arthroplasty with a long-stem prosthesis. Multiple systems have been proposed for classifying periprosthetic fractures. According to the Johannson classification, this would be a type B fracture. According to the classification proposed by Duncan, this would be a type B_2 lesion.

The Johannson classification is given in Table 4.2, and the Duncan classification is given in Table 4.3.

The optimum form of treatment for a periprosthetic fracture associated with a loose stem is femoral revision with adjunctive fixation (including plates, cerclage wires, and/or onlay cortical strut allograft). The length of the revision stem should bypass the fracture site. Given the prefracture symptoms attributed to the putative acetabular wear, conversion to a total hip arthroplasty would also be appropriate for this patient.

TABLE 4.2. PERIPROSTHETIC FRACTURES: JOHANNSON CLASSIFICATION

Fracture Type	Description
A	Proximal to the stem tip
B	Long spiral fracture spanning the stem tip
C	Entirely distal to the stem tip

TABLE 4.3. PERIPROSTHETIC FRACTURES: DUNCAN CLASSIFICATION

Fracture Type	Description
A	Well above the tip of the stem
(A_G)	(At the greater trochanter)
(A_L)	(At the lesser trochanter)
B	At or just below the tip of the stem
(B_1)	(With well fixed stem)
(B_2)	(With loose stem)
(B_3)	(With poor proximal femoral bone stock)
C	Well below the tip of the stem

Nonoperative treatment of periprosthetic fractures is associated with increased rates of malunion and nonunion, as well as the myriad complications associated with prolonged recumbence. This is a particularly inappropriate option in the setting of a loose stem (which would require later revision even if the fracture healed without complication).

Note: If the stem is loose, it should be revised.

References

Duncan C, Masri BA: Fractures of the Femur After Hip Replacement. Instr Course Lect 44:293–304, 1995.

Johannson JE, et al.: Fracture of the Ipsilateral Femur in Patients with Total Hip Replacement. J Bone Joint Surg Am, 63:1435–1442, 1981.

18. **b** Valgus-flexion osteotomy. The goal of osteotomy in this situation would be to remove the affected portion of the femoral head from a weight-bearing location and to rotate healthy articular tissue into the key weight-bearing positions.

Valgus reorientation of the proximal femur would shift the diseased portion of the head laterally (into a nonarticulating position). A varus osteotomy would shift the diseased zone of the head medially into a more cephalad position, where it would be in direct contact with the weight-bearing dome of the acetabulum.

Flexion at the osteotomy site would shift the affected portion of the femoral head further anteriorly and would deliver it away from a position where it would be loaded. Extension at the osteotomy would shift the affected zone of the head posteriorly into a more cephalad, weight-bearing position.

Reference

Scher MA: Intertrochanteric Osteotomy and Autogenous Bone Grafting for Avascular Necrosis of the Femoral Head. J Bone Joint Surg Am, 75:1119–1133, 1993.

19. **a** Polymethylmethacrylate is stronger under compression than under tension. Hand mixing of the constituents (liquid monomer and polymer powder) entraps air voids. Evaporation of monomer also creates

air voids in the mixture. Voids act as stress risers, and, thus, porosity compromises the strength of the polymethylmethacrylate. Decreasing the porosity of the mixture of monomer and polymer will increase its strength. This can be accomplished either (1) by mixing the monomer and polymer in a vacuum or (2) by centrifuging after mixing.

Polymethylmethacrylate itself is radiolucent. The addition of 10% barium sulfate to before polymerization renders the cement radiopaque, but this does not significantly alter its strength.

Polymethylmethacrylate functions more as a grout than as an adhesive. It will, however, adhere strongly to the surface of a polymethylmethacrylate-precoated stem.

The elastic modulus of polymethylmethacrylate is less than that of cobalt chromium alloy, titanium, and cortical bone, but it is greater than that of cancellous bone (see question 5).

20. **c** Active foot and ankle motion has been shown to produce a 22% mean increase in lower extremity venous outflow. Using venous occlusion strain-gauge plethysmography, McNally et al. found that 1 minute of active cyclic dorsiflexion and plantarflexion of the toes and ankle produced a significant increase in venous outflow in each of 22 patients studied after total hip arthroplasty. The mean maximum increase from baseline lower extremity venous outflow was 22% (range, 7% to 53%). This increase was detectable 2 minutes after exercise. The flow had increased further at 7 and 12 minutes after exercise, and it had returned to baseline by 30 minutes after exercise.

Decreased venous stasis should theoretically aid in the prevention of deep venous thrombosis. Thus, it would be logical to infer that active foot and ankle motion should decrease deep venous thrombosis. However, despite the beneficial hemodynamic consequences of active foot and ankle exercise, a prophylactic effect of such exercise on venous thrombogenesis has not yet been scientifically proven.

Reference

McNally MA, et al.: The Effect of Active Movement of the Foot on Venous Blood Flow after Total Hip Replacement. J Bone Joint Surg Am, 79: 1198–1201, 1997.

21. **b** The semitendinosus. The musculature of the posterior thigh is divisible into a lateral half (biceps femoris) and a medial half (semitendinosus and semimembranosus). As the semitendinosus and semimembranosus travel down the posteromedial thigh, the semitendinosus lies posterolateral to the semimembranosus.

In Fig. 4.3, the semimembranosus is marked by the *white square.* It lies anteromedial to the semitendinosus. The *arrow* is superimposed on the biceps femoris and points to the sciatic nerve. Note the multifasciculated ("bundle of grapes") appearance of the nerve. The large muscle belly directly anterior to the semimembranosus is the adductor magnus (marked by the letter *K*). The smaller (unlabeled) muscle directly medial to the adductor magnus in the figure is the gracilis.

22. **b** A 22-year-old woman with juvenile rheumatoid arthritis. The major risk factors for developing heterotopic ossification after total hip arthroplasty include ankylosing spondylitis, hypertrophic osteoarthritis, diffuse idiopathic skeletal hyperostosis, Paget disease, and a history of prior heterotopic ossification. Rheumatoid arthritis is not considered a risk factor for heterotopic ossification after total hip arthroplasty. Heterotopic ossification of the hip has been classified by Brooker (Table 4.4).

Note: Excision of symptomatic heterotopic ossification should not be considered until after it has biologically matured. Biologic maturity is indicated by a return to normal signal on bone scan. This typically requires approximately 6 months.

References

Goel A, Sharp DJ: Heterotopic Bone Formation After Hip Replacement: The Influence of the Type of Osteoarthritis. J Bone Joint Surg Br, 73:255–257, 1991.

Thomas BJ: Heterotopic Ossification Following Total Hip Arthroplasty. Orthop Clin North Am, 23:347–358, 1992.

Warren SB, Brooker AF Jr: Excision of Heterotopic Bone Followed by Irradiation After Total Hip Arthroplasty. J Bone Joint Surg Am, 74:201–210, 1992.

23. **d** Approximately 70%. At an average 10.1-year follow-up, DeLee and Charnley found bone-cement interface radiolucencies in 69.5% of the acetabular components. However, only 9.2% of the patients with demarcation demonstrated progressive socket migration. Most patients with demarcation were asymptomatic. On average, patients with demarcation were 9 years younger than those without demarcation. Demarcation was also more likely among patients with an underlying diagnosis of rheumatoid arthritis.

The authors invoked three principal technical explanations for the prevalence of acetabular radiolucencies:

TABLE 4.4. HETEROTOPIC OSSIFICATION OF THE HIP CLASSIFIED BY BROOKER

Class I	Islands of bone within soft tissues
Class II	Spurs at pelvis and/or proximal femur with residual nonossified gap >1 cm
Class III	Spurs at pelvis or proximal femur with residual nonossified gap <1 cm
Class IV	Bony ankylosis of the hip

(1) holding the socket for too long with the socket holder during polymerization (inducing socket motion during polymerization); (2) suboptimal socket hemostasis at the time of cement insertion; and (3) suboptimal cement pressurization.

Reference

DeLee JG, Charnley J: Radiologic Demarcation of Cemented Sockets in Total Hip Replacement. Clin Orthop, 121:20–32, 1976.

24. **b** Decreased joint compressive forces. Femoral component offset is defined as the distance between the center of rotation of the femoral head and the axis of the stem. Increasing the offset lateralizes the insertion of the hip abductors. This increases the moment arm of the hip abductors. Thus, *less* abductor force will be required to produce the same torque at the hip joint, and joint compressive forces will be *decreased* during single leg stance.

    Increased offset provides greater clearance between the greater trochanter and acetabulum and is therefore associated with a lower chance of impingement. Increased offset is associated with *higher* bending stresses on the femoral component.

25. **d** Lumbosacral trunk traction injury. Pelvic fractures with posterior instability have been associated with an incidence of lumbosacral nerve injury of up to 50%. Huittinen and colleagues investigated the patterns of associated lumbosacral nerve injury in 42 cadaveric specimen that had sustained pelvic fractures in association with their demise. The most common associated form of neurologic damage was traction injury to the lumbosacral trunk (29% of the specimen).

    The lumbosacral trunk crosses over the anterior sacral ala as it descends into the true pelvis. It is extremely vulnerable to traction injury in this location. Neuropraxia of the lumbosacral trunk is the most common deficit when the stability of the ipsilateral hemipelvis is grossly disrupted. Associated neurologic deficits are manifested in the L4 and L5 dermatomes and myotomes. The *superior gluteal nerve* runs in close proximity to the lumbosacral trunk, and it is also commonly subjected to traction injury (26%).

    For self-evident reasons, the anterior primary rami of the sacral nerve roots are commonly injured in association with compression fractures that propagate through the sacral foramina. Disruption of the L5 nerve root by the sharp edge of a vertical sacral fracture is an unusual injury. The *obturator nerve* originates from the lumbar plexus (L2, L3, and L4). When obturator nerve injury occurs at the time of pelvic fracture, it is typically associated with fracture dislocations of the posterior pelvic ring. The obturator nerve is rarely injured by pubic rami fragments at the disrupted obturator foramen.

Note: The L5 nerve root is vulnerable to iatrogenic injury during exposure and retraction for anterior approaches to the sacroiliac joint.

References

Helfet D, Koval K: Intra-Operative Somatosensory Evoked Potential Monitoring During Acute Pelvic Fracture Surgery. J Orthop Trauma, 9:28–34, 1995.

Huittinen VM, et al.: Lumbo-Sacral Nerve Injury in Fractures of the Pelvis. Acta Chir Scand, 429:3–43, 1972.

26. **b** Ductility. Examples of ductile materials include metal and polymethylmethacrylate in the "dough stage" of hardening.

    Toughness is a material property that refers to the total amount of energy required to stress a material to the point of failure (both elastic and plastic deformation). It is quantified by measuring the total area under the stress-strain curve. *Brittleness* is the opposite of ductility. It describes materials that undergo little permanent deformation before failure (e.g., ceramics or solidified polymethylmethacrylate). *Fatigue strength* refers to the ability of a material to endure cyclic loading. The yield point refers to the transitional point on the stress strain curve between elastic (linear) and plastic (permanent) deformation.

References

Frankel VH, Burstein AH: Orthopaedic Biomechanics. Philadelphia, Lea & Febiger, 1970.

Nordin M, Frankel VH: Basic Biomechanics of the Musculoskeletal System, 2nd Ed. Philadelphia, Lea & Febiger, 1989.

27. **a** Approximately 12%. In a canine model, Leggon et al. reported that femora with a 50% circumferential cortical defect demonstrated only 12.7±3.8% of intact torsional strength.

    Edgerton et al. found that femora with a 20% circumferential cortical defect demonstrated a 72% reduction in torsional strength. Brooks and colleagues demonstrated that a single 2.8 or 3.6-mm diaphyseal drill hole weakened the torsional strength of canine long bones by a mean of 55.2%.

References

Brooks DB, Burstein AH, Frankel VH: The Biomechanics of Torsional Fractures. J Bone Joint Surg Am, 52:507–514, 1970.

Burstein AH, et al.: Bone Strength: The Effect of Screw Holes. J Bone Joint Surg Am, 54:1143–1156, 1972.

Leggon RE, et al.: Strength Reduction and the Effects of Treatment of Long Bones with Diaphyseal Defects Involving 50% of the Cortex. J Orthop Res, 6:540–546, 1988.

28. **c** Rotational corrections can produce undesirable linear translations of the center of rotation of the hip joint. The Bernese (Ganz) periacetabular osteotomy

has many advantages: (1) it can be performed through a single incision, most commonly through the Smith-Peterson approach; (2) it does not significantly alter the dimensions of the true pelvis, and, thus, it does not preclude vaginal child delivery; (3) it does not sacrifice the continuity of the posterior column of the pelvis, and, thus, early weight bearing is possible; (4) it can provide large improvements in both lateral and anterior femoral head coverage; and (5) it does not significantly complicate subsequent total hip arthroplasty.

However, because of the angled bone cuts (nonconcentric osteotomy), rotation of the acetabular fragment can cause undesired linear translations. Specifically, adduction of the acetabular fragment may cause lateral translation of the joint center of rotation (which would increase joint reaction forces by lengthening the lever arm between the hip center of rotation and the body's center of gravity). This potential problem can be avoided by shifting the inferomedial corner of the acetabular fragment in a cephalad direction, rather than allowing it to translate laterally, as the acetabular fragment is adducted.

Reference

McGrory BJ, et al.: Bernese Periacetabular Osteotomy. J Orthop Tech, 1(4):179–191, 1993.

29. **c** The gluteus medius. All the listed muscles serve (either primarily or secondarily) as hip external rotators except the gluteus medius. In addition to abducting the hip, the gluteus medius is the principal internal rotator of the hip.

    Additional external rotators of the hip include the piriformis, the superior gemellus, the obturator externus, the inferior gemellus, and the quadratus femoris. Additional *internal* rotators of the hip include the tensor fasciae latae and the adductor magnus (posterior head).
30. **a** The obturator oblique view is the best view for assessing the integrity of the anterior column. The *obturator oblique view* is the best view for assessing the integrity of the anterior column (the *iliopubic line*) and the posterior wall of the acetabulum. The iliac oblique view is the best view for assessing the integrity of the posterior column (the *ilioischial line*) and the anterior wall of the acetabulum. The pelvic inlet view is the best view for detecting rotational instability at a sacroiliac joint. The *pelvic outlet view* is the best view for detecting vertical instability at a sacroiliac joint.

Reference

Judet R, Judet J, Letournel E: Fractures of the Acetabulum: Classification and Surgical Approaches for Open Reduction. J Bone Joint Surg Am, 46: 1615–1646, 1964.

31. **a** Two decades after fusion, the incidence of low back pain is approximately 60%. Two decades after hip arthrodesis, the incidence of low back pain is 57% to 60%. The incidence of ipsilateral knee pain is 45% to 60%. Hips fused in abduction result in a higher incidence of low back pain and ipsilateral knee pain than those fused in neutral to slight adduction. Back symptoms are relieved more than ipsilateral knee symptoms by conversion to total joint arthroplasty. The outcomes of conversion arthroplasty procedures are roughly equivalent to revision arthroplasties (worse than for primary total hip arthroplasties of nonfused joints). A malaligned arthrodesis is best managed by corrective osteotomy, rather than by takedown of the arthrodesis.

References

Callaghan JJ, et al.: Hip Arthrodesis: J Bone Joint Surg Am, 67:1328–1335, 1985. Sponseller PD, et al.: Hip Arthrodesis in Young Patients. J Bone Joint Surg Am, 66:853–859, 1984.

32. **d** Uncemented, fully porous-coated cobalt-chromium stem. Stress shielding occurs as bone adaptively remodels according to the Wolff law. As stresses are transferred through the prosthesis to more distal regions of the femur, the more proximal regions of the femur see relatively less load. This results in proximal femoral bone loss.

    Stress shielding is seen with all types of prostheses (including cemented stems). However, current analytic models and clinical data suggest that stress shielding effects are greater with stiffer stems and stems with extensive porous coating. These two factors increase the amount of load that is transferred distally. Cobalt-chromium is stiffer than titanium.

    The long-term clinical significance of this bone loss has yet to be determined. Clinical evidence suggests that the amount of proximal femoral bone loss eventually reaches a plateau. However, extensive proximal bone atrophy is a risk factor for iatrogenic femur fracture during revision situations.

References

Cohen B, Rushton N: Bone Remodeling in the Proximal Femur After Charnley Total Hip Arthroplasty. J Bone Joint Surg Br, 77(5):815–819, 1995.
Engh CA, Bobyn JD: The Influence of Stem Size and Extent of Porous Coating on Femoral Bone Resorption After Primary Cementless Hip Arthroplasty. Clin Orthop, 231:7–28, 1988.
Weinaus H, et al.: The Effect of Material Properties of Femoral Hip Components on Bone Remodelling. J Orthop Res, 10:845–853, 1992.

33. **c** The femoral nerve–superior gluteal nerve plane. The superficial dissection of the Smith-Petersen approach to the hip develops the interval between the sartorius muscle (femoral nerve) and the tensor fasciae latae muscle (superior gluteal nerve). The deep dissection of the approach develops the interval between the rectus

femoris muscle (femoral nerve) and the gluteus medius muscle (superior gluteal nerve).

The *anterolateral* approach (Watson-Jones) involves no true internervous plane. This approach proceeds between the gluteus medius and the tensor fasciae latae muscles (both of which are innervated by the superior gluteal nerve). The posterior (Moore or "southern") approach also employs no true internervous plane. In this approach, the gluteus maximus (inferior gluteal nerve) is split in line with its fibers.

Reference

Hoppenfeld S: Surgical Exposures in Orthopaedics, 2nd Ed. Philadelphia, JB Lippincott, 1994.

34. **c** Synovial chondromatosis. The plain radiograph (Fig. 4.4A) reveals nonspecific findings including mild joint space narrowing and marginal subcapital articular erosions. The T1 magnetic resonance image (Fig. 4.4B) demonstrates a distended joint space with a proliferative intrasynovial process. The T2 magnetic resonance image (Fig. 4.4C) reveals an effusion with discrete foci of intermediate signal intensity. These foci could represent either intraarticular loose bodies or cross sections of villous synovial projections. Pigmented villonodular synovitis produces villous synovial projections, but it does not typically form loose bodies. Synovial chondromatosis may produce both loose bodies as well as villous synovial projections. The presence of loose bodies and their cartilage composition confirm the diagnosis of synovial chondromatosis.

The loose bodies are formed by a process of multifocal subsynovial metaplasia. Histologic demonstration of subsynovial metaplasia is necessary to confirm the diagnosis of primary synovial chondromatosis. The hyaline nodules of synovial chondromatosis often undergo secondary enchondral ossification; hence the corollary term synovial osteochondromatosis.

Synovial chondromatosis most frequently presents as a monoarticular arthropathy of the knee (in more than 50% of cases). Involvement of the hip, shoulder, and elbow is less common.

Note: Atypical histologic features can sometimes be encountered in the chondrocytes of synovial chondromatosis. However, the process remains benign, and the diagnosis should not be mistaken for chondrosarcoma.

References

Hardacker J, Mindell ER: Synovial Chondromatosis with Secondary Subluxation of the Hip. J Bone Joint Surg Am, 73:1405–1407, 1991.
Okada Y, et al.: Arthroscopic Surgery For Synovial Chondromatosis of the Hip. J Bone Joint Surg Br, 71:198–199, 1989.

35. **d** Sterilization with γ irradiation and shelf aging in the presence of air. Sterilization with γ irradiation is believed to produce free radicals that subsequently lead to oxidative degradation of polyethylene. The white band represents a region of highly oxidized material. It is found in components that were γ sterilized in air. Oxidative degradation progresses with time. The oxidization alters the mechanical properties of the polyethylene and renders it more susceptible to wear in vivo.

Machining and molding have no effect on the presence of the white band. Sterilization in ethylene oxide gas has not been shown to affect the mechanical properties of ultrahigh-molecular weight polyethylene.

Note: Calcium stearate reduces friction between polymer particles. Lowered viscosity decreases the energy required for processing.

Reference

Rimnac CM, et al.: Post-Irradiation Aging of Ultra-High Molecular Weight Polyethylene. J Bone Joint Surg Am, 76(7):1052–1056, 1994.

36. **b** Press-fit fixation is associated with an increased incidence of gaps in this location (compared with screw fixation with line-to-line reaming). A polar (zone II) gap at the bone-prosthesis interface, as in this case, has been attributed to the tight peripheral fit and resultant incomplete seating of press-fit acetabular components.

The mode of uncemented cup fixation affects gap distribution. Unlike *line-to-line reaming with supplemental screw fixation* (which has a tendency to create peripheral gaps), *underreaming with press-fit fixation* inherently prevents peripheral gaps but has a tendency to produce polar gaps.

Gap distribution, in turn, influences gap fate. In their analysis of *line-to-line reaming with screws,* Schmalzried and Harris found that patients with peripheral gaps (zones I and/or III) on initial postoperative radiographs were far more likely to develop progressive radiolucent lines within the first 5 years than patients without initial peripheral gaps (39% versus 14%). Conversely, in their analysis of 122 *press-fit acetabular components without screws,* Schmalzried and colleagues found that most (63%) of the radiolucencies that were present in the apical region (zone II) of acetabular components on initial postoperative radiographs were no longer visible at 2-year follow-up. No acetabular fractures occurred during implantation. No loosening or osteolysis had occurred at 5-year follow-up.

Note: Some experts attribute the relative infrequency of progression of zone II gaps to the tight peripheral bone-prosthesis interface that is obtained with press-fit fixation. Theoretically, this tight fit may form a barrier between isolated zone II gaps apical gaps and the effective joint space. This "barrier" may restrict access of particulate wear debris and thus may exclude the stimulus for bone resorption.

References

Schmalzried TP, Harris WH: The Harris-Galante Porous-Coated Acetabular Component with Screw Fixation. J Bone Joint Surg Am, 74:1130–1139, 1992.

Schmalzried TP, Jasty M, Harris WH: Periprosthetic Bone Loss in Total Hip Arthroplasty: Polyethylene Wear Debris and the Concept of the Effective Joint Space. J Bone Joint Surg Am, 74:849–863, 1992.

Schmalzried TP, et al.: Harris-Galante Porous Acetabular Component Press-Fit Without Screw Fixation. J. Arthroplasty, 9:235–242, 1994.

37. **b** Pistoning (cement within bone) (type IB). In the classic study by Gruen et al., mode IB was the most common mechanism of failure (Fig. 4.20). Among the 56 stems that demonstrated radiographic signs of progressive loosening, this mechanism accounted for 35%.

Of the radiolucencies at the cement-bone interface, 81.3% occurred in zone 7. Radiolucencies at the cement-prosthesis interface were most frequently encountered in zone 1. A high percentage (approximately 50%) of the radiolucencies in both groups (bone-cement interface and stem-cement interface) were noted on the initial postoperative films, and these were attributed to intraoperative technical shortcomings.

Note: This study is frequently quoted, yet the results of first-generation cement technique should be extrapolated to contemporary cementing methods with caution.

Reference

Gruen TA, et al.: Modes of Failure of Cemented Stem Type Femoral Components. Clin Orthop, 141:17–27, 1978.

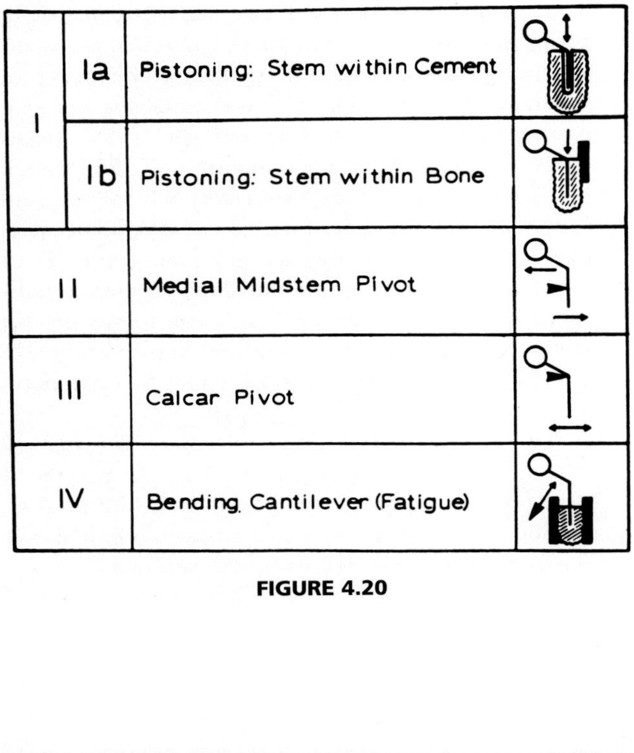

I	Ia	Pistoning: Stem within Cement	
	Ib	Pistoning: Stem within Bone	
II		Medial Midstem Pivot	
III		Calcar Pivot	
IV		Bending Cantilever (Fatigue)	

FIGURE 4.20

38. **b** Motion of up to 28 μm is compatible with bone ingrowth, but motion greater than 150 μm produces fibrous ingrowth. In a canine model, motion of less than 28 μm did not preclude bone ingrowth. Motion of greater than 150 μm produced fibrous ingrowth.

Reference

Pilliar RM, et al.: Observations on the Effect of Movement on Bone Ingrowth into Porous-Surfaced Implants. Clin Orthop, 208,108–113, 1986.

39. **b** Inadequate overall length of the prosthesis. Circumduction is the process by which the involved extremity follows a laterally curved path during the swing phase of gait. This gait pattern can arise in the context of an above-knee prosthesis for two basic reasons: (1) if the prosthesis is too long (for any reason), then it must be swung laterally to clear the ground; and (2) if the residual limb is seated too far into the socket, then the medial brim of the prosthesis may irritate the ischium and/or groin.

During *swing* phase, this irritation can be relieved by circumduction. During stance phase, this irritation can be relieved by a wide walking base or by ipsilateral lateral trunk bending.

The functional length of the prosthesis may be excessive (long) for a variety of reasons. These include (1) insufficient knee flexion, (2) excessive ankle plantarflexion, (3) inadequate prosthesis suspension (pistoning), (4) an excessively tight knee-extension aid, and (5) incomplete seating of the residual limb in the socket.

Reference

Lower Extremity Prosthetics Syllabus. New York, Prosthetic-Orthotic Publications, 1996.

40. **e** Open reduction and internal fixation with revision of the femoral component of the total hip arthroplasty using a longer stem. Periprosthetic fractures around loose implant necessitate revision of the implant with placement of a longer femoral component, plus or minus bone graft and additional internal fixation. Skeletal traction is not usually a good option given its associated morbidity and long convalescence. Occasionally, fractures occur between ipsilaterally joint replacements and are particularly challenging situations because of stress riser effects. A total femoral replacement would eliminate concerns regarding insufficient bone stock, malunion, and stress riser effects, but it should be reserved for severe cases with poor bone stock and fractures between ipsilateral prostheses.

Reference

Buly RL: Personal Communication, Hospital For Special Surgery, New York, New York, 1998.

41. **b** Compensation for excessive retroversion of the acetabular shell. The use of a liner with a posterior elevation has been associated with a decreased incidence of *posterior* dislocation. Such a liner may be employed to compensate for malposition of a modular shell that has been implanted in excessive retroversion.

A liner with a posterior elevation will limit the amount of external rotation that can be achieved because it will impinge against the posterior femoral neck. Levering of the posterior neck of the prosthesis against the elevated posterior wall with extreme external rotation may, in fact, increase the likelihood of anterior dislocation.

Note: A modular head with a skirt around its base (over its attachment to the neck of the femoral component) will widen the neck and hence will decrease the effective head-to-neck ratio. This will exacerbate the potential for impingement between the socket and the posterior femoral neck during external rotation.

Reference

Cobb TK, et al.: The Elevated-Rim Acetabular Liner in Total Hip Arthroplasty: Relationship to Postoperative Dislocation. J Bone Joint Surg Am, 78(1):80–86, 1996.

Krushell RJ, Burke DW, Harris WH: Elevated-Rim Acetabular Components: Effect on Range of Motion and Stability in Total Hip Arthroplasty. J Arthroplasty, 6:S53–S58, 1991.

42. **e** The adductor longus. The key landmark in this image (Fig. 4.5) is the superficial femoral artery. At the bifurcation of the femoral artery, the *superficial* branch continues anterior to the adductor longus, and the *deep* branch diverges to travel *posterior* to the adductor longus. Throughout the midthigh, the superficial femoral artery travels directly anterior to the adductor longus.

The terminal portion of the deep femoral artery is evident directly posterior to the femur in this image. Further proximally, the deep femoral artery lies further medially (anterior to the adductor *brevis*). The adductor brevis terminates proximal to the level of this image.

43. **a** Increased femoral retroversion. Anatomic alterations associated with developmental hip dysplasia include increased femoral anteversion, a narrow acetabulum, deficient anterior and/or superior acetabular bone stock, a false acetabulum, a narrow proximal femoral intramedullary canal, and a shallow true acetabulum.

Reference

Morrey BF, ed: Reconstructive Surgery of the Joints, 2nd Ed. Churchill Livingstone, p. 1014, 1996.

44. **d** The superior gemellus. The *arrow* in Fig. 4.6 marks the obturator internus. The obturator internus is innervated by the nerve to the obturator internus. This nerve also innervates the superior gemellus.

The tendon of the obturator internus exits the pelvis through the lesser sciatic notch. Thus, the obturator internus has been referred to as "the key to the lesser sciatic notch."

The obturator externus is innervated by a branch of the obturator nerve. The inferior gemellus and the quadratus femoris are innervated by the nerve to the quadratus femoris. The piriformis is innervated by the nerve to the piriformis.

45. **d** Intraarticular glucocorticoid injection. Although systemic glucocorticoid exposure is one of the more common risk factors for avascular necrosis of the femoral head, intraarticular glucocorticoid administration has not been linked with this disease.

Other clinical entities that are commonly associated with the development of avascular necrosis of the femoral head include alcoholism, Gaucher disease, radiation, trauma (hip dislocation and fractures of the femoral neck), dysbaric phenomena (Caisson disease), systemic lupus erythematosus, pancreatitis, and sickle cell anemia.

Note: Most (approximately 90%) cases of atraumatic avascular necrosis of the femoral head are attributed to alcoholism or exposure to systemic corticosteroids.

Reference

Mont MA Hungerford DS: Non-Traumatic Avascular Necrosis of the Femoral Head. J Bone Joint Surg Am, 77:459–474, 1995.

46. **a** Provide increased offset. The radiograph demonstrates a "swan-neck" prosthesis. The intent of such a design is to increase offset without increasing leg length. One of the most frequent applications for this design is developmental hip dysplasia (DDH) associated with a pseudoacetabulum. In such a situation, the swan-neck design allows the hip center of rotation to be brought down to its proper anatomic location in spite of the associated shortening of the hip abductors.

The increased offset increases the moment arm of the abductors, and this reduces the hip joint reaction force. However, the increased offset increases the bending moment on the implant. The increased bending moment, in turn, increases the risk of stem fracture and augments the strain in the medial cement mantle.

McGrory and colleagues provided clinical documentation of enhanced range of abduction and abduction strength after the use of femoral components with increased offset.

References

Davey JR, et al.: Femoral Component Offset. Its Effect on Strain in Bone Cement. J Arthroplasty, 8(1):23–26, 1993.

McGrory BJ, et al.: Effect of Femoral Offset on Range of Motion and Abductor Muscle Strength After Total Hip Arthroplasty. J Bone Joint Surg Br, 77(6):865–869, 1995.

47. **a** Preoperative antibiotics. The use of prophylactic antibiotics is generally considered to be the single most effective prophylactic measure against acute deep wound infection after total hip arthroplasty. A preoperative dose of a first-generation cephalosporin should be administered within 2 hours before the skin incision. This should be followed by two to three postoperative doses. Longer durations of postoperative prophylactic antibiotics have not been proven to be of benefit.

   Theoretically, laminar flow may decrease postoperative infection rates by decreasing bacterial counts in the air. Body exhaust suits may also decrease airborne contamination. However, the efficacy of these devices has yet to be conclusively demonstrated. In fact, in one study, horizontal laminar flow was associated with a paradoxically increased infection rate.

   Double gloving has not been proven to decrease the incidence of wound infection. However, frequent perforations during orthopaedic procedures have been demonstrated. Thus, double gloves (and periodic intraoperative glove changes) are recommended to protect both the patient and the surgeon.

References

Classen DC, et al.: The Timing of Prophylactic Administration of Antibiotics and the Risk of Surgical Wound Infection. New Engl J Med, 326:281–286, 1992.

Hanssen, et al.: Prevention of Deep Periprosthetic Joint Infection. J Bone Joint Surg Am, 78:458–471, 1996.

48. **e** If an intertrochanteric fracture is associated with comminution of the medial cortex, the medial translation of the shaft fragment will decrease the bending moment on the implant. Varus reductions of intertrochanteric fractures lengthen the lever arm between the femoral shaft and the body's weight-bearing axis. Thus, a varus reduction will subject the implant to a larger bending moment. If the medial femoral cortex is intact, it can share the bending load with the implant. Comminution of the medial cortex heightens the load on the implant.

   The bending moment on an implant can be *reduced* by translating the implant closer to the weight-bearing axis of the body. This can be accomplished in several ways, including (1) a valgus reduction, (2) moving the implant from the lateral femoral cortex [dynamic hip screw (DHS)] to the intramedullary canal (γ nail), or (3) medial translation of the distal fragment.

   Increasing the angle of inclination of a sliding hip screw (valgus reduction) is associated with decreased internal friction because the axis of weight bearing is more parallel to the axis of sliding. With lower (more varus) angles of inclination, there is a larger compressive vector between the sliding metallic surfaces and hence greater internal friction.

49. **d** Lateral trunk bending (to the ipsilateral side). During normal single stance phase, the two areas of maximal pressure between the prosthesis and the limb are at the medial socket brim and the distal lateral residual limb. Contact vectors on the contained portion of the limb in these two areas prevent varus rotation of the limb.

   Lateral bending to the *ipsilateral* side will unload the irritated area by bringing the body's center of gravity over the ipsilateral foot. This decreases the torque on the residual femur.

Reference

Lower Extremity Prosthetics Syllabus. New York, Prosthetic-Orthotic Publications, 1996.

50. **b** Recurrent dislocation. Posttraumatic arthritis is the most common deleterious long-term sequela of native hip dislocation (approximately 20% incidence). Articular cartilage can be damaged on a macroscopic level at the time of dislocation. Chondrocyte injury from compression has also been demonstrated. The incidence of avascular necrosis after hip dislocation varies according to the time elapsed to reduction. If reduction is accomplished within the first 6 hours, the incidence of avascular necrosis is approximately 2% to 10%.

   The incidence of sciatic nerve injury varies from approximately 8% to 19% and is more frequently observed after fracture dislocations (versus pure dislocations). The peroneal division of the sciatic nerve is most commonly affected, and dysfunction typically resolves.

   The incidence of irreducibility (necessitating open reduction) is approximately 2% to 15%. Failure of closed reduction of a posterior dislocation typically stems from interposition of the posterior capsule, the labrum, the ligamentum terres, the piriformis, or a fragment of bone. A computed tomography scan (with 1- to 2-mm cuts) should be obtained to confirm concentric reduction and rule out intraarticular fragments of bone or cartilage to prevent third-body wear. Redislocation after successful reduction is uncommon (approximately 1%) in the absence of a large posterior wall fragment causing gross instability.

Reference

Tornetta P, Mostafavi HR: Hip Dislocation. J Am Acad Orthop Surg, 5(1): 27–36, 1997.

51. **b** The obturator nerve. The obturator nerve exits the pelvis through the obturator foramen (not the greater

sciatic notch). Structures that exit the greater sciatic notch below the piriformis include the inferior gluteal nerve and vessels, the pudendal nerve and vessels, the posterior femoral cutaneous nerve, the sciatic nerve, the nerve to the quadratus femoris, and the nerve to the obturator internis.

Note: The only structures that exit the greater sciatic notch above the piriformis are the superior gluteal nerve and vessels. The sacrospinous ligament defines the boundary between the greater and lesser sciatic notches.

52. **c** (1) definitely loose and (2) probably loose. Harris defined the following radiographic classification for assessing the presence of femoral loosening. *Definite* loosening is present when there is cement fracture or prosthetic migration or subsidence. Probable loosening is present when there is a complete radiolucent line at the cement-bone interface (on any single view). There is *possible* loosening when a lucent line surrounds more than 50% but less than 100% of the femoral component.

Because of the documented subsidence in Fig. 4.8, the stem is definitely loose. Because of the complete radiolucency along the bone-cement interface of the acetabular component, it is probably loose.

Reference

Harris WH, McCarthy JC, O'Neill DA: Femoral Component Loosening Using Contemporary Techniques of Femoral Cement Fixation. J Bone Joint Surg Am, 64:1063–1067, 1982.

53. **c** (1) fully coated uncemented long stem and (2) uncemented cup. Revision arthroplasty is not an exact science. However, given the markedly attenuated femoral cortex spanning the entire length of the loose prosthesis, all standard-length implants (cemented or uncemented) would be suboptimal. One may infer from the cortical ectasia that no cancellous bone remains for cement intrusion. Thus, components requiring cement fixation in this region would be suboptimal. The attenuation of the proximal bone stock is also too far advanced to support a standard-length bone-ingrowth component securely. An optimal femoral implant for this situation would be one that bypassed the jeopardized proximal bone stock to achieve fixation in the untainted diaphyseal region.

Current trends in acetabular revision favor uncemented implants for situations when a bony rim remains intact and intraoperative stability can be achieved. High rates of loosening have been reported for cemented acetabular revisions (17% to 71%). Short-term results of uncemented acetabular revisions appear favorable.

Note: Some authorities would advocate the Ling technique (intramedullary cancellous allografting followed by cementing) as a means of addressing the bone loss in this situation. Bypassing the region of cortical ectasia would still be advisable.

Reference

Buly RL, Nestor BJ: Revision Total Hip Replacement. In Craig EV, ed: Clinical Orthopaedics. Philadelphia, Lippincott Williams & Wilkins, 1999.

54. **e** The nerve to the obturator internus and the pudendal nerve. The nerve to the obturator internus and the pudendal nerve both exit the pelvis through the greater sciatic notch (inferior to the piriformis) and reenter the pelvis through the lesser sciatic notch.
55. **c** Use of titanium femoral heads. Particulate wear debris incites an inflammatory response that results in osteolysis. This process has been implicated as a major cause of implant failure. Factors that have been associated with higher rates of wear include (1) the use of thin polyethylene liners (less than 6 mm), (2) the use of titanium heads, and (3) the use of larger (32-mm) heads.

Titanium is softer and therefore is not as resistant to abrasion as cobalt-chromium. Because of their susceptibility to surface damage, titanium articular surfaces produce significantly more wear debris than those composed of cobalt-chromium.

One should not use 32-mm heads for several reasons. For a given outer acetabular shell diameter, a larger head requires a thinner polyethylene liner. Furthermore, the larger head produces greater volumetric wear. Third-body particulate contamination of the articulating surfaces from any source (bone, cement, or metal debris) increases wear significantly. Both the head-neck junction of modular femoral components and the liner-shell interface of modular acetabular components have been implicated in the production of wear debris.

Note: Ceramics surfaces are harder than metal. Thus, they are less vulnerable to surface damage by third-body wear.

References

Agins HJ, et al.: Metallic Wear in Failed Titanium-Alloy Total Hip Replacements: A Histologic and Quantitative Analysis. J Bone Joint Surg Am, 70:347–356, 1988.
Harris WH: Osteolysis and Particle Disease. Acta Orthop Scand 65(1):113–123, 1994.
Livermore J, et al.: Effect of Femoral Head Size on Wear of the Polyethylene Acetabular Component. J Bone Joint Surg Am, 72:518–528, 1990.
Nasser S, et al.: Cementless Total Joint Arthroplasty Prostheses with Articular Surfaces of Titanium-Alloy. Clin Orthop, 261:171–185, 1990.

56. **e** Adjustment of the fit of his weight belt. Recognition of the symptoms of lateral femoral cutaneous nerve entrapment *(meralgia paresthetica)* can prevent the performance of multiple unnecessary diagnostic tests.

Removing tight garments or other identifiable potential sources of external compression (such as a weight-lifting belt) may completely relieve this condition.

57. **e** Excessive flexion. Ankylosing spondylitis is associated with loss of lumbar lordosis. Loss of lumbar lordosis, in turn, flexes the pelvis. The resultant functional flexion of the acetabuli poses a risk for anterior dislocation when total hip arthroplasty is performed in the context of this disease. In this setting, the surgeon should be particularly careful to avoid excessive anteversion of the component.

    Anterior instability is assessed with the hip adducted, extended, and externally rotated. *Posterior instability* is assessed with the hip adducted, flexed, and internally rotated.

    Note: Because of the associated pelvic flexion, the obturator foramen will appear more wide open on an anteroposterior pelvis film of a patient with ankylosing spondylitis.

58. **a** The presence of a metal-oxide coating on the surface of an implant will prevent fretting. The presence of a metal-oxide coating on the surface of an implant is referred to as passivation. A passified surface serves as a kinematic barrier to the migration of metal ions. Thus, a passified surface is relatively resistant to electrochemical (galvanic) corrosion. However, passivation provides *no* resistance to *mechanical* forms of corrosion such as fretting. In fact, mechanical disruption of a passified surface coating will render the underlying nonoxidized metal vulnerable to galvanic corrosion.

    Debris particles from any type of metal corrosion (mechanical or electrochemical) may migrate to the articulating surfaces of an implant and may accelerate polyethylene debris production through third-body wear.

    Elevated serum levels of chromium and titanium have been detected in patients with total hip arthroplasty components composed of these substances. Serum levels of these metals have been noted to be even higher among patients with loose prostheses (see question 63).

Reference

Jacobs J, et al.: Corrosion of Metal Implants. J Bone Joint Surg Am, 80: 268–282, 1998.

59. **b** Hip arthroscopy and débridement. The magnetic resonance image reveals an acetabular labral tear. The anterosuperior portion of the acetabular rim is typically involved. Labral tears occur more commonly in the setting of acetabular dysplasia (overt or occult). Labral disease may be associated with periacetabular ganglion cyst formation. After lack of response to an adequate course of conservative treatment, arthroscopic evaluation and débridement of the involved portion of labrum are appropriate.

    Torn acetabular labrum was a commonly overlooked pathologic entity until the advent of magnetic resonance imaging. Thus, long-term results of arthroscopic intervention for this condition do not yet exist. Biopsy of the associated cyst is unwarranted. Repair is not typically attempted, and arthrotomy would be too invasive in this situation. When there is associated hip dysplasia, the degree of associated articular cartilage degeneration should be assessed because it is a superimposed potential source of pain.

Reference

McCarthy JC, et al.: Hip Arthroscopy: Applications and Technique. J Am Acad Orthop Surg, 3:115–122, 1995.

60. **b** The superior gluteal nerve. The superficial dissection of the direct lateral approach to the hip uses the interval between the tensor fasciae latae and the gluteus maximus (employing the internervous plane between the superior gluteal and inferior gluteal nerves). However, the *deep* dissection splits the fibers of the gluteus medius and thus uses no true internervous plane.

    If the gluteus medius is split more than approximately 3 cm proximally to its insertion on the greater trochanter and/or if excessive retraction is applied to this muscle, the superior gluteal nerve may be damaged.

    Note: Abitbol and colleagues documented that electromyographic evidence of subclinical injury to the superior and inferior gluteal nerves was present in most patients immediately after total hip arthroplasty (regardless of whether a lateral or posterior approach was used). These electromyographic abnormalities universally improved after 1 year.

References

Abitbol JJ, et al.: Gluteal Nerve Damage Following Total Hip Arthroplasty: A Prospective Analysis. J Arthroplasty, 5:319, 1990.

Hardinge: The Direct Lateral Approach to the Hip. J Bone Joint Surg Br, 64:17–19, 1982.

Hoppenfeld S: Surgical Exposures in Orthopaedics, 2nd Ed. Philadelphia, JB Lippincott, 1994.

61. **c** Non–weight bearing, crutches, and close observation. Fatigue fractures of the femoral neck occur primarily in persons involved in repetitive impact activities (e.g., marching in military recruits or long-distance running). In contradistinction to insufficiency fractures, which occur in *abnormal* bone, fatigue fractures occur in *normal* bone that is subjected abnormal stresses. They are usually related to an abrupt increase in training.

    Patients typically present with activity-related groin pain. However, some patients may remain asymptomatic until a true fracture occurs. Other potential causes of hip pain such as infection, neoplasm, synovitis, tendinitis, and avascular necrosis should be excluded. Plain radiographs are initially negative. Bone scan and magnetic resonance imaging are more sensitive modalities.

Treatment depends on the type of fatigue fracture. Shin and Gillingham described a useful classification system based on radiographic and magnetic resonance findings (Table 4.5).

Compression fractures are subdivided according to the severity of the fatigue line. If the fatigue line extends less than 50% across the diameter of the neck, recommended treatment consists of non–weight bearing and close follow-up to confirm that the fracture does not progress. Percutaneous pinning is recommended when the fatigue line extending greater than 50% across the neck.

Reference

Shin AY, Gillingham BL: Fatigue Fractures of the Femoral Neck in Athletes. J Am Acad Orthop Surg, 5:293–302, 1997.

62. **c** Paget disease. The radiograph in Fig. 4.9 reveals femoral bowing in association with coxa vara, thickened cortices, and coarse trabeculae. These features are characteristic of Paget disease. The visible portion of the pelvis reveals no stigmata of Paget disease despite advanced involvement of the ipsilateral proximal femur. Contiguous bones are not necessarily affected.

63. **b** Stainless steel and cobalt alloy. Galvanic corrosion occurs because different metals exhibit different tendencies for oxidation in solution. When two different metals are in close proximity to one another in solution, electrons will flow from the more reactive metal (anode) to the more noble metal (cathode). Under static conditions, the couple between titanium alloy and cobalt alloy is fairly stable. Conversely, stainless steel is susceptible to galvanic attack. Therefore, combinations of stainless steel with titanium alloy (or stainless steel with cobalt alloy) should be avoided.

    Zirconium is a ceramic (not a metal). Thus, it cannot participate in galvanic corrosion.

References

Jacobs J, et al.: Corrosion of Metal Implants. J Bone Joint Surg Am, 80:268–282, 1998.

TABLE 4.5. FATIGUE FRACTURE CLASSIFICATION

Fracture Type	Injury Location	Recommended Treatment
Compression	Inferomedial neck	(see below)
Tension	Superolateral neck	Internal fixation (pinning)
Displacement	Complete	Open reduction and internal fixation (emergency)

Kummer FJ, Rose RM: Corrosion of titanium/cobalt-chronium alloy couples. Bone Joint Surg Am, 65:1125, 1983.

64. **c** The ischiofemoral ligament. The posterior capsule is formed by the ischiofemoral ligament. The iliofemoral ligament (or Y ligament of Bigelow) forms the anterior capsule. The indirect head of the rectus femoris originates cephalad to the acetabulum. The direct head of the rectus femoris originates from the anterior inferior iliac spine.

65. **d** Factor Xa. *Heparin* enhances the activity of antithrombin III. Dextran decreases blood viscosity and platelet aggregation. Aspirin affects platelet aggregation by inhibiting cyclooxygenase.

    Warfarin (Coumadin) inhibits the posttranslational activation (γ-carboxylation) of the vitamin-K–dependent factors (II, VII, IX, and X). *Low-molecular-weight heparin* (like standard heparin) enhances the endogenous anticoagulant antithrombin III. However, it exerts its main anticoagulant effect through inhibiting factor Xa.

Reference

Colwell CW, et al.: Use of Enoxaparin, a Low Molecular Weight Heparin, and Unfractionated Heparin for the Prevention of Deep Venous Thrombosis After Total Hip Arthroplasty. J Bone Joint Surg Am, 76:3–14, 1994.

66. **d** An increased incidence of deep venous thrombosis. Paget disease may lead to hip degeneration by affecting the femur, the acetabulum, or both. Total hip arthroplasty in this setting is associated with an elevated incidence of heterotopic ossification (ranging from 37% to 65%). Protrusio acetabuli is present in 22% to 35% of affected hips.

    Regions of active pagetoid bone are hyperemic. Reaming this bone may provoke excessive hemorrhage. Pretreatment with antipagetoid medications (disphosphonates or calcitonin) has been advocated to diminish intraoperative blood loss. Excessive bleeding from the prepared osseous surfaces during implantation may impair cemented fixation. Reaming may be difficult because of the sclerotic quality of the affected bone.

    Involvement of the femoral neck often produces a varus deformity. Diseased femoral shafts typically assume an exaggerated anterolateral bow. These two deformities create a risk of varus malalignment of the femoral component and potential perforation of the lateral femoral cortex.

References

Ludkowski P, Wilson-MacDonald J: Total Arthroplasty in Paget's Disease of the Hip: A Clinical Review and Review of the Literature. Clin Orthop, 255:160–167, 1990.

Merkow RL, Pellicci PM, Hely DP, Salvati EA: Total Hip Replacement for Paget's Disease of the Hip. J Bone Joint Surg Am, 66:752–758, 1984.

67. **b** The gracilis. The anterior branch of the obturator nerve innervates the gracilis and the adductor longus. The posterior branch innervates the adductor magnus and the adductor brevis. The rectus femoris is innervated by the femoral nerve. The semitendinosus is innervated by the tibial division of the sciatic nerve.

68. **a** Primary total hip arthroplasty. The principal goals of management of this injury are (1) prompt mobilization to avoid the morbidity associated with prolonged bed rest (e.g., deep venous thrombosis, pulmonary embolism, pneumonia), (2) minimizing of the potential morbidity from the fracture itself (malunion, nonunion, avascular necrosis), and (3) minimizing of the need for repeat procedures.

Nonoperative management of femoral neck fractures has virtually no role in contemporary adult orthopaedics, except in baseline nonambulators who are gravely ill and who experience little pain from the fracture when they are transferred. Open reduction and internal fixation of displaced femoral neck fractures are associated with a very high complication rate and the need for subsequent operative salvage. Lu-Yao et al. reported a combined 49% rate of avascular necrosis or malunion with an associated 20% to 36% rate of reoperation.

The long-term functional outcome of hemiarthroplasty in physiologically young, active patients is suboptimal compared with total hip arthroplasty because of acetabular erosion. At 2 years, Koefed found that 37% of all hemiarthroplasties needed to be (or already had been) converted to total hip arthroplasties. Phillips et al. found a very high failure rate (44%) for hemiarthroplasty in active, younger patients because of accelerated acetabular erosion; these investigators differentiated the poor results in this population from the satisfactory long-term results of hemiarthroplasty in their comparison group of physiologically older, inactive patients.

For a physiologically young, active patient who sustains a displaced femoral neck fracture, total hip arthroplasty offers a lower complication rate, a lower revision rate, and predictably superior long-term functional results than either open reduction and internal fixation or hemiarthroplasty. The diagram in Fig. 4.21 represents an algorithm proposed by Papandrea and Fromison for the treatment of displaced femoral neck fractures.

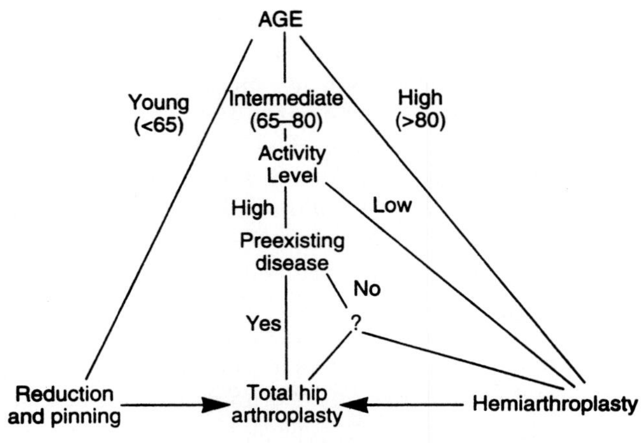

FIGURE 4.21

References

Asnis SF, Wanek-Scaglione L: Intracapsular Fractures of the Femoral Neck. J Bone Joint Surg Am, 76:1793–1803, 1994.

Gebhard JS, et al.: A Comparison of Total Hip Arthroplasty and Hemiarthroplasty for Treatment of Acute Fracture of the Femoral Neck. Clin Orthop, 282:123–131, 1992.

Koefed H: Moore Prosthesis in the Treatment of Fresh Femoral Neck Fractures: A Critical Review with Special Attention to Secondary Acetabular Degeneration. Injury, 14:531–540, 1983.

Lee BP, et al.: Total Hip Arthroplasty for the Treatment of Acute Fracture of the Femoral Neck. J Bone Joint Surg Am, 80:70–75, 1998.

Lu-Yao GL, et al.: Outcomes After Displaced Fractures of the Femoral Head. J Bone Joint Surg Am, 76:15–15, 1994.

Papandrea RF, Fromison MI: Total Hip Arthroplasty After Acute Displaced Femoral Neck Fractures. Am J Orthop, 25:85–88, 1996.

Phillips TW, et al.: Thompson Hemiarthroplasty and Acetabular Erosion. J Bone Joint Surg Am, 71:913–917, 1989.

Skinner P, et al.: Displaced Subcapital Fractures of the Femur: A Prospective, Randomized Comparison of Internal Fixation, Hemiarthroplasty, and Total Hip Replacement. Injury, 20:291–293, 1989.

69. **d** Greater than primary total hip arthroplasty performed for osteoarthritis for the first 4 months and, thereafter, approximately equivalent to the risk of dislocation after total hip arthroplasty performed for osteoarthritis. Total hip arthroplasty is commonly avoided in the setting of acute femoral neck fracture because of its perceived high risk of dislocation. The risk of dislocation in this setting is not trivial. Indeed, based on a review of nine separate studies (601 total hip arthroplasties performed for acute femoral neck fractures), 10.1% of the patients had dislocations at some point. This is considerably higher than the 2% to 3% rate of dislocation for primary total hip arthroplasties performed for osteoarthritis. However, when acute, one-time dislocations (occurring within the first 4 months after fracture) were excluded, the dislocation rate fell to 2.5%. This rate of dislocation is approximately equal to the 2% to 3% overall incidence of dislocation after primary total hip arthroplasty for osteoarthritis or rheumatoid arthritis. This rate of dislocation is also approximately equal to the 2.1% to 2.9% overall risk of hemiarthroplasty dislocation reported by Lu-Yao et al. Dislocation precautions must be vigilantly adhered to after all total hip arthroplasties, but particularly during the first 4 months after total hip arthroplasty in the setting of acute femoral neck fracture.

References

Lu-Yao GL, et al.: Outcomes After Displaced Fractures of the Femoral Head. J Bone Joint Surg Am, 76:15–25, 1994.

Papandrea RF, Fromison MI: Total Hip Arthroplasty After Acute Displaced Femoral Neck Fractures. Am J Orthop, 25:85–88, 1996.

70. **e** 10 μm and smaller. Phagocytosis of particles by macrophages has been implicated as the initiator of the inflammatory response that produces osteolysis. To be phagocytized by macrophages, particles must be less than 10 μm.

Note: Not only do wear particles stimulate bone resorption (by macrophages), but evidence also suggests that they can inhibit bone formation by a direct effect on osteoblasts.

References

Allen MJ, Brett F, Millett PJ, Rushton N: The Effects of Particulate Polyethylene at a Weight-Bearing Bone-Implant Interface. J Bone Joint Surg Br, 78(1):32–37, 1996.

Allen MJ, Myer BJ, Millett PJ, Rushton N: The Effects of Particulate Cobalt, Chromium, and Cobalt-Chromium Alloy on Human Osteoblast-like Cells In Vitro. J Bone Joint Surg Br, 79(3):475–482, 1997.

Harris WH: Osteolysis and Particle Disease. Acta Orthop Scand 65(1): 113–123, 1994.

71. **a** External rotation and hyperextension. The hip apprehension test is performed with combined adduction, external rotation, and hyperextension. This maneuver attempts to reproduce symptomatic anterior subluxation of the femoral head in patients with hip dysplasia. The test attempts to exploit the deficient anterolateral femoral head coverage that is commonly encountered in dysplastic hips.

Reference

McGrory BJ, et al.: Bernese Periacetabular Osteotomy. J Orthop Tech, 1(4):179–191, 1993.

72. **b** A clinical line between the anterior superior iliac spine and the ipsilateral ischial tuberosity. The *Nelaton line* is a clinical line between the anterior superior iliac spine and the ipsilateral ischial tuberosity. Ordinarily, this line should intersect the tip of the greater trochanter. If the tip of the trochanter lies above this line, the clinician should suspect potential hip dislocation.

The *Klein line* is a radiographic line that projects along the superior femoral neck. Failure of this line to intersect a portion of the femoral head suggests a diagnosis of slipped capital femoral epiphysis.

The *Hilgenreiner line* is a horizontal radiographic line through the two triradiate cartilages. Its intersection with the *Perkin line* (a vertical line through the lateral osseous margin of the acetabulum) defines four quadrants. The femoral head ossification center should lie in the inferomedial quadrant. If the femoral head ossification center lies outside of this quadrant, one should suspect hip dislocation.

The *Shenton line* is a curvilinear radiographic line along the inferior femoral neck that continues along the superior obturator foramen (inferior margin of the superior pubic ramus). Discontinuity of this line suggests hip dislocation.

The clinical line from the anterior superior iliac spine to the umbilicus has no relevance to orthopaedics, but (if you wish to resurrect fond memories of general surgery) the McBurney point lies two-thirds of the way to the anterior superior iliac spine on this line.

Note: The acetabular index is defined by the angle subtended by (1) the Hilgenreiner line and (2) a line drawn from the triradiate cartilage to the lateral ossified margin of the acetabulum. The normal acetabular index is less than 30 degrees in newborns and less than 20 degrees by the age of 2 years.

The center-edge angle *(the Wiberg angle)* is subtended by (1) the Perkins line and (2) a line from the center of the ossific nucleus of the femoral head to the lateral ossified margin of the acetabulum. The normal value for the Wiberg angle is less than 20 degrees.

73. **e** 1.5 femoral diameters past the screw hole. In a cadaveric model, Panjabi and colleagues demonstrated that strain was minimized when the stem length extended 1.5 femoral diameters past a drill hole in the lateral femoral cortex. The stress raiser effect was partially relieved (albeit to a lesser extent) when the stem barely bypassed the defect. Bypassing the defect by more than 1.5 femoral diameters did not provide additional benefit.

Reference

Panjabi MM, et al.: Effect of Femoral Stem Length on Stress Raisers Associated with Revision Hip Arthroplasty. J Orthop Res, 3:447–455, 1985.

74. **d** The femoral component and acetabular shell are both well-fixed. The radiographs reveal polyethylene failure (either extreme wear or fracture). This is indicated by the eccentric position (Fig. 4.10) of the femoral head within the acetabular shell. Predisposing factors for this can include large femoral heads (32 mm) and thin polyethylene liners.

Both the acetabular shell and the femoral stem appear well fixed. Radiographic signs of loosening (e.g., component migration, pedestal formation, and radiolucency at the bone-component interfaces) are all absent.

References

Berry DJ, et al.: Catastrophic Failure of the Polyethylene Liner of Uncemented Acetabular Components. J Bone Joint Surg Br, 76:575–578, 1994.

Engh CA, et al.: The Case for Porous Coated Implants. Clin Orthop, 261:63–81, 1990.

75. **c** Observe. The answer is obvious. Never operate on an asymptomatic patient, unless you have a very good reason. If the components were modular, this question would be more controversial because some clinicians

could advocate prophylactic polyethylene exchange. In this case, there is obvious wear of the polyethylene liner, however, it is a cemented all-polyethylene component. The entire component would have to be removed and revised. Furthermore, the stem is a monoblock design that would also necessitate revision if there were any damage to the bearing surfaces. Given that both components are well fixed and the patient is asymptomatic, observation is warranted.

As an aside, for a given acetabular shell size, larger femoral heads require that the polyethylene liner be thinner. Thin polyethylene liners have been correlated with increased wear rates. In addition, 32-mm diameter femoral heads have been associated with increased volumetric wear compared with 22- and 28-mm heads. Wear debris production should be minimized to prevent osteolysis and premature component loosening.

Note: The 32-mm diameter heads are associated with greater volumetric wear production but less linear wear compared with smaller head sizes.

References

Bartel DL, Bicknell VL, Wright TM: The Effect of Conformity, Thickness, and Material on Stresses in Ultra-High Molecular Weight Components for Total Joint Replacement. J Bone Joint Surg Am, 68(7):1041–1051, 1986.

Maxian TA, et al.: Adaptive Finite Element Modeling of Long-Term Polyethylene Wear in Total Hip Arthroplasty. J Orthop Res, 14(4):668–675, 1996.

76. **b** Leg length discrepancy (right leg longer). Under ordinary circumstances, the right hip abductors prevent pelvic tilt to the left during right stance phase. *Weak right hip abductors* may produce pelvic tilt to the contralateral side during stance phase. This pattern is referred to as a *Trendelenburg sign.* Alternatively, the center of gravity of the torso may be shifted toward the right hip joint (ipsilateral trunk lean). Reducing the distance (lever arm) between the right hip (fulcrum) and the center of gravity of the body will reduce the demand on the weak abductors. This pattern is referred to as the *Duchenne sign* or an *abductor lurch.*

The same lever arm is lengthened in the presence of scoliosis that is decompensated to the contralateral side. Ipsilateral trunk lean can compensate for the resultant increased demand on the ipsilateral hip abductors.

By decreasing the abductor force necessary to maintain single leg stance, ipsilateral trunk lean will decrease the joint reaction force across the ipsilateral hip. Decreasing compression will lessen discomfort in an *osteoarthritic joint.* The pattern of shortened ipsilateral stance phase secondary to hip pain is referred to as a *coxalgic gait.* In the presence of a leg length discrepancy (with the contralateral leg longer), trunk lean will assist the contralateral foot to clear the floor during contralateral swing phase.

Note: Ipsilateral hip arthrodesis is another potential source of trunk lean.

Reference

Perry J: Gait Analysis: Normal and Pathological Function. Thorofare, NJ, Slack, p. 276, 1992.

77. **c** The gluteus minimus. The *gluteus minimus* is the most medial structure in the abductor region. It runs obliquely along the outer table of the ilium to the greater trochanter. The prominent fat plane between *the gluteus medius* and the gluteus minimus is seen directly lateral to the labeled muscle. The fat plane between the gluteus medius and the gluteus maximus is characteristically less pronounced than the fat plane between the gluteus medius and the gluteus minimus. The gluteus minimus is directly adjacent to the acetabular dome and the superior femoral neck.

The tensor fasciae latae is a more superficial structure. Unlike the gluteus minimus, it does not insert on the greater trochanter. Furthermore, the tensor fasciae latae is a relatively anterior structure. (The relatively posterior position of this image can be inferred from the presence of the lesser trochanter.) The *reflected head of the rectus femoris* originates from the superolateral aspect of the acetabulum. However, its origin is anterior to this image, and its fibers run orthogonally to the fibers of the minimus (out of the plane of this image).

Note: The tensor fasciae latae, the gluteus medius, and the gluteus minimus are innervated by the superior gluteal nerve.

78. **d** Porosity reduction decreases volume expansion during polymerization. Changes in cement volume during the polymerization process are a function of two variables: (1) molecular alterations and (2) temperature. Polymerization of the polymethylmethacrylate monomer causes volume shrinkage. However, the polymerization reaction is an exothermic reaction. Increased temperature induces a thermal expansion of entrapped gas bubbles. A three-stage concept of polymerization helps to clarify the interplay of these two conflicting variables (Fig. 4.22).

During *stage I,* thermal effects are negligible. Polymerization of the monomer causes volume contraction. During *stage II,* increased temperature drives volume expansion. The magnitude of this thermal expansion is decreased by porosity reduction. During *stage III,* polymerization is complete, but further volume contraction occurs as the cement cools.

Note: The shear strength of the metal-cement interface is markedly improved when the metal is precoated with polymethylmethacrylate.

Reference

Chan KH et al.: In Morrey BF, ed: Reconstructive Surgery of the Joints, 2nd Ed. Churchill Livingston, pp. 37–40, 1996.

79. **c** Iliotibial band contracture. The variation in passive hip extension with different amounts of abduction

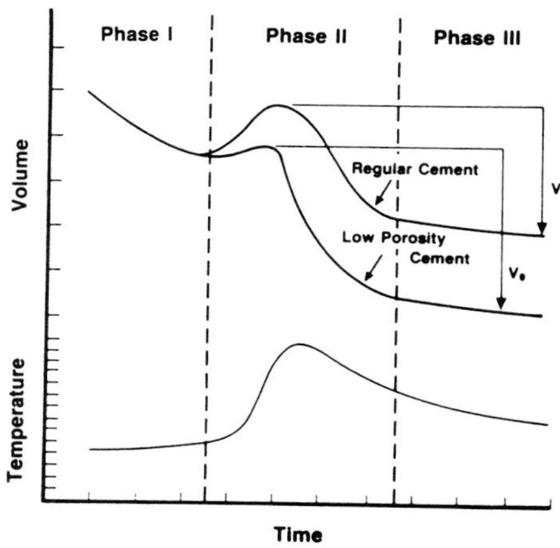

FIGURE 4.22

localizes the contracture to the iliotibial band. The resultant limitation in extension is most evident when the hip is adducted, as it is during late single-leg stance. The effect of iliotibial band tension is eliminated with relative abduction of the extremity.

Other potential causes of limited hip extension (such as iliopsoas contracture or a tight anterior joint capsule) would not be eliminated by abduction.

Note: The classic test for detecting iliotibial band tightness is the *Ober test.* This test is performed with the patient in the lateral decubitus position with the upward hip in extension. Limited adduction in this position indicates iliotibial band tightness.

Reference

Perry J: Gait Analysis: Normal and Pathological Function. Thorofare, NJ, Slack, p. 251, 1992.

80. **a** Multiple myeloma. Figure 4.12 reveals multiple lytic lesions around the hips. The margin is not sclerotic. Multiple myeloma characteristically produces lytic osseous lesions in marrow-containing bones such as the pelvis and vertebral bodies. Osseous foci of myeloma are frequently "cold" on bone scan because their aggressiveness precludes an osteoblastic response. (Labeled phosphate must be incorporated into reactive bone for a bone scan to be positive.)

The biopsy reveals multiple small plasma cells with minimal intervening stroma. Bland sheets of homogeneous plasma cells are often pictured in textbook examples of multiple myeloma.

The diagnosis of multiple myeloma is substantiated by the presence of Bence Jones proteins in her urine. These represent the light chains of the immunoglobulins produced by the monoclonal B-cell proliferation. Serum protein electrophoresis would confirm the presence of a monoclonal spike.

Given the history of carcinoma, the potential for a metastatic focus should immediately be considered. However, *colon carcinoma* cells are characteristically larger and tend to assume glandular patterns. *Chondrosarcoma* is an unlikely diagnosis because of the absence of a cartilaginous matrix.

Note: Solitary myeloma (plasmacytoma) has a better prognosis than multiple myeloma.

81. **c** 800 cGy in a single dose. The current radiation protocol for prophylaxis against heterotopic ossification is 700 to 800 cGy delivered in a single dose 1 to 4 days postoperatively. Previously recommended protocols consisted of a cumulative dose of 2,000 cGy administered in fractions. This was effective but time consuming.

Healy et al. compared early postoperative single doses of 700 cGy to doses of 550 cGy. They reported an unacceptably high rate of failure of prophylaxis with the lower dosage.

Indomethacin and aspirin have also been shown to have prophylactic efficacy. Pellegrini et al. showed that *pre*operative radiation can provide sufficient prophylaxis as well. This finding suggests that the culpable osteogenic precursor cells are derived from local tissues.

Note: The porous ingrowth surfaces of noncemented components should be shielded from the irradiated field. The beam should be limited to the capsule and abductor regions.

References

Fingeroth RJ, Ahmed AQ: Single Dose Prophylaxis for Heterotopic Ossification after Total Hip Arthroplasty. Clin Orthop, 317:131–140, 1995.

Healy WL, et al.: Single-Dose Irradiation for the Prevention of Heterotopic Ossification after Total Hip Arthroplasty: A Comparison of Doses of Five Hundred and Fifty and Seven Hundred Centigray. J Bone Joint Surg Am, 77(4):590–595, 1995.

Kjaersgaard-Andersen P, Ritter MA: Short-Term Treatment with Nonsteroidal Antiinflammatory Medications to Prevent Heterotopic Bone Formation after Total Hip Arthroplasty: A Preliminary Report. Clin Orthop, 279:157–162, 1992.

Pellegrini VD, et al.: Prevention of Heterotopic Ossification with Irradiation After Total Hip Arthroplasty: Radiation Therapy with Single Dose of 800 Centigray Administered to a Limited Field. J Bone Joint Surg Am, 74:186–200, 1992.

Pellegrini VD Jr, Gregoritch SJ: Preoperative Irradiation for Prevention of Heterotopic Ossification Following Total Hip Arthroplasty. J Bone Joint Surg Am, 78(6):870–881, 1996.

82. **c** Smaller (unnamed) vessels and fractured cancellous osseous surfaces. Identification of major torn arteries in association with pelvic fractures is seldom possible. It is estimated that named arterial sources of hemorrhage can be identified in only 5% to 10% of complex pelvic fractures.

Huittinen and Slatis performed postmortem pelvic angiograms on 27 trauma victims with pelvic fractures. Only three named arterial sources of hemorrhage were found among these specimens (two obturator and one hypogastric). Most of the bleeding occurred through fractured cancellous osseous surfaces and disrupted pelvic floor soft tissues. This study supports the notion of prompt fracture reduction to tamponade the fractured bony surfaces. This study does not lend credence to routine arterial embolization or hypogastric artery ligation.

References

Agnew SG: Hemodynamically Unstable Pelvic Fractures. Orthop Clin North Am, 25(4):715–721, 1994.

Huittinen V, Slatis P: Postmortem Angiography and Dissection of the Hypogastric Artery in Pelvic Fractures. Surgery, 73(3):454–462, 1973.

83. **b** Ankylosing spondylitis. Figure 4.13 demonstrates bilateral joint space narrowing. The narrowing is concentric, suggesting an inflammatory arthropathy. In addition, the sacroiliac joints appear autofused. The spine also demonstrates the presence of syndesmophytes.

    The *epiphyseal dysplasias* produce short stature. They are associated with coxa vara and premature degenerative joint disease.

    The hip joint is the most common joint affected by hemochromatosis. Its radiographic appearance is similar to that of osteoarthritis. Chondrocalcinosis is often present in association with this disease.

84. **a** Nonoperative management. Despite the patient's moderate symptoms, the radiograph (Fig. 4.14A) demonstrates advanced osteonecrosis involving more than 30% of the femoral head. The head is collapsed, and there is secondary acetabular degeneration. (Note the medial and superolateral acetabular osteophytes.)

    By the classification system of Ficat and Arlet, the patient has stage IV disease. Core decompression and vascularized allografts have demonstrated minimal efficacy for patients with stage IV osteonecrosis.

    Treatment of stage IV lesions is dictated by patient age and clinical symptoms. The patient described in this case is young, with relatively mild symptoms. Therefore, nonoperative management is indicated (nonsteroidal antiinflammatory drugs, use of a cane, activity modification, and physical therapy). It would be appropriate to consider hip arthrodesis or total hip arthroplasty if his pain and disability were more severe.

    The Ficat and Arlet classification of osteonecrosis is given in Table 4.6.

TABLE 4.6. FICAT AND ARLET CLASSIFICATION OF OSTEONECROSIS

Stage	Pain	Radiographic Findings
I	Yes	None (but positive magnetic resonance imaging)
II	Yes	Subchondral cysts or sclerosis
III	Yes	Subchondral collapse (loss of sphericity)
IV	Yes	Arthrosis with reciprocal acetabular changes

Reference

Mont MA, Hungerford DS: Non-Traumatic Avascular Necrosis of the Femoral Head. J Bone Joint Surg Am, 77:459–474, 1995.

85. **d** The obturator artery. The artery of the ligamentum terres (foveal artery) is a branch of the obturator artery.

    Note: The lateral ascending cervical vessels give rise to the lateral epiphyseal arteries, which provide the majority of the blood supply to the femoral head.

References

Crock HV: An Atlas of the Arterial Supply of the Head and Neck of the Femur in Man. Clin Orthop, 152:17–27, 1980.

Trueta J, Harrison MH: The Normal Vascular Anatomy of the Femoral Head in Adult Man. J Bone Joint Surg Br, 35:442, 1953.

86. **c** 100 to 300 μm. In a canine model, Bobyn and colleagues demonstrated that pore sizes 50 to 400 μm provided maximal bone-implant interface shear strength (17 MPA). Smaller pore sizes did not permit uniform tissue mineralization. The strength of fixation with pore sizes larger than 400 μm approached the strength of pore sizes 50 to 400 μm, but this strength was not achieved as predictably or as rapidly.

References

Bobyn JD, et al.: The Optimum Pore Size for the Fixation of Porous-Surfaced Metal Implants by the Ingrowth of Bone. Clin Orthop, 150:263–270, 1980.

Callaghan JJ: The Clinical Results and Basic Science of Total Hip Arthroplasty with Porous-Coated Prostheses. J Bone Joint Surg Am, 75:299–310, 1993.

87. Answers **a** through **d** are all correct. Answer **e** is unacceptable. The rationale is self-evident.

Reference

Crockett H, et al.: J Common Sense, 19:94–98, 1998.

FIGURE CREDITS

Figure 4.9. From Greenfield GB: Radiology of Bone Diseases, p. 126, Lippincott, with permission.

Figure 4.13. From Greenspan A: Orthopedic Radiology. Philadelphia, Lippincott Williams & Wilkins, p. 467, 2000, with permission.

Figure 4.15. From Craig EV, ed: Clinical Orthopaedics. Philadelphia, Lippincott Williams & Wilkins, p. 580, 1999, with permission.

Figure 4.16. From Rockwood CA, Green DP, eds: Fractures in Adults, 4th Ed. Philadelphia, Lippincott–Raven, p. 1667, 1996, with permission.

Figure 4.17. From J Bone Joint Surg Am, 62:1065, 1980, with permission.

Figure 4.18. From J Bone Joint Surg Am, 72:504, 1990, with permission.

Figure 4.19. From Rockwood CA, Green DP, eds: Fractures in Adults, 4th Ed. Philadelphia, Lippincott–Raven, p. 1662, 1996, with permission.

Figure 4.20. From Gruen TA, et al.: Failure of Femoral Components. Clin Orthop, 14:18, 1979, with permission.

Figure 4.21. From Papandrea RF, Fromison MI: Total Hip Arthroplasty After Acute Displaced Femoral Neck Fractures. Am J Orthop, 25:85–88, 1996, with permission.

Figure 4.22. From Chan KH, et al. In Morrey BF, ed: Reconstructive Surgery of the Joints, 2nd Ed. Churchill Livingstone, pp. 37–40, 1996, with permission.

5

ADULT KNEE

QUESTIONS

1. The patient whose radiographs and magnetic resonance imaging scan are shown in Fig. 5.1 has which of the following problems?
   (a) Patellar tilt
   (b) Bipartite patella
   (c) Fracture of patella
   (d) Chondromalacia patellae
   (e) Patellar maltracking
2. The *patellar clunk syndrome* is the result of what phenomenon?
   (a) Hypertrophic scar tissue at the inferior pole of the patella impinges on the femoral component during extension.
   (b) Hypertrophic scar tissue at the superior pole of the patella impinges on the femoral component during flexion.
   (c) Patellar component loosening occurs.
   (d) Hypertrophic scar tissue at the inferior pole of the patella impinges on the femoral component during flexion.
   (e) Hypertrophic scar tissue at the superior pole of the patella impinges on the femoral component during extension.
3. High tibial osteotomy for varus gonarthrosis has most commonly been associated with the subsequent development of which of the following abnormalities of the patella?
   (a) Patella alta
   (b) Patella infera
   (c) Patella fracture
   (d) Patella dislocation
   (e) Chondromalacia patellae
4. During early stance phase, the ground reaction force vector
   (a) Passes through the knee center of rotation
   (b) Is orthogonal to the plane of the floor
   (c) Is equal in magnitude to the force being transmitted by the patellar ligament
   (d) Is antiparallel to the knee joint reaction force
   (e) Passes posterior to the knee center of rotation
5. Which of the following conditions is the most significant risk factor for peroneal nerve palsy after a total knee arthroplasty?
   (a) Preoperative severe valgus deformity
   (b) Preoperative biplanar (flexion and valgus) deformity
   (c) Excessive tourniquet time
   (d) Pressure on the nerve from the postoperative dressing
   (e) Intraoperative exposure of the nerve
6. In total knee arthroplasty, the *extension gap* refers to
   (a) The distance between the medial and lateral femoral condyles
   (b) The distance between the proximal tibial cut and the anterior femoral cut
   (c) The distance between the distal femoral cut and the proximal tibial cut
   (d) The distance between the posterior femoral cut and the proximal tibial cut
   (e) The depth of the intercondylar box cut in a posterior cruciate ligament–substituting design
7. An 85-year-old man undergoes revision of the femoral component of his posterior cruciate ligament–substituting total knee arthroplasty for aseptic loosening. The patellar and tibial components are confirmed to be well fixed and well positioned during surgery, and, thus, neither is revised. After revision of the femur with an identical component, soft tissue tension is fine in flexion but lax in extension. To address this laxity, the surgeon exchanges the tibial polyethylene for a thicker insert. What effect will this maneuver have on the joint line?
   (a) The joint line will be unchanged.
   (b) The joint line will be translated posteriorly.
   (c) The joint line will be raised.
   (d) The joint line will be translated anteriorly.
   (e) The joint line will be lowered.
8. Based on the surgeon's solution to the soft tissue balancing problem in question 7, what would be the most likely effect on the motion and/or stability of the revised knee?
   (a) Decreased varus-valgus stability in flexion

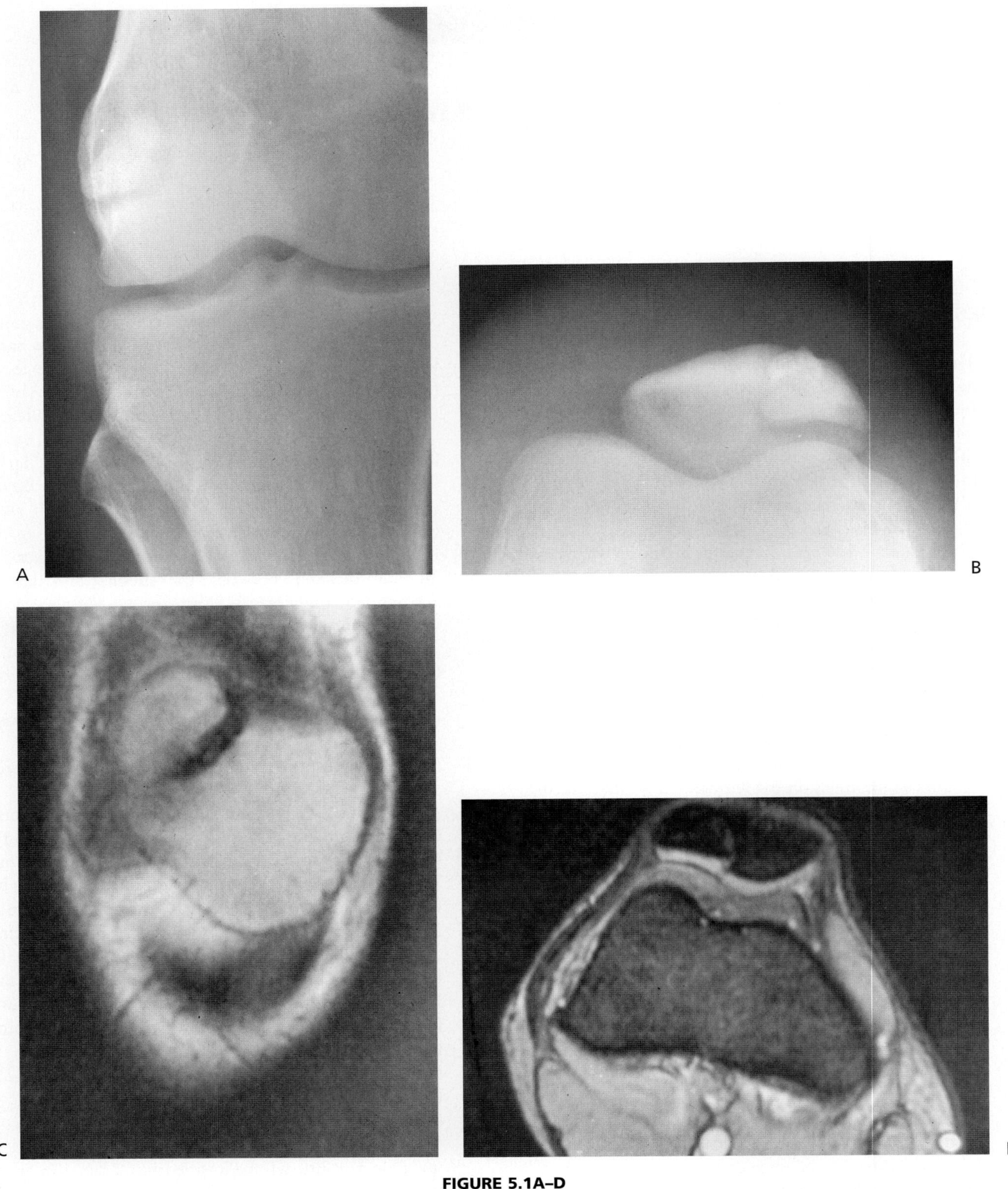

FIGURE 5.1A–D

(b) Increased flexion
(c) Posterior instability in extension
(d) Decreased flexion
(e) Posterior instability in flexion

9. What would have been the best alternative means to perform the revision of the total knee arthroplasty in question 7?
   (a) Revision of the femoral component with exchange of the tibial polyethylene (as described; there is no better alternative)
   (b) Revision of the femoral component (as described) with concomitant tibial component revision and resection of additional proximal tibia to lower the position of the tibial component
   (c) Revision of the femoral component with exchange of the tibial polyethylene (as described) followed by revision of the patellar component to move it more proximally and thus correct its malposition relative to the new joint line
   (d) Revision of the femoral component with exchange of the tibial polyethylene (as described) with the addition of posterior femoral augments
   (e) Revision of the femoral component with the addition of distal femoral augments and use of a polyethylene insert comparable to the original
10. What is the normal alignment of the shafts of the tibia and femur in the coronal plane during stance?
   (a) 10 degrees valgus
   (b) 5 degrees valgus
   (c) 2 degrees valgus
   (d) Neutral (0 degrees)
   (e) 2 degrees varus
11. A 58-year-old-postal worker undergoes a cemented posterior cruciate ligament–sacrificing total knee arthroplasty with lateral release for rheumatoid arthropathy with an associated 20-degree valgus deformity. On release of the tourniquet, brisk hemorrhage is encountered from the lateral aspect of the joint. What is the most likely source of hemorrhage?
   (a) The infrapatellar branch of the saphenous vein
   (b) The lateral superior genicular artery
   (c) The popliteal artery or vein
   (d) The middle genicular artery
   (e) The exposed cut osseous surfaces not tamponaded by cement
12. A 25-year-old man presents with diffuse knee pain and swelling. Physical examination reveals an effusion, diffuse tenderness, and a mass in the popliteal fossa. A lateral plain radiograph is shown in Fig. 5.2A. A magnetic resonance imaging scan was also obtained (Fig. 5.2B and C). Arthroscopy was performed, during which the tissue specimen (Fig. 5.2D) was obtained. What is the most likely diagnosis?
   (a) Septic arthritis
   (b) Pigmented villonodular synovitis
   (c) Clear cell chondrosarcoma
   (d) Synovial osteochondromatosis
   (e) Synovial sarcoma
13. Which of the following patients would be the most ideal candidate for a high tibial osteotomy?
   (a) A 41-year-old construction worker with isolated medial compartmental osteoarthritis and 8 degrees of varus alignment
   (b) A 67-year-old woman with isolated, medial compartmental osteoarthritis, and 8 degrees of varus alignment
   (c) A 38-year-old professional mountain climber with moderate medial compartmental osteoarthritis and neutral alignment
   (d) A 40-year-old farmer with advanced, isolated medial compartment osteoarthritis, 12 degrees of varus alignment, and 5 mm of lateral tibial subluxation
   (e) A 37-year-old school-teacher with rheumatoid arthropathy, 5 degrees of varus alignment, and pain limited to the medial side of the knee
14. A 27-year-old physical therapist presents with right knee pain and swelling. She reports malaise with inconsistent aches and pains in her arms and legs over the preceding several days. There is no history of trauma or fever. Physical examination reveals a knee effusion with warmth and diffuse tenderness. Plain radiographs are unremarkable. An aspiration reveals cloudy fluid that is sent for routine culture and cell count. The cell count reveals a white blood cell count of 60,000, but the Gram stain reveals no organisms. She is treated with empiric antibiotics, and her condition seems to improve rapidly. However, the final culture is negative. What is the most likely diagnosis?
   (a) Juvenile rheumatoid arthritis
   (b) Reiter syndrome
   (c) Lyme disease
   (d) Gout
   (e) Gonococcal arthritis
15. A 33-year-old postal worker complains of chronic anterior knee pain that has not responded to multiple courses of supervised physical therapy and activity modification. Her pain is aggravated when she rises from watching television and when she ascends stairs. She has lateral facet tenderness and a negative apprehension sign. Medial glide is less than one quadrant. Quadriceps motor strength is 5/5. Standing anteroposterior and lateral radiographs are normal. On tangential radiographs, the Merchant angle and the Laurin lateral patellofemoral angle both measure 0 degrees. A midpatellar computed tomography image demonstrates patellar tilt without subluxation. What would be the most appropriate form of surgical intervention for this patient?
   (a) Proximal realignment
   (b) Lateral retinacular release

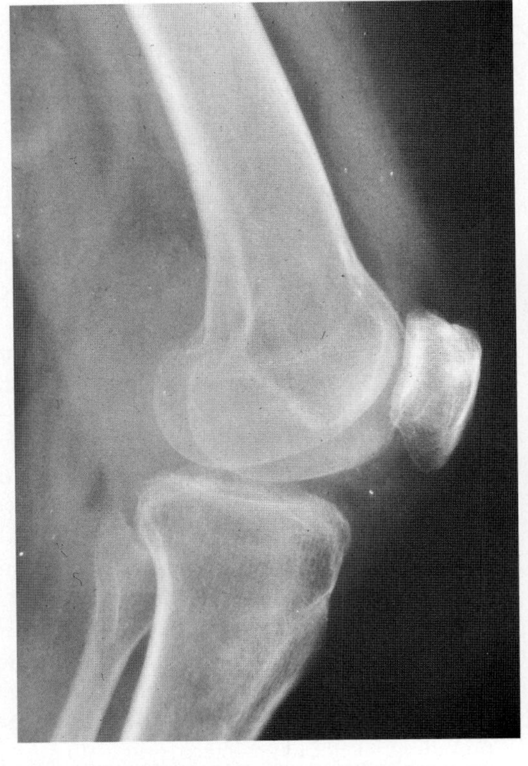
A

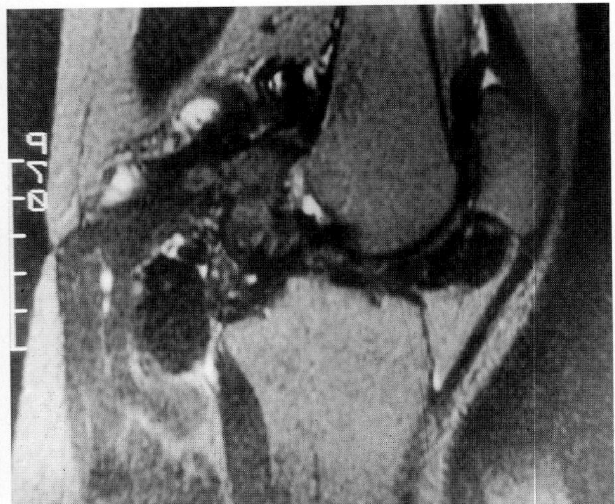

B

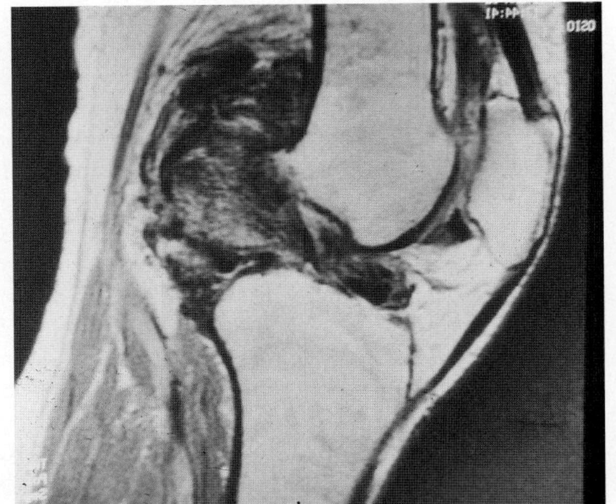
C

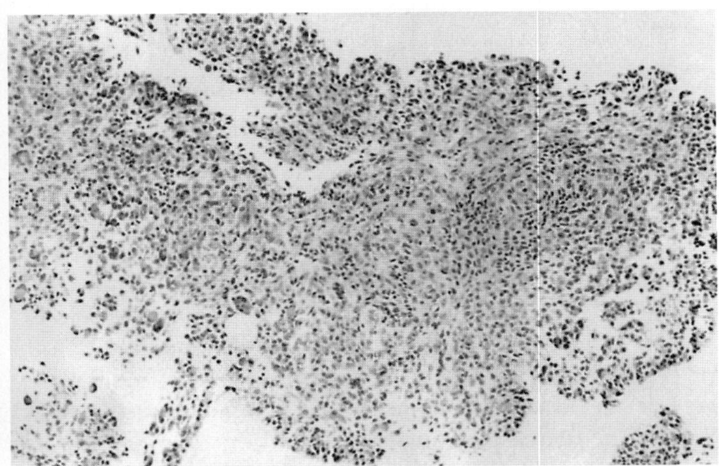
D

FIGURE 5.2A–D

(c) Distal realignment
(d) Patellectomy
(e) Distal realignment with lateral retinacular release

16. Which of the following statements regarding lower extremity alignment is correct?
    (a) When alignment is normal, the femoral shaft axis is colinear with the tibial shaft axis.
    (b) When alignment is normal, the femoral shaft axis is colinear with the mechanical axis of the lower extremity.
    (c) When alignment is normal, the mechanical axis of the femur is colinear with the tibial shaft axis.
    (d) When a varus knee deformity exists, the mechanical axis of the femur projects medially to the tibial shaft axis.
    (e) When a varus knee deformity exists, the mechanical axis of the lower extremity passes laterally to the mechanical axis of the femur.
17. Under which of the following conditions would retention of the posterior cruciate ligament (rather than sub-

stitution for the posterior cruciate ligament) be most appropriate during total knee arthroplasty?
(a) Rheumatoid arthritis
(b) Prior high tibial osteotomy
(c) Prior patellectomy
(d) Chronic anterior cruciate ligament insufficiency
(e) Combined flexion and varus deformity greater than 20 degrees

18. A 62-year-old woman presents with acute right knee pain, which she localizes to the medial side of the joint. She has been limping since she woke with the discomfort 4 weeks ago. There is no history of trauma, fever, or weight loss. The pain is worse at night. Physical examination is remarkable for medial joint line tenderness and a trace effusion. She is otherwise healthy, with the exception of psoriasis. Laboratory data reveal a white blood cell count of 5,000 and an erythrocyte sedimentation rate of 20. Plain radiographs and a magnetic resonance imaging scan are obtained. What is the most likely diagnosis?
(a) Idiopathic osteonecrosis
(b) Osteoid osteoma
(c) Metastatic breast cancer
(d) Osteochondritis dissecans
(e) Psoriatic arthritis

19. What would be the most appropriate treatment plan for the patient described in question 18?
(a) Analgesics and protected weight bearing
(b) High tibial osteotomy
(c) Total knee arthroplasty
(d) Arthroscopic débridement and allografting
(e) Unicompartmental knee replacement

20. Which of the following statements is not a theoretic advantage of a posterior cruciate ligament–retaining implant (as compared with a posterior cruciate ligament–substituting implant)?
(a) More bone is removed from the distal femur in posterior cruciate ligament–substituting designs, and, thus, there is an increased chance of iatrogenic fracture and less bone stock available if revision is ever necessary.
(b) Ligament-retaining designs have traditionally used less conforming tibial polyethylene inserts that permit mixing of femoral and tibial components of different sizes.
(c) The decreased articular conformity of the tibial polyethylene in traditional posterior cruciate ligament–retaining designs reduces peak stresses in the polyethylene, and thus may decrease wear debris generation.
(d) The incidence of patellar clunk syndrome is lower in posterior cruciate ligament–retaining designs.
(e) The posterior cruciate ligament contains nerve endings that may provide significant proprioceptive feedback.

21. Which of the following is false regarding knee arthrodesis with antegrade intramedullary nail fixation for septic failure of a total knee arthroplasty?
(a) The procedure permits early postoperative full weight bearing.
(b) Prior ipsilateral total hip arthroplasty is a contraindication to the procedure.
(c) The procedure is contraindicated in the presence of a prior failed fusion attempt with external fixation because of potential contamination of the intramedullary cavity by pin tracts.
(d) The procedure does not preserve the normal mechanical axis of the lower extremity.
(e) Massive bone loss is associated with a lower rate of fusion.

22. Gait analysis of a patient with a below-knee amputation reveals excessive knee flexion between heel strike and midstance. All the following are potential explanations for this phenomenon except
(a) Excessive anterior tilt of the socket
(b) Quadriceps weakness
(c) Excessive anterior displacement of the socket over the foot
(d) Excessively soft heel cushion or excessively flexible plantar-flexion bumper
(e) Excessive dorsiflexion of the foot

23. A total knee arthroplasty femoral component articulates with the tibial polyethylene. The condyles of the femoral component have a coronal radius of curvature of 12 mm. The tibial polyethylene has a thickness of 8 mm, an elastic modulus of 1, and a coronal radius of curvature of 14 mm. Which of the following statements about the contact stresses in the polyethylene is correct?
(a) If the polyethylene thickness is changed to 5 mm, then the peak contact stresses will not change.
(b) If the elastic modulus of the polyethylene is doubled, then the peak contact stresses will increase.
(c) If the coronal radius of curvature of the polyethylene is changed to 16 mm, then the peak contact stresses will decrease.
(d) If the coronal radius of curvature of the polyethylene is changed to 12 mm, then the peak contact stresses will increase.
(e) If the polyethylene thickness is changed to 10 mm and the coronal radius of curvature of the polyethylene is changed to 13 mm, then the peak contact stresses will increase.

24. A 21-year-old badminton enthusiast presents with "shin splints" and pain over the medial calf. What sensory nerve innervates this dermatome?
(a) The tibial nerve
(b) The sural nerve
(c) The deep peroneal nerve
(d) The saphenous nerve

(e) The superficial peroneal nerve

25. What is the blood supply to the anterior cruciate ligament?
    (a) The medial geniculate
    (b) The middle geniculate
    (c) The superolateral geniculate
    (d) The inferolateral geniculate
    (e) The recurrent geniculate

26. A pediatric resident sustains a knee dislocation when he collides with the orthopaedic resident on call. This injury is most commonly associated with which of the following?
    (a) Major vascular injury
    (b) Neurologic injury
    (c) Intraarticular fracture
    (d) Open injury
    (e) Compartment syndrome

27. Which of the following statements is correct regarding the biomechanics of a total knee arthroplasty design with a highly conforming polyethylene insert?
    (a) When a prosthetic knee is loaded into extreme valgus (creating a 3-mm gap at the medial joint line), a femoral component with a flat coronal condylar contour will increase peak polyethylene contact stresses less than a femoral component with a constant coronal radius of curvature.
    (b) When a prosthetic knee is loaded into extreme valgus, peak polyethylene contact stresses are greater when both femoral condyles remain in contact with the polyethylene than when there is unilateral (medial condyle) liftoff.
    (c) When a prosthetic knee is loaded into extreme varus (creating a 3-mm gap at the lateral joint line), a femoral component with a constant coronal radius of curvature will increase peak polyethylene contact stresses more than a femoral component with a flat coronal contour.
    (d) When a prosthetic knee is loaded into extreme varus, peak polyethylene contact stresses are less when there is unilateral (lateral condyle) liftoff than when both femoral condyles remain in contact with the polyethylene.
    (e) When a prosthetic knee is loaded into extreme valgus (creating a 3-mm gap at the medial joint line), a femoral component with a constant coronal radius of curvature will increase peak polyethylene contact stresses less than a femoral component with a flat coronal contour.

28. A 33-year-old man presents with isolated, posttraumatic lateral compartmental degenerative joint disease and a 12-degree valgus deformity. This affliction has begun to compromise his ability to operate the family farm. He does not wish to consider a change in occupation or activity level until his twin 13-year-old sons are old enough to take over for him. He asks for your opinion. Which of the following surgical recommendations would be most appropriate?
    (a) Posterior cruciate ligament–retaining total knee arthroplasty
    (b) Lateral closing wedge high tibial osteotomy
    (c) Posterior cruciate ligament–substituting total knee arthroplasty
    (d) Medial closing wedge high tibial osteotomy
    (e) Medial closing wedge supracondylar femoral osteotomy

29. Which of the following statements most accurately describes the prognosis for a patient who undergoes high tibial osteotomy for varus gonarthrosis?
    (a) Approximately 50% survivorship of the osteotomy at 6 years is expected.
    (b) Overcorrection of the varus deformity (past neutral) leads to a worse prognosis.
    (c) Approximately 80% survivorship of the osteotomy at 6 years is expected.
    (d) If the patient fares well for the first 6 years, then clinical deterioration over the subsequent 6 years is extremely unlikely.
    (e) Approximate 10% survivorship of the osteotomy at 6 years is expected.

30. Which of the following statements regarding patellar component design in total knee arthroplasty is correct?
    (a) Metal-backed components have been associated with a decreased amount of polyethylene deformation and wear.
    (b) Anatomically shaped components are less constrained than dome-shaped components.
    (c) Designs that incorporate a single large central peg have been associated with a greater risk for patella fracture than designs with multiple smaller, more peripheral pegs.
    (d) Other components rarely need to be revised at the time of revision of a failed metal-backed patellar component.
    (e) Despite theoretic concerns about metal-backed components, dissociation between the polyethylene and the metal backing has not proven to be a clinical problem.

31. In the treatment of varus gonarthrosis, advantages of performing a lateral-based, closing wedge, high tibial osteotomy above (versus below) the level of the tibial tubercle include all the following except
    (a) The broad bone surface heals more rapidly.
    (b) Compressive force is placed across the osteotomy by the quadriceps mechanism.
    (c) The fibula or proximal tibial-fibular joint does not need to be released or divided.
    (d) Malalignment is corrected closer to the point of actual deformity.
    (e) Patellar tracking can be altered if necessary when the osteotomy is performed proximal to the tubercle.

32. A 47-year-old used car salesman presents with severe, medial compartmental osteoarthrosis 10 years after total medial meniscectomy. He has not responded to nonoperative treatment. The most predictable single intervention for long-term improvement in pain and function in this patient is which of the following?
    (a) Arthroscopic débridement
    (b) Knee arthrodesis
    (c) Meniscal allograft
    (d) Total knee arthroplasty
    (e) High tibial osteotomy
33. A 51-year-old chain saw operator complains of right knee pain, clicking, and locking. He undergoes arthroscopic débridement of a complex, degenerative medial meniscal tear. Preoperative anteroposterior radiographs are shown in Fig. 5.3. The patient presents to the emergency room on postoperative day 3 with acute right knee swelling, warmth, and pain. Aspiration reveals hazy synovial fluid, but Gram stain reveals no organisms. He is afebrile and has no other complaints. The patient is admitted and started on empiric antibiotics. Three days later, all culture results are negative, but the patient continues to have severe knee pain. He denies having taken any postoperative antibiotics. What is the most likely diagnosis?
    (a) Postoperative septic arthritis with false-negative cultures
    (b) Reflex sympathetic dystrophy
    (c) Pseudogout

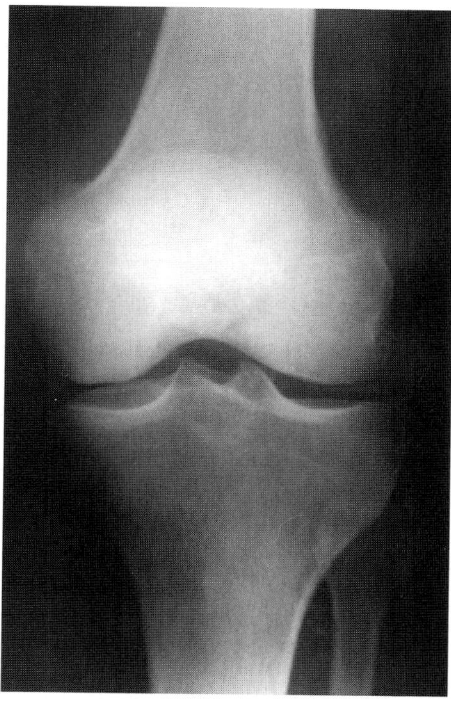

FIGURE 5.3

    (d) Palindromic rheumatism
    (e) Lyme disease
34. A 37-year-old man inadvertently discharges a nail gun into his knee while repairing the deck of his beach house. He presents to the emergency room with his soiled blue jeans tacked to the medial aspect of his knee by the head of the nail. The skin is dimpled by the nail head. He is holding his knee in 10 degrees of flexion, but he can flex to 30 degrees, at which point guarding precludes further assessment. Radiographs of the knee are shown in Fig. 5.4. What is the most appropriate treatment based on the radiographic and clinical findings?
    (a) Removal of the nail with irrigation and wound closure in the emergency room; tetanus prophylaxis and 5 days of oral antibiotics
    (b) Removal of the nail with irrigation in the emergency room, with the wound left open; tetanus prophylaxis and 5 days of oral antibiotics
    (c) Removal of the nail in the operating room with diagnostic arthroscopy of the knee plus knee irrigation and débridement if necessary; tetanus prophylaxis and intravenous antibiotics
    (d) Magnetic resonance imaging or computed tomography scan of the knee to determine whether there is articular penetration, followed by (1) removal of the nail in the emergency room if the wound is extraarticular or (2) arthroscopic irrigation and débridement if there is articular violation
    (e) Removal of the screw head and countersinking of the nail
35. Which of the following structures always pass anterior to the posterior cruciate ligament?
    (a) The insertion of the posterior horn of the lateral meniscus
    (b) The ligament of Wrisberg
    (c) The popliteus origin
    (d) The posterior oblique ligament
    (e) The ligament of Humphry
36. A car strikes a 26-year-old man while he is standing on a street corner. You are called to evaluate the knee as the neurosurgeons are attending to his subdural hematoma in the operating room. The anteroposterior radiograph demonstrates a bony proximal avulsion of the medial collateral ligament and a bony distal avulsion of the anterior cruciate ligament. Based on this information, what findings would you anticipate when you examine this knee under anesthesia? (You may assume that the injury is closed and that the knee did not dislocate.)
    (a) 2+ valgus instability at 30 degrees of flexion, stable to valgus in full extension; 1A Lachman, stable to varus at 30 degrees and in full extension
    (b) 2+ valgus instability at 30 degrees of flexion, stable to valgus in full extension, 2B Lachman, stable to varus at 30 degrees and in full extension

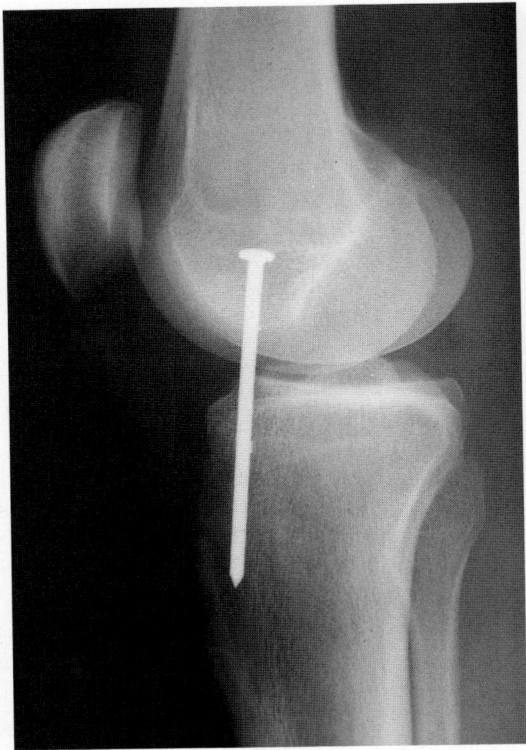

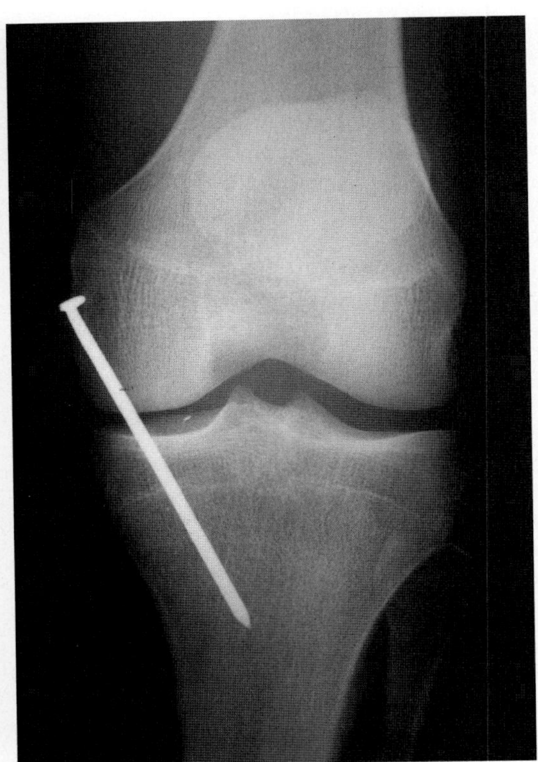

FIGURE 5.4A and B

(c) 2+ valgus instability at 30 degrees of flexion and in full extension, 1A Lachman, stable to varus at 30 degrees and in full extension
(d) 2+ varus and valgus instability at 30 degrees of flexion and in full extension, 2B Lachman, 2+ posterior drawer
(e) 2+ valgus instability at 30 degrees of flexion and in full extension, 2B Lachman, stable to varus at 30 degrees and in full extension

37. Which of the following intraoperative steps is most useful in preventing patellofemoral tracking problems in total knee arthroplasty?
    (a) Internal rotation of the tibial component
    (b) Internal rotation of the femoral component
    (c) Use of an oversized femoral component
    (d) Medialization of the patellar component
    (e) Medialization of the femoral component
38. A 58-year-old man is found 7 hours after sustaining a comminuted fracture of his left tibia secondary to a close-range shotgun blast. He is hypotensive in the field (systolic blood pressure less than 90 mm Hg), but he responds well to intravenous fluids. He has a weak left dorsalis pedis pulse, with good capillary refill. What is the patient's Mangled Extremity Severity Score, and should limb salvage be attempted?
    (a) 7; attempt salvage
    (b) 7; perform primary amputation
    (c) 8; attempt salvage
    (d) 8; perform primary amputation
    (e) 6; attempt salvage
39. A 40-year-old postal worker presents with a complaint of posterior knee "fullness" with mild associated medial knee pain. A magnetic resonance imaging scan was obtained by the referring primary caregiver. Selected sagittal and axial T2-weighted magnetic resonance images are shown in Fig. 5.5. What is the most likely diagnosis?
    (a) Meniscal cyst
    (b) Synovial sarcoma
    (c) Pigmented villonodular synovitis
    (d) Popliteal cyst
    (e) Fibrosarcoma
40. Which of the following is the most appropriate initial step in the workup and management of the lesion in question 39?
    (a) Excisional biopsy
    (b) Bone scan
    (c) Diagnostic and therapeutic arthroscopy
    (d) Open excision and capsular reinforcement with a gastrocnemius pedicle graft
    (e) Nonsteroidal antiinflammatory drugs and a compression sleeve
41. The lesion in Fig. 5.5 is typically interposed between which of the following two structures?

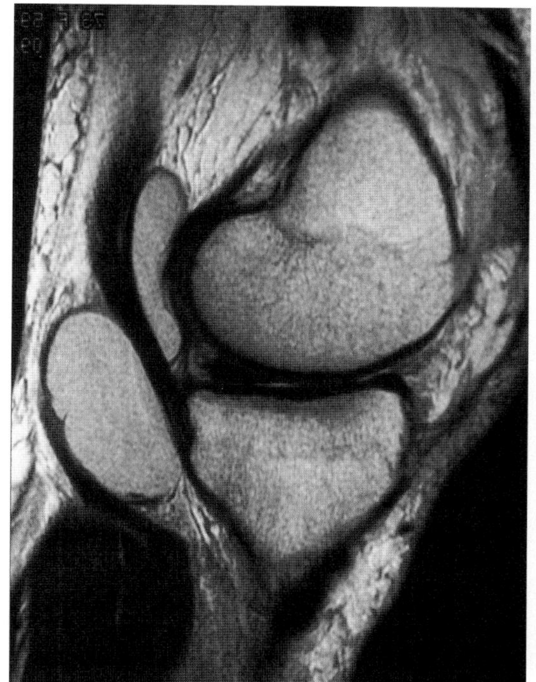

A

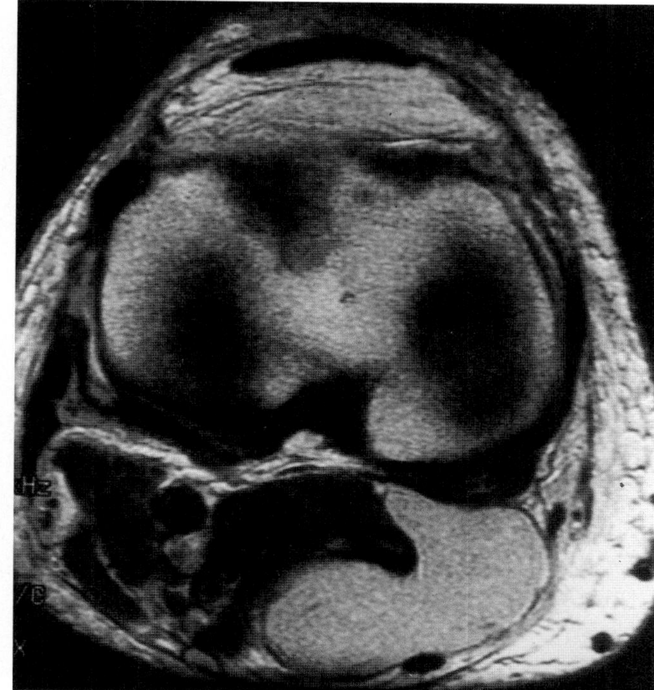

B

FIGURE 5.5A and B

(a) The sartorius and the medial head of the gastrocnemius
(b) The semimembranosus and the medial head of the gastrocnemius
(c) The sartorius and the semimembranosus
(d) The semitendinosus and the semimembranosus
(e) The medial head of the gastrocnemius and the popliteal artery

42. A 41-year-old mechanic presents with progressive mechanical knee pain and intermittent swelling. He states that he has no known medical problems except for chronic low back pain. A lateral film of his spine is shown in Fig. 5.6. At the time of arthrotomy for a total knee arthroplasty, dark pigmentation is noted throughout the meniscal remnants and residual articular cartilage. What is the most likely diagnosis?
(a) Hemochromatosis
(b) Homocystinuria
(c) Pigmented villonodular synovitis
(d) Alkaptonuria
(e) Ankylosing spondylitis

43. What is the enzymatic defect associated with alkaptonuria?
(a) Glucocerebrosidase
(b) Homogentisic acid oxidase
(c) Hypoxanthine-guanine phosphoribosyltransferase
(d) Heparin-*N*-sulfatase
(e) *N*-Acetylgalactosamine-6-sulfatase

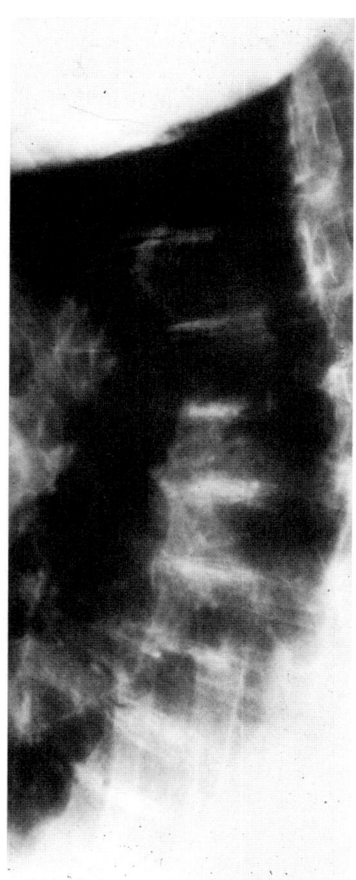

FIGURE 5.6

44. The radiograph in Fig. 5.7 is most consistent with which of the following diagnoses?
    (a) Osteonecrosis
    (b) Neuropathic arthropathy
    (c) Hemophilic arthropathy
    (d) Osteoarthritis
    (e) Synovial osteochondromatosis
45. A primary posterior stabilized total knee arthroplasty is performed on an osteoarthritic knee with neutral preoperative alignment. The tibial cut is made at 90 degrees to the tibial axis, and the anterior and posterior distal femoral cuts are inadvertently performed in excessive external rotation. All other cuts are performed in appropriate standard fashion. What would be the most likely resultant soft tissue imbalance during the trial reduction?
    (a) Medial laxity in extension and flexion
    (b) Lateral laxity in extension and flexion
    (c) Medial laxity in flexion; balanced in extension
    (d) Lateral laxity in flexion; balanced in extension
    (e) Lateral laxity in flexion; medial laxity in extension
46. Which of the following statements regarding tibial shaft fracture fixation is false?
    (a) Intramedullary nailing is capable of providing absolute stability.
    (b) A lag screw is capable of providing greater interfragmentary compression than a dynamic compression plate.
    (c) Failure to use pretension in a dynamic compression plate can lead to gapping of the cortex opposite the plated cortex.
    (d) A uniplanar external fixator construct is stiffest in the plane of the pins.
    (e) A well-molded cast is incapable of providing absolute stability.
47. What is the most common diagnosis precipitating below-knee amputations in the United States?

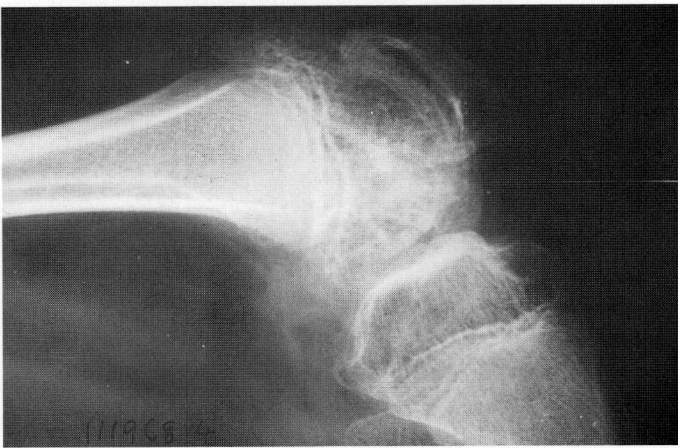

FIGURE 5.7

    (a) Trauma
    (b) Tumor
    (c) Congenital malformation
    (d) Peripheral vascular disease
    (e) Failed total knee arthroplasty
48. Which of the following is not a classic postmeniscectomy Fairbank sign?
    (a) A peripheral ridge osteophyte
    (b) Subchondral cyst formation
    (c) Joint space narrowing
    (d) Squaring of the femoral condyle
49. What is the most common location of myositis ossificans?
    (a) The popliteal fossa
    (b) The hip abductors
    (c) The quadriceps
    (d) The hip adductors
    (e) The deep posterior compartment of the calf
50. Stance phase constitutes what percentage of the normal gait cycle?
    (a) 30%
    (b) 40%
    (c) 50%
    (d) 60%
    (e) 70%
51. A patient with rheumatoid arthritis undergoes a posterior cruciate ligament–substituting total knee arthroplasty with instrumentation that references the distal femoral cut off an intramedullary guide and references the anterior and posterior femoral cuts off the posterior femoral condyles. The patient has a preoperative 10-degree flexion contracture and an associated 10-degree valgus deformity. What is the most likely resultant form of component malalignment?
    (a) Medial patellar subluxation
    (b) Medial displacement of the femoral component
    (c) Internal rotation of the femoral component
    (d) Flexion of the femoral component
    (e) Excessive valgus orientation of the femoral component
52. A grade IIIC open tibia fracture is treated with an external fixator. The stiffness of the construct would be increased by all of the following except
    (a) Increasing the number of pins in each fragment
    (b) Increasing the distance between the pins in each fragment
    (c) Moving the central pins further from the fracture
    (d) Decreasing the distance between the bar and the bone
    (e) Increasing the number of connecting bars
53. Which of the following is not a contraindication to unicompartmental knee arthroplasty?
    (a) Anterior cruciate ligament insufficiency
    (b) Mild patellofemoral chondromalacia
    (c) Posterior cruciate ligament insufficiency

(d) An osteoarthritic knee with a fixed 12-degree varus deformity and a "kissing" lesion on the medial (non–weight-bearing) portion of the lateral femoral condyle
(e) Rheumatoid arthritis

54. One of your medical school roommates, a disability doctor, asks you to review the radiographic studies in Fig. 5.8 of a 16-year-old patient with knee pain and a mass. What is the most likely diagnosis?
(a) Synovial sarcoma
(b) Meniscal cyst
(c) Pigmented villonodular synovitis
(d) Early rheumatoid arthritis with pannus formation
(e) Ganglion cyst

55. The term "Foucher sign" refers to
(a) The tendency for popliteal cysts to become firm during knee *extension* and soft with knee *flexion*
(b) Lateral translation of the patella in terminal knee extension
(c) An instinctive attempt to stabilize the affected knee with the contralateral foot when the patient is asked to stand on the affected leg and flex the involved knee
(d) Anterior translation of the tibia on the femur during resisted knee extension with the knee flexed to 90 degrees
(e) Production of joint line pain by abrupt internal or external rotation of the tibia with the knee flexed to 90 degrees

56. Which of the following is not a cause of limited knee flexion after total knee arthroplasty with a posterior cruciate ligament–retaining prosthesis?
(a) An oversized femoral component
(b) An anterior tibial slope
(c) Insufficient patella resection
(d) Anterior translation of the femoral component
(e) Excessive posterior cruciate ligament tension

57. Which of the following is the least significant factor in predicting ultimate postoperative flexion after total knee arthroplasty?
(a) Lack of aggressive early postoperative physical therapy
(b) Preoperative range of motion
(c) Postoperative joint line level
(d) Preoperative status of the anterior cruciate ligament
(e) Postoperative patellar thickness

58. A trial reduction is performed on a posterior cruciate ligament–retaining total knee arthroplasty with a flat tibial trial component that does not have undersurface fixation. Varus-valgus balance is excellent in extension. However, the tibial component lifts off anteriorly with flexion. What does this finding signify?

A
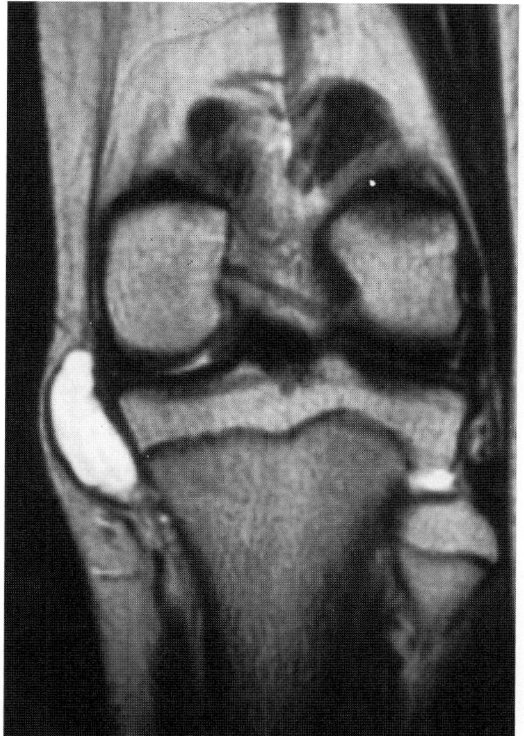
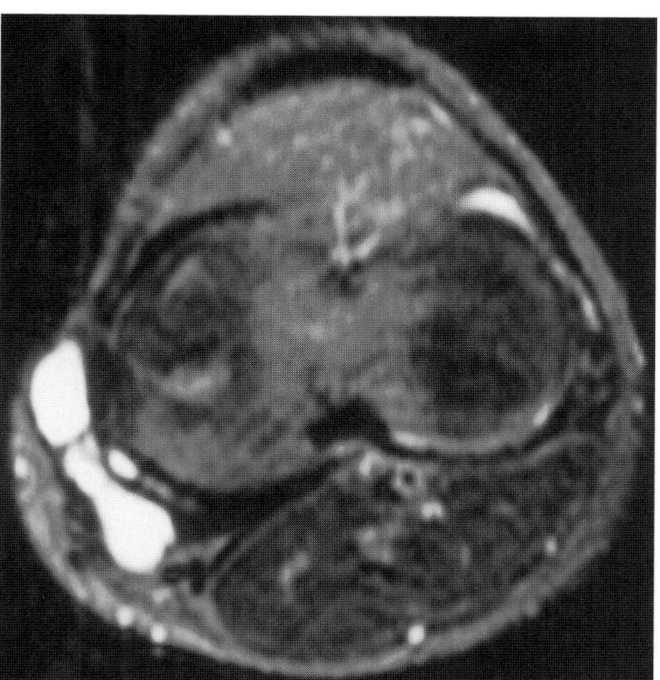
B

FIGURE 5.8A and B

(a) Insufficient femoral rollback
(b) Excessive polyethylene thickness
(c) Insufficient proximal tibial resection
(d) Oversizing of the femoral component
(e) Excessive posterior cruciate ligament tension

59. The "four-bar linkage" mechanism refers to
(a) Biplanar external fixator format with bridged sets of double bars
(b) The intrinsic axial rotation mechanism in certain meniscal-bearing total knee arthroplasty designs
(c) The relationship between the cruciate ligaments and their osseous attachments that defines sagittal knee motion
(d) The interrelationship between the mechanical and anatomic axes of the tibial and femur
(e) A covert method of bar-hopping at the American Academy of Orthopedic Surgeons

60. Which of the following arteries does not contribute to the peripatellar anastomotic ring?
(a) The supreme genicular artery
(b) The medial inferior genicular artery
(c) The lateral inferior genicular artery
(d) The anterior tibial recurrent artery
(e) The fibular circumflex artery

61. Which of the following statements is false regarding the effects of surgically induced defects in bone?
(a) When a screw is removed from a hole in the proximal tibial metaphysis, the torsional strength of the tibia as a whole will not be reduced.
(b) A unicortical drill hole will have the greatest effect on a tubular bone's ability to withstand a bending load if it is positioned in the center of the tensile cortex.
(c) If the shape of a diaphyseal defect is elongated in the direction of the long axis of a bone without increasing the area of the defect, then the torsional strength of the bone will *not* change.
(d) A larger hole causes greater weakening than a smaller hole of similar shape.

62. Which of the following statements is most accurate regarding primary, posterior stabilized total knee arthroplasty in obese patients?
(a) Moderately and severely obese patients have a significantly higher incidence of postoperative patellofemoral symptoms.
(b) Moderately and severely obese patients have a significantly lower incidence of thrombophlebitis.
(c) Moderately and severely obese patients have a significantly higher incidence of wound infections.
(d) Moderately and severely obese patients have a significantly higher incidence of thrombophlebitis.
(e) Moderately and severely obese patients have a significantly lower incidence of wound infections.

63. Which of the following statements regarding femoral rollback is incorrect?
(a) It increases the quadriceps moment arm.
(b) Sagittal shifting of the contact point between the femur and the tibia may precipitate tibial loosening over time.
(c) Posterior cruciate ligament–substituting implant designs prevent posterior tibial translation but do not cause femoral rollback.
(d) "Total condylar" prosthesis design is associated with negligible femoral rollback.
(e) In a posterior cruciate ligament–substituting design, the resultant joint reaction force vector always points along the tibial peg.

64. Which of the following is not a cause of excessive medial tightness in extension during trial reduction of a total knee arthroplasty in a patient with varus osteoarthritis?
(a) Inadequate medial tibial osteophyte resection
(b) Excessive valgus cut of the proximal tibia
(c) Excessive valgus cut of the distal femur
(d) Inadequate medial soft tissue release
(e) Impacting of the medial portion of the femoral component into soft bone

65. Which of the following confers the greatest risk of infection after a total knee arthroplasty?
(a) Rheumatoid arthritis
(b) Prior sepsis of the knee
(c) Current steroid use
(d) Open skin lesions on the affected extremity
(e) Obesity

66. A 67-year-old man presents with acute knee pain and fever 10 days after constrained revision total knee replacement with an extensor mechanism allograft. His knee is diffusely warm, swollen, and tender. There is no drainage. He is hemodynamically stable with no signs of systemic sepsis. Radiographs do not demonstrate fracture or loosening of any components; however, some air is noted in the soft tissues. What is the most appropriate next step in management?
(a) Arthrocentesis followed by culture-guided intravenous antibiotics
(b) Technetium scan
(c) Irrigation and débridement
(d) Indium scan
(e) Immediate commencement of broad-spectrum antibiotics

67. A 44-year-old man sustains a grade IIIC open tibia fracture when he is run over by a car. Limb salvage attempts are unsuccessful, and he ultimately requires a below-knee amputation. By how much will his energy expenditure during gait (oxygen consumed per meter traveled) be increased over his baseline? (You may assume that he is fitted with a standard below-knee prosthesis and that he walked on two feet before the accident.)
(a) 10%

(b) 25%
(c) 50%
(d) 75%
(e) 100%

68. A 20-year-old rollerblader trips over a fire hydrant and sustains a closed tibial shaft fracture. The fibula remains intact. Which of the following statements is incorrect regarding this injury?
    (a) It is associated with an increased risk of nonunion.
    (b) It is associated with an increased incidence of valgus malunion.
    (c) It is associated with an increased incidence of delayed union.
    (d) It is associated with a conversion of the strain pattern of the lateral tibial cortex from compressive to tension.
    (e) It is associated with an increased risk of posttraumatic degeneration of the ipsilateral ankle.
69. The trial reduction of a total knee arthroplasty reveals good ligamentous tension in flexion. However, excessive tension prevents full extension. When the tibial insert thickness is decreased enough to allow full extension, there is excessive ligamentous laxity in flexion. What is the best solution to this problem?
    (a) Resect additional proximal tibia.
    (b) Resect additional posterior femur.
    (c) Resect additional proximal tibia and posterior femur.
    (d) Downsize the femoral component.
    (e) Resect additional distal femur.
70. A 31-year-old electrician presents for evaluation of "sciatica." He is unable to perform a unilateral active straight leg raise on the affected side. He states that his affected leg feels "paralyzed." The examiner places his hands beneath the patient's heels and detects no downward pressure from the contralateral heel during the attempted straight leg raise. These findings constitute
    (a) A positive Hoover test
    (b) A positive Beevor sign
    (c) A positive Holmgren sign
    (d) A positive Homans sign
    (e) A positive Gower sign
71. Cadence refers to
    (a) The velocity of gait
    (b) The distance between heel strike and the next ipsilateral heel strike
    (c) The number of steps per unit time
    (d) The distance between heel strike and the next contralateral heel strike
    (e) The horizontal translation of the center of gravity during gait
72. What is the most common presentation of periprosthetic patellar fracture after total knee arthroplasty?
    (a) Asymptomatic coincidental finding on routine follow-up radiograph
    (b) Fall onto a flexed knee
    (c) Painful giving way precipitating a fall
    (d) Insidious onset of progressive extensor weakness
    (e) Sudden onset of pain during continuous passive motion (CPM) use postoperatively
73. In which of the following patients would a formal arteriogram be least appropriate after a knee dislocation?
    (a) A patient who presents without distal pulses in whom distal pulses return after the knee is relocated
    (b) A patient who presents without distal pulses in whom distal pulses remain absent when the knee is relocated
    (c) A patient with no history of compromised distal pulses for whom you intend to perform a ligament reconstruction with the use of a tourniquet 3 weeks after dislocation
    (d) A patient with an ipsilateral femur fracture and transiently diminished distal pulses
    (e) A patient who presents with distal pulses intact in whom distal pulses remain intact after the knee is relocated
74. Routine postoperative radiographs after an uncomplicated cemented posterior stabilized total knee arthroplasty reveal a nondisplaced, sagittal, intercondylar split periprosthetic femur fracture. What is the most appropriate management for this finding?
    (a) Revision of the femoral component to a cemented, stemmed component to bypass the defect
    (b) Protected weight bearing for 6 to 8 weeks
    (c) Revision of the femoral component to an uncemented, fluted stemmed component to bypass the defect
    (d) Stabilization with a retrograde intramedullary nail
    (e) Stabilization with cerclage wires
75. Which of the following statements is not correct regarding wear characteristics in total knee arthroplasty?
    (a) Particle number correlates inversely with polyethylene thickness.
    (b) Particles tend to be larger than those associated with total hip arthroplasty.
    (c) Polyethylene surface damage is more severe in thin components and in components with relatively flat tibial articulating surfaces.
    (d) Delamination is a more common mechanism of wear in total knee arthroplasty than in total hip arthroplasty.
    (e) Oxidative degradation of polyethylene occurs during γ irradiation in the presence of air, but it does not continue after sterilization.
76. A posterior cruciate ligament–sacrificing total knee arthroplasty is performed on an osteoarthritic knee with no preoperative coronal plane deformity and no preoperative collateral ligament insufficiency. The dis-

tal femoral cut is made in 5 degrees of valgus orientation relative to the perpendicular to the femoral shaft axis. On trial reduction, soft tissue imbalance is encountered. Specifically, the medial soft tissues are noted to be excessively lax in both extension and flexion. Lateral soft tissue tension is appropriate in both flexion and extension. Which of the following is the best explanation for this finding?

(a) An excessively thick trial tibial polyethylene insert
(b) A varus tibial cut
(c) An excessively valgus distal femoral cut
(d) A valgus tibial cut
(e) Excessive external rotation of the anterior and posterior cuts on the distal femur

77. An identical bending force is applied to two solid intramedullary tibial nails (1 and 2). The lengths of the rods are equivalent, and they are made of the same material. The radius of rod 1 is twice the radius of rod 2. How many times will rod 2 bend compared with rod 1?

(a) 2 times
(b) 4 times
(c) 8 times
(d) 0.5 times
(e) 16 times

ANSWERS

1. **b** Bipartite patella. Bipartite patellae are generally incidental findings with no clinical significance. The pattern shown (separation of the superolateral pole) accounts for 75% of bipartite patellae. Lateral margin detachment accounts for 20%, and inferior pole detachment accounts for the remaining 5%.

Note: Fifty percent of bipartite patellae are bilateral.

Reference

Green WT: Painful Bipartite Patellae. Clin Orthop, 110:197–200, 1975.

2. **e** Hypertrophic scar tissue at the superior pole of the patella impinges on the femoral component during extension. The *patellar clunk syndrome* is a form of soft tissue impingement that occurs after total knee arthroplasty as a result of formation of a fibrous nodule in the *suprapatellar* synovium adjacent to the quadriceps tendon insertion. This nodule becomes transiently entrapped against the intercondylar recess of the femoral component during active *extension.* This phenomenon has been associated with certain posterior cruciate ligament–substituting femoral component designs in which there is an abrupt transitional ridge between the prosthetic intercondylar notch and the prosthetic femoral trochlea. Riding of the fibrous nodule over this ridge leads to a sensation of "clunking." The patellar clunk syndrome can be cured by arthroscopic resection of the nodule. The syndrome has been obviated by modified component designs that incorporate a more gradual transitional zone at the anterior femur for smoother patellar tracking.

Reference

Insall J, ed: Surgery of the Knee, 2nd Ed. New York, Churchill Livingstone, 1993.

3. **b** Patella infera. High tibial osteotomy remains an appropriate procedure for the relatively young, active patient with unicompartmental varus gonarthrosis. A steady functional decline over time is commonly seen after high tibial osteotomy, and many patients ultimately require conversion to total knee arthroplasty. Radiographic follow-up has shown that approximately 80% of knees develop patella infera (patella baja) after high tibial osteotomy. The average Insall-Salvati and Blackburn-Peel indices are both lowered. This factor may contribute to the less satisfactory results of total knee arthroplasty after high tibial osteotomy as compared with total knee arthroplasty without prior high tibial osteotomy.

At the time of conversion total knee arthroplasty, the patellar ligament is typically found to be scarred and contracted. As a result, the extensor mechanism is often difficult to evert. Early range of motion and continuous passive motion after high tibial osteotomy have been advocated to prevent the development of postoperative infrapatellar scarring and contracture.

References

Scuderi GR, Windsor RE, Insall JN: Observations on Patellar Height After Proximal Tibial Osteotomy. J Bone Joint Surg Am, 71(2):245–248, 1989.
Windsor RE, Insall JN, Vince KG: Technical Considerations of Total Knee Arthroplasty After Proximal Tibial Osteotomy. J Bone Joint Surg Am, 70(4):547–555, 1988.

4. **e** Passes posterior to the knee center of rotation. During early stance, the ground reaction force passes posterior to the knee center of rotation. The significance of this finding lies in the knee flexion moment that the ground reaction force creates after heel strike. During normal gait, this flexion moment is resisted by the eccentric contraction of the quadriceps. However, in the patient with an above-knee amputation, there is no functional extensor mechanism. Thus, many above-knee prostheses incorporate an intrinsic braking mechanism to prevent inadvertent excessive flexion *(buckling)* of the prosthetic knee articulation after heel strike.

Reference

Burstein AH, Wright TM: Fundamentals of Orthopaedic Biomechanics. Philadelphia, Williams & Wilkins, 1994.

5. **b** Preoperative biplanar (flexion and valgus) deformity. A preoperative complex biplanar (flexion and valgus) deformity is the most significant risk factor for peroneal nerve palsy after total knee arthroplasty. Other associated conditions include (1) valgus deformity of any magnitude, (2) flexion contracture greater that 20 degrees, and (3) pressure on the nerve from the postoperative dressing. Excessive tourniquet time could, theoretically, jeopardize the nerve, but clinical studies have not identified tourniquet time to be a significant risk factor. Intraoperative exposure of the nerve in high-risk cases has not been definitively proven to have a protective effect.

Reference

Asp JP, Rand JA: Peroneal Nerve Palsy After Total Knee Arthroplasty. Clin Orthop, 261:233–237, 1990.

Insall J, ed: Surgery of the Knee, 2nd Ed. New York, Churchill Livingstone, 1993.

Rose HA, Hood RW, Otis, JC, et al.: Peroneal Nerve Palsy Following Total Knee Arthroplasty: A Review of the Hospital for Special Surgery Experience. J Bone Joint Surg Am, 64:347–351, 1982.

6. **c** The distance between the distal femoral cut and the proximal tibial cut. The *flexion gap* is the distance between the posterior femoral cut and the proximal tibial cut (measured in flexion). The *extension gap* is the distance between the distal femoral cut and the proximal tibial cut (measured in extension).

Reference

Insall J, ed: Surgery of the Knee, 2nd Ed. New York, Churchill Livingstone, 1993.

7. **c** The joint line will be raised. Because of the loss of distal femoral bone stock in this case, the extension gap was widened, and the new femoral component was implanted in a more cephalad position than the initial femoral component. Compensatory insertion of a thicker polyethylene will *raise* the joint line. This will produce relative patella infera (patella baja).

   Note: Aseptic loosening of the femoral component is extremely uncommon. In total knee arthroplasty, aseptic loosening most frequently involves the patellar component and least commonly affects the femoral component.

8. **d** Decreased flexion. Using a thicker polyethylene insert effectively corrected the ligamentous laxity in extension, but ligamentous tension in flexion (which was satisfactory before the polyethylene adjustment) would also be increased. Excessive ligamentous tension in flexion would likely limit flexion (Fig. 5.9).

   With a posterior cruciate ligament–substituting component, compromised posterior stability would not be encountered unless there was sufficiently excessive laxity of the soft tissues to permit subluxation of the cam mechanism. Because satisfactory soft tissue tension was established in extension (and because excessive soft tissue tension was created in flexion), there would be no posterior instability in this situation.

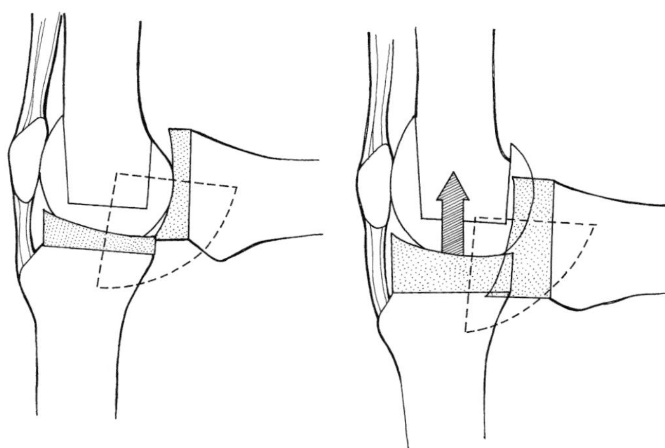

FIGURE 5.9

9. **e** Revision of the femoral component with the addition of distal femoral augments and use of a polyethylene insert comparable to the original. Option a (the previously described revision approach) is suboptimal because of two reasons: (1) the joint line has been raised and (2) the thicker polyethylene insert will limit flexion. Option b is not a valid solution to the problem because it does not correct the asymmetry between the flexion and extension gaps. Cutting more tibia to lower the position of the tibial component would widen the extension gap even further. An even thicker polyethylene insert would be required to fill the extension gap and to establish ligamentous stability in extension. Despite distal repositioning of the tibial component, the joint line would still be raised because of the proximal position of the femoral component and the thicker polyethylene insert. Option c also fails to address the asymmetry between the flexion and extension gaps. Although this proposed solution would theoretically correct the relative patella baja, patellar bone stock is limited. Component removal would risk compromising bone stock further. The position of the implant could not be altered significantly, and fixation in the new position would be jeopardized. Furthermore, even if the patella baja could be adequately corrected, the joint line would remain high relative to the contralateral knee. In the absence of infection, there is virtually no justification for removing a well-fixed patellar component. Option d solves neither of the two identified problems. The joint line would remain high, and the posterior augmentation on the femur would limit flexion even further.

Option e would reestablish appropriate soft tissue balance in both flexion and extension. Thus, flexion would not be restricted. Furthermore, this solution would preserve the level of the joint line, and it would not require removal of either of the two well-fixed components.

Note: A simple rule of thumb in revision total knee arthroplasty is that one should replace what has been taken away. Hence, distal femoral bone loss requires distal femoral augmentation.

10. **b** 5 degrees valgus. The normal coronal alignment between the shafts of the femur and tibia during stance is 4.9±0.7 degrees valgus.

References

Hsu RW, et al.: Normal Axial Alignment of the Lower Extremity and Load-bearing Distribution at the Knee. Clin Orthop, 255:215–227, 1990.
Moreland JR, et al.: Radiographic Analysis of the Axial Alignment of the Lower Extremity. J Bone Joint Surg Am, 69:745, 1987.

11. **b** The lateral superior genicular artery. The *superior lateral genicular artery* is commonly severed during the course of performing a thorough lateral release. A conscientious effort should be made to identify and cauterize this vessel.

The *infrapatellar branch of the saphenous vein* is a medial structure, and, therefore, it would not cause hemorrhage in the lateral side of the joint. Direct trauma to either of the popliteal vessels is a grave complication, but, fortunately, it is extremely rare.

The *middle genicular artery* is the principal blood supply to the anterior and posterior cruciate ligament (both of which were resected in this case). However, the middle genicular artery branches to the cruciate ligaments are typically cauterized at the time of excision, and they are not a significant source of bleeding. *Cut osseous surfaces* that are not tamponaded by the cemented components can produce hemorrhage of a slow, steady, oozing type, but brisk focal bleeding from this source is uncharacteristic.

Note: Several studies have suggested an association between division of the superior lateral geniculate artery (during lateral release) and avascular necrosis of the patella after total knee arthroplasty.

Reference

McMahon MS, et al.: Scintigraphic Determination of Patellar Viability After Excision of the Infrapatellar Fat Pad and/or Lateral Retinacular Release After Total Knee Arthroplasty. Clin Orthop, 260:10–16, 1990.

12. **b** Pigmented villonodular synovitis. The clinical, radiographic, and histologic features of this case are typical of this disease. Pigmented villonodular synovitis characteristically presents in adolescence or early adulthood. The clinical swelling is driven by proliferative synovium with both villous and nodular features. Histologic characteristics include sheets of plump, hyperplastic, polyhedral synovial cells with scattered giant cells. Hemosiderin deposition is typically seen as a result of recurrent hemarthroses. Hemosiderin deposits appear as a signal voids on magnetic resonance imaging. This true synovial tumor is benign but locally aggressive, with a one-third incidence of erosion into adjacent osseous structures, as demonstrated by this case. Pigmented villonodular synovitis is also noted for its proclivity for local recurrence.

Synovial sarcoma is not a true tumor of synovium. It is malignant, and its histiogenesis is unknown. It typically arises in the vicinity of a joint but not within the joint. In fact, it rarely directly involves synovium at all. It presents with a well-circumscribed mass. Histologically, a biphasic pattern is characteristic with both spindle and epithelioid populations, although, rarely, a monophasic pattern is encountered (spindle cells only). Soft tissue calcifications are present approximately 25% of the time.

The histologic features of this case are also inconsistent with the diagnoses of septic arthritis, clear cell chondrosarcoma, and synovial osteochondromatosis.

13. **a** A 41-year-old construction worker with isolated medial compartmental osteoarthritis and 8 degrees of alignment. With the long-term success of total knee arthroplasty, the indications for high tibial osteotomy have become progressively more limited. However, high tibial osteotomy remains a reliable, temporizing procedure in certain specific situations. The ideal patient has unicompartmental (medial compartment) osteoarthritis. He or she should be relatively young, with a physically demanding occupation or lifestyle (e.g., farming or construction). An appropriate candidate must also demonstrate abnormal tibiofemoral alignment. If alignment is normal, a realignment procedure will *not* be efficacious.

Patients with inflammatory arthritides (e.g., rheumatoid arthritis) are inappropriate for the procedure because, by definition, they have diffuse joint involvement. Other relative contraindications to high tibial osteotomy include (1) age greater than 60 to 65 years, (2) tibiofemoral angle greater than 10 to 15 degrees (on standing radiograph), (3) flexion contracture greater than 10 to 15 degrees, (4) lateral tibial subluxation (knee instability), (5) flexion less than 90 degrees, and (6) lack of patient acceptance of the anticipated cosmetic appearance of an appropriately corrected (valgus-aligned) knee.

The patient in option b, despite having unicompartmental osteoarthritis, is too old for high tibial osteotomy. Given her age and the excellent long-term results of total knee arthroplasty, it would be difficult to justify a temporizing procedure such as high tibial osteotomy. She would have a better, more predictable long-term result from a total knee arthroplasty. The patient in option c does not have pathologic alignment. The patient in option d has an excessive deformity with associated tibial subluxation. The patient in option e presents with inflammatory arthritis. Despite prevailing medial compartment involvement, she has tricompartmental disease by definition.

References

Coventry MB: Current Concepts Review: Upper Tibial Osteotomy for Osteoarthritis. J Bone Joint Surg Am, 67:1136–1140, 1985.

Insall JN: High Tibial Osteotomy for Varus Gonarthrosis. J Bone Joint Surg Am, 66:1040–1048, 1984.

14. **e** Gonococcal arthritis. This is a stereotypical presentation of gonococcal arthritis. Prodromal migratory polyarthralgias are characteristic. A few affected patients will have genitourinary symptoms, and many patients are not febrile. Even when the arthrocentesis reveals frank purulence, Gram stains and cultures are notoriously negative in the setting of gonococcal arthritis, as demonstrated by this case. *Neisseria gonorrhoeae* is a fastidious organism that requires inoculation in *Thayer-Martin medium* (which contains chocolate agar) and incubation in carbon dioxide at 37°C. The joint culture is positive in fewer than half of affected patients.

    Unlike nongonococcal bacterial arthritis, which tends to affect immunocompromised persons at the extremes of age, gonococcal septic arthritis tends to affect young, healthy persons. However, deficiencies in complement factors C5 to C9 have been associated with an increased susceptibility to *Neisseria* organisms. *N. gonorrhoeae* propagates as gram-negative diplococci. Unlike patients with nongonococcal bacterial arthritis, patients with gonococcal septic arthritis rarely demonstrate concurrent positive blood cultures. None of the other listed answers (including the arthritis associated with Lyme disease) would demonstrate a rapid resolution with antibiotics.
15. **b** Lateral retinacular release. This patient demonstrates anterior knee pain with patellar tilt. There is no associated subluxation (Merchant angle is 0 degrees). Fulkerson et al. demonstrated the efficacy of releasing the tight lateral retinaculum under these circumstances. Proximal and distal extensor mechanism realignment procedures are not necessary to correct isolated patellar tilt.

    The results of lateral retinacular release are less consistent and less satisfactory when there is associated patellar subluxation or instability. In cases of combined tilt and subluxation, a formal extensor mechanism realignment procedure should be considered. Advanced patellofemoral arthrosis is a contraindication to lateral release.

    Note: Lateral release should be employed with trepidation when patellar alignment and tracking are normal.

Reference

Fulkerson JP, et al.: Computerized Tomography of the Patellofemoral Joint Before and After Lateral Retinacular Release. Arthroscopy, 3(1):19–24, 1987.

16. **c** When alignment is normal, the mechanical axis of the femur is colinear with the tibial shaft axis. The *mechanical axis of the femur* is defined by a line drawn from the center of the femoral head to the center of the knee. The *mechanical axis of the lower extremity* is defined by a line drawn from the center of the femoral head to the center of the ankle. When alignment is normal, the mechanical axis of the femur and the mechanical axis of the lower extremity are colinear with one another and with the tibial shaft axis, but none of these are colinear with the femoral shaft axis. When a varus knee deformity exists, the mechanical axis of the femur projects *laterally* to the tibial shaft axis, and the mechanical axis of the lower extremity passes *medially* to the mechanical axis of the femur.
17. **d** Chronic anterior cruciate ligament insufficiency. Four essential contraindications to posterior cruciate ligament retention during total knee arthroplasty have been identified: (1) fixed flexion and angular deformity greater than 20 degrees, (2) prior patellectomy, (3) prior high tibial osteotomy, and (4) rheumatoid arthritis.

    Fixed flexion and angular deformities greater than 20 degrees cannot be properly corrected without posterior cruciate ligament release because the contracted posterior cruciate ligament is an integral part of such a deformity.

    In the setting of *prior patellectomy,* the results of posterior cruciate ligament–retaining designs are inferior to those of posterior cruciate ligament–substituting designs with respect to (1) the development of late anteroposterior instability, (2) stair climbing ability, and (3) the incidence of recurvatum deformity.

    High tibial osteotomy induces a fibrotic response in the posterior cruciate ligament and changes its length and orientation. Thus, in the setting of prior high tibial osteotomy, the posterior cruciate ligament should be sacrificed, and a posterior-stabilized implant should be used.

    The persistent synovitis produced by *rheumatoid arthritis* causes the posterior cruciate ligament to attenuate over time. Such attenuation is associated with a significant incidence of posterior instability, recurvatum deformity, and revision requirement.

    Chronic anterior cruciate ligament insufficiency may precipitate premature degenerative joint disease and may necessitate total knee arthroplasty, but it does not compromise the status of the posterior cruciate ligament or contraindicate a posterior cruciate ligament–retaining implant.

Reference

Laskin RS: The Posterior Cruciate Ligament in Total Knee Replacement. Knee, 2:139–144, 1995.
Laskin RS, O'Flynn H: Total Knee Replacement with Posterior Cruciate Ligament Retention in Rheumatoid Arthritis. Clin Orthop, 345:24–28, 1997.
Paletta GA, Laskin RS: Total Knee Arthroplasty after a Previous Patellectomy. J Bone Joint Surg Am, 77:1708–1712, 1995.

18. **a** Idiopathic osteonecrosis. This is a characteristic presentation of idiopathic osteonecrosis of the knee. The disease typically affects women who are more than 60 years old. The female-to-male ratio is approximately 3:1. Under most circumstances, the disease is usually located at the weight-bearing portion of the medial femoral condyle. There is often an associated nonspecific mild elevation of the erythrocyte sedimentation rate. A history of increased pain at night is common and should not be mistaken for an osteoid osteoma, which (despite a similar appearance on bone scan) occurs in a much younger population. The bone scan shows intense focal uptake at the involved region. Later in the course of osteonecrosis, complementary signal uptake may be seen on the medial plateau if secondary arthritis has developed.

    Plain radiographs are initially unremarkable *(stage 1),* but they subsequently reveal flattening of the weight-bearing portion of the medial femoral condyle *(stage 2).* Later in the disease course, a subchondral radiolucency with a surrounding sclerotic halo will become evident *(stage 3).* In *stage 4* disease, subchondral collapse has occurred, and in *stage 5,* there is secondary degenerative joint disease.

    On T1-weighted magnetic resonance imaging, normal marrow signal is replaced by a well-circumscribed area of decreased signal intensity. T2-weighted magnetic resonance imaging typically reveals a central signal void surrounded by marginal high signal uptake (which presumably represents reactive edema). This is in contrast to the high T2 signal that would be expected throughout a metastatic breast lesion.

    Osteochondritis dissecans characteristically affects a much younger age group, and it usually involves the region of the medial femoral condyle immediately adjacent to the intercondylar notch, as opposed to the central weight-bearing portion. The presentation of psoriatic arthritis of the knee is similar to that of rheumatoid arthritis. Like all inflammatory arthropathies of the knee, it characteristically produces symmetric joint space involvement. Thus, the focal lesion at the medial femoral condyle in this case should not be attributed to psoriatic arthritis.

Reference

Ecker ML, Lotke PA: Spontaneous Osteonecrosis of the Knee. J Am Acad Orthop Surg, 2(3):173–178, 1994.

19. **a** Analgesics and protected weight bearing. The prognosis for idiopathic osteonecrosis of the knee depends on the size of the initial lesion. Conservative management is more successful for smaller lesions (lesions that involve less than 50% of the width of the condyle). Smaller lesions display a greater tendency to resolve after a relatively benign course. Larger lesions tend to produce persistent, progressive symptoms with ultimate evolution into disabling degenerative joint disease. Options for patients in this category include arthroscopic débridement, high tibial osteotomy, core decompression, allografting, and prosthetic replacement (total knee arthroplasty) or unicompartmental arthroplasty). Débridement has not been shown to alter the natural history of the disease. Core decompression has a high degree of efficacy for stage 1 and 2 involvement. Allografting is currently an experimental option for younger patients, in whom this disease is less common. High tibial osteotomy is a viable option for an affected younger active patient; again, this disease is relatively uncommon in the young population. Prosthetic replacement is the procedure of choice for the majority of patients with large lesions and/or recalcitrant symptoms. Good results have been reported for both unicompartmental arthroplasty and total knee arthroplasties.

    Despite the absence of collapse, this patient's magnetic resonance imaging scan manifests involvement of a significant portion of the condyle, a finding suggesting a low likelihood of a benign course. Although a total knee arthroplasty may ultimately be required, a trial of conservative management is still warranted. Four weeks of discomfort is *not* an indication for total knee arthroplasty.

    Note: According to Ritter et al., the results of total knee arthroplasty for osteonecrosis are not statistically significantly different from the results of total knee arthroplasty for osteoarthritis.

Reference

Lotke P, et al.: The Treatment of Osteonecrosis of the Medial Femoral Condyle. Clin Orthop, 171:109–116, 1982.
Ritter MA, et al.: The Survival of TKA in Patients with Osteonecrosis of the Medial Femoral Condyle. Clin Orthop, 267:108–114, 1991.

20. **c** The decreased articular conformity of the tibial polyethylene in traditional posterior cruciate ligament–retaining designs reduces peak stresses in the polyethylene and thus may decrease wear debris generation. Statement c is false. In fact, decreased articular confor-

mity *increases* peak polyethylene stresses and consequently may increase wear debris generation (Fig. 5.10A). Posterior cruciate ligament–retaining designs have traditionally incorporated relatively flat tibial articular surfaces to permit femoral rollback (Fig. 5.10B). The intentional lack of articular conformity in traditional posterior cruciate ligament–retaining designs conveniently permits mixing of femoral and tibial components of various sizes.

The box cut in posterior cruciate ligament–substituting designs sacrifices a considerable amount of bone stock (approximately 3 cm^3). This may compromise the amount of bone available in a subsequent revision situation and may predispose the patient to iatrogenic fracture. The patellar clunk syndrome has not been reported in association with posterior cruciate ligament–retaining femoral components. Theoretically, the nerve endings in the posterior cruciate ligament may serve a clinically significant proprioceptive function. However, no such role has been documented to date.

Note: Manufacturers of more recent posterior cruciate ligament–retaining designs have responded to concerns regarding wear by adopting more conforming polyethylene geometry. This adaptation has been likened to "total condylar" designs and may theoretically compromise femoral rollback.

Reference

Laskin RS: The Posterior Cruciate Ligament in Total Knee Replacement. Knee, 2:139–144, 1995.

21. **c** The procedure is contraindicated in the presence of a prior failed fusion attempt with external fixation because of potential contamination of the intramedullary cavity by pin tracts. Knee arthrodesis with intramedullary nail fixation is an effective salvage option for severely infected total knee arthroplasties when reimplantation is deemed inappropriate. The procedure confers excellent stability to compromised bones and allows immediate weight bearing. A staged procedure (débridement followed by 4 to 6 weeks of intravenous antibiotics before fusion) is advisable. Massive bone loss is associated with higher rates of delayed union and nonunion. However, even in the presence of massive bone loss, successful union is obtained in most cases.

Ipsilateral total hip arthroplasty precludes antegrade intramedullary nail fixation. Insertion of an intramedullary device of any type in the setting of knee sepsis raises concern for potential dissemination of infection. Pin tract contamination of the intramedullary canal is another theoretic concern. However, intramedullary rod fixation remains the best salvage

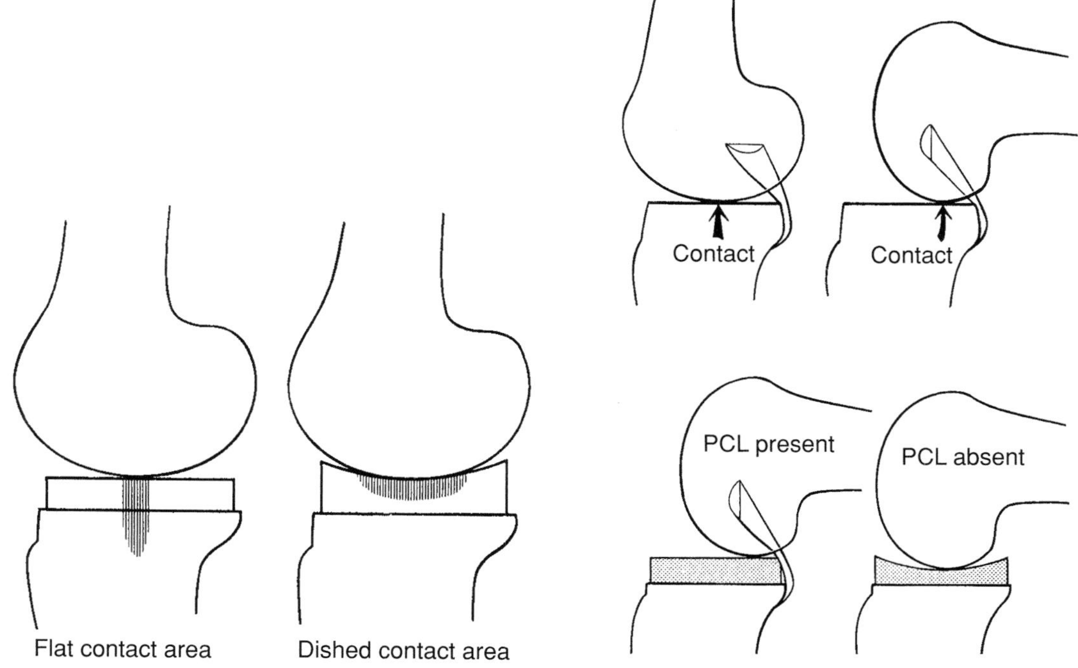

FIGURE 5.10A and B

option after failed compression arthrodesis with an external fixator.

References

Puranen J, et al.: Arthrodesis of the Knee with Intramedullary Nailing. J Bone Joint Surg Am, 72:433–442, 1990.

Wilde AH, et al.: Intramedullary Fixation for Arthrodesis of the Knee After Infected Total Knee Arthroplasty. Clin Orthop, 248:87–92, 1989.

22. **d** Excessively soft heel cushion or excessively flexible plantar-flexion bumper. During normal gait, the knee flexes between heel strike (in which the knee is close to full extension) and midstance (in which the knee reaches approximately 15 to 20 degrees of flexion). Under normal conditions, the eccentric contraction of the quadriceps prevents further knee flexion.

If gait analysis of a patient with a below-knee amputation reveals excessive knee flexion during this phase of gait (early stance), then one must consider two categories of possible causes: (1) intrinsic patient factors and (2) prosthetic factors. Potential intrinsic patient factors would include a knee flexion contracture or quadriceps weakness.

If the prosthetic foot is too dorsiflexed or if the socket is tilted too far anteriorly, then the knee must flex farther to allow the entire foot to contact the floor. An excessively *stiff* (not soft) heel cushion and/or an excessively *rigid* plantar-flexion bumper may also necessitate an increased range of knee flexion, to bring the plantar surface of the prosthetic foot flat on the ground.

Excessive anterior displacement of the socket over the foot increases the flexion moment arm of the ground reaction force acting across the knee through the heel. This increased flexion moment will tend to drive the knee into further flexion during early stance. Compromised quadriceps strength would exacerbate this problem. Conversely, this effect may be dampened by the use of a softer heel cushion or a more flexible plantar-flexion bumper.

Reference

Lower Extremity Prosthetics Syllabus. New York, Prosthetic-Orthotic Publications, 1996.

23. **b** If the elastic modulus of the polyethylene is doubled, then the peak contact stresses will increase. Prosthesis contact stresses are affected by component geometry and material properties. Increasing the elastic modulus of the polyethylene, such as by increasing polyethylene density, will make the polyethylene stiffer (less conforming). Thus, when the components are loaded, the peak polyethylene contact stresses will increase.

If the coronal radius of curvature of the polyethylene is increased to 16 mm, one has, in effect, flattened the polyethylene and hence decreased the conformity between the components. Thus, the peak contact stresses will *increase*.

If the coronal radius of curvature of the polyethylene is decreased to 12 mm, one has, in effect, matched the geometry of the components (increased the conformity). Thus, the peak contact stresses will *decrease*. Finite element analysis has demonstrated that reducing the polyethylene thickness to 5 mm will increase peak contact stresses.

Reference

Burstein AH, Wright TM: Fundamentals of Orthopaedic Biomechanics. Philadelphia, Williams & Wilkins, 1994.

24. **d** The saphenous nerve. The saphenous nerve runs along the medial aspect the leg and provides sensation to this region. This is also the L4 dermatome.
25. **b** The middle geniculate. The middle geniculate artery supplies the anterior cruciate ligament. It is commonly encountered in total knee arthroplasty during excision of the anterior cruciate ligament and should be cauterized to prevent excessive bleeding.
26. **a** Major vascular injury. Dislocation of the knee is a serious injury with a high rate of associated injuries. Vascular injuries are the most common (30% incidence). Injuries to the popliteal artery are the most frequent, followed by the popliteal vein. With anterior or posterior dislocation, the popliteal artery is tethered between the adductor hiatus (proximally) and the origin of the soleus muscle (distally).

Neurologic injuries are also commonly associated (23% incidence). The peroneal nerve is typically injured by lateral displacement of the femoral condyle. There is a 10% incidence of associated fracture with knee dislocation. Open injury to the joint occurs only 5% of the time.

Reference

Levine AM, ed: Orthopaedic Knowledge Update: Trauma. Rosemont, IL, American Academy of Orthopedic Surgeons, 1996.

27. **e** When a prosthetic knee is loaded into extreme valgus (creating a 3-mm gap at the medial joint line), a femoral component with a constant coronal radius of curvature will increase peak polyethylene contact stresses less than a femoral component with a flat coronal contour. Stress equals force divided by area. Hence, decreasing contact area increases stress.

If a prosthetic knee is loaded into extreme varus or valgus, peak polyethylene contact stresses are greater when there is unilateral condylar liftoff than when both femoral condyles remain in contact with the polyethylene. When a prosthetic knee is loaded into extreme varus or valgus producing unilateral condylar liftoff, a femoral component with a flat coronal condylar contour will increase peak polyethylene contact stresses *more* than a femoral component with a constant coronal radius of curvature.

Reference

Burstein AH, Wright TM: Fundamentals of Orthopaedic Biomechanics. Philadelphia, Williams & Wilkins, 1994.

28. **e** Medial closing wedge supracondylar femoral osteotomy. This patient's young age and physically demanding occupation render him a suboptimal candidate for a total knee arthroplasty of any type. Given his unicompartmental disease and tibiofemoral malalignment, he would be an appropriate candidate for osteotomy.

A medial closing wedge osteotomy would be able to correct the valgus malalignment of his knee and thus, unload the degenerated lateral compartment. A lateral closing wedge procedure would worsen his malalignment.

Medial proximal tibial and medial distal femoral closing wedge osteotomies would have opposite effects on joint line obliquity. The proximal tibial procedure would make the joint line more oblique to the floor, whereas the distal femoral procedure would keep the joint line more parallel to the floor and thus would minimize shear forces across an already degenerative joint. Thus, the best recommendation for this patient would be to undergo a distal femoral medial closing wedge osteotomy as a temporizing procedure, with later conversion to a total knee arthroplasty when necessary.

References

Aglietti P: Correction of Valgus Knee Deformity With a Supracondylar V Osteotomy. Clin Orthop, 217:214–220, 1987.
Healy W: Distal Femoral Varus Osteotomy. J Bone Joint Surg Am, 70:102–109, 1988.

29. **c** Approximately 80% survivorship at 6 years. The results of high tibial osteotomy are known to deteriorate with time, and the procedure should be considered to be a temporizing modality from the outset. Using survivorship analysis, Ritter concluded that the reliable longevity of high tibial osteotomy is approximately 6 years. Specifically, he noted approximately 80% survival at 6 years; failure was defined as either (1) an Hospital for Special Surgery (HSS) knee score of less than 70 points or (2) conversion to a total knee arthroplasty. The most abrupt deterioration in survival was between 6 and 7 years; by 7 years, survival rates had fallen to approximately 60%.

Ritter's results are consistent with those of Insall, who demonstrated 85% good to excellent results at 5 years. However, only 63% good to excellent results were observed at 8 to 9 years. More recently, Coventry reported a 94% survival rate at 5 years. Most authorities agree that superior results are achieved when overcorrection (8 degrees or more valgus) is obtained at surgery.

References

Coventry MB: Proximal Tibial Osteotomy: A Critical Long-Term Study of 87 Cases. J Bone Joint Surg Am, 75:196–201, 1993.
Insall JN: High Tibial Osteotomy for Varus Gonarthrosis. J Bone Joint Surg Am, 66:1040–1048, 1984.
Ritter MA: Proximal Tibial Osteotomy: A Survivorship Analysis. J Arthroplasty, 3:309–311, 1988.

30. **c** Designs that incorporate a single large central peg have been associated with a greater risk for patella fracture than designs with multiple smaller, more peripheral pegs. Multiple small, peripheral peg holes have been shown to increase anterior patellar strain less than a single large central peg hole. Accordingly, designs that incorporate a single, large central peg have been associated with a greater risk for patella fracture than designs with multiple smaller, more peripheral pegs.

Metal-backed patellar components have had atrocious results and have essentially been abandoned. The metal backing critically compromises polyethylene thickness. Thinner polyethylene produces accelerated polyethylene deformation and wear. Frank polyethylene fracture or detachment from the metal backing has also been commonly encountered. In this setting, contact between exposed metal backing and the prosthetic femoral trochlea has severely damaged femoral implants. Metal debris, in turn, becomes imbedded in tibial polyethylene. Thus, revision of multiple components is frequently necessary at the time of revision of a failed metal-backed patella procedure.

Anatomically shaped components are more conforming and more constrained than their dome-shaped counterparts. Therefore, the anatomically shaped components are less forgiving and require greater surgical precision, particularly with regard to rotational alignment.

Reference

Callaghan JJ, et al., eds: Orthopaedic Knowledge Update: Hip and Knee Reconstruction. Rosemont, IL, American Academy of Orthopedic Surgeons, 1995.

31. **c** The fibula does not need to be released or divided when the osteotomy is performed proximal to the

tubercle. High tibial osteotomy can be performed *distal* to the tibial tubercle. Performing the high tibial osteotomy *proximal* to the tibial tubercle has several advantages. First, an osteotomy through the proximal tibial metaphysis creates a broader cancellous interface that enhances the inherent stability and the speed of healing at the osteotomy site. Second, the extensor mechanism places a distractive force across an osteotomy that is distal to the tubercle. This potential impediment to healing is converted to a compressive force when the osteotomy is performed proximal to the tubercle. Third, correction of malalignment closer to the point of actual deformity (the joint line) more accurately reproduces normal anatomy. Finally, patellar tracking can be improved when the osteotomy is performed proximal to the tubercle (i.e., internal rotation of the distal tibial fragment is a form of distal realignment of the extensor mechanism that would unload the lateral patellar facet). The relationship between the patella and femur remains constant when the osteotomy is performed distal to the tubercle.

An intact fibula and proximal tibial syndesmosis can exert a tethering effect and can prevent osteotomy closure. The fibula's tethering effect on the osteotomized tibia is *not* averted by making the osteotomy proximal to the tubercle because tibial osteotomy at this level is *still* distal to the tibiofibular syndesmosis. Thus, regardless of the position of the tibial osteotomy in relation to the tubercle, the surgeon must (1) release the proximal tibiofibular ligaments, (2) resect the fibular head and reattach the biceps tendon and lateral collateral ligament (LCL) to the fibular neck, (3) obliquely osteotomize the fibular shaft, or (4) resect a segment of the fibular shaft.

References

Coventry MB: Current Concepts Review: Upper Tibial Osteotomy for Osteoarthritis. J Bone Joint Surg Am, 67:1136–1140, 1985.

Jackson JP, Waugh W: Tibial Osteotomy for Osteoarthritis of the Knee. J Bone Joint Surg Br, 43:746–751, 1961.

32. **d** Total knee arthroplasty. In patients with gonarthrosis, total knee arthroplasty has been shown to be effective for the relief of pain, correction of deformity, and improvement in function. Long-term survivorship (longer than 15 years) has been shown to exceed 90%. Diduch and Insall and their colleagues reported their results in a group of younger patients (all less than 55 years old, with a mean of 51 years) treated with a cemented, posterior cruciate-substituting design. Concern over the potential for a significantly increased failure rate in younger, more active patients was not realized. These authors demonstrated excellent functional outcomes, with survivorship of approximately 87% at 18 years; failure was defined as revision of any of the three components or the polyethylene insert.

None of the remaining options provides such good, predictable, long-term results for the described situation. *Arthroscopic débridement* may be therapeutic for select patients with degenerative meniscal tears and mechanical symptoms. However, these results are less predictable and are often transient. The underlying arthritic process tends to progress, and many of these patients eventually require total knee arthroplasty. Despite the excellent pain relief provided by *arthrodesis*, few patients are pleased with the resultant functional limitations.

High tibial osteotomy provides good short-term results in appropriately selected patients and buys time for younger patients. However, the short-term improvements after osteotomy tend to deteriorate with time. Furthermore, conversion to a total knee arthroplasty is technically more difficult and yields less satisfactory clinical results than primary total knee replacement.

Meniscal allografting is not a treatment for osteoarthrosis. This procedure remains an experimental option for the prevention of osteoarthrosis in young patients who have lost a significant percentage of their meniscus. The long-term results of meniscal allografting are unknown, but the short-term results are superior in patients in whom osteoarthritic change is minimal or absent.

Reference

Diduch D, Insall JN, et al.: Total Knee Replacement in Young, Active Patients: Long-Term Follow-up and Functional Outcome. J Bone Joint Surg Am, 79:575–582, 1997.

33. **c** Pseudogout. The patient's preoperative radiographs demonstrate chondrocalcinosis involving both menisci, but particularly the lateral side. Acute pseudogout attacks are commonly provoked by surgery.

In the postoperative setting, infection must be excluded. The negative cultures and the circumstantial clinical and radiographic evidence suggest the diagnosis of pseudogout. Of course, this diagnosis is not made based on circumstantial evidence. Crystal analysis is required, and it should have been performed in this case. Anticipated findings would include rod-shaped crystals of *calcium pyrophosphate dihydrate.* Crystal analysis would also be necessary to differential pseudogout from true gout, which could present in an identical manner. Monosodium urate crystals are needle shaped and are negatively birefringent on polarizing light microscopy.

Inflammation is produced when calcium pyrophosphate dihydrate crystals are shed from host cartilage deposits and are phagocytized by polymorphonuclear leukocytes inducing the release of lysosomal enzymes and chemotactic factors. Treatment of acute attacks consists of aspiration, nonsteroidal antiinflammatory drugs, colchicine, or intraarticular corticosteroids.

34. **c** Removal of the nail in the operating room with diagnostic arthroscopy of the knee plus knee irrigation and débridement if necessary; tetanus prophylaxis and intravenous antibiotics. The position of nail on the plain radiographs is strongly indicative of intraarticular penetration.

Neither magnetic resonance imaging nor computed tomography would be sensitive for detecting joint violation in this situation because imaging would be compromised by metal artifact. Consideration could be given to joint injection with a methylene blue dye solution to prove the presence of joint penetration. However, in this particular case, dye extravasation may not have occurred because of the skin dimpling (tamponade) effect of the nail head.

Because of the strong clinical suspicion for the existence of a contaminated intraarticular foreign body, diagnostic and therapeutic arthroscopy is warranted. The capsule, coronary ligament, and femoral condyle were contaminated (by metal debris and residue of the thermal glue with which such nails are coated). This residue was débrided, as were the coronary ligament defect and the chondral trough that the nail had created on the medial aspect of the femoral condyle.

Note: It is crucial to be cognizant of the distal reflection of the knee joint capsule when one places external fixator pins in the proximal tibia. To avoid violation of the joint space, it is recommended that pins not be placed further proximally than 1.5 cm distal to the tibial articular surface.

Reference

Murphy CP, et al.: The Small Pin Circular Fixator for Proximal Tibial Fractures with Soft Tissue Compromise. Orthopedics, 14: 273–280, 1991.

35. **e** The ligament of Humphry. The meniscofemoral ligaments *(of Humphry and Wrisberg)* can be differentiated from the posterior cruciate ligament by their smaller bulk and their more cephalad origin. Although the ligaments of Humphry and Wrisberg travel with the posterior cruciate ligament to the anterolateral aspect of the medial femoral condyle, they originate from the posterior horn of the lateral meniscus. By definition, the ligament of Humphry passes anterior and that of Wrisberg posterior to the posterior cruciate ligament. Whereas the posterior cruciate ligament ascends across the joint line at the midline of the knee, the *popliteus tendon* crosses the joint line at the lateral compartment posterior to the lateral meniscus (at the popliteus hiatus).

36. **e** 2+ valgus instability at 30 degrees of flexion and in full extension, 2B Lachman, stable to varus at 30 degrees and in full extension. The radiograph reveals a bony proximal avulsion of the medial collateral ligament and a bony distal avulsion of the anterior cruciate ligament. Isolated medial cruciate ligament insufficiency would produce valgus instability at 30 degrees only because an intact anterior cruciate ligament would prevent gross valgus opening in full extension. The combined medial and anterior cruciate ligament insufficiency would produce valgus instability at both 30 degrees and in full extension.

The observed fractures suggest a valgus mechanism of injury. It would be highly unlikely for the restraints to varus opening to be disrupted in the absence of a concomitant penetrating injury or knee dislocation.

37. **d** Medialization of the patellar component. Intraoperative steps to improve patellofemoral tracking include (1) external rotation of the femoral component, (2) avoidance of internal rotation of the tibial component (Fig. 5.11A), (3) avoidance of an oversized femoral component (Fig. 5.11B), (4) joint line preservation, (5) medialization of the patellar component (Fig. 5.11C), (6) avoidance of medialization of the femoral component (Fig. 5.11D), and (7) secure repair of the medial retinaculum during closure of the arthrotomy. Most of these steps are designed to avoid the inherent tendency for lateral patellar tracking. Steps 2, 3, 5, and 6 decrease tension in the lateral retinaculum. Steps 1, 5, and 6 will prevent an increase in the Q-angle and will thereby decrease the tendency for lateral subluxation.

References

Callaghan JJ, et al., eds: Orthopaedic Knowledge Update: Hip and Knee Reconstruction. Rosemont, IL, American Academy of Orthopedic Surgeons, 1995.

Scuderi GR, Insall JN, Scott WN: Patellofemoral Pain After Total Knee Arthroplasty. J Am Acad Orthop Surg, 2(5):239–246, 1994.

38. **d** 8; perform primary amputation. The Mangled Extremity Severity Score (MESS) was designed to assist in the evaluation and management of patients with lower extremity injury. This scoring system uses early objective criteria to assist in discriminating patients with salvageable limbs from those who should undergo primary amputation. The MESS score is a point-based system that is derived from the four categories given in Table 5.1.

This patient suffered a close-range shotgun blast to his leg (three points), had a leg with diminished pulses for more than 6 hours (one times two equals two points), was transiently hypotensive in the field (one point), and was more than 50 years of age (two points), giving him a total of eight points. A MESS value of seven points or more has been associated with an

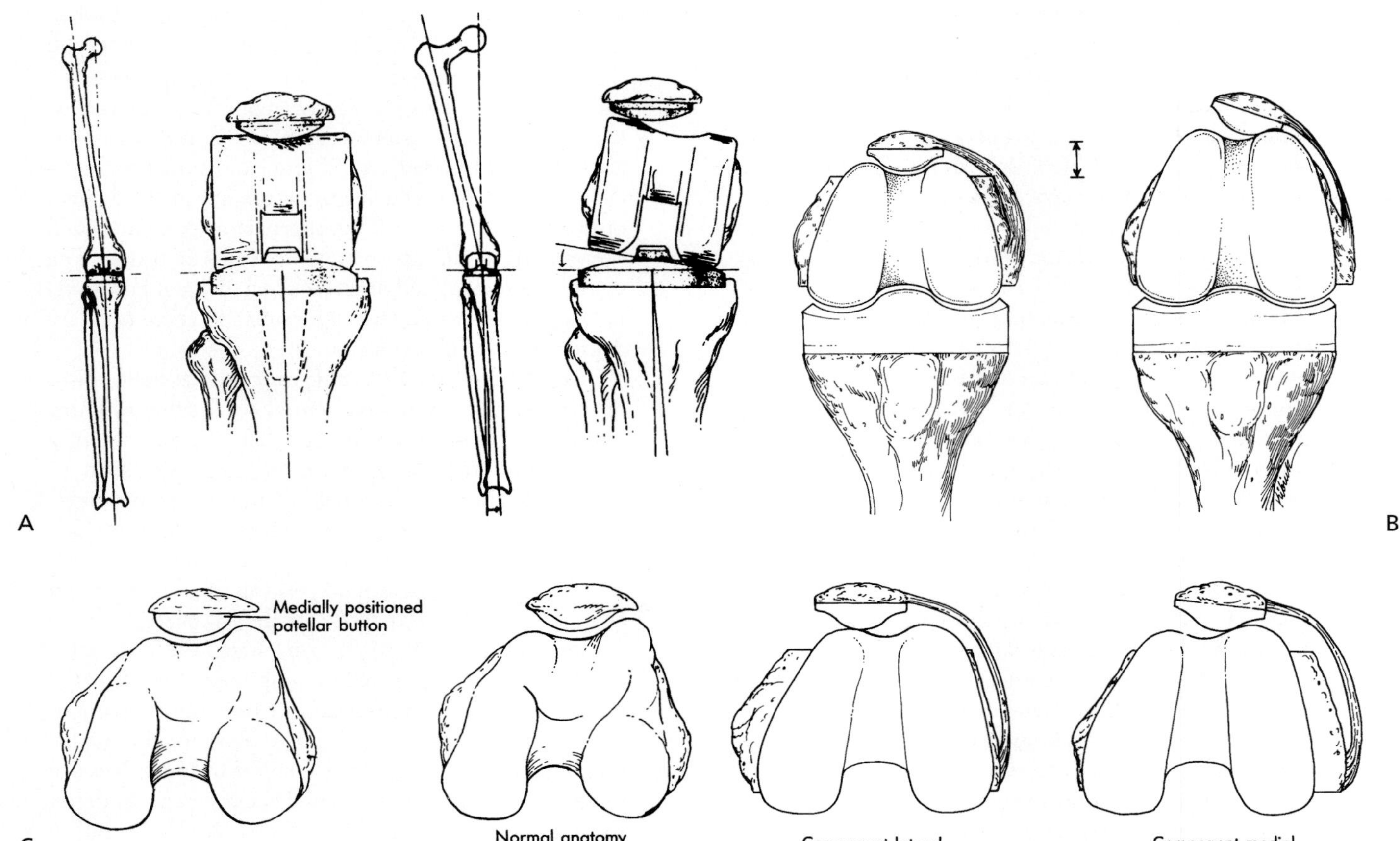

FIGURE 5.11A–D

TABLE 5.1. MANGLED EXTREMITY SEVERITY SCORE (MESS)

Status	Points
I: Skeletal or soft tissue injury	
Low-energy (stab, simple fracture, low-velocity gunshot wound)	1
Medium-energy (open or multiple fractures, dislocation)	2
High-energy (close-range shotgun wound, high-velocity gunshot wound, or crush injury)	3
Very high-energy (as above plus gross contamination or soft tissue avulsion)	4
II: Limb ischemia (score doubled for ischemia >6 h)	
Pulse reduced or absent but perfusion normal	1
Pulseless; paresthesias, diminished capillary refill	2
Cool, paralyzed, insensate	3
III: Shock	
Systolic blood pressure always >90 mm Hg	0
Hypotension transiently	1
Persistent hypotension	2
IV: Age	
<30 yr	0
30–50 yr	1
>50 yr	2

amputation rate of 100%. Conversely, a MESS score of less than four points is associated with a 100% salvage rate. Scores of four to six points constitute a gray area, and, therefore, salvage should be attempted in most of these circumstances. A surgeon contemplating amputation should maintain meticulous documentation of the clinical facts (including photographs) in the event that decisions are later called into question.

References

Helfet DL, et al.: Limb Salvage Versus Amputation: Preliminary Results of the Mangled Extremity Severity Score. Clin Orthop, 256:80–86, 1990.

McNamara MG, Heckman JD, Corley FG: Severe Open Fractures of the Lower Extremity: A Retrospective Evaluation of the Mangled Extremity Severity Score (MESS). J Orthop Trauma, 8(2):81–87, 1994.

39. **d** Popliteal cyst. The magnetic resonance images provide a textbook example of a popliteal cyst. The well-circumscribed region of high signal intensity on the T2-weighted images signifies a fluid-filled cavity. Although lateral lesions do occur, popliteal cysts characteristically arise at the posteromedial aspect of the knee.

Certain sarcomas (e.g., synovial sarcoma, malignant fibrous histiocytoma, or fibrosarcoma) may occur in the popliteal fossa and have been mistaken for popliteal cysts. However, sarcomas would display a solid (rather than fluid) composition on magnetic resonance imaging scans.

The homogeneous extraarticular appearance of this lesion would not be typical of pigmented villonodular synovitis, which generally manifests as a nonhomogeneous, proliferative *intra*articular disorder. Although meniscal cysts can mimic popliteal cysts, they virtually all communicate directly with a tear at the periphery of the meniscus. Popliteal cysts such as this communicate with the knee joint, but they do not communicate directly with meniscal tears. Furthermore, cysts of the lateral meniscus occur far more commonly than cysts of the medial meniscus. In the rare instances that meniscal cysts arise medially, they tend to communicate with a more anterior portion of the knee capsule than popliteal cysts.

Reference

Curl WW: Popliteal Cysts: Historical Background and Current Knowledge. J Am Acad Orthop Surg, 4(3):129–133, 1996.

40. **e** Nonsteroidal antiinflammatory drugs and a compression sleeve. Most popliteal cysts are associated with intraarticular disease. The cyst is formed as pressure from a synovial effusion drives fluid from the knee joint through the valvelike connection with the gastrocnemius-semimembranosus bursa. Although most popliteal cysts tend to recur until the responsible intraarticular lesion is addressed, a trial of conservative management is warranted in most circumstances. Popliteal cysts themselves rarely produce significant discomfort or disability unless they rupture and produce a *pseudothrombophlebitis syndrome.* Conversely, the associated intraarticular disease may produce significant discomfort.

Conservative measures include nonsteroidal antiinflammatory drugs and compression sleeves. Arthroscopic intervention may be warranted when the associated intraarticular disease fails to respond to conservative measures. Open excision is indicated in the rare circumstances that a cyst fails to respond to arthroscopic management. Cyst excision should be accompanied by resection of its stalk

Reference

Curl WW: Popliteal Cysts: Historical Background and Current Knowledge. J Am Acad Orthop Surg, 4(3):129–133, 1996.

41. **b** The semimembranosus and the medial head of the gastrocnemius. Popliteal cysts typically occur at the posteromedial aspect of the knee, where they communicate with the knee capsule. They characteristically occupy the potential space between the semimembranosus tendon and the medial head of the gastrocnemius (Fig. 5.11). They are believed to arise from the gastrocnemius-semimembranosus bursae.

Note: Under the rare circumstances that popliteal cysts occur on the lateral side of the knee, they arise from the bursa of the popliteal tendon.

Reference

Curl WW: Popliteal Cysts: Historical Background and Current Knowledge. J Am Acad Orthop Surg, 4(3):129–133, 1996.

42. **d** Alkaptonuria. Alkaptonuria is an uncommon hereditary metabolic disorder characterized by the accumulation of a dark pigment that has a high affinity for connective tissue macromolecules. Chronic pigment deposition in articular cartilage produces a form of degenerative arthritis called *ochronotic arthropathy.*

Affected patients commonly develop lumbar pain and stiffness. Calcification and narrowing of the intervertebral disc spaces are the most characteristic radiographic findings, as seen in Fig. 5.6. Associated bridging mineral deposition may mimic the "bamboo spine" of ankylosing spondylitis.

Peripheral joint involvement typically occurs several years after the onset of spine symptoms. The knee is the most commonly affected peripheral joint. Ochronotic arthropathy of the knee cannot be definitively distinguished from standard degenerative joint disease on the basis of radiographs. Subtle distinguishing features of ochronotic arthropathy include (1) its greater tendency for symmetric involvement of the medial and lateral compartments or isolated involvement of the lateral compartment (versus the tendency for ordinary osteoarthritis to involve the medial compartment asymmetrically), (2) its proclivity to produce tendinous calcification, and (3) its association with the presence of multiple loose intraarticular osteochondral fragments. Clinical features that differentiate ochronotic knee arthropathy from standard degenerative joint disease include (1) earlier onset (approximately fourth to fifth decades) and (2) characteristic intraarticular pigment deposition.

Hemochromatosis and *pigmented villonodular synovitis* are also capable of producing intraarticular pigment deposition within the knee. However, the pigment accumulation in hemachromatosis and pigmented villonodular synovitis (hemosiderin) is different from the pigment associated with ochronosis (see question 43). Unlike ochronosis, pigmented villonodular synovitis is associated with characteristic proliferative synovial changes and does not affect the spine. *Homocystinuria* is a disorder of amino acid catabolism that is associated with multiple skeletal manifestations (scoliosis, enlarged epiphyses, and fragile bones) but is not associated with intraarticular pigment deposition.

Note: Hemochromatosis produces characteristic degenerative changes in metacarpophalangeal joints 2 to 4 and chondrocalcinosis of the triangular fibrocartilage complex (TFCC).

43. **b** Homogentisic acid oxidase. The lack of homogentisic acid oxidase activity causes an accumulation of homogentisic acid in the urine, plasma, and connective tissues. The conversion of homogentisic acid to a melanin-like substance accounts for the ochronotic pigmentation of affected tissues (Table 5.2).

Note: Lesch-Nyhan syndrome is a cause of secondary gout. Morquio syndrome is distinguished from the other mucopolysaccharidoses by the associated accumulation of keratan sulfate. The others are associated with accumulation of heparan sulfate and dermatan sulfate.

44. **c** Hemophilic arthropathy. The radiographs manifest symmetric obliteration of the medial and lateral joint spaces. This is the hallmark of an inflammatory arthropathy. Hemophilic arthropathy is the only inflammatory arthropathy listed in the question. Other inflammatory arthropathies include rheumatoid arthritis, the seronegative spondyloarthropathies, and arthropathies related to calcium pyrophosphate dihydrate.

Characteristic radiographic features associated with hemophilic arthropathy include epiphyseal overgrowth, squaring of the inferior pole of the patella, and widening of the intercondylar notch. The knee is the most commonly afflicted joint. The severity of joint destruction varies according to the extent of the patient's underlying coagulation defect and the control thereof.

Osteoarthritis characteristically produces asymmetric joint space narrowing. *Osteonecrosis* typically produces isolated destruction of the medial compartment (see question 18). The hallmark of *synovial osteochondromatosis* is the presence of multiple intraarticular calcified loose bodies. *Neuropathic arthropathy* produces a distinctively bizarre pattern of joint destruction, fragmentation, and subluxation.

TABLE 5.2. ENZYMATIC DEFECTS

Disease	Enzymatic Defect
Alkaptonuria	Homogentisic acid oxidase
Gaucher disease	Glucocerebrocidase
Hunter syndrome (MPS II)	l-Iduronosulfate sulfatase
Hurler syndrome (MPS I)	α-l-Iduronidase
Morquio syndrome (MPS IV)	*N*-Acetylgalactosamine-6-sulfatase
Sanfilippo syndrome (MPS III)	Heparin-*N*-sulfatase
Homocystinuria	Cystathione β-synthase
Lesch-Nyhan syndrome	Hypoxanthine guanine

MPS, mucopolysaccharidosis.

45. **c** Medial laxity in flexion; balanced in extension. Making the anterior and posterior femoral cuts in excessive external rotation will lead to resection of a disproportionate amount of the posterior medial femoral condyle and insufficient resection of the posterior lateral femoral condyle. This will produce an asymmetric flexion gap (medial laxity). The extension gap is not affected by the anterior and posterior femoral condyle cuts.

46. **a** Intramedullary nailing is capable of providing absolute stability. With *absolute* stability, there is rigid interfragmentary compression and no motion between fragments under load. Absolute stability fosters primary bone healing. With *relative* stability, motion between fragments is proportional to applied load. Relative stability fosters secondary bone healing. Intramedullary nailing (reamed and unreamed) is a form of internal splinting that provides *relative* stability (*not* absolute stability). Forms of fixation that provide *relative* stability include casting, external fixation, and intramedullary nailing (none of which provide rigid interfragmentary compression). Forms of fixation that can accomplish *absolute* stability include the lag screw and compression plating. A lag screw is capable of generating significantly greater compressive forces than a dynamic compression plate (3,000 N versus 600 N). Compression plating with a straight plate induces compression of the cortex closest to the plate and gapping of the opposite cortex. This phenomenon can be avoided by "pretensioning" the plate (contouring a bow into the plate and applying the plate with the concave surface against the bone). A uniplanar external fixator construct is stiffest in the plane of the pins. Thus, to be most effective at preventing sagittal bending of a tibia fracture, the bar should be placed directly anterior to the leg, so the pins and bar lie in the sagittal plane.

47. **d** Peripheral vascular disease. This question is a recurrent offender on the orthopaedic in-training examination (OITE). Peripheral vascular disease (with or without diabetes) accounts for approximately 85% of all lower extremity amputations. Injury is the second most common cause of amputation overall, but it is the leading indication in young adulthood.

Note: If nothing else, our general surgery internships have taught us that punishment and leprosy are not common indications for amputation in contemporary Western society.

48. **b** Subchondral cyst formation. The three classic Fairbank signs are (1) joint space narrowing, (2) squaring of the femoral condyle, and (3) formation of a peripheral ridge osteophyte (Fig. 5.12). Although subchondral cyst formation is a classic characteristic of osteoarthritis, it was not one of the classic postmeniscectomy radiographic alterations described by Fairbank.

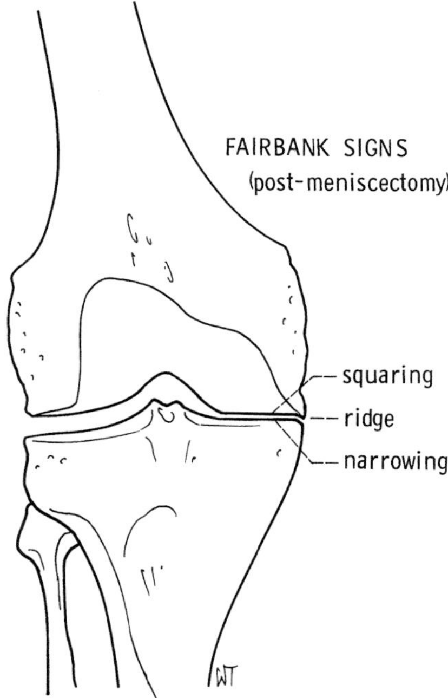

FIGURE 5.12

Reference

Fairbank TJ: Knee Joint Changes After Meniscectomy. J Bone Joint Surg Br, 30:664–670, 1948.

49. **c** The quadriceps. Myositis ossificans typically presents as a rapidly evolving soft tissue mass. A history of antecedent trauma is characteristically elicited. Although myositis ossificans most commonly occurs in the quadriceps, it may arise in the popliteal fossa (where it may be mistaken for parosteal osteosarcoma) or in many other extraosseous locations (where it may be difficult to distinguish from extraosseous osteosarcoma).

   Note: The zonal architecture of myositis ossificans aids in radiographically distinguishing this lesion from extraosseous osteogenic sarcoma. Myositis ossificans initially forms a peripheral rim of calcification. Mineral deposition subsequently proceeds from the periphery toward the center, but the perimeter remains the region with the highest density. In most cases of osteogenic sarcoma, the zonal gradation and propagation of mineral deposition are reversed, from central to peripheral.

Reference

Huvos AG: Bone Tumors: Diagnosis, Treatment, and Prognosis, 2nd Ed. Philadelphia, WB Saunders, 1991.

50. **d** 60%. Under normal circumstances, stance phase constitutes approximately 60% of the gait cycle; swing phase accounts for the remaining 40%. In an antalgic gait pattern, swing phase is accelerated on the contralateral (unaffected) limb in an effort to minimize the duration of single leg stance on the affected limb.

51. **c** Internal rotation of the femoral component. Advanced rheumatoid arthritis of the knee is commonly associated with a valgus deformity, in contrast to the varus deformity that is commonly associated with advanced osteoarthritis. The varus deformity in osteoarthritis is typically associated with bone loss from the medial *tibia*, whereas the valgus deformity in rheumatoid arthritis is characteristically accompanied by bone loss from the posterolateral *femur*. Bone loss from the posterolateral femoral condyle is typically accentuated in the presence of a flexion contracture.

   When performing total knee arthroplasty in this setting, the surgeon must be cognizant of this pattern of bone loss. Specifically, extreme caution must be exercised when using instrumentation systems that reference the rotation of the anterior and posterior femoral cuts on the posterior femoral condyles. If the surgeon is oblivious to the posterolateral femoral bone loss, then the anterior and posterior femoral cuts will be made in excessive internal rotation. The resultant internal rotation of the femoral component will promote lateral patellar subluxation. The transepicondylar axis is a more reliable rotational reference than the posterior femoral condyles in this setting. The varus-valgus and flexion-extension alignment of the distal femoral cut will not be deleteriously affected in this situation because the distal femoral cut is referenced off the intramedullary guide.

52. **c** Moving the central pins farther from the fracture. The stiffness of an external fixator construct is increased by (1) increasing the number of pins in each fragment, (2) increasing the distance between the pins in each fragment, (3) increasing the number of connecting bars, (4) decreasing the distance between the bar and the bone, (5) moving the central pins closer to the fracture, and (6) increasing the radius of the pins.

   Statement c is false. In fact, moving the central pins farther from the fracture will decrease the stiffness of the bone-frame construct by increasing the effective moment arm acting across the construct. With further separation of two pins in a single fragment, that fragment has greater resistance to rotational deformation (increased stiffness).

   Note: Pin stiffness is proportional to the fourth power of the pin radius (r^4).

53. **b** Mild patellofemoral chondromalacia. A knee with a fixed varus deformity greater than 10 degrees is not amenable to unicompartmental knee arthroplasty because of the associated difficulty correcting the contracture.

   Although advanced degeneration of the patellofemoral joint constitutes a contraindication to unicompartmental knee arthroplasty, mild chondromalacia is permissible, provided the patient has no patellofemoral symptoms. The absence of either cruciate ligament is a contraindication to unicompartmental knee arthroplasty because the associated instability serves as a diathesis for degeneration of the opposite compartment as well as premature implant failure.

The presence of an inflammatory arthropathy (e.g., such as rheumatoid arthritis or arthritis related to calcium pyrophosphate dihydrate) precludes unicompartmental knee arthroplasty because of the associated likelihood of deterioration of the opposite compartment. Unicompartmental knee arthroplasty is not ideal in patients with an obese body habitus because excessive stress concentration on the tibial component may lead to subsidence of the implant.

Note: The lateral femoral condyle "kissing" lesion is produced by tibial spine impingement. This defect is a marker for lateral subluxation of the tibia. If small, this lesion should not preclude unicompartmental knee arthroplasty. However, advanced lateral tibial subluxation signifies gross ligamentous insufficiency that cannot be stabilized by unicompartmental knee arthroplasty and that may subject a unicompartmental knee arthroplasty implant to abnormal loading and premature failure.

References

Padgett DE: Unicompartmental Knee Arthroplasty. In Craig EV, ed: Clinical Orthopaedics. Philadelphia, Lippincott Williams & Wilkins, 1999.

Scott RD: Unicompartmental Total Knee Arthroplasty. In Insall J, ed: Surgery of the Knee, 2nd Ed. New York, Churchill Livingstone, pp. 805–808, 1993.

54. **b** Meniscal cyst. The coronal and axial magnetic resonance images (Fig. 5.8) manifest a homogeneous cystic collection directly abutting the medial joint line. An adjacent horizontal cleavage tear of the medial meniscus is present. These findings are characteristic of a meniscal cyst. Although meniscal cysts occur more frequently on the lateral side of the knee, medial meniscal cysts may also occur. These lesions are virtually always contiguous with horizontal cleavage tears, which are believed to "pump" fluid into the cyst by a "bellows" mechanism.

Popliteal cysts typically arise more posteriorly from the medial compartment. They may also be associated with meniscal tears but are not directly contiguous with them. *Pigmented villonodular synovitis* may sometimes present in a unifocal form, but it characteristically occurs as a more diffuse process. Pigmented villonodular synovitis typically has a heterogeneous appearance on magnetic resonance imaging, unlike the uniform appearance of the lesion in this case. In contrast to the extraarticular lesion in this question, pigmented villonodular synovitis (like the pannus of rheumatoid arthritis) is a proliferative intraarticular process.

Reference

Mills CA, Henderson IPJ: Cysts of the Medial Meniscus. J Bone Joint Surg Br, 75:293–298, 1993.

55. **a** The tendency for popliteal cysts to become firm during knee *extension* and soft with knee *flexion*. Option a is the definition of the *Foucher sign*. Option b describes the *J-sign*, an indication of a deficient vastus medialis obliquus, overpull of the vastus lateralis, an increased Q-angle, or a combination of these factors. Option c describes a positive *Helfet test*, a manifestation of proximal tibiofibular joint instability. Option d describes a positive *quadriceps active test*, a sign of posterior cruciate ligament insufficiency. Option e describes a positive Steinmann test, a sign of meniscal disease.

Reference

Canoso JJ, et al.: Foucher's Sign of the Baker's Cyst. Ann Rheum Dis, 46: 228–232, 1987.

56. **d** Anterior translation of the femoral component. The proximal tibial cut should be made in slight (approximately 3 to 5 degrees) flexion. Posterior tibial slope facilitates femoral rollback by widening the flexion space. Conversely, placing the tibial component in extension (anterior tibial slope) will limit flexion by compromising femoral rollback. Excessive posterior cruciate ligament tension will also compromise the flexion space.

If the femoral component is oversized, its increased sagittal dimension will "overstuff" the flexion space (Fig. 5.13). Posterior translation of the femoral component will have a similar effect. Anterior translation of the femoral component, conversely, will widen the flexion space.

Excessive patellar thickness (from insufficient patella resection) creates increased tension in the quadriceps. This "overstuffing" of the patellofemoral space is another potential source of limited knee flexion.

References

Anouchi Y, et al.: Range of Motion in Total Knee Replacement. Clin Orthop, 331:87–92, 1996.

Walker PS, Garg A: Range of Motion in Total Knee Arthroplasty: A Computer Analysis. Clin Orthop, 262:227–235, 1991.

57. **d** Preoperative status of the anterior cruciate ligament. Lack of aggressive early postoperative physical therapy has been identified as a significant risk factor for suboptimal range of motion (less than 90 degrees). Other risk factors include joint line elevation, preoperative

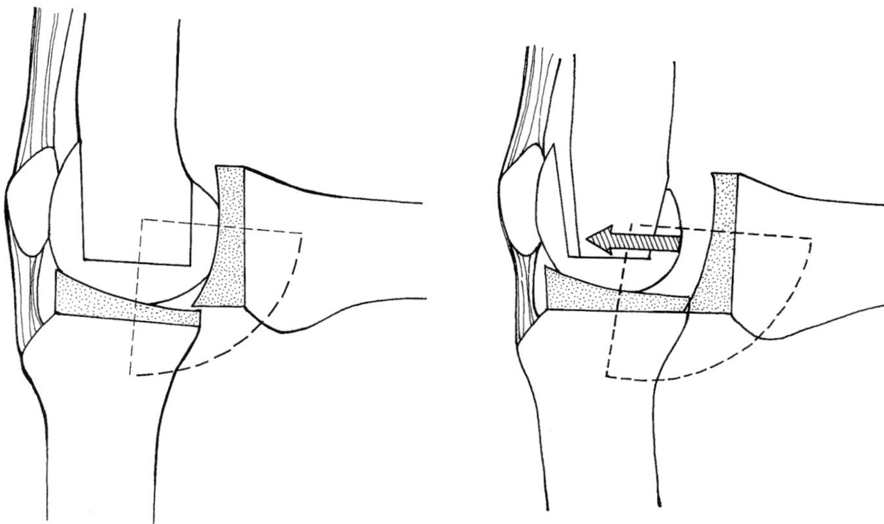

FIGURE 5.13

range of motion, and increased patellar thickness. Age, gender, and the posterior cruciate ligament status of the implant design have not been found to be significant predictors of ultimate range of motion.

References

Papagelopoulos PJ, Sim FH: Limited Range of Motion After Total Knee Arthroplasty. Orthopedics, 20(11):1061–1065, 1997.

Ritter M, Stringer E: Predictive Range of Motion After Total Knee Replacement. Clin Orthop, 143:115–119, 1979.

Shoji H: Factors Affecting Postoperative Flexion in Total Knee Arthroplasty. Orthopedics, 13(6):643–649, 1990.

58. **e** Excessive posterior cruciate ligament tension. Anterior liftoff of the tibial trial component during knee flexion indicates excessive tension in the posterior cruciate ligament. Inordinate posterior cruciate ligament tension causes the femur to roll back too far on the tibial tray. Compression of the posterior lip of the tray causes anterior tray liftoff (Fig. 5.14). With correct posterior cruciate ligament balance, the femur will roll back, but not far enough to induce anterior liftoff.

Oversizing of the femoral component may limit flexion, but this would prevent the femur from rolling

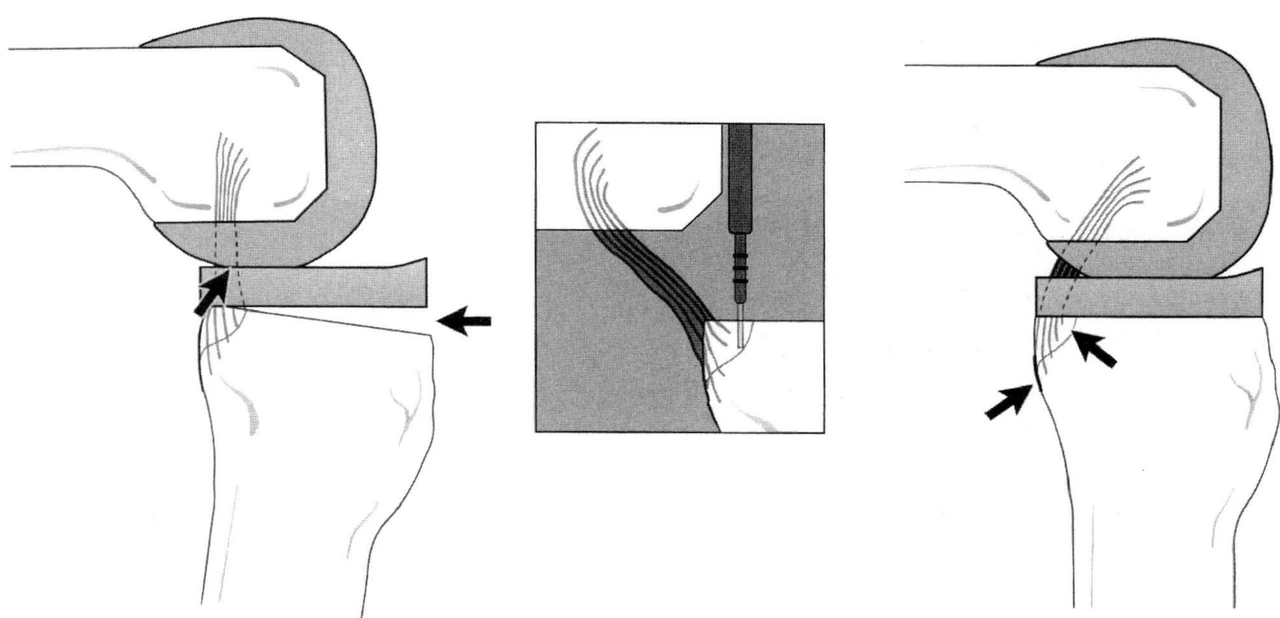

FIGURE 5.14

back far enough on the tibia to induce liftoff. Excessive polyethylene thickness and/or insufficient proximal tibial resection would narrow both the flexion and the extension gaps, but this would not affect the extent of femoral rollback.

Reference

Fu FH, Harner CD, Vince KG, eds: Knee Surgery. Philadelphia, Williams & Wilkins, p. 1389, 1994.

59. **c** The relationship between the cruciate ligaments and their osseous attachments that defines sagittal knee motion. The *four-bar linkage* mechanism describes the constant anatomic lengths of the cruciate ligaments and the fixed distances between their respective femoral and tibial attachments (Fig. 5.15A). These four constant distances define the changing center of rotation of the knee and the sagittal translation of the femur on the tibia during flexion (Fig. 5.15B).

During anterior cruciate ligament reconstruction, the graft must be placed in an isometric position to ensure that appropriate four-bar linkage is reestablished to ensure proper knee kinematics.

Reference

Dye SF: Anatomy and Biomechanics of the Anterior Cruciate Ligament. Clin Sports Med, 7:715–725, 1988.

60. **e** Fibular circumflex artery. The extraosseous peripatellar anastomotic ring receives contributions from the following arteries: (1) the medial and lateral inferior genicular, (2) the medial and lateral superior genicular, (3) the supreme genicular (descending genicular), and (4) the anterior tibial recurrent (Fig. 5.16). *The fibular circumflex artery* supplies the proximal portion of the lateral compartment of the leg.

Note: The supreme genicular artery (descending genicular) arises from the superficial femoral artery proximal to Hunter canal.

Reference

Scapinelli R: Blood Supply of the Human Patella: Its Relation to Ischaemic Necrosis After Fracture. J Bone Joint Surg Br, 49:564, 1967.

61. **c** If the shape of a diaphyseal defect is elongated in the direction of the long axis of a bone without increasing the area of the defect, then the torsional strength of the bone will *not* change. When a defect is made in a uniform material, strain is increased in its immediate vicinity. The location, size, and orientation of defects in bone affect the resultant compromise in the strength of the bone. Iatrogenic holes may occur in low-stress regions of a bone without significantly altering the bone's strength. For example, an emptied screw hole in the proximal tibial metaphysis will not reduce the overall torsional strength of the tibia. This is so because of

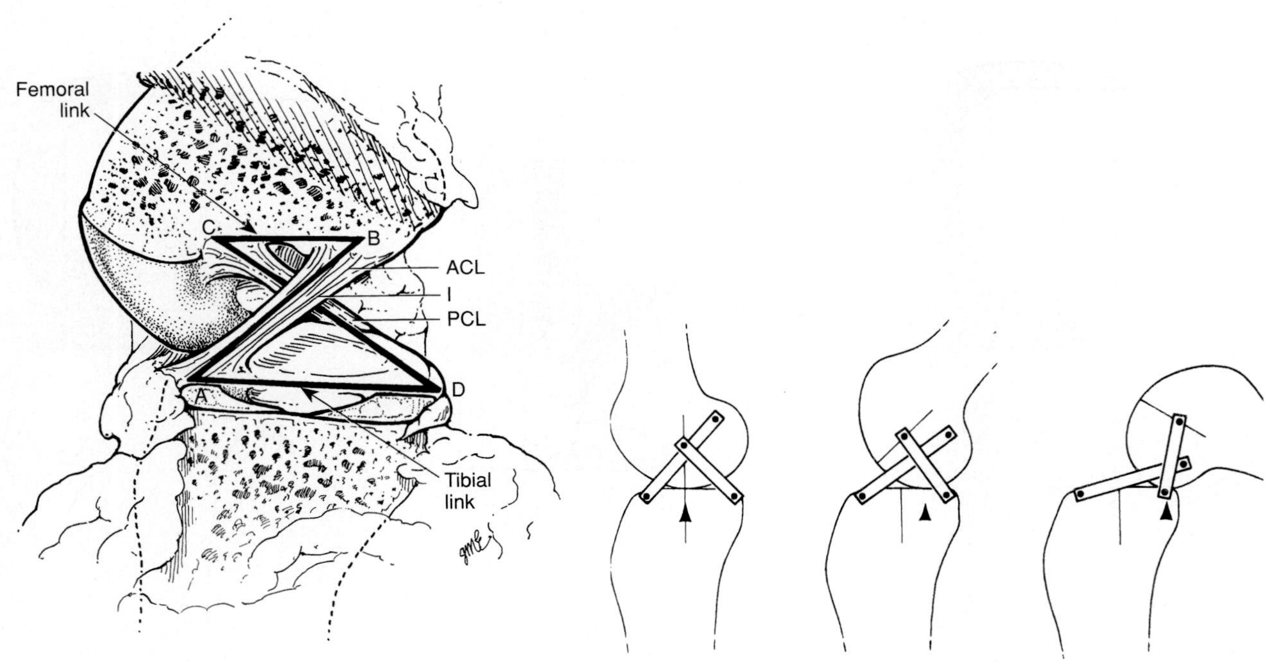

FIGURE 5.15A and B

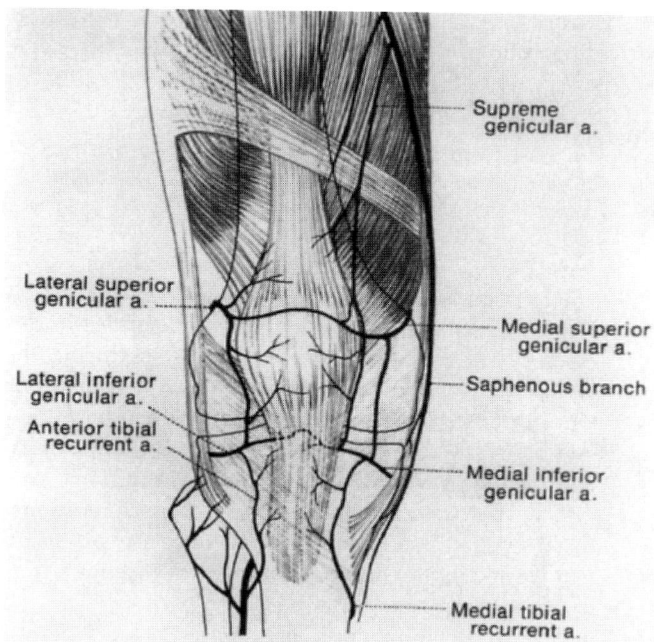

FIGURE 5.16

the large torsional *section modulus* of this region of the tibia compared with the diaphysis. Much greater strains are induced in the diaphysis (specifically, at the junction of middle and distal thirds). Despite the presence of a metaphyseal hole, the tibial diaphysis would still be the first to fail.

Under bending loads, a unicortical drill hole will weaken a tubular bone the most if it is made in the center of the tensile cortex because the yield stress of bone is much less under tension than compression. If the shape of a diaphyseal defect is elongated in the direction of the long axis of a bone without increasing the area of the defect, then the torsional strength of the bone will be *decreased*. Larger holes cause greater weakening than smaller holes of similar shapes.

Reference

Burstein A, Wright T: Fundamentals of Orthopaedic Biomechanics. Philadelphia, Williams & Wilkins, 1994.

62. **a** Moderately and severely obese patients have a significantly higher incidence of postoperative patellofemoral symptoms. In a series of 257 primary, posterior stabilized total knee arthroplasties, Stern and Insall found no discernible difference in the overall knee scores among five different weight classes. However, moderately and severely obese patients were found to have a twofold higher incidence of postoperative patellofemoral symptoms (30% versus 14%; $p < .03$). The same investigation found no definite correlation between extreme body weight and thrombophlebitis or wound complications.

Reference

Stern S, Insall J: Total Knee Arthroplasty in Obese Patients. J Bone Joint Surg Am, 72:1400, 1990.

63. **c** Posterior cruciate ligament–substituting implant designs prevent posterior tibial translation but do not cause femoral rollback. In a knee with a competent posterior cruciate ligament, the posterior cruciate ligament causes the femur to translate posteriorly on the tibia during knee flexion. This phenomenon increases the moment arm of the quadriceps. In a posterior cruciate ligament–retaining knee prosthesis, this sagittal shifting of the contact point between the femur and tibia may precipitate tibial loosening through a "see-saw" effect.

    The cam of posterior cruciate ligament–substituting (posterior stabilized) designs induces femoral roll back. However, these designs do not induce a similar "see-saw" effect because the resultant vector always passes through the tibial peg.

    The *total condylar design* relied on neither the native posterior cruciate ligament nor a prosthetic cam to prevent posterior tibial translation. Rather, this progenitor design relied on appropriate collateral ligament tension and the roller-in-trough effect of a highly conforming, "dished" tibial articular surface. Negligible femoral rollback occurs with such a design. Hence, flexion of total condylar prostheses was limited (to approximately 90 to 100 degrees) because of impingement between the posterior femur and the posterior rim of the tibial tray.

Reference

Garino JP, Lotke PA. In Fu FH, Harner CD, Vince KG, eds: Knee Surgery. Philadelphia, Williams & Wilkins, p. 1329, 1994.

64. **e** Impacting the medial portion of the femoral component into soft bone. Impacting the medial portion of the femoral component into the medial femoral condyle will produce relative varus (less valgus) alignment of the distal femoral articular surface. This will widen the medial side of the extension gap. Overzealous impaction technique should be conscientiously avoided in patients with compromised bone density.

    Inordinately valgus bone cuts on either side of the joint will narrow the medial side of the extension gap. Osteophytes on the medial joint line should be thoroughly excised to remove their tethering effect on the medial soft tissues and to minimize the required amount of medial soft tissue release.
65. **b** Prior sepsis of the knee. Rheumatoid arthritis, previous skin incisions about the knee, diabetes mellitus,

systemic steroid use, obesity, advanced age, malnutrition, and concomitant infection at remote sites have all been associated with an increased risk of postoperative infection after total knee replacement. The greatest risk, however, is from previous sepsis of the knee, which confers an approximately 7% rate of deep infection after knee arthroplasty.

References

Hanssen AD, et al.: Prevention of Deep Periprosthetic Joint Infection. J Bone Joint Surg Am, 78:458–471, 1996.

Wilson MG, et al.: Infection as a Complication of Total Knee Replacement Arthroplasty. J Bone Joint Surg Am, 72:878–883, 1990.

66. **c** Irrigation and débridement. The clinical situation is highly suggestive of infection. A revision and the use of an allograft should increase one's suspicion of infection. The radiographs reveal air in the joint and in the surrounding soft tissues, findings that suggest infection by a highly virulent organism (specifically, *Clostridium perfringens* or mixed gram-negative species). Antibiotic suppression has no role in the presence of such a virulent organism, and emergency irrigation and débridement are indicated. Preoperative nuclear medicine studies would serve no role in this situation other than to delay appropriate intervention.
67. **b** 25%. In general, higher levels of amputation are associated with less efficient energy expenditure. Using the rate of oxygen consumption per meter walked as an index of the energy cost of gait, the energy expenditure of a patient with a standard *below-knee amputation* will be increased approximately *25%* above baseline. The energy expenditure of a patient with a standard *above-knee amputation* will be increased approximately *50% to 65%* above baseline.

    Note: For a given level of amputation, the efficiency of energy expenditure is less for vascular amputees than for traumatic amputees. Amputees tend to adjust their ambulatory velocity to keep their rate of energy expenditure within normal limits.

Reference

Waters RL, et al.: Energy Cost of Walking of Amputees: The Influence of Level of Amputation. J Bone Joint Surg Am, 58:42–46, 1976.

68. **b** It is associated with an increased incidence of valgus malunion. Tibial shaft fractures without concomitant fibula fractures have been associated with an increased incidence of nonunion, delayed union, and *varus* malunion.

    When the lower limb is loaded after isolated division of the tibia, the normal tibial strain pattern (lateral compression and medial tension) is reversed to medial compression and lateral tension. This biomechanical alteration explains the tendency for varus angulation in this setting. Resultant disturbances in ankle joint load distribution have been associated with ankle degeneration.

Reference

Teitz CC, et al.: Problems Associated with Tibial Fractures with Intact Fibulae. J Bone Joint Surg Am, 62:770–776, 1980.

69. **e** Resect additional distal femur. When the extension gap is smaller than the flexion gap (as described in this case), a flexion contracture will result. Reducing the polyethylene thickness or resecting more proximal tibia will not correct the gap asymmetry; rather, both gaps will be widened. Although this will correct the flexion contracture, it will produce instability in flexion.

    The solution to this situation is to resect additional distal femur. This maneuver will widen the extension gap (correcting the flexion contracture) without affecting the flexion gap.
70. **a** A positive Hoover test. The *Hoover test* is a sign of malingering or hysteria. When an individual attempts a supine straight leg raise, downward pressure should be involuntarily exerted by the contralateral heel.

    The *Beevor sign* (translation of the umbilicus away from the affected region during a situp) is a sign of unilateral rectus abdominis muscle weakness. The *Holmgren sign* (layering of a lipohemarthrosis in the suprapatellar pouch detected on lateral radiograph) is a sign of an intraarticular fracture of the knee.

    The *Homans sign* (calf pain elicited by passive ankle dorsiflexion with the knee extended) is a nonspecific sign of deep venous thrombosis. The *Gower sign* ("walking" one's hands up one's legs in an effort to stand up from a prone position) is a clinical sign of proximal muscle weakness that is commonly associated with muscular dystrophy (as well as other myopathies that affect the hip extensors, quadriceps, and trunk extensors).
71. **c** The number of steps per unit time. *Cadence* refers to the number of steps per unit time. *Stride length* refers to the forward distance traveled between heel strike of one foot and the next ipsilateral heel strike. *Step length* refers to the forward distance traveled between heel strike of one foot and the next contralateral heel strike. *Gait velocity* is a function of cadence and step length.
72. **a** Asymptomatic coincidental finding on routine follow-up radiograph. The most common presentation of periprosthetic patellar fracture after total knee arthroplasty is as a coincidental finding on routine follow-up radiographs. In this setting, the integrity of the extensor mechanism should be thoroughly evaluated by palpation and straight leg raising. An asymptomatic, nondisplaced periprosthetic patellar fracture requires no specific treatment.

Reference

Engh GA, Ammeen DJ: Periprosthetic Fractures Adjacent to Total Knee Implants: Treatment and Clinical Results. J Bone Joint Surg Am, 79: 1100–1113, 1997.

73. **b** A patient who presents without distal pulses; distal pulses remain absent when the knee is relocated. Knee dislocation is associated with a high incidence of popliteal artery injury (approximately 30%). Distal pulses should be evaluated before and after reduction of a dislocated knee. However, significant vascular injury may be present even in the absence of overt clinical signs of ischemia or diminished pulses. For these reasons, many authors advocate routine arteriograms for all patients who have sustained a knee dislocation.

Selected studies in the general surgical literature have proposed that close clinical observation (without arteriography) may be acceptable for patients in whom distal pulses and perfusion were not compromised. Expectant management without arteriography in this setting is a controversial proposition predicated on the immediate availability of a vascular surgeon if intervention becomes necessary.

It is generally accepted that an arteriogram should be performed on all patients who manifest diminished distal pulses before or after reduction. The one caveat to this generalization is the patient with a clear arterial injury in whom distal perfusion remains unequivocally compromised after reduction. Formal preoperative arteriography is contraindicated in this setting because delayed repair increases the risk of amputation; the average delay for a formal preoperative arteriogram is approximately 3 hours.

Preoperative arteriography serves two essential purposes: (1) to detect arterial injury and (2) to localize arterial injury. When pulses are absent after an isolated knee dislocation, neither the presence nor the location of the lesion is typically in dispute. However, when the location of the source of a transiently diminished pulse is less obvious (e.g., when knee dislocation occurs with concomitant ipsilateral femur or tibial fracture), preoperative arteriography is useful.

Tourniquet stasis combined with exposed subintimal tissue may precipitate thrombosis. For this reason, arteriography is recommended before the elective use of a tourniquet on a previously dislocated limb.

References

Kendall RW, et al.: The Role of Arteriography in Assessing Vascular Injuries Associated with Dislocations of the Knee. J Trauma, 35:875–878, 1993.
Stain SC, et al.: Selective Management of Nonocclusive Arterial Injuries. Arch Surg, 124:1136–1141, 1989.
Treiman GS, et al.: Examination of the Patient with a Knee Dislocation: The Case for Selective Arteriography. Arch Surg, 127:1056–1062, 1992.

74. **b** Protected weight bearing for 6 to 8 weeks. Intraoperative periprosthetic sagittal intercondylar split fractures typically occur during total knee arthroplasty while either (1) making the box cut or (2) impacting the femoral component into an insufficiently cut box.

If such a fracture is recognized intraoperatively and is not displaced, it can be stabilized with one or two transcondylar cancellous screws. Additional stability is conferred by the cement and by the femoral component itself. If this fracture is noted to be displaced intraoperatively, a stemmed femoral component should be used (cement should be kept away from the fracture interface). When a nondisplaced fracture of this variety is noted on postoperative radiographs, the accepted management consists of protected weight bearing for 6 to 8 weeks to permit healing without displacement.

Note: However, evidence in the literature indicates that protected weight bearing may not be necessary. Lombardi et al. reported a series of 35 incidental nondisplaced intercondylar fractures, all of which healed without modification of the standard postoperative physical therapy protocol.

References

Engh GA, Ammeen DJ: Periprosthetic Fractures Adjacent to Total Knee Implants. Treatment and Clinical Results. J Bone Joint Surg Am, 79: 1100–1113, 1997.
Lombardi AV, et al.: Intercondylar Distal Femoral Fracture: An Unreported Complication of Posterior-Stabilized Total Knee Arthroplasty. J Arthroplasty, 10:643–650, 1995.

75. **e** Oxidative degradation of polyethylene occurs during γ irradiation in the presence of air, but it does not continue after sterilization. Not only does oxidative degradation of polyethylene occur during γ irradiation, but also it continues during the shelf life of the implant and *in vivo*. Oxidation decreases the molecular weight of the polyethylene chains.

Wear debris generated in total knee replacements tends to be larger than the particles associated with total hip arthroplasty. Some authors have hypothesized that the higher percentage of smaller (submicrometer) debris associated with total hip arthroplasty may impart a greater inflammatory stimulus on the macrophage and may therefore evoke more osteolysis.

Polyethylene thickness is a major determinant of contact stress distribution. Polyethylene surface damage and particle number correlate inversely with polyethylene thickness. Surface damage is more severe in thin components and in components with relatively flat tibial articulating surfaces. Recommended minimum polyethylene thickness is 8 to 10 mm.

Delamination is a more common mechanism of wear in total knee arthroplasty than in total hip arthroplasty. This form of degradation is propagated by subsurface shear stresses, and it is initiated at intergranular fusion defects. Delamination is minimized when the contact point between the femoral condyles and the polyethylene remains constant. Sagittal translation of the condyles intensifies subsurface shear stresses and exacerbates delamination.

References

Blunn GW, et al.: The Dominance of Cyclic Sliding in Producing Wear in Total Knee Replacements. Clin Orthop, 273:253–260, 1991.

Chiba J, et al.: A Biomechanical, Histologic, and Immunohistologic Analysis of Membranes Obtained from Failed Cemented and Cementless Total Knee Arthroplasty. Clin Orthop, 299:114–124, 1994.

Hirakawa K, et al.: Characterization of Debris Adjacent to Failed Knee Implants of Three Different Designs. Clin Orthop, 331:151–158, 1996.

Wright TM, Bartel DL: The Problem of Surface Damage in Total Knee Components. Clin Orthop, 205:67–74, 1986.

76. **b** Varus tibial cut. The standard proximal tibial cut should be perpendicular to the tibial shaft axis. A varus tibial cut would widen the medial joint space in both flexion and extension. Another potential explanation for the medial laxity would be iatrogenic medial collateral ligament insufficiency. Excessive external rotation of the anterior and posterior cuts on the distal femur would produce relative medial laxity, but only in *flexion.*

A valgus proximal tibial cut would widen the *lateral* side of both the flexion and extension gaps. An excessively valgus distal femoral cut (more than the standard 5 degrees) would produce relative lateral laxity (in extension only). An excessively thick trial tibial polyethylene insert would lead to symmetrically increased soft tissue tension (medial and lateral) in both flexion and extension.

77. **e** 16 times. A structure's resistance to bending (rigidity) is referred to as its *moment of inertia.* The moment of inertia of a *rod* is proportional to the fourth power of its radius (r^4). Thus, if the radius of a rod is doubled, then its moment of inertia will increase by 16 times.

In contrast to a rod, the moment of inertia of a *plate* is proportional to the third power of its thickness. Thus, if the thickness of a plate is doubled, then its moment on inertia will increase by eight times.

The rigidity of a plate or rod is inversely proportional to the third power of its length. Hence, a rod will bend eight times as much if its length is doubled.

Note: The area moment of inertia of a rod refers to its resistance to torsion. Like the moment of inertia of a rod, the area moment of inertia of a rod is also proportional to the fourth power of its radius.

Reference

Nordin M, Frankel VH: Basic Biomechanics of the Musculoskeletal System, 2nd Ed. Philadelphia, Lea & Febiger, 1989.

FIGURE CREDITS

Figure 5.2D. From Unni KK: Bone Tumors. Philadelphia, Lippincott–Raven, p. 426, 1996, with permission.

Figure 5.9. From Fu FH, Harner CD, Vince KG, eds: Knee Surgery. Philadelphia, Williams & Wilkins, p. 1556, 1994, with permission.

Figure 5.10A and B. From Fu FH, Harner CD, Vince KG, eds: Knee Surgery. Philadelphia, Williams & Wilkins, pp. 1324–1325, 1994, with permission.

Figure 5.11A. From Fu FH, et al.: Knee Surgery. Philadelphia, Lippincott Williams & Wilkins, p. 1476, 1994, with permission.

Figure 5.11B–D. From Fu FH, et al.: Knee Surgery. Philadelphia, Lippincott Williams & Wilkins, p. 79, 1994, with permission.

Figure 5.12. From Fu FH, et al.: Knee Surgery. Philadelphia, Lippincott Williams & Wilkins, p. 616, 1994, with permission.

Figure 5.13. From Fu FH, et al.: Knee Surgery. Philadelphia, Lippincott Williams & Wilkins, p. 1557, 1994, with permission.

Figure 5.14. From Fu FH, et al.: Knee Surgery. Philadelphia, Lippincott Williams & Wilkins, p. 1389, 1994, with permission.

Figure 5.15A. From Fu FH, et al.: Knee Surgery. Philadelphia, Lippincott Williams & Wilkins, p. 1325, 1994, with permission.

Figure 5.15B. . From Fu FH, et al.: Knee Surgery. Philadelphia, Lippincott Williams & Wilkins, p. 683, 1994, with permission.

Figure 5.16. . From Fu FH, et al.: Knee Surgery. Philadelphia, Lippincott Williams & Wilkins, p. 932, 1994, with permission.

6

SPORTS KNEE

QUESTIONS

1. A 24-year-old professional dancer presents with recurrent right knee instability 10 months after anterior cruciate ligament reconstruction with a cadaveric patellar tendon allograft. She denies recurrent trauma. Examination reveals full range of motion, a 2+ pivot shift, and a 2B (5- to 10-mm excursion with no end point) Lachman test. A lateral radiograph is shown in Fig. 6.1. What is the most likely explanation for graft failure in this situation?
   (a) Malpositioned tibial tunnel
   (b) Immunologic graft rejection
   (c) Failure of tibial fixation
   (d) Malpositioned femoral tunnel
   (e) Failure of femoral fixation
2. Which of the following statements regarding knee biomechanics is correct?
   (a) In early flexion, the iliotibial band translates anteriorly relative to the lateral femoral condyle.
   (b) The lateral cruciate ligament and arcuatecapsular ligament complex are the primary restraints to external tibial rotation from 0 to 30 degrees of knee flexion; at greater angles of knee flexion, the posterior cruciate ligament becomes the primary restraint to external tibial rotation.
   (c) The lateral cruciate ligament and arcuatecapsular ligament complex are the primary restraints to valgus knee instability.
   (d) With a positive pivot shift test, the lateral tibial plateau begins in an anteriorly subluxated position.
   (e) The pivot shift phenomenon is appreciated as the knee is extended from a flexed position.
3. What structure is marked by the arrow in Fig. 6.2?
   (a) The origin of the lateral collateral ligament
   (b) The insertion of the popliteus tendon
   (c) The insertion of the semimembranosus tendon
   (d) The origin of the deep medial collateral ligament
   (e) The insertion of the biceps femoris tendon
4. Which of the following statements regarding knee anatomy is incorrect?
   (a) Knee flexion is polycentric.
   (b) Both tibial plateaus are concave in the sagittal plane.
   (c) During terminal knee extension, there is obligatory internal rotation of the femur with respect to the tibia.
   (d) Both tibial plateaus are sloped posteriorly with respect to the tibial shaft.
   (e) The sulcus terminalis is a region of the lateral femoral condyle.
5. A 23-year-old snowboarder loses control while achieving big air off a 60-foot cliff and sustains a diaphyseal femur fracture. What is the incidence of associated ipsilateral knee ligament injury (grade II or greater)?
   (a) Less than 1%
   (b) 5%
   (c) 50%
   (d) 75%
   (e) More than 90%
6. The radiographic line along the roof of the intercondylar notch is referred to as
   (a) The Insall-Salvati line
   (b) The line of Schneider
   (c) The Blumensaat line
   (d) The Blackburn-Peel line
   (e) The Klein line
7. The lateral side of the knee has been divided into three distinct anatomic layers. Layer I is composed of
   (a) The iliotibial tract and the biceps femoris tendon
   (b) The lateral geniculate fascia and its anterior expansion
   (c) The lateral patellar retinaculum
   (d) The lateral collateral and fabellofibular ligaments
   (e) The arcuate ligament
8. Figure 6.3 is a sagittal magnetic resonance image of an in-line skater who sustained an internal rotation injury to his knee while he was jumping a fire hydrant. He denies history of prior knee surgery or trauma. This isolated image is most consistent with which of the following types of meniscal injury?
   (a) Displaced bucket handle tear of the lateral meniscus
   (b) Radial tear of the medial meniscus
   (c) Horizontal cleavage tear of the lateral meniscus

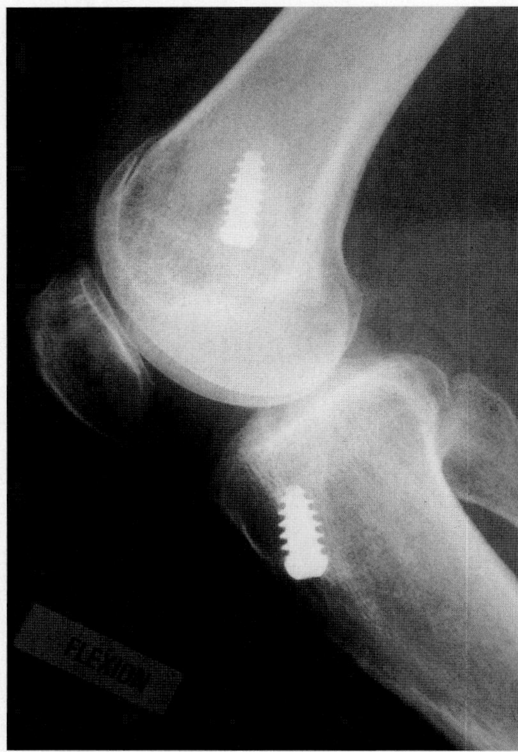

FIGURE 6.1

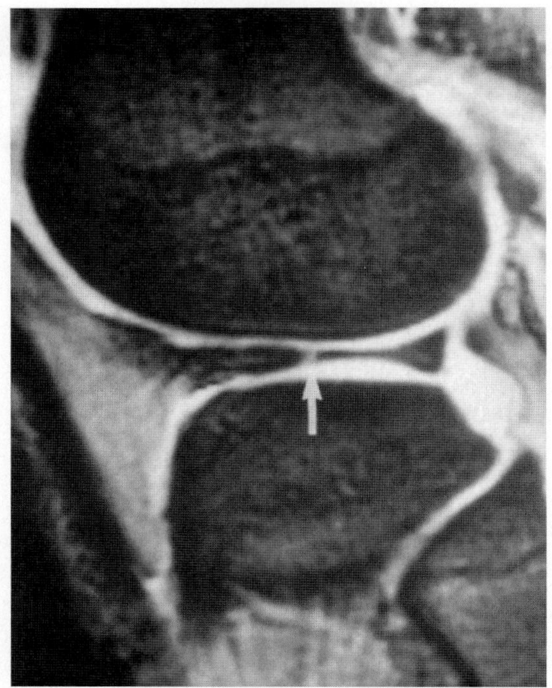

FIGURE 6.3

(d) Displaced buckethandle tear of the medial meniscus
(e) Radial tear of the lateral meniscus

9. Meniscal tissue contains all of the following types of collagen except
   (a) I
   (b) II
   (c) IV

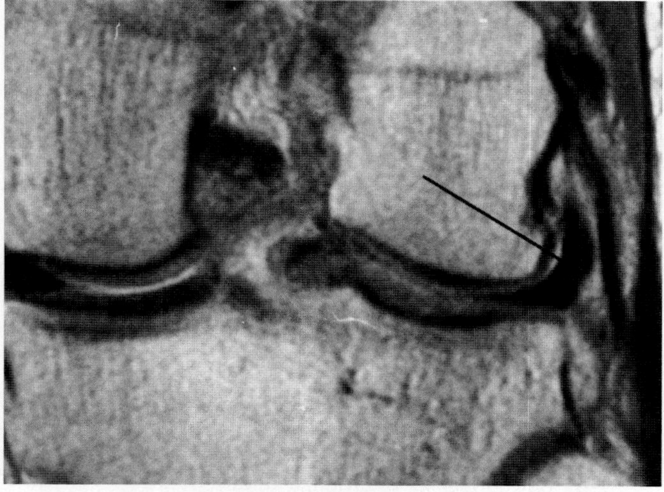

FIGURE 6.2

   (d) V
   (e) VI
10. The principal blood supply to the anterior cruciate ligament is
   (a) The descending geniculate artery
   (b) The superior medial and superior lateral geniculate arteries
   (c) The inferior medial and inferior lateral geniculate arteries
   (d) The middle geniculate artery
   (e) The posterior tibial recurrent artery
11. What is the most common location for osteochondritis dissecans of the knee?
   (a) The lateral aspect of the medial tibial plateau
   (b) The lateral aspect of the medial femoral condyle
   (c) The medial aspect of the lateral femoral condyle
   (d) Centrally on the lateral femoral condyle
   (e) The medial aspect of the lateral tibial plateau
12. Total medial meniscectomy decreases the static standing contact area between the weight-bearing surfaces in the medial compartment by
   (a) 10% to 30%
   (b) 30% to 50%
   (c) 50% to 70%
   (d) 70% to 90%
   (e) 100%
13. Which of the following has the most anterior insertion?
   (a) The semimembranosus tendon
   (b) The biceps femoris tendon

(c) The iliotibial band
(d) The lateral collateral ligament
(e) The semitendinosus tendon

14. A 30-year-old man complains of acute right knee swelling after a weekend of tennis. He denies recollection of trauma to the knee. He has experienced four similar, self-limited episodes of painful knee swelling during the previous year. His recent past medical history is significant for tobacco use, Bell palsy, recreational cocaine use, and chronic temporomandibular joint pain. What serologic test would be most appropriate to order?
    (a) Antinuclear antibody
    (b) Rheumatoid factor
    (c) Uric acid
    (d) HLA-B27
    (e) Lyme titer
15. Which of the following statements is false?
    (a) A displaced meniscal tear may create a false-negative Lachman test.
    (b) A complete medial collateral ligament tear may produce a false-negative pivot shift test.
    (c) A posterior cruciate ligament tear may produce a false-positive 2A Lachman test.
    (d) Hamstring tone may produce a false-negative pivot shift test.
    (e) An isolated grade II lateral cruciate ligament tear may produce a false-positive 2B Lachman test.
16. Which of the following statements is false regarding the reverse pivot shift test?
    (a) It may be a normal bilateral finding in physiologically normal persons.
    (b) It is performed with the foot externally rotated.
    (c) It is performed with varus stress.
    (d) The starting position is knee flexion.
    (e) With a positive test, the reduction should occur at 20 to 30 degrees of flexion.
17. A 29-year-old man undergoes anterior cruciate ligament reconstruction with a central third patellar tendon autograft. Full range of motion is achieved on the operating room table after graft fixation. One month postoperatively, he has full flexion, but he lacks 10 degrees of terminal extension (actively and passively), and terminal extension is painful. A lateral radiograph is obtained and demonstrates good tunnel position (Fig. 6.4). The most likely explanation for this patient's loss of motion is
    (a) Graft failure
    (b) Excessive tensioning of the graft
    (c) An anterior cruciate ligament nodule
    (d) Placement of the femoral tunnel too far posteriorly
    (e) Arthrofibrosis
18. Which of the following structures has the greatest *in vitro* tensile strength?
    (a) The gracilis tendon

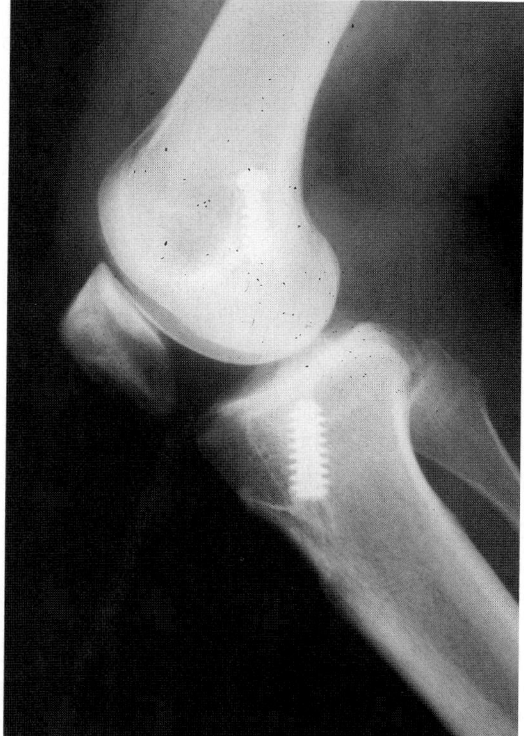

FIGURE 6.4

    (b) The native anterior cruciate ligament
    (c) The semitendinosus tendon
    (d) The central third patellar tendon allograft (15-mm width)
    (e) The distal iliotibial tract (18-mm width)
19. A 28-year-old internal medicine resident decides to run the New York City marathon. During his fourth week of training, he starts to experience lateral knee pain. The discomfort is aggravated by stair climbing and running downhill. His physical examination is significant for mild genu varum, tenderness over the lateral femoral condyle, and a positive Ober test. Radiographs of the knee are normal. The most likely diagnosis is
    (a) Stress fracture of lateral femoral condyle
    (b) Popliteal tendinitis
    (c) Lateral synovial plica syndrome
    (d) Iliotibial band friction syndrome
    (e) Lateral meniscal tear
20. Which of the following recommendations would be most appropriate in the initial management of a patient with the condition described in question 19?
    (a) Medial wedge orthotic
    (b) Magnetic resonance imaging of the knee to confirm the diagnosis
    (c) Bone scan to confirm the diagnosis
    (d) Knee arthroscopy
    (e) Rigid foot orthotic to prevent hyperpronation

21. What imaging test should be ordered to determine whether the articular cartilage overlying a region of osteochondritis dissecans is intact?
    (a) Positron emission tomography
    (b) Plain radiography
    (c) Magnetic resonance imaging
    (d) Technetium scintigraphy
    (e) Ultrasonography
22. In which of the following orientations should the lower extremity be positioned to minimize the chance of a false-negative pivot shift test?
    (a) Hip adducted; leg internally rotated
    (b) Hip abducted; leg internally rotated
    (c) Hip abducted; leg externally rotated
    (d) Hip adducted; leg externally rotated
    (e) Neutral hip adduction and abduction; leg internally rotated
23. Which of the following statements regarding knee stability is most accurate?
    (a) The anterior horn of the medial meniscus is a secondary restraint to anterior tibial translation.
    (b) The posterior horn of the medial meniscus is a primary restraint to anterior tibial translation.
    (c) The anterior horn of the medial meniscus is a primary restraint to anterior tibial translation.
    (d) The posterior horn of the medial meniscus is a secondary restraint to anterior tibial translation.
    (e) The medial meniscus has no role in controlling anterior to posterior translation of the tibia.
24. Which of the following statements regarding the menisci is false?
    (a) Most of the collagen fibers in the menisci are oriented radially.
    (b) Approximately 70% of the meniscus is avascular.
    (c) The lateral meniscus has approximately twice the excursion of the medial meniscus.
    (d) A greater percentage of the lateral plateau is covered by the lateral meniscus as compared with the medial plateau's coverage by the medial meniscus.
    (e) The menisci contain neural tissue.
25. A professional wrestler drops from the top ropes in an attempt to drive his knee into his opponent's back. His opponent quickly moves and strikes his flexed knee on the mat. He subsequently forfeits the match because of knee pain and swelling. One week later he presents to your office for evaluation. Clinical examination reveals a mild effusion, a IA Lachman test, a positive posterior sag, a grade II posterior drawer, and a positive 90-degree quadriceps active test. The posterior drawer test with the foot in external rotation reveals no additional excursion. Varus and valgus stress at 30 reveals no instability. Prone external rotation at 30 degrees is symmetric. Reverse pivot shift is negative. Radiographs reveal no fracture. KT-1000 demonstrates 8 mm of posterior translation. Magnetic resonance imaging reveals no meniscal or articular cartilage injury. The most appropriate management of this injury is
    (a) Quadriceps rehabilitation
    (b) Return to the ring as soon as the effusion has completely resolved and full motion has been regained
    (c) Posterior cruciate ligament reconstruction with central third patellar tendon autograph
    (d) Combined posterior cruciate ligament and posterolateral corner reconstruction
    (e) Posterior cruciate ligament reconstruction with Achilles tendon allograft
26. Which of the following is the most accurate statement regarding anatomic considerations in harvesting the semitendinosus and gracilis tendons for anterior cruciate ligament reconstruction?
    (a) The gracilis and sartorius tendons insert as a conjoined structure at the pes anserinus.
    (b) The gracilis inserts at the level of the apex of the tibial tubercle.
    (c) The semitendinosus inserts deep to the superficial medial collateral ligament.
    (d) The gracilis tendon is distal to the semitendinosus tendon.
    (e) The inferior fibers of the semitendinosus diverge to form an accessory insertion.
27. Which of the following is not an insertion of the semimembranosus?
    (a) The posteromedial tibia (posterior to the medial collateral ligament)
    (b) The fascia of the popliteus
    (c) The medial tibia (deep to the superficial medial collateral ligament)
    (d) The oblique popliteal ligament
    (e) The conjoined tibial insertion with the sartorius
28. A 14-year-old model presents with painless swelling at the medial side of her knee. Her past medical history is unremarkable. Her agent sends her to a plastic surgeon for evaluation. A magnetic resonance image is obtained. T1 and T2 images are shown in Fig. 6.5 A and B, respectively. The patient's plastic surgeon requests your opinion. What is the most likely diagnosis?
    (a) Popliteal cyst
    (b) Pigmented villonodular synovitis
    (c) Aneurysmal bone cyst
    (d) Meniscal cyst
    (e) Epidermal inclusion cyst
29. What is the most abundant component of articular cartilage (by weight)?
    (a) Type I collagen
    (b) Water
    (c) Type II collagen
    (d) Proteoglycans
    (e) Type III collagen

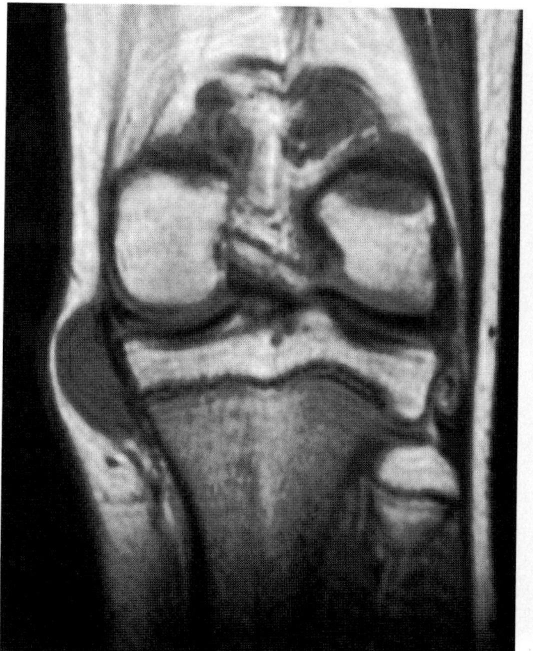

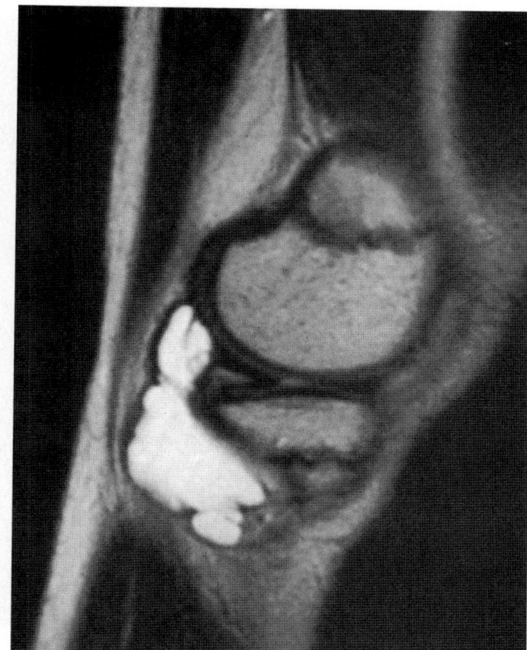

FIGURE 6.5A and B

30. Which of the following statements is false regarding the Maquet procedure (anteriorization) for anterior translation of the tibial tubercle?
    (a) The patella is translated distally.
    (b) The greater the magnitude of anterior tubercle translation, the larger is the decrease in patellofemoral contact area.
    (c) The patella rotates in the sagittal plane around a horizontal axis.
    (d) For a given anterior translation of the tibial tubercle, a longer tibial osteotomy will produce a greater vertical translation of the patella.
    (e) The patellofemoral contact area moves proximally with anterior translation of the tubercle.
31. Which of the following statements regarding the posterior cruciate ligament is true?
    (a) When the knee is extended, the anterolateral fibers tighten.
    (b) The femoral origin of the posterior cruciate ligament is longer in the anteroposterior dimension than in the vertical dimension.
    (c) The meniscofemoral ligament of Humphry originates from the posterior horn of the lateral meniscus. It runs posteriorly to the posterior cruciate ligament and inserts on the lateral wall of the medial femoral condyle.
    (d) The fibers of the posteromedial posterior cruciate ligament are stronger, stiffer, and larger than the anterolateral fibers.
    (e) A single-bundle posterior cruciate ligament graft should be tensioned in extension.
32. A 12-year-old soccer player complains of vague right knee pain associated with activity. He denies swelling, clicking, locking, and giving way. Physical examination reveals no focal tenderness, no effusion, no instability, but a positive Wilson sign. A plain radiograph is shown in Fig. 6.6A. A sagittal magnetic resonance image is shown in Fig. 6.6B. What is the most appropriate treatment?
    (a) Activity modification
    (b) Arthroscopic débridement with abrasion chondroplasty
    (c) Arthroscopic débridement with chondral flap fixation
    (d) Arthroscopic débridement with osteochondral allograft
    (e) Retrograde drilling
33. Which of the following is the least likely finding to be associated with an acute combined anterior cruciate ligament/medial collateral ligament rupture?
    (a) Lateral meniscal tear
    (b) Lateral femoral condyle bone contusion

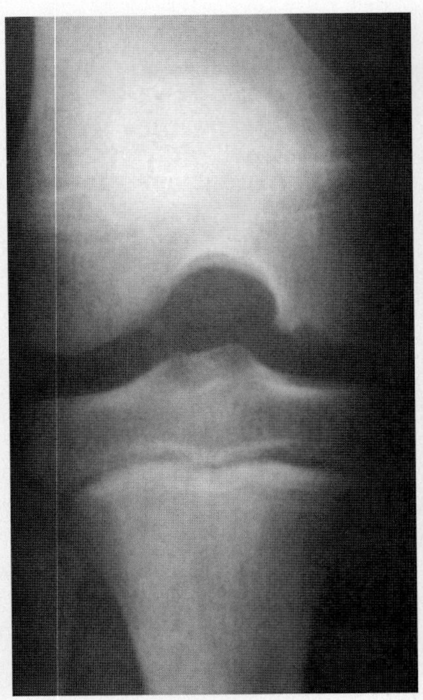

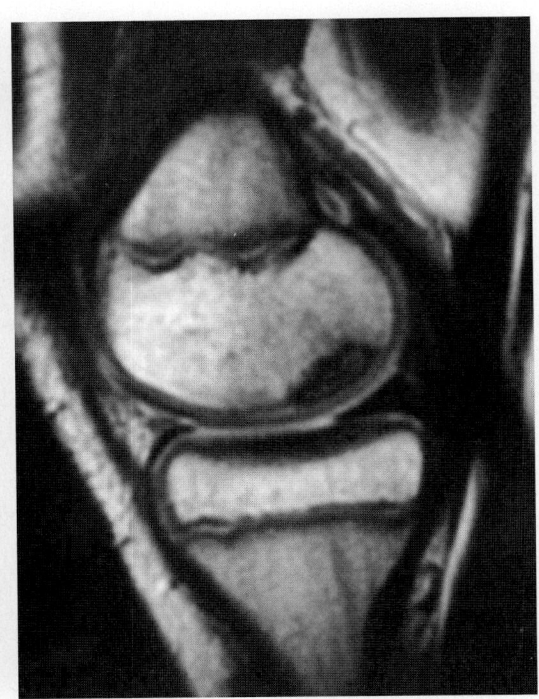

FIGURE 6.6A and B

(c) Hemarthrosis
(d) Lateral tibial plateau contusion
(e) Medial meniscal tear

34. The radiograph in Fig. 6.7 is consistent with which of the following diagnoses?
    (a) Anterior cruciate ligament injury
    (b) Iliotibial band friction syndrome
    (c) Pelligrini-Stieda lesion
    (d) Lateral cruciate ligament injury
    (e) Biceps femoris avulsion
35. Which of the following statements regarding the anterior cruciate ligament is correct?
    (a) The anteromedial fibers are under less tension when the knee is extended.
    (b) The average length of the adult anterior cruciate ligament is greater than 40 mm.
    (c) The posterolateral fibers are under uniform tension between 0 and 90 degrees of flexion.
    (d) The tibial attachment of the ligament is broader in the medial to lateral direction than in the anterior to posterior direction.
    (e) Most tears occur in the distal half of the ligament.
36. A 60-year-old nurse presents with several months of "aching" in her right knee. In addition, she has recently noticed a posterior knee mass. Her primary care physician ordered a magnetic resonance imaging scan to evaluate the mass. Select images are shown in Figs. 6.6 to 6.8. What is the most likely diagnosis?
    (a) Synovial sarcoma

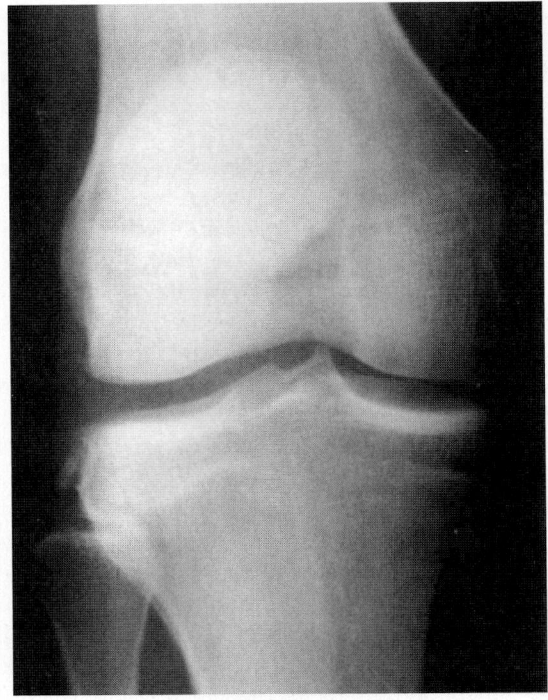

FIGURE 6.7

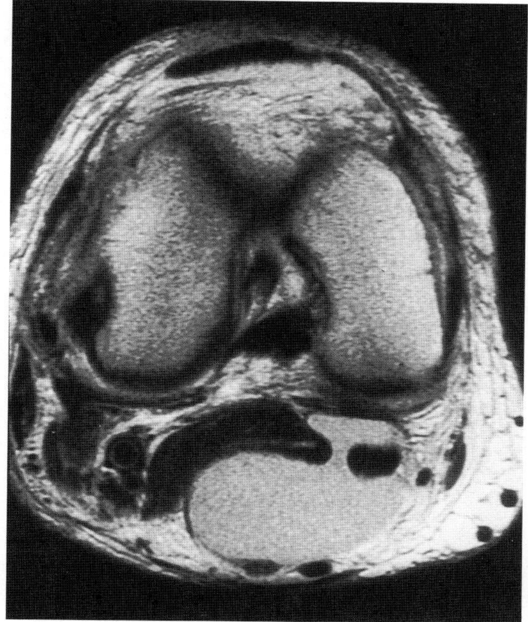

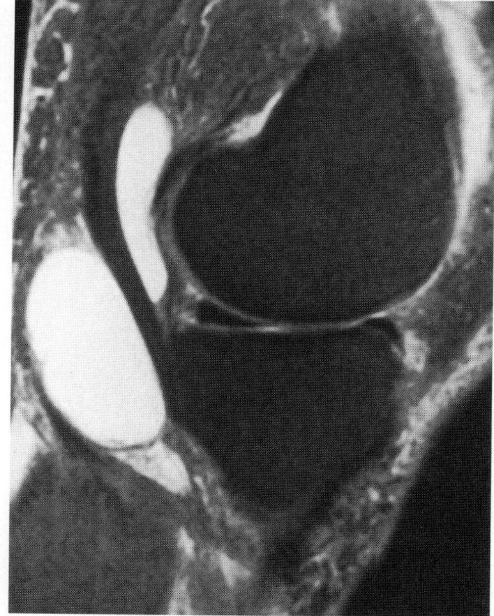

FIGURE 6.8A and B

(b) Meniscal cyst
(c) Liposarcoma
(d) Pigmented villonodular synovitis
(e) Popliteal cyst

37. A 21-year-old aerobics instructor presents for evaluation 1 week after injuring her left knee when she fell off a stair-climbing machine. Examination of the involved knee at 30 degrees of flexion reveals increased posterior translation, increased varus rotation, and increased external tibial rotation. These changes are significantly less pronounced when the knee is examined at 90 degrees of flexion. Her Lachman test is a 1A. What is the most likely diagnosis?
    (a) Combined posterior cruciate ligament and medial collateral ligament injuries
    (b) Isolated posterolateral corner injury
    (c) Combined anterior cruciate ligament and lateral cruciate ligament injuries
    (d) Isolated posterior cruciate ligament injury
    (e) Combined posterior cruciate ligament and posterolateral corner injuries
38. A constant load is applied to an armadillo ligament, and the deformation curve is generated. Deformation over time under a constant load occurs. What property does this curve demonstrate?
    (a) Stress relaxation
    (b) Hysteresis
    (c) Anisotropism
    (d) Creep
    (e) Normalization
39. Which of the following patients is the most ideal candidate for meniscal repair?
    (a) An 18-year-old man with an acute 1.5-cm longitudinal peripheral tear of the lateral meniscus who is undergoing a concurrent anterior cruciate ligament reconstruction
    (b) A 25-year-old woman with an intact anterior cruciate ligament and an acute radial tear extending to the periphery of the medial meniscus
    (c) A 22-year-old man with a chronic flap tear of the posterior horn of the lateral meniscus who is undergoing a concurrent anterior cruciate ligament reconstruction
    (d) A 19-year-old woman with an acute anterior cruciate ligament disruption and an acute 2.0-cm longitudinal tear of the peripheral lateral meniscus who wishes to postpone anterior cruciate ligament reconstruction until a later date
    (e) A 25-year-old man with an intact anterior cruciate ligament and a chronic 3.5-cm longitudinal tear within the central third of the medial meniscus
40. What structure is labeled by the arrow in the coronal magnetic resonance image in Fig. 6.9?
    (a) The sural nerve
    (b) The peroneal artery
    (c) The inferior lateral geniculate artery
    (d) The saphenous vein
    (e) The peroneal nerve
41. Sudden cardiac death in young athletes is most commonly associated with which of the following conditions?

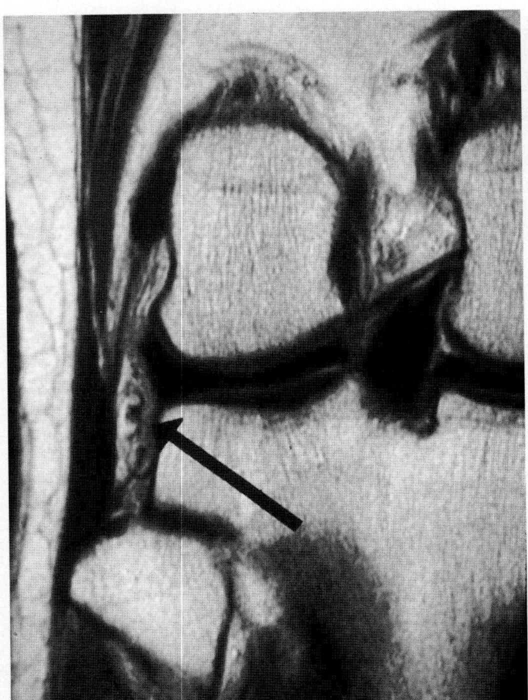

FIGURE 6.9

(a) Congenital abnormalities of the coronary arteries
(b) Mitral valve prolapse
(c) Hypertrophic cardiomyopathy
(d) Premature atherosclerosis
(e) Subacute viral myocarditis

42. Which of the following is the most common knee injury associated with alpine skiing?
(a) Anterior cruciate ligament tear
(b) Posterior cruciate ligament tear
(c) Medial collateral ligament tear
(d) Lateral collateral ligament tear
(e) Tibial plateau fracture

43. Which of the following is the most significant risk factor for septic arthritis after arthroscopic anterior cruciate ligament reconstruction?
(a) The presence of severe patellofemoral chondromalacia
(b) Prior intraarticular injection
(c) Acute anterior cruciate ligament reconstruction (less than 1 week after injury)
(d) A concomitant open procedure
(e) Inadequate notchplasty

44. Changes in articular cartilage resulting from normal aging include all the following except
(a) Decreased chondrocyte synthetic activity
(b) Localized superficial cartilage fibrillations
(c) Increased water concentration
(d) Decreased stability of large proteoglycan aggregates
(e) Increased collagen crosslinking

45. Abuse of anabolic steroids by college athletes has been associated with all the following side effects except
(a) Testicular atrophy
(b) Alopecia
(c) Hypercholesterolemia
(d) Gigantism
(e) Gynecomastia

46. What structure is labeled by the "O" in the coronal magnetic resonance image in Fig. 6.10?
(a) The plantaris muscle
(b) The lateral head of the gastrocnemius muscle
(c) The soleus muscle
(d) The medial head of the gastrocnemius muscle
(e) The popliteus muscle

47. While relaxing on call at the local Veterans Affairs hospital, the urology team decides to play a round of golf. En route to the back nine, the second-year postgraduate resident is ejected from the cart during an abrupt turn. He lands on his right foot with the ipsilateral knee flexed as his body continues to turn clockwise. He complains of right lateral knee pain and is unable to walk. After completing a hemipelvectomy, you receive a page from the Veterans Affairs radiologist, who states that the second-year urology postgraduate resident has an anterior dislocation of his proximal tibiofibular joint. What should you recommend?

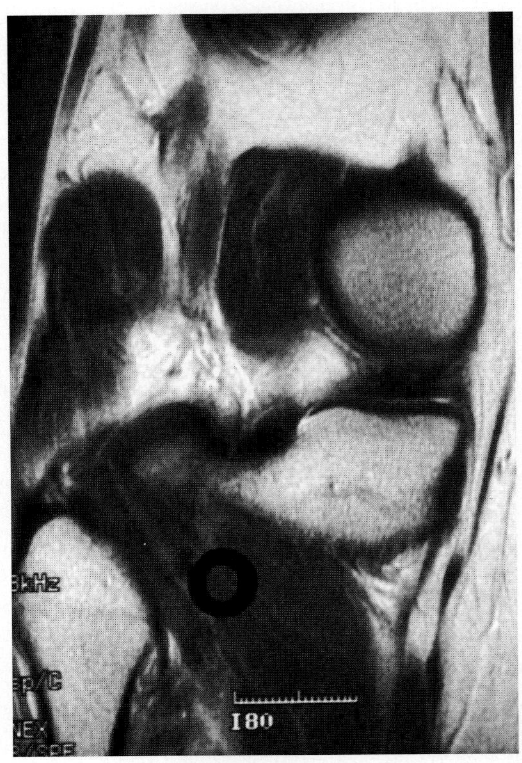

FIGURE 6.10

(a) Open reduction and primary arthrodesis of the proximal tibiofibular joint
(b) Open reduction and internal fixation of the proximal tibiofibular joint
(c) Open reduction followed by a long-leg cast for 4 to 6 weeks
(d) Closed reduction followed by a long-leg cast for 2 to 3 weeks
(e) Fibular head resection

48. Proteoglycan content is highest in which of the following regions of articular cartilage?
(a) The zone of calcified cartilage
(b) The superficial zone
(c) The middle zone
(d) The deep zone
(e) The subchondral zone

49. Which of the following correctly describes the reverse pivotshift maneuver?
(a) The patient is positioned prone with the knee in extension and internal rotation, valgus stress is applied, and the knee subluxates as it is flexed.
(b) The patient is positioned supine with the knee in extension and external rotation, varus stress is applied, and the knee reduces as it is flexed.
(c) The patient is positioned supine with the knee externally rotated at 90 degrees of flexion, valgus stress is applied, and the knee reduces as it is extended.
(d) The patient is positioned supine with the knee internally rotated at 90 degrees of flexion, varus stress is applied, and the knee subluxates as it is extended.
(e) The patient is positioned supine with the knee externally rotated at 90 degrees of flexion, valgus stress is applied, and the knee subluxates as it is extended.

50. Which of the following statements regarding meniscal cysts is false?
(a) Meniscal cysts are typically associated with intrameniscal disease and are directly attached to the meniscus.
(b) Meniscal cysts occur more commonly on the medial side of the knee than on the lateral side.
(c) Medial meniscal cysts tend to be larger than lateral meniscal cysts.
(d) Cyst content is histochemically similar to that of synovial fluid.
(e) Most associated meniscal tears are horizontal.

51. Endurance training has all the following effects on slow-twitch (type I) skeletal muscle except
(a) Increased number of slow-twitch muscle fibers
(b) Increased number of mitochondria
(c) Increased oxidative capacity
(d) Increased capillary density
(e) Decreased local accumulation of lactate in response to exercise

52. A 31-year-old woman who tore her anterior cruciate ligament 6 months previously complains of loss of extension and anterior knee pain. She denies further trauma to the knee. Imaging is shown in Fig. 6.11. What is the most likely diagnosis?
(a) Pigmented villonodular synovitis
(b) Osteochondritis dissecans
(c) Idiopathic osteonecrosis
(d) Bony impingement
(e) Instability

53. The predominant types of collagen in (a) articular cartilage and (B) menisci are
(a) (A) type I; (b) type II
(b) (A) type II; (b) type II
(c) (A) type II; (b) type I
(d) (A) type I; (b) type III
(e) (A) type II; (b) type III

54. What structure is marked by the arrow in Fig. 6.12?
(a) The ligament of Humphry
(b) The posterior cruciate ligament
(c) The arcuate ligament
(d) The oblique popliteal ligament
(e) The ligament of Wrisberg

55. Congenital absence of the anterior cruciate ligament is associated with all the following except
(a) Thrombocytopenia-absent radius syndrome
(b) Congenital knee dislocation
(c) Discoid lateral meniscus
(d) Infantile Blount disease
(e) Congenital absence of the menisci

56. A 22-year-old female basketball player has a syncopal episode during practice. She immediately awakens and has no complaints. She is taken to a local emergency room, where a workup (including cardiac enzymes and an electrocardiogram) is negative. As the emergency room physician prepares her discharge papers, the oncall orthopaedic surgery resident overhears her story and immediately notices her height (6 feet, 6 inches), long fingers, and mild scoliosis. He recommends a cardiac echocardiogram, which reveals a dilated aortic root. After referring the patient to a cardiothoracic surgeon, the orthopaedic resident explains that the cause of her probable underlying medical condition is
(a) A defect in the type III collagen gene
(b) A defect in the fibrillin gene
(c) Decreased synthesis of type I collagen
(d) A defect in the osteocalcin gene
(e) Myofibroblast dysfunction

57. Anterior cruciate ligament reconstruction with a Gore-Tex graft has been associated with an increased rate of all the following complications except
(a) Recurrent sterile effusions
(b) Graft loosening
(c) Infection
(d) Graft resorption

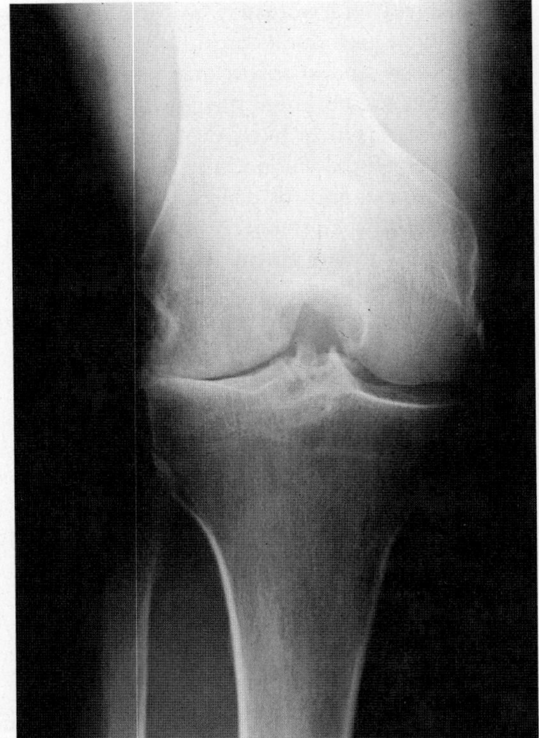

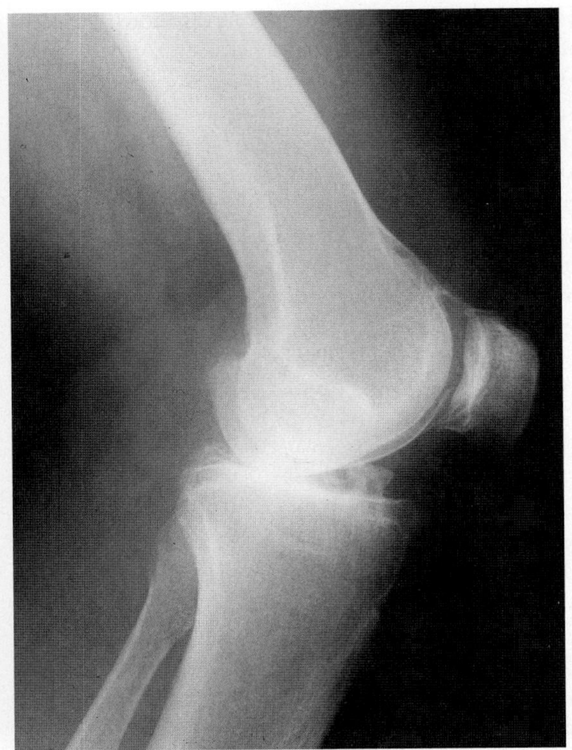

FIGURE 6.11A and B

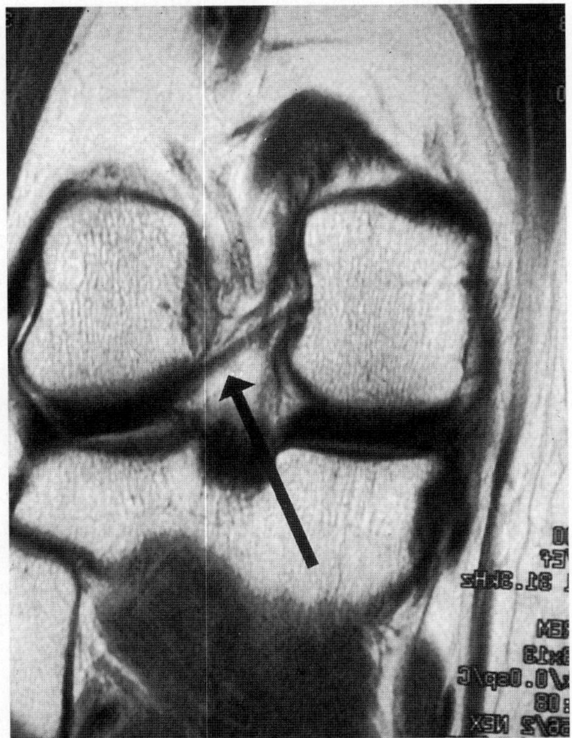

FIGURE 6.12

(e) Graft rupture

58. The lateral meniscus is seen in three consecutive 5-mm sagittal magnetic resonance imaging sections. Such images support which of the following diagnoses?
    (a) Tear of the lateral head of the gastrocnemius
    (b) Posterolateral corner insufficiency
    (c) Patellar tendon rupture
    (d) Tear of the popliteomeniscal fasciculi
    (e) Discoid lateral meniscus
59. A 19-year-old woman has magnetic resonance imaging performed 48 hours after a windsurfing mishap. Sagittal images demonstrate a bone contusion on the anterior portion of the lateral femoral condyle. What is the most likely diagnosis?
    (a) Anterior cruciate ligament tear
    (b) Lateral meniscal tear
    (c) Patellar tendon rupture
    (d) Posterior cruciate ligament tear
    (e) Patellar dislocation with spontaneous reduction
60. After reaming the femoral tunnel during an endoscopic anterior cruciate ligament reconstruction, you realize that the reamer has violated the posterior cortex. You have already prepared a patellar tendon autograft. How should you proceed?
    (a) Continue the procedure and insert the femoral interference screw anterior to the bone plug.
    (b) Ream the femoral tunnel again at a different angle and use a larger interference screw.

(c) Tie the femoral bone plug tensioning sutures over a button on the lateral femoral cortex through a separate incision.
(d) Ream the femoral tunnel again with a smaller diameter reamer and use a larger interference screw.
(e) Abort the procedure, freeze the graft for later implantation, and return to the operating room in 6 months to complete the procedure (after the posterior wall has healed).

61. A 35-year-old nurse complains of chronic left anterior knee pain. All conservative measures have failed. Examination reveals lateral facet tenderness and decreased medial patellar mobility. Her standing Q-angles are 10 degrees bilaterally. The range of motion of her hips and knees is normal. A midpatella computed tomography image demonstrates tilt and subluxation. Arthroscopy demonstrates grade IV chondromalacia of the lateral facet. Which of the following surgical procedures would be most appropriate?
(a) Lateral retinacular release alone
(b) External rotation osteotomy of the femur
(c) Proximal extensor mechanism realignment (advancement of the vastus medialis obliquus) and lateral retinacular release
(d) Anterior displacement of the tibial tubercle (Maquet procedure) and lateral retinacular release
(e) Anteromedialization of the tibial tubercle (Fulkerson procedure) and lateral retinacular release

62. A 27-year-old man complains of knee pain after he catches a wheel in the gutter while he is in-line skating. Examination reveals a 2+ Lachman test and a negative posterior drawer test. The knee is stable to varus stress. Valgus stress produces 12 mm of joint line opening. What would be the most appropriate form of surgical intervention for this patient?
(a) Medial collateral ligament reconstruction
(b) Combined lateral cruciate ligament and anterior cruciate ligament reconstruction
(c) Anterior cruciate ligament reconstruction
(d) Combined medial collateral ligament and anterior cruciate ligament reconstruction
(e) Lateral cruciate ligament reconstruction

63. Which of the following is least likely to be associated with limited knee extension after anterior cruciate ligament reconstruction?
(a) Anterior malposition of the femoral tunnel
(b) Inadequate notchplasty
(c) Arthrofibrosis
(d) Anterior malposition of the tibial tunnel
(e) Cyclops lesion

64. A 32-year-old motocross racer presents for a second opinion regarding pain in his right foot (just a warmup for Chapter 7, Foot and Ankle). His past orthopaedic history includes open reduction and internal fixation of a talar neck fracture and a comminuted plafond fracture 4 years ago. He has undergone 12 unspecified subsequent procedures. Inspection of his foot reveals a draining hindfoot sinus. A radiograph is shown in Fig. 6.13. Which of the following procedures should you recommend?
(a) Arthroscopy of the subtalar joint
(b) Triple arthrodesis
(c) Arthroscopy of the ipsilateral knee
(d) Subtalar arthrodesis
(e) Frontal lobotomy
(f) Tibiotalocalcaneal fusion

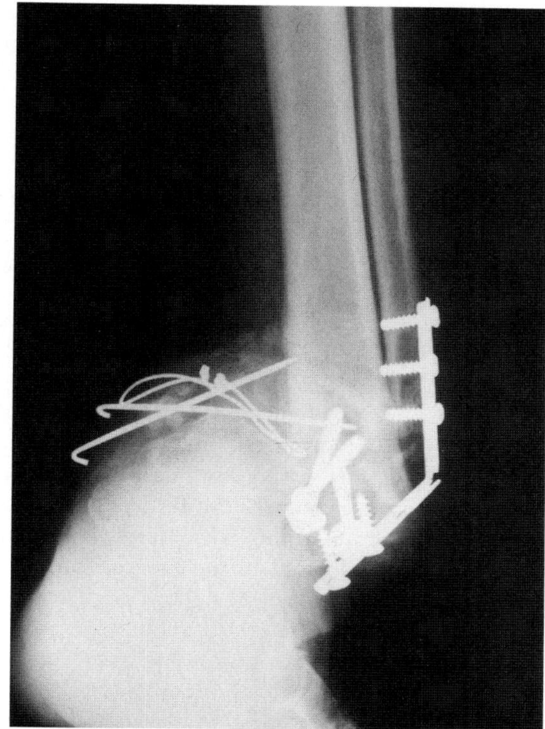

FIGURE 6.13

ANSWERS

1. **d** Malpositioned femoral tunnel. According to several studies, errors in surgical technique are the most common reasons for anterior cruciate ligament failure. The radiograph in Fig. 6.1 demonstrates a malpositioned femoral tunnel. Specifically, the tunnel is too anterior. The femoral origin of an anterior cruciate ligament graft should mimic the origin of the native anterior cruciate ligament. Thus, it should be positioned adjacent to the posterior femoral cortex ("the posterior wall").

   Excessively anterior placement of the femoral tunnel is a nonisometric position. If the femoral tunnel is malpositioned anteriorly and the graft is tensioned in *flexion,* it will be lax in extension. If the femoral tunnel is malpositioned anteriorly and the graft is tensioned in *extension*, it will subsequently either limit flexion or stretch out as flexion is regained over time and thus will become incompetent.

References

Penner DA, et al.: An In-Vitro Study of Anterior Cruciate Ligament Graft Placement and Isometry. Am J Sports Med, 16:238–243, 1988.

Vergis A, Gillquist J: Graft Failure in IntraArticular Anterior Cruciate Ligament Reconstructions: A Review of the Literature. Arthroscopy, 11:312–321, 1995.

Thompson W, Distefano V: IntraArticular ACL Reconstruction: Mechanism of Failure Analyzed at Revision. Arthroscopy, 11: 349–350, 1995.

2. **d** With a positive pivot shift test, the lateral tibial plateau begins in an anteriorly subluxated position. *Posterior* translation of the iliotibial band (relative to the lateral femoral condyle) during early flexion contributes to reduction of the lateral tibial plateau during a positive pivot shift test. In such a situation, anterior cruciate ligament insufficiency allows the lateral tibial plateau to start in an anteriorly subluxated and internally rotated position. As the knee is flexed, the iliotibial band translates posteriorly, becomes taut, and exerts an external rotation and posterior force on the tibia.

   The posterolateral structures (lateral cruciate ligament and arcuatecapsular ligament complex) are the primary restraints to external tibial rotation in all ranges of knee flexion. The posterior cruciate ligament is a *secondary* restraint to external tibial rotation in the higher range of knee flexion. Cutting the posterior cruciate ligament (subsequent to the posterolateral structures) will further increase external tibial rotation. However, cutting the posterior cruciate ligament alone (leaving the posterolateral structures intact) will not increase external tibial rotation. The posterolateral structures are the primary restraints to *varus* (not valgus) knee instability in *all* ranges of knee flexion.

Reference

Galway RD, et al.: Pivot Shift: A Clinical Sign of Symptomatic ACL Insufficiency. J Bone Joint Surg Br, 54:763–776, 1972.

3. **b** The insertion of the popliteus tendon. Fig. 6.2 is a coronal T1-weighted magnetic resonance image of a right knee. The arrow is superimposed on the lateral femoral condyle. Two factors that assist in determining that this is the lateral side of the knee are as follows: (1) the anterior calf musculature, which originates from the lateral side of the tibia, is seen in the lower left corner of the image; (2) the anterior cruciate ligament is seen running from its origin on the medial aspect of the lateral femoral condyle to its insertion along the tibial spine. The *semimembranosus* tendon inserts on the medial side of the femur.

   The *biceps femoris* tendon and the *lateral collateral ligament* insert on the fibular head, which is posterior to the plane of this image. As depicted in this image, the *popliteus tendon* inserts on the femur within a groove that is deep to the lateral cruciate ligament.

   Note: In cases of putative posterolateral corner injury, this location must be closely examined for evidence of popliteus tendon avulsion.

4. **b** Both tibial plateaus are concave in the sagittal plane. The medial plateau is concave in the sagittal plane. However, the lateral plateau is convex in the sagittal plane. This difference in sagittal contour is a useful means of identifying which compartment one is viewing during an evaluation of sagittal magnetic resonance images. The sulcus terminalis is a distinguishing feature of the lateral femoral condyle. It is best visualized on plain lateral radiographs or sagittal magnetic resonance images.

   The knee does not function as a simple hinge. Knee flexion is polycentric. There is obligatory internal rotation of the femur with respect to the tibia during terminal knee extension. This is referred to as the *screw home mechanism.*

5. **b** 5%. Moore et al. retrospectively reviewed 309 consecutive patients with 320 diaphyseal femur fractures and noted a 5.3% incidence of ipsilateral knee ligament injuries (grade II or greater).

   Note: The Hansen rule dictates that after successful completion of intramedullary nailing of the femur, two duties must be performed and documented: (1) a thorough ligamentous examination of the ipsilateral knee and (2) radiographic confirmation of the absence of an ipsilateral femoral neck fracture.

Reference

Moore TM, Patzakis MJ, Harvey JP: Ipsilateral Diaphyseal Femur Fractures and Knee Ligament Injuries. Clin Orthop, 232:182–189, 1988.

6. **c** The Blumensaat line. On a lateral knee film, the roof of the intercondylar notch appears as a discrete sclerotic line. This line is referred to as the *Blumensaat line.* The extension of this line should intersect the inferior pole of the patella when the knee is flexed to 30 degrees. Patella alta is present when the Blumensaat line intersects the extensor mechanism distally to the inferior pole of the patella. Other radiographic indicators of patella alta include (1) an Insall-Salvati ratio of greater than 1.2 and (2) a Blackburn-Peel ratio of greater than 1.0.

   Note: The *Insall-Salvati* ratio is the ratio of patellar tendon length to patellar length. The *Blackburn-Peel ratio* is the ratio of (1) the perpendicular distance between the anterior extension of the tibial plateau and the lower end of the patellar articular surface to (2) the length of the patellar articular surface. (Both these ratios are measured on lateral radiographs.)

References

Blackburn JS, Peel TE: A New Method for Determining Patellar Height. J Bone Joint Surg Br, 59:241–242, 1977.
Insall J, Salvati E: Patella Position in the Normal Knee Joint. Radiology, 101: 101–104, 1971.

7. **a** The iliotibial tract and the biceps femoris tendon. Seebacher et al. described a three layer concept of the posterolateral aspect of the knee in their classic article. *Layer I* consists of the iliotibial tract, the biceps femoris tendon, and their fascial expansions. *Layer II* includes the lateral patellar retinaculum. *Layer III* consists of superficial and deep laminae. The superficial lamina includes the fabellofibular and lateral collateral ligaments; the deep lamina includes the arcuate ligament and joint capsule.

Reference

Seebacher JR, Inglis AE, Marshall JL, Warren RF: The Structure of the Posterolateral Aspect of the Knee. J Bone Joint Surg Am, 64:536–541, 1982.

8. **e** Radial tear of the lateral meniscus. Two factors indicate that this image intersects the lateral compartment: (1) the presence of the fibular head and (2) the convex contour of the tibial articular surface (the medial tibial plateau is concave).

   The posterior horn of the lateral meniscus is entirely absent in this image, and the anterior horn is normal. Bucket handle tears typically propagate within the substance of the meniscus, and, thus, a peripheral rim of intact meniscus would remain intact. No peripheral remnant of the posterior horn remains in this image. Furthermore, if a bucket-handle fragment had displaced medially, then its connecting limb should be seen traversing the plane of this image. The most reasonable explanation for the complete absence of the posterior horn in Fig. 6.3 is that the plane of the image lies within the plane of a radial tear that extends all the way to the capsule.
9. **c** IV. Many different types of collagen have been identified within the meniscus. The most prevalent form is type I (approximately 90%). The menisci also contain type I, type II, type V, and type VI collagen.

   Type IV collagen is associated with basement membranes (lamina densa), but it has not been isolated from meniscal tissue. Unlike most other forms of collagen, basement membrane collagen is not fibrillar.

References

Arnoczky S, et al.: Meniscus. In Woo S, Buckwalter JA, eds: Injury and Repair of the Musculoskeletal Soft Tissues. Rosemont, IL, American Academy of Orthopedic Surgeons, pp. 483–548, 1988.
Eyre DR, et al.: Biochemistry of the Meniscus: Unique Profile of Collagen Types and Site Dependent Variations in Composition. Orthop Trans, 8:56, 1983.

10. **d** The middle geniculate artery. The middle geniculate artery is the principal blood supply to the anterior and posterior cruciate ligaments. The middle geniculate artery is a direct branch of the popliteal artery.

Reference

Arnoczky SP: Blood Supply to the Anterior Cruciate Ligament and Supporting Structures. Orthop Clin North Am, 16:15–28, 1985.

11. **b** The lateral aspect of the medial femoral condyle. Osteochondritis dissecans of the knee classically occurs at the *lateral* aspect of the medial femoral condyle. Standard anteroposterior radiographs of the knee may miss this lesion because the lesion is often located relatively posteriorly on the condyle. Thus, an intercondylar notch view *(tunnel view)* is more sensitive. The lateral radiograph typically demonstrates that the affected segment of the medial femoral condyle is contained within a region defined by the intersection of the Blumensaat line and the continuation of a line along the posterior femoral cortex. This region is referred to as the *Harding area* (Fig. 6.14).

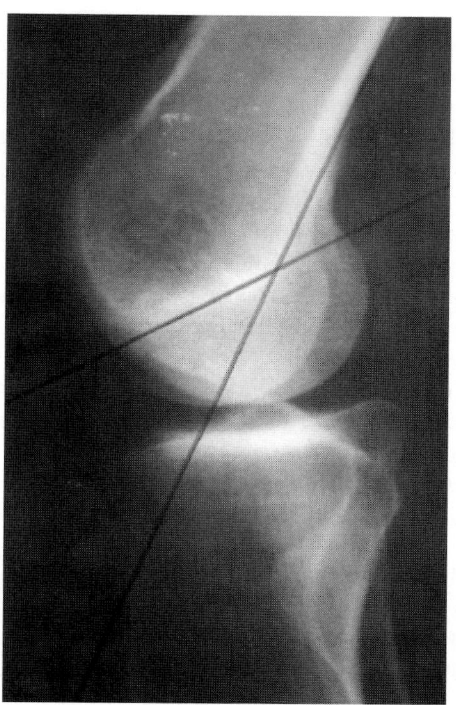

FIGURE 6.14

Note: Osteochondritis dissecans lesions on the lateral femoral condyle are more likely to be located on the central portion of the condyle.

Reference

Aichroth P: Osteochondritis Dissecans of the Knee: A Clinical Survey. J Bone Joint Surg Br, 53:440–447, 1971.

12. **c** 50% to 70%. Krause and colleagues demonstrated that the menisci transmit 30% to 55% of the load across the knee in the standing position.

    Ahmed and Burke demonstrated that medial meniscectomy reduced the contact area between the weight-bearing surfaces in the medial compartment by 50% to 70%. Thus, stress on the involved articular surfaces is increased. The increased stress is a function of a constant load applied across a decreased contact area.

    Note: Stress = Force/Area.

References

Ahmed AM, Burke DL: *In-Vitro* Measurement of Static Pressure Distribution in Synovial Joints. I. Tibial Surface of the Knee. J Biomech Eng, 105: 216–225, 1983.

Krause WR, et al.: Mechanical Changes in the Knee After Meniscectomy. J Bone Joint Surg Am, 58:599–604, 1976.

13. **e** The semitendinosus tendon. The semitendinosus is part of the per anserinus (sartorius, gracilis) and inserts anteromedially on the tibia. The *iliotibial band* inserts on the Gerdy tubercle. *The lateral collateral ligament* and *biceps femoris* insert on the fibular head.

    Both the *semitendinosus* and the *semimembranosus* insert on the *medial* side of the tibia. These two tendons run obliquely (posterior to anterior) and therefore would not appear as robust, vertically oriented structures in a single coronal image.

    Note: The lateral collateral ligament is oriented obliquely (proximal anterior to distal posterior). Thus, it is not typically completely visualized on a single coronal magnetic resonance image. Visualization of the entire length of the lateral collateral ligament on a single coronal image is a secondary sign of anterior cruciate ligament insufficiency. Anterior subluxation of the lateral side of the knee produces vertical orientation (loss of sagittal plane obliquity) of the lateral cruciate ligament.

14. **e** Lyme titer. The clinical manifestations of Lyme disease have been grouped into three stages: (I) localized erythema migrans, (II) disseminated infection, and (III) persistent infection.

    Stage III disease often demonstrates an intermittent asymmetric oligoarthritis with a predilection for large joints, particularly the knee. The symptoms of stage II disease include fatigue, malaise, migratory musculoskeletal pain, cardiac dysfunction, and many different neurologic abnormalities (e.g., cerebellar ataxia, meningitis, encephalopathy, and cranial neuropathy).

    Note: The organism responsible for Lyme disease is *Borrelia burgdorferi*. The associated tick vector is *Ixodes dammini.*

References

Schmidli J, et al.: Cultivation of *Borrelia burgdorferi* from Joint Fluid 3 Months After Treatment of Facial Nerve Palsy. J Infect Dis, 158:905, 1988.

Steere AC, et al.: The Clinical Evolution of Lyme Arthritis. Ann Intern Med, 107:725, 1987.

15. **e** An isolated grade II lateral cruciate ligament tear may produce a false-positive 2B Lachman test. A displaced meniscal tear may block anterior tibial translation and thus may create a false-negative Lachman or pivot shift test.

    Posterior cruciate ligament insufficiency may yield a false impression of abnormal anterior tibial translation when a Lachman test is performed because the tibia starts in a posteriorly subluxated position. Yet the Lachman end point should be solid in this setting. Patient apprehension may decrease the sensitivity of the pivot shift maneuver because hamstring guarding may prevent anterior tibial subluxation.

    Medial collateral ligament insufficiency is another potential source of a false-negative pivot shift because the pivot shift requires an intact medial hinge on which to pivot. Although the medial collateral ligament is a significant secondary restraint to anterior tibial translation in a medial collateral ligament–deficient knee, neither the medial collateral ligament nor the lateral cruciate ligament provides significant restraint to anterior tibial translation in an anterior cruciate ligament–competent knee. Thus, an isolated lateral cruciate ligament injury could not yield a false-positive Lachman test.

Reference

Torg JS, et al.: Clinical Diagnosis of ACL Instability in the Athlete. Am J Sports Med, 4:84–91, 1976.

16. **c** It is performed with varus stress. The pivot shift test is a sign of posterolateral rotatory instability. With a positive reverse pivot shift test, the lateral tibial plateau begins in a posteriorly subluxated position and reduces at approximately 20 to 30 degrees of flexion as the knee is extended with concomitant valgus and axial loads.

    Note: Approximately one-third of physiologically normal persons may manifest bilateral positive reverse pivot shift tests during an examination performed while these persons are under anesthesia. Thus, the contralateral knee should always be examined as an internal control. The presence of a reverse pivot shift should not be considered abnormal unless this finding is absent in the contralateral knee.

Reference

Cooper DE: Tests for Posterolateral Instability of the Knee in Normal Subjects. J Bone Joint Surg Am, 73:30–36, 1991.

17. **c** An anterior cruciate ligament nodule. The most likely explanation for this patient's loss of extension is the development of an anterior cruciate ligament nodule *(cyclops lesion).* This lesion consists of a nodule of hypertrophic fibrous tissue that presumptively originates from residual tissue anterior to the tibial tunnel. This nodule produces a mechanical block to terminal extension, but it does not limit flexion.

    Arthrofibrosis is a more generalized intraarticular scarring process that typically produces a loss of both flexion and extension. The finding that full motion was achieved on the operating room table renders the other choices (excessive graft tensioning and graft malposition) unlikely explanations. The radiograph demonstrates good tunnel position. Graft failure usually does not result in loss of motion.

Reference

Marzo JM, et al.: Intra-Articular Fibrous Nodule as a Cause of Loss of Extension Following Anterior Cruciate Ligament Reconstruction. Arthroscopy, 8: 10–18, 1992.

18. **d** The central third patellar tendon allograft (15-mm width). Many donor tissues have been used as grafts to reconstruct the anterior cruciate ligament. In their classic article, Noyes et al. compared the tensile strengths of various autograft materials in an *in vitro* model using young adult tissues. The maximal tensile loads were as shown in Table 6.1. The tensile strength of the central third patellar tendon bone-patella-tendon-bone (BTB) autograft contributed to its widespread popularity in anterior cruciate ligament reconstruction.

    Note: This *in vitro* study pertains only to the initial tensile strength of various graft tissues. It does not address graft fixation strength or the *in vivo* changes of graft tensile strength with remodeling over time.

Reference

Noyes F, et al.: Biomechanical Analysis of Human Ligament Grafts Used in Knee Ligament Repairs and Reconstructions. J Bone Joint Surg Am, 66: 344–352, 1984.

TABLE 6.1. MAXIMAL TENSILE LOADS

Tissue	Maximal Load (n)
Central one-third patellar tendon	2,900
Medial one-third patellar tendon	2,734
Native anterior cruciate ligament	*1,725*
Semitendinosus	1,216
Gracilis	838
Distal iliotibial tract	769
Fascia lata	628

19. **d** Iliotibial band friction syndrome. This history and physical examination are characteristic of iliotibial band friction syndrome. Affected patients are typically involved in activities that require repetitive knee flexion (e.g., longdistance running or cycling). The lateral knee pain is often exacerbated by running downhill or climbing stairs. Maximum pain is typically experienced at 30 degrees of flexion. The pain is believed to originate from friction between the iliotibial band and the lateral femoral condyle. Physical examination typically demonstrates tenderness over the lateral condyle approximately 3 cm proximal to the joint line.

    Note: A positive Ober test is indicative of iliotibial band tightness. This is a predisposing factor for iliotibial band friction syndrome.

Reference

Noble CA: Iliotibial Band Friction Syndrome in Runners. Am J Sports Med, 8:232–234, 1980.

20. **e** Rigid foot orthotic to prevent hyperpronation. The diagnosis of iliotibial band syndrome is made clinically. Given a classic history and physical examination, a magnetic resonance imaging scan or bone scan would be unwarranted. Arthroscopy would be an inappropriate intervention in this setting from both a diagnostic and a therapeutic perspective.

    Initial treatment of iliotibial band friction syndrome should always consist of conservative modalities such as nonsteroidal antiinflammatory drugs, activity modification, and iliotibial band stretching. Correctable biomechanical diatheses should also be addressed. Specifically, rigid orthotics should be prescribed for patients who hyperpronate, and *lateral* wedge orthotics should be prescribed for patients with tight iliotibial bands or functional genu varum.

    Patients with iliotibial band friction syndrome who fail to respond to conservative measures may require local steroid injection or (in particularly recalcitrant circumstances) surgical treatment to decompress the involved portion of the iliotibial band.

References

Cox JS, Blanda JB: Peripatellar Pathologies. In Delee JC, Drez D, eds: Orthopaedic Sports Medicine. Philadelphia, WB Saunders, pp. 1251–1252, 1994.
Noble CA: Iliotibial Band Friction Syndrome in Runners. Am J Sports Med, 8:232–234, 1980.

21. **c** Magnetic resonance imaging. If the articular cartilage over an osteochondritis dissecans fragment is discontinuous, then synovial fluid will be permitted to

track around the perimeter of the fragment. This *fluid sign* is readily apparent on T2-weighted magnetic resonance imaging sequences.

Reference

Mesgarzadeh M, et al.: Osteochondritis Dissecans: Analysis of Mechanical Stability with Radiography, Scintigraphy, and MRI Imaging. Radiology, 165: 775, 1987.

22. **c** Hip abducted; leg externally rotated. Classically, the foot is held in internal rotation while a valgus stress is placed on the knee. Gradual flexion results in reduction of the tibia from the anteriorly subluxated position, with a consequent shift at approximately 20 to 30 degrees of flexion. Testing with the foot internally rotated, as originally described, is less sensitive for detecting anterior cruciate ligament deficiency. External rotation of the foot with abduction of the hip confers greater sensitivity.

Reference

Bach BR, et al.: The Pivot Shift Phenomenon. Am J Sports Med, 16:571–576, 1988.

23. **d** The *posterior* horn of the medial meniscus is a *secondary* restraint to anterior tibial translation. The anterior cruciate ligament is the primary restraint to anterior tibial translation. When the anterior cruciate ligament is intact, the medial meniscus does not affect anterior to posterior translation of the knee. However, in an anterior cruciate ligament–deficient knee, the posterior horn of the medial meniscus limits anterior tibial translation by becoming wedged between the tibial plateau and the medial femoral condyle. Thus, excision of the posterior horn of the medial meniscus in an anterior cruciate ligament–deficient knee will further compromise knee stability. Furthermore, this phenomenon explains why the posterior horn of the medial meniscus may be at risk of injury when the anterior cruciate ligament is incompetent.

Reference

Levy IM, Torzilli PA, Warren RF: The Effect of Medial Meniscectomy on Anterior-Posterior Motion of the Knee. J Bone Joint Surg Am, 64:883–888, 1982.

24. **a** Most of the collagen fibers in the menisci are oriented radially. The menisci are composed of fibrocartilage; 70% of their dry weight is collagen (90% of which is type I collagen). Most of the collagen fibers are oriented *circumferentially,* and this corresponds to their purpose of resisting hoop stresses. Smaller numbers of radial fibers serve as "ties" to prevent longitudinal splitting of the more prevalent circumferential fibers. The lateral meniscus covers a higher percentage of the lateral tibial plateau (approximately 70%), as compared with the medial meniscus' coverage of the medial plateau (approximately 30%). Only the peripheral third of the menisci has a vascular supply. The implication of the vascular anatomy of the menisci is that only tears of the peripheral third have potential to heal. Most of the meniscus receives its nutrition from the synovial fluid by either passive diffusion or by the mechanical pumping induced by weight bearing and motion.

    The lateral meniscus has approximately twice the excursion (approximately 12 mm) of the medial meniscus (approximately 6 mm). This finding is frequently invoked to account for the higher incidence of tears in the medial meniscus. Histologic studies have demonstrated neural elements in the peripheral third of the menisci. The presence of mechanoreceptors suggests that the meniscal neural tissue potentially plays a significant sensory feedback role.

Reference

Bullough PG, et al.: The Strength of the Menisci of the Knee as it Relates to Their Fine Structure. J Bone Joint Surg Br, 52:564–570, 1970.

25. **a** Quadriceps rehabilitation. The patient's mechanism of injury and physical examination are characteristic of an *isolated* posterior cruciate ligament tear. Most authorities agree that isolated acute posterior cruciate ligament deficiency should be treated nonoperatively. The focus of nonoperative management is restoration of full motion followed by aggressive quadriceps strengthening.

    Examination while the patient is under anesthesia is often useful to rule out associated ligamentous disease. It is crucial to exclude associated ligamentous damage definitively because acute combined ligament injuries of all types warrant surgical intervention. It has been suggested that more than 10 mm of posterior drawer excursion in the setting of a suspected "isolated" posterior cruciate ligament tear may represent an occult combined injury rather than a true isolated posterior cruciate ligament injury, and such injuries are often managed operatively.

Reference

Veltri DM, Warren RF: Isolated and Combined PCL Injuries. J Am Acad Orthop Surg, 1(2):67–75, 1993.

26. **e** The inferior fibers of the semitendinosus diverge to form an accessory insertion. The semitendinosus and gracilis tendons are readily available for harvesting as autograft material with little donor site morbidity provided that the local anatomy is well understood.

The semitendinosus and gracilis tendons have a conjoined insertion on the tibia. The proximal point of this insertion is approximately 2 cm distal and 2 cm medial to the apex of the tibial tubercle. The semitendinosus and gracilis pass superficial to the medial collateral ligament. The semitendinosus runs on the distal side of the gracilis tendon.

The inferior fibers of the semitendinosus diverge from the main tendon (approximately 5.5 cm proximal to the main insertion) to form an accessory insertion on the tibia approximately 3 cm distal to the conjoined tendon insertion. This accessory insertion should be divided to facilitate graft harvest and to minimize damage to the tendon during retrograde harvesting with a tendon stripper.

Reference

Pagnani MJ, et al.: Anatomic Considerations in Harvesting the Semitendinosus and Gracilis Tendons and a Technique of Harvest. Am J Sports Med, 21(4):565–571, 1993.

27. **e** Conjoined tibial insertion with the sartorius. The principal insertion of the semimembranosus is at the posteromedial tibia just distal to the joint line. A second insertion onto the tibia extends further anteriorly (deep to the medial collateral ligament). Additional fibers extend to the oblique popliteal ligament, the posteromedial knee capsule and posterior oblique ligament (over the medial meniscus), and the fascia of the popliteus muscle. The sartorius inserts further anteriorly and more superficially than any of the expansions of the semimembranosus.

The semimembranosus is innervated by the tibial division of the sciatic nerve. The tibial portion of the sciatic nerve also innervates the posterior portion of the adductor magnus (which, despite its name, functions as a medial hamstring). Aside from its primary function as a knee flexor, the semimembranosus functions as a hip extender and internal rotator of the tibia.

Note: The medial hamstrings are innervated by L5, and the lateral hamstrings and gluteus maximus are innervated by S1.

References

Jobe CM, Wright: Anatomy of the Knee. In Fu FH, et al., eds: Knee Surgery. Baltimore, Williams & Wilkins, p. 27, 1994.

Warren LF, Marshal JL: The Supporting Structures and Layers on the Medial Side of the Knee. J Bone Joint Surg Am, 61:56–62, 1979.

28. **d** Meniscal cyst. Fig. 6.5 reveals a wellcircumscribed, homogeneous subcutaneous mass resting on the medial surface of the medial collateral ligament. The intermediate signal intensity on T1-weighted imaging (Fig. 6.5A) and the high signal intensity on T2-weighted imaging (Fig. 6.5B) suggest high water content. The cyst appears to track posteriorly along the medial joint line, with continuity between the cyst and a horizontal cleavage tear of the posterior horn of the medial meniscus.

29. **b** Water. Water accounts for most of the weight of both articular cartilage and meniscus tissue (60% to 85%). Most of this water is extracellular. Proteoglycans comprise 5% to 10% of the wet weight of articular cartilage. Type II collagen is the most abundant form of collagen in articular cartilage.

References

Mankin HJ, Thrasher AZ: Water Content and Binding in Normal and Osteoarthritic Human Articular Cartilage. J Bone Joint Surg Am, 57: 76–80, 1975.

Mow VC, et al.: Structure and Function of Articular Cartilage and Meniscus. In Mow VC, Hayes WC, eds: Basic Orthopaedic Biomechanics. New York, Raven, pp. 143–198, 1991.

30. **d** For a given anterior translation of the tibial tubercle, a longer tibial osteotomy will produce a greater vertical translation of the patella. The Maquet procedure is a technique for displacing the tibial tubercle anteriorly in an effort to decrease patellofemoral compressive forces. This is accomplished by an opening wedge coronal tibial osteotomy. The tubercle is translated anteriorly as it is rotated on an intact distal soft tissue hinge. A wedge of iliac crest autograft is inserted to maintain the displacement.

Because of the intact distal hinge, anterior translation of the tubercle is coupled to distal translation of the patella. There is concomitant rotation of the patella around a horizontal axis as the inferior pole of the patella is displaced further anteriorly than the proximal pole. This rotation in the sagittal plane decreases patellofemoral contact area and shifts the point of patellofemoral contact proximally. The greater the magnitude of anterior tubercle translation, the larger is the decrease in patellofemoral contact area. For a given anterior displacement of the tibial tubercle, a longer tibial osteotomy will produce a *smaller* vertical translation of the patella.

Note: Although the Maquet procedure is intended to decrease patellofemoral contact pressure, the associated decrease in patellofemoral contact area ultimately offsets the decrease in compressive force. Thus, excessive anterior translation of the tubercle can cause abnormally high focal contact pressures (Pressure = Force/Area).

References

Hayes WC, et al.: Patellofemoral Contact Pressures and the Effects of Surgical Reconstructive Procedures. In Articular Cartilage and Knee Joint Function: Basic Science and Arthroscopy. New York, Raven, p. 57, 1990.

Nakamura N, et al.: Advancement of the Tibial Tuberosity: A Biomechanical Study. J Bone Joint Surg Br, 67:255, 1985.

31. **b** The femoral origin of the posterior cruciate ligament is longer in the anteroposterior dimension than in the vertical dimension. The posterior cruciate ligament is composed of two principal fiber bundles: (1) the anterolateral bundle, which becomes taut in *flexion;* and (2) the posteromedial bundle, which tightens in extension. The femoral attachment of the posterior cruciate ligament is positioned high and anteriorly on the medial side of the intercondylar notch. The footprint of the femoral attachment has an oblong shape that is longer in the anteroposterior dimension than in the vertical dimension.

The meniscofemoral ligaments of Humphry and Wrisberg connect the posterior horn of the lateral meniscus to the lateral aspect of the medial femoral condyle. The *ligament of Humphry* runs *anteriorly* to the posterior cruciate ligament. The *ligament of Wrisberg* runs *posteriorly* to the posterior cruciate ligament.

The *anterolateral* portion of the posterior cruciate ligament is stronger, stiffer, and larger than the posteromedial segment of the ligament. Because the anterolateral bundle is structurally and functionally more significant, a single-bundle posterior cruciate ligament reconstruction aims to reconstruct this portion of the native ligament. Thus, a single-bundle posterior cruciate ligament graft should be tensioned in approximately 70 to 80 degrees of flexion. If one were to tension the anterolateral bundle in extension, then flexion could be restricted because these fibers typically tighten further as the knee flexes.

Note: Some authorities currently advocate a double-bundle graft as a means of more precisely reconstructing the normal anatomy and function of both the anterolateral and the posteromedial segments of the posterior cruciate ligament.

Reference

Van Dommelen BA, Fowler PR: Anatomy of the Posterior Cruciate Ligament: A Review. Am J Sports Med, 17:24–29, 1989.

32. **a** Activity modification. The history, examination, and radiographs suggest a diagnosis of juvenile osteochondritis dissecans. This condition has a relatively benign natural history compared with its adult counterpart. If symptoms are mild, then most patients' symptoms will resolve spontaneously with activity modification alone, and the longterm prognosis is good. The intact articular cartilage over the lesion (Fig. 6.6B) is another favorable prognostic sign.

Note: The *Wilson* sign refers to the induction of pain as the knee is passively extended while the tibia is held in internal rotation. The patient experiences discomfort as the tibial spine contacts the region of osteochondritis dissecans on the lateral aspect of the medial femoral condyle at approximately 30 degrees of flexion. (This sign is neither perfectly sensitive nor perfectly specific for osteochondritis dissecans.)

References

Linden B: Osteochondritis Dissecans of the Femoral Condyles: A Long-Term Follow-Up Study. J Bone Joint Surg Am, 59:769–776, 1977.
Wilson JN: A Diagnostic Sign in Osteochondritis Dissecans of the Knee. J Bone Joint Surg Am, 49:477–480, 1967.

33. **e** Medial meniscal tear. An acute combined disruption of the anterior cruciate ligament and the medial collateral ligament is typically the result of a combined valgus and rotational deformation. The valgus component of the force creates compression across the lateral compartment. Distinct contusion signals may be evident (by magnetic resonance imaging) in the subchondral bone at the point of impact between the lateral femoral condyle and the lateral tibial plateau. The compression and shear across the lateral compartment may produce a tear of the lateral meniscus. There is relative distraction across the medial compartment rendering medial femoral condyle contusion unlikely.

Note: Despite the classic concept of O'Donoghue's "unhappy triad" (anterior cruciate ligament tear, medial collateral ligament tear, and medial meniscal tear), research has reported that there is a much higher incidence of lateral meniscus tears (versus medial) in the setting of acute combined anterior cruciate ligament–medial collateral ligament injuries.

References

Shelbourne KD, Nitz PA: The O'Donoghue Triad Revisited: Combined Injuries Involving the Anterior Cruciate Ligament and Medial Collateral Ligament. Am J Sports Med, 19:474–477, 1991.

Vellet AD, et al.: Occult Post-Traumatic Injuries of the Knee: Prevalence, Classification, and Shortterm Sequelae Evaluated with MRI Imaging. Radiology, 178:271–276, 1991.

34. **a** Anterior cruciate ligament injury. The plain anteroposterior radiograph (Fig. 6.7) reveals an avulsion fracture from the tibia at the lateral joint line. This lesion had been referred to as a "Segond fracture." It indicates avulsion of the lateral capsule from the tibia, and it is commonly associated with anterior cruciate ligament injury.

Note: A *Pellegrini-Stieda* lesion refers to calcification at the femoral attachment of the medial collateral ligament. It is indicative of prior trauma to the medial collateral ligament.

References

Segond P: Recherches Cliniques et Experimentales sur les Epanchements Sanguines du Genou par Entorse. Prog Med, 1879.
Woods GW, et al.: Lateral Capsular Sign: X-Ray Clue to a Significant Knee Instability. Am J Sports Med, 7:27–33, 1979.

35. **a** The anteromedial fibers are under less tension when the knee is extended. The anteromedial portion of the

anterior cruciate ligament is under greater tension when the knee is flexed than when it is extended. The opposite is true for the posterolateral fibers of the anterior cruciate ligament. Cadaveric studies have consistently demonstrated that the average length of the adult anterior cruciate ligament is less than 40 mm. (The classic investigation by Girgus et al. reported an average length of 38 mm.) The anterior cruciate ligament inserts on the anterior aspect of the intercondylar eminence of the tibia. The dimensions of this attachment are greater in the anterior to posterior direction than in the medial to lateral direction. Most tears occur in the *proximal* half of the ligament.

References

Girgis FG, et al.: The Cruciate Ligaments of the Knee Joint. Clin Orthop, 106:222–231, 1975.

Sherman MF, et al.: The LongTerm Followup of Primary ACL Repair. Am J Sports Med, 19:243–255, 1991.

36. **e** Popliteal cyst. The T1-weighted and fat-suppressed T2-weighted sagittal magnetic resonance images in Figs. 6.6 to 6.8 reveal a bilobed, well-circumscribed homogeneous mass in the popliteal fossa. The two lobes are separated by the semimembranosus tendon. The signal intensity of the contents of the lesion (intermediate on T1 and bright on T2) is consistent with fluid. Solid tumors (such as synovial sarcoma or liposarcoma) would not yield as bright and homogeneous a signal. These signal characteristics could be consistent with either a popliteal cyst or a meniscal cyst.

Pigmented villonodular synovitis is capable of producing a juxtaarticular mass. However, the absence of an effusion or intrasynovial proliferative changes in this case renders pigmented villonodular synovitis an unlikely diagnosis. Furthermore, the signal intensity within regions of pigmented villonodular synovitis is characteristically heterogeneous because of the signal void effect within regions of hemosiderin deposition.

Popliteal cysts characteristically communicate with the posteromedial aspect at the normal orifice between the knee joint and the gastrocnemius-semimembranosus bursa. As they fill with synovial fluid, they expand between the medial head of the gastrocnemius and the semimembranosus tendon. The images are not consistent with a meniscal cyst given the absence of a meniscal tear at the location where the cyst communicates with the knee joint.

Reference

Burk DL, et al.: Meniscal and Ganglion Cysts of the Knee: MR Evaluation. AJR Am J Roentgenol, 150:331–336, 1988.

37. **b** Isolated posterolateral corner injury. The two principal components of the posterolateral corner are the lateral collateral ligament and the arcuate popliteus complex. The arcuate popliteus complex consists of the arcuate ligament, the popliteus tendon, the posterolateral capsule, and the fabellofibular ligament. Selective ligament cutting studies have demonstrated that the lateral cruciate ligament and arcuate popliteus complex are the primary restraints to varus rotation and external tibial rotation at all angles of knee flexion. Isolated cutting of the lateral cruciate ligament and arcuate popliteus complex will produce increased varus rotation and increased external tibial rotation at all angles of knee flexion (with the greatest increase at 30 degrees of flexion). Insufficiency of these structures also produces a slight increase in posterior tibial translation at 30 degrees. Sectioning the posterior cruciate ligament in addition to the posterolateral corner will lead to a significant increase in posterior tibial translation and varus rotation at all angles of flexion.

Isolated posterior cruciate ligament disruption leads to increased posterior tibial translation at all angles of knee flexion. Maximal posterior translation after isolated posterior cruciate ligament sectioning occurs at 90 degrees. Isolated sectioning of the posterior cruciate ligament does not produce increased varus rotation or external tibial rotation at any angle of flexion. Sectioning the posterolateral corner in addition to the posterior cruciate ligament will lead to a further increase in external tibial rotation at 90 degrees.

References

Gollehon DL, Torzilli PA, Warren RF: The Role of the Posterolateral and Cruciate Ligaments in the Stability of the Human Knee. J Bone Joint Surg Am, 69:233–242, 1987.

Veltri DM, Warren RF: Isolated and Combined PCL Injuries. J Am Acad Orthop Surg, 1:67–75, 1993.

38. **d** Creep. Viscoelastic materials (such as tendons and ligaments) have both viscous and elastic properties. They demonstrate time-dependent stress-strain behavior (creep and stress relaxation). *Stress relaxation* refers to decreasing stress over time under a constant deformation. *Creep* refers to increasing deformation over time under a constant load. *Hysteresis* refers to a variation between the load-elongation curves during loading versus unloading. An *anisotropic* structure is one that exhibits different mechanical properties depending on the direction of testing relative to its geometric form.

Note: Bone is an anisotropic material.

Reference

Taylor DC, et al.: Viscoelastic Properties of Muscle-Tendon Units. Am J Sports Med, 18:300–309, 1990.

39. **a** An 18-year-old man with an acute 1.5-cm longitudinal peripheral tear of the lateral meniscus who is

undergoing a concurrent anterior cruciate ligament reconstruction. The optimal circumstances for meniscal repair include (1) young patient age, (2) acute meniscal disease (versus chronic), (3) a longitudinal pattern (versus radial or flap), and (4) peripheral tear location (within the vascular portion of the meniscus). The healing potential of a meniscal tear is worse in the setting of anterior cruciate ligament insufficiency that is not concurrently addressed. Cannon and Vittori demonstrated that patients undergoing concomitant anterior cruciate ligament reconstruction have a better chance of a successful meniscal repair (93%) compared with patients undergoing isolated meniscal repairs in anterior cruciate ligament–competent knees (50%).

Reference

Cannon WD, Vittori JM: The Incidence of Healing in Arthroscopic Meniscal Repairs in Anterior Cruciate Ligament Reconstructed Knees Versus Stable Knees. Am J Sports Med, 20:176–181, 1992.

40. **c** The inferior lateral geniculate artery. The arrow marks the cross-sectional image of a tubular structure running in the anterior to posterior direction immediately distal to the lateral joint line. The structure is extracapsular but deep to the lateral collateral ligament and the biceps tendon.

Note: The inferolateral geniculate artery runs between the superficial and deep laminae of layer III.

Reference

Seebacher JR, Inglis AE, Marshall JL, Warren RF: The Structure of the Posterolateral Aspect of the Knee. J Bone Joint Surg Am, 64:536–541, 1982.

41. **c** Hypertrophic cardiomyopathy. The most condition that is most frequently associated with sudden cardiac death in young athletes is hypertrophic cardiomyopathy. Less common associated conditions include viral myocarditis, mitral valve prolapse, congenital coronary artery anomalies, Marfan syndrome, premature coronary atherosclerosis, QT interval prolongation syndromes, and right ventricular dysplasia.

Patients with hypertrophic cardiomyopathy may participate in strenuous athletics for many years without significant symptoms. Sudden death in these persons typically occurs during or immediately after a period of strenuous exertion. The structural defect is believed to predispose the athlete to a fatal arrhythmia.

Echocardiography is the most sensitive screening tool for this condition. However, universal screening is not economically feasible.

References

Maron BJ: Sudden Death in Athletes: Risk Factors and Screening. J Musculoskel Med, 8(7):63–78, 1991.

Van Camp SP: Exercise-Related Sudden Deaths: Risks and Causes. Physician Sports Med, 16:97–112, 1988.

42. **c** Medial collateral ligament tear. Knee injuries account for 20% to 30% of all alpine skiing injuries. Medial collateral ligament tears account for 60% of knee injuries in skiers and 15% to 20% of all skiing injuries.

Note: The incidence of lateral meniscal tears is greater than that of medial meniscal tears among alpine skiers.

Reference

Paletta GA, Warren RF: Knee Injuries and Alpine Skiing. Sports Med, 17: 411–423, 1994.

43. **d** A concomitant open procedure. In a study by Williams et al., seven postoperative infections were discovered in a review of 2,500 consecutive arthroscopic anterior cruciate ligament reconstructions using patellar tendon or hamstring autografts. Most patients presented with increasing knee pain or persistent drainage. The most consistent physical finding was a large persistent effusion. Laboratory studies revealed an elevated erythrocyte sedimentation rate in all cases. However, the average white blood cell count was within normal limits. Knee aspirates done in the office isolated the organism in each case. *Staphylococcus aureus* was the most common pathogen. These patients required multiple irrigations and débridements to eradicate the infection. The original autografts were retained in three of the seven cases. Six of the seven patients who developed septic arthritis had undergone a concomitant open secondary procedure, including medial collateral ligament reconstruction, meniscus repair, or posterolateral corner reconstruction.

Reference

Williams X, Laurencin X, Warren X, et al.: Am J Sports Med, 25(2):261–267, 1997.

44. **c** Increased water concentration. During normal aging, there is a *decrease* in the water content of articular cartilage. This is in contrast to osteoarthritis, in which there is an initial increase in water content. Other changes associated with normal aging include decreased chondrocyte synthetic activity, decreased stability of large proteoglycan aggregates, localized superficial cartilage fibrillations, and increased collagen crosslinking.

Reference

Buckwalter JA, Mankin HJ: Articular Cartilage. J Bone Joint Surg Am, 79: 612–632, 1997.

45. **d** Gigantism. Anabolic steroids are synthetic derivatives of testosterone that have been engineered to preserve the anabolic effects but eliminate the androgenic effects. Anabolic steroids produce their desired effects by inducing protein synthesis in muscle cells. Side effects include an altered cholesterol profile (increased low-density lipoprotein and decreased high-density lipoprotein); accelerated male-pattern baldness, disturbed menstrual cycle, hypertension, altered mental status (psychotic episodes and aggressive behavior), and impaired spermatogenesis. Testicular atrophy occurs because the exogenous steroids suppress endogenous androgen production through a negative feedback loop. Aromatization of the exogenous steroids to estradiol is responsible for gynecomastia.

Gigantism refers to excessive stature caused by excessive growth hormone secretion before skeletal maturity. Although anabolic steroids exert some of their effect by stimulating secretion of endogenous growth hormone, they have not been associated with gigantism. In fact, exogenous anabolic steroids have been associated with premature physeal closure.

Reference

Haupt HA: Anabolic Steroids and Growth Hormone. Am J Sports Med, 21: 468–474, 1993.

46. **e** The popliteus muscle. The popliteus muscle is the most anterior muscle in the proximal aspect of the deep posterior compartment of the leg. Its fibers are oriented obliquely (from the inferomedial to proximal lateral) as they cross the posterior knee capsule.

47. **d** Closed reduction followed by a long-leg cast for 2 to 3 weeks. Proximal tibiofibular joint dislocations are rare. Three types are seen: (1) anterolateral, (2) posteromedial, and (3) superior. Anterolateral dislocations are the most common variety. A violent indirect mechanism (e.g., internal tibial rotation with the knee flexed) is characteristically responsible for anterolateral dislocations. Posteromedial dislocations are typically produced by direct trauma. Superior (proximal) dislocations are usually associated with tibial shaft fractures.

Recommended treatment for *anterolateral* dislocations includes closed reduction followed by temporary immobilization. Open reduction is rarely necessary. Delayed excision may be appropriate when symptomatic chronic subluxation occurs. Arthrodesis has been associated with secondary ankle complaints. Closed reduction is accomplished by direct pressure applied to the anterior aspect of the fibular head as the tibia is externally rotated. The reduction is facilitated by flexion of the knee (to relax the lateral collateral ligament), pronation of the foot (to relax the musculature of the lateral compartment), and dorsiflexion of the ankle (to relax the musculature of the anterior compartment).

The recommended treatment for *posteromedial* dislocations consists of open reduction and temporary screw fixation. A superior dislocation of the proximal tibiofibular joint commonly reduces spontaneously on reduction of the associated tibial shaft fracture.

References

Ogden JA: J Bone Joint Surg Am, 56:145–154, 1974.

Trafton PG: Injuries to the Proximal Tibio-Fibular Joint. In From Browner BD, et al., eds: Skeletal Trauma, 2nd Ed. Philadelphia, WB Saunders, pp. 2279–2280, 1998.

48. **d** The deep zone. Articular cartilage can be divided into four zones: (1) superficial, (2) middle (transitional), (3) deep, and (4) zone of calcified cartilage. The *superficial zone* has relatively low proteoglycan content. It is rich in collagen, most of which is arranged parallel to the joint surface. Collagen fibers increase in diameter and become less organized within the *middle zone.* The *deep zone* has the highest proteoglycan concentration. This coincides with its function, which is to resist compression. The zone of calcified cartilage is replete with hydroxyapatite salts.

Note: Proteoglycans consist of multiple glycosaminoglycan chains linked to a protein core. Chondroitin sulfates are the predominant form of glycosaminoglycan found within articular cartilage.

Reference

Simon SR, ed: Orthopaedic Basic Science. Rosemont, IL, American Academy of Orthopedic Surgeons, 1994.

49. **c** The patient is positioned supine with the knee externally rotated at 90 degrees of flexion, valgus stress applied, and the knee reduces as it is extended. The reverse pivot shift test is performed with the patient supine. The hip and knee of the affected leg are flexed to 90 degrees. The examiner places an external rotation force on the tibia to cause posterolateral subluxation in the posterior cruciate ligament–deficient knee. The knee is then extended while a valgus force is maintained. The reduction occurs as the knee is brought into extension.

50. **b** Meniscal cysts occur more commonly on the medial side of the knee than on the lateral side. By definition, meniscal cysts are associated with intrameniscal disease and are directly attached to the meniscus. If there is no continuity with the meniscus, then alternative diagnoses should be considered (i.e., ganglion cyst or popliteal cyst). Associated horizontal meniscal tears are present in most cases (some authorities believe in all cases). Horizontal tears are believed to contribute to the formation and perpetuation of the cysts. Communication between the cyst and the meniscal tear can usually be demonstrated. Lateral meniscal cysts are

more common than their medial counterparts, but medial meniscal cysts tend to be larger. Cyst content is histochemically similar to synovial fluid.

Note: Popliteal cysts are also often associated with meniscal disease, but unlike meniscal cysts, they do not directly communicate with the associated meniscal disease.

Reference

Lantz B, Singer KM: Meniscal Cysts. Clin Sports Med, 9(3):707–725, 1990.

51. **a** Increased number of slow-twitch muscle fibers. The distribution and quantity of slow-twitch (type I) and fast-twitch (type II) myocytes are genetically determined. Endurance training (high repetitions, low resistance) can have many effects on muscle tissue, but it does not increase the number of type I myocytes. Endurance training increases the efficiency of type I myocytes by increasing the number of mitochondria, increasing oxidative capacity, increasing capillary density, and decreasing the local accumulation of lactate in response to exercise. Strength training (low repetitions, high resistance) produces selective hypertrophy of type II myocytes. (Some evidence suggests that a minimal amount of type II myocyte hyperplasia may also occur in response to strength training.)

Reference

Orthopaedic Knowledge Update 3. Rosemont, IL, American Academy of Orthopedic Surgeons, 1990.

52. **d** Bony impingement. The image demonstrates an osteophyte in the intercondylar notch that acts as a mechanical block to extension.

    The images reveal no evidence of a proliferative intrasynovial process such as *pigmented villonodular synovitis* or *synovial chondromatosis.* Chondroblastoma commonly affects the distal femoral epiphysis; however, it occurs before skeletal maturity and it does not present this way. This patient's age is also inconsistent with a diagnosis of *idiopathic osteonecrosis,* which characteristically affects older persons. Furthermore, idiopathic osteonecrosis characteristically occurs at the *central* portion of the weightbearing surface of the medial femoral condyle.

53. **c** (A) type II; (b) type I. The menisci are composed of fibrocartilage. The predominant type of collagen in the menisci is type I (approximately 90%). The predominant type of collagen in articular (hyaline) cartilage is type II. Collagen accounts for approximately 60% to 70% of the dry weight of the menisci. Chondroitin sulfate is the predominant type of glycosaminoglycan found in both articular cartilage and meniscal tissue.

Reference

Simon SR, ed: Orthopaedic Basic Science. Rosemont, IL, American Academy of Orthopedic Surgeons, 1994.

54. **e** The ligament of Wrisberg. The plane of this coronal magnetic resonance image (Fig. 6.12) can be localized to the posterior portion of the intercondylar notch by virtue of the presence of the posterior femoral condyles and the absence of the femoral shaft. The identified structure runs obliquely from the lateral meniscus toward the lateral aspect of the medial femoral condyle. Both the meniscofemoral ligaments (Humphry and Wrisberg) attach to the posterior horn of the lateral meniscus and traverse the knee in this orientation.

    Distinguishing the ligament of Humphry from the ligament of Wrisberg depends on discerning the structure's relationship to the posterior cruciate ligament. *The ligament of Humphry runs anterior to the posterior cruciate ligament; the ligament of Wrisberg runs posteriorly to the posterior cruciate ligament.* The plane of this image intersects the tibial attachment of the posterior cruciate ligament. Thus, because the posterior cruciate ligament traverses the joint obliquely (from posterodistal to anteroproximal), the plane of the image must be posterior to the remainder of the posterior cruciate ligament.

Reference

Heller L, Langman J: The Menisco-Femoral Ligaments of the Human Knee. J Bone Joint Surg Br, 46:307–313, 1964.

55. **d** Infantile Blount disease. Congenital absence of the anterior cruciate ligament has been associated with a wide variety of conditions including proximal femoral focal deficiency, tibial hemimelia, congenital knee dislocation, discoid lateral meniscus, congenital absence of the menisci, thrombocytopenia-absent radius syndrome, congenital patellar dislocation, and congenital ring meniscus.

    Congenital anterior cruciate ligament absence has *not* been associated with Blount disease. Affected patients often do not require anterior cruciate ligament reconstruction because of the low demand on the affected knee imparted by the associated anomalies.

Reference

Thomas NP, et al.: Congenital Absence of the Anterior Cruciate Ligament. J Bone Joint Surg Br, 67:572, 1985.

56. **b** A defect in the fibrillin gene. *Marfan syndrome* is an autosomal dominant disorder that has been attributed to a defect in the fibrillin gene. This defect results in abnormal collagen cross-linkage and flawed elastin fibers.

Musculoskeletal features of the Marfan phenotype include arachnodactyly, ligamentous laxity, increased height, scoliosis, pectus excavatum, protrusio acetabuli, pes planovalgus, and an abnormally high ratio of arm span to height. Nonmusculoskeletal features include myopia, ectopia lentis, a predilection for spontaneous pneumothorax, mitral valve prolapse, aortic root dilatation, and a predilection for aortic dissection. The associated cardiac abnormalities can be life-threatening. Patients with Marfan syndrome who experience a syncopal episode should undergo urgent echocardiography.

Osteocalcin is a noncollagenous protein found in bone that is believed to play a role in osteoclast chemotaxis. *Dermal myofibroblasts* are normally found in the palmar fascia and are believed to play a role in the origin of Dupuytren contracture.

References

Dietz HC, et al.: Marfan Syndrome Caused by a Recurrent *de Novo* Missense Mutation in the Fibrillin Gene. Nature, 352:337, 1991.

Joseph KN, et al.: Orthopaedic Aspects of the Marfan Phenotype. Clin Orthop, 277:251–261, 1992.

57. **d** Graft resorption. The results of anterior cruciate ligament reconstruction with synthetic ligament grafts have been discouraging. Various materials have been used, including Dacron, carbon fiber, and Gore-Tex. Despite reports of successful short-term outcomes, the durability of synthetic grafts is suboptimal, and results deteriorate over time.

With continued cyclic loading, synthetic ligaments shed wear debris, which, in turn, is responsible for synovitis and recurrent sterile effusions. Osteolysis and graft loosening have been attributed to the particle load.

Phagocytized graft particles can induce release of degradative enzymes into the knee. However the graft itself cannot be enzymatically degraded. Graft failure is a function of fatigue and attrition.

The experience of Paulos and colleagues revealed a 56% incidence of unacceptable results. Complications included a 2.7% infection rate, loosening of more than 3 mm in 34%, loosening of more than 8 mm in 5%, and a 12% rate of graft rupture.

Reference

Paulos LE, et al.: The GoreTex Anterior Cruciate Ligament Prosthesis: A Long-Term Followup. Am J Sports Med, 20:246–252, 1992.

58. **e** Discoid lateral meniscus. That the three sagittal magnetic resonance images demonstrating the anterior and posterior horns of the lateral meniscus are in continuity with one another is a reliable sign of a discoid lateral meniscus. No more than two consecutive 5-mm sagittal sections should demonstrate continuity between the anterior and posterior horns of a normal lateral meniscus.

Reference

Silverman JM, et al.: Discoid Menisci of the Knee: MRI Appearance. Radiology, 173:351–354, 1989.

59. **a** Anterior cruciate ligament tear. Although the anterior cruciate ligament is not mentioned in the question, its incompetence can be inferred based on the contusion signal on the anterior aspect of the lateral femoral condyle. This contusion is created when the lateral tibial plateau subluxates anteriorly and impacts the femoral condyle.

Reference

Rosen MA, et al.: Occult Osseous Lesions Documented by Magnetic Resonance Imaging Associated with Anterior Cruciate Ligament Ruptures. Arthroscopy, 7:45–51, 1991.

60. **c** Tie the femoral bone plug tensioning sutures over a button on the lateral femoral cortex through a separate incision. A properly placed femoral tunnel should preserve a posterior cortical thickness of approximately 2 to 3 mm. If the posterior femoral cortex is inadvertently violated, interference screw fixation should be abandoned, but the procedure need not be aborted. Adequate femoral fixation can still be obtained. The tensioning sutures from the proximal portion of the graft are passed in the standard retrograde fashion and are delivered through a drill hole in the lateral femoral cortex, where they are tied over a button.

Reference

Hunter RE: Avoiding Complications of ACL Surgery: Arthroscopy Association of North America (AANA) Specialty Day. New Orleans, 1998.

61. **e** Anteromedialization of the tibial tubercle (Fulkerson procedure) and lateral retinacular release. The axial computed tomography image confirms the presence of both lateral patellar subluxation and severe patellar tilt. Although lateral retinacular release may yield a good clinical result in the setting of isolated patellar tilt, the presence of concomitant lateral facet arthrosis and patellar subluxation warrants an additional procedure. Anteromedial transfer of the tubercle would effectively restore patellofemoral congruence and would unload the lateral facet.

References

Fulkerson JP, Schutzer SF: After Failure of Conservative Treatment for Painful Patellofemoral Malalignment: Lateral Retinacular Release or Realignment. Orthop Clin North Am, 17:283, 1986.

Fulkerson JP, et al.: Computerized Tomography of the Patellofemoral Joint

Before and After Lateral Release or Realignment. Arthroscopy, 3(1):19–24, 1987.

62. **c** Anterior cruciate ligament reconstruction. Shelbourne and Porter demonstrated the efficacy of anterior cruciate ligament reconstruction alone in the setting of acute combined anterior cruciate ligament–medial collateral ligament insufficiency. Reconstruction of the anterior cruciate ligament is sufficient to restore stability in this setting. The medial collateral ligament will heal itself. The addition of an open medial collateral ligament repair may increase the likelihood of postoperative knee stiffness and may deter rehabilitation.

Reference

Shelbourne KD, Porter DA: Anterior Cruciate LigamentMedial Collateral Ligament Injury: Nonoperative Management of Medial Collateral Ligament Tears with Anterior Cruciate Ligament Reconstruction. Am J Sports Med, 20:283–286, 1992.

63. **a** Anterior malposition of the femoral tunnel. There are many potential sources of impaired extension after anterior cruciate ligament reconstruction. These include arthrofibrosis, anterior cruciate ligament nodules, and impingement of the graft with the roof of the intercondylar notch. Roof impingement may be the result of an inadequate notchplasty or anterior malposition of the tibial tunnel. When the knee is extended, the tibial tunnel should project parallel and posterior to the Blumensaat line.

    Anterior malposition of the femoral tunnel is associated with impaired *flexion* after anterior cruciate ligament reconstruction, but it is not usually associated with compromised extension. Anterior malposition of the femoral tunnel cannot produce roof impingement because the graft will be behind the Blumensaat line regardless of where in the notch the femoral tunnel is drilled.

    Note: Roof impingement is associated with regional increased signal intensity within the distal two-thirds of the graft on magnetic resonance imaging. The proximal third of the graft will manifest normal signal intensity in the setting of roof impingement. This putative injury signal can progress to graft rupture.

Reference

Howell SM, Taylor MA: Failure of Reconstruction of the Anterior Cruciate Ligament due to Impingement by the Intercondylar Roof. J Bone Joint Surg Am, 75:1044–1055, 1993.

64. **f** Tibiocalcaneal fusion. The only possible salvage procedure may be a tibiotalocalcaneal fusion. None of the other listed options would be appropriate. Multiple studies have shown that arthroscopy and fusion of the subtalar joint are technically impossible in the absence of a subtalar joint. Amputation may be another alternative.

FIGURE CREDITS

Figure 6.3. From Stoller DW: Magnetic Resonance Imaging in Orthopaedics & Sports Medicine. Philadelphia, Lippincott–Raven, p. 278, 1997 with permission.

Figure 6.6. From Fu F, et al.: Knee Surgery. Baltimore, Williams & Wilkins, pp. 385–386, 1994, with permission.

Figure 6.7. From Fu F, et al.: Knee Surgery. Baltimore, Williams & Wilkins, p. 797, 1994, with permission.

Figure 6.14. From Fu F, et al.: Knee Surgery. Baltimore, Williams & Wilkins, p. 385, 1994, with permission.

7

FOOT AND ANKLE

QUESTIONS

1. Which of the following is the best indication for first metatarsocuneiform joint fusion?
   (a) Adolescent bunion deformity
   (b) Hypermobile metatarsus primus varus
   (c) Hallux valgus with an intermetatarsal angle of 13 degrees
   (d) Transfer metatarsalgia
   (e) "Cock-up" deformity of the great toe
2. A transfer lesion is most likely to result after which of the following procedures?
   (a) Proximal metatarsal osteotomy for hallux valgus fixed in 20 degrees of dorsiflexion
   (b) Flexor digitorum longus transfer to the navicular for posterior tibial tendon insufficiency
   (c) Girdlestone-Taylor procedure (flexor to extensor tendon transfer) for flexible hammer toe deformity
   (d) Arthrodesis of the first metatarsophalangeal joint in 5 degrees of plantar flexion
   (e) Arthrodesis of the first metatarsophalangeal joint in 5 degrees of dorsiflexion
3. A 45-year-old postal worker with diabetes presents with a 4-cm ulcer beneath his first metatarsal head. There is no purulence. Flexor tendons are visible in the wound, but no erythema, swelling, or fluctuance is present beyond the edges of the ulcer. Radiographs reveal no evidence of bony involvement. According to the Wagner classification, what grade is this ulcer?
   (a) Grade I
   (b) Grade II
   (c) Grade III
   (d) Grade IV
   (e) Grade V
4. What is the most appropriate treatment for the lesion described in question 3?
   (a) Oral antibiotics and elevation
   (b) Total contact cast
   (c) Intravenous antibiotics
   (d) Leech therapy
   (e) Surgical débridement and intravenous antibiotics
5. What is the most common mechanism responsible for fractures of the talar neck?
   (a) Inversion
   (b) Eversion
   (c) Axial compression
   (d) Plantar flexion
   (e) Dorsiflexion
6. Which of the following statements regarding coupled motion in the foot and ankle is true?
   (a) Dorsiflexion of the metatarsophalangeal joints is coupled with a decrease in height of the longitudinal arch of the foot.
   (b) Tibiotalar dorsiflexion is coupled with proximal migration and external rotation of the fibula.
   (c) Foot pronation is coupled with divergence of the talonavicular and calcaneocuboid joint axes.
   (d) Subtalar eversion is coupled with external rotation of the tibia.
   (e) During terminal stance, the tibia internally rotates.
7. A 22-year-old ballet dancer presents with complaints of chronic left ankle instability. You obtain the stress radiograph shown in Fig. 7.1. If conservative management fails, what surgical procedure should you recommend?
   (a) Watson-Jones
   (b) Chrisman-Snook
   (c) Lapidus
   (d) Modified Brostrom
   (e) Evans
8. A 17-year-old high school football player complains of pain in his right great toe. He relates the onset of his symptoms to a tackle in last week's game. He has moderate swelling and resolving ecchymosis over the metatarsophalangeal joint. Active dorsiflexion and plantar flexion are 20 and 10 degrees, respectively (both are limited by pain). Radiographs are normal. What would be the most appropriate recommendation to this athlete?
   (a) Ice, antiinflammatory drug use, and immediate return to play
   (b) Gradual return to play over the next 2 weeks with taping to restrict extension

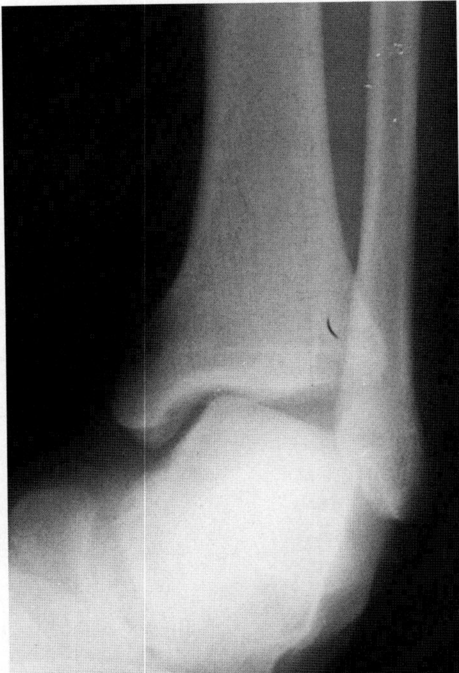

FIGURE 7.1

(c) Short-leg walking cast for 4 weeks followed by a gradual return to competition
(d) Steroid injection into the first metatarsophalangeal joint
(e) Reconstruction of the flexor hallucis brevis tendon

9. When one performs ankle arthroscopy, which of the following structures is at greatest risk during establishment of the anterolateral portal?
   (a) The peroneus tertius tendon
   (b) The sural nerve
   (c) The dorsal intermediate cutaneous nerve
   (d) The artery of the sinus tarsi
   (e) The dorsalis pedis artery
10. Which of the following techniques is inappropriate during placement of an ankle syndesmotic screw?
   (a) Orientation of the screw parallel to the tibial plafond
   (b) Use of a lag screw to ensure adequate compression of the syndesmosis
   (c) Dorsiflexion of the ankle to 10 to 15 degrees during screw placement
   (d) Angulation of the screw 30 degrees anterior to the coronal plane
   (e) Placement of the screw 2 to 3 cm proximal to the tibial plafond
11. Radiographic follow-up 8 weeks after open reduction and internal fixation of a displaced talus fracture reveals the presence of a Hawkins sign. What does this finding signify?
   (a) An occult subtalar dislocation
   (b) Nonunion of the fracture
   (c) Talar beaking (indicating early posttraumatic arthritis)
   (d) Revascularization of the talus
   (e) Avascular necrosis of the talus
12. A 27-year-old woman presents with complaints of heel pain while jogging. Her pain is exacerbated by running uphill. Palpable fullness and tenderness are present immediately anterior to the Achilles tendon. Her pain is reproduced with dorsiflexion. Radiographs reveal a prominence of the posterior superior calcaneus. What would be the most appropriate form of treatment at this time?
   (a) Antiinflammatory drugs, heel lift, and activity modification
   (b) Retrocalcaneal steroid injection
   (c) Short-leg cast
   (d) Excision of the calcaneal prominence
   (e) Vulpius lengthening of the Achilles tendon
13. What musculotendinous unit is identified by the double arrow at the lower left of the axial T1-weighted magnetic resonance image in Fig. 7.2?
   (a) The tibialis posterior
   (b) The peroneus longus
   (c) The flexor hallucis longus
   (d) The peroneus tertius
   (e) The flexor digitorum longus
14. What is the optimal position for first metatarsophalangeal joint arthrodesis?
   (a) 0 to 5 degrees of valgus and 30 degrees of dorsiflexion in relation to the floor

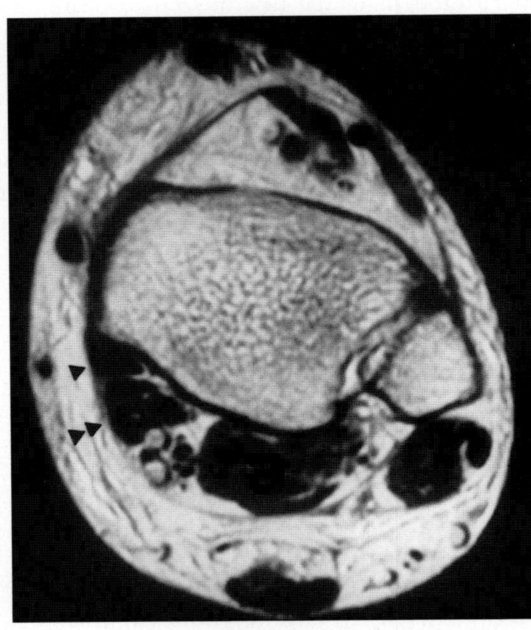

FIGURE 7.2

(b) 15 degrees of valgus and 30 degrees of dorsiflexion in relation to the floor
(c) 15 degrees of valgus and 15 degrees of dorsiflexion in relation to the floor
(d) 0 to 5 degrees of valgus and 0 degrees of dorsiflexion in relation to the floor
(e) 0 to 5 degrees of valgus and 30 degrees of dorsiflexion in relation to the metatarsal shaft

15. The origin and insertion of the flexor digitorum brevis are
(a) Origin: the medial tubercle of the calcaneus; insertion: the middle phalanges
(b) Origin: the lateral tubercle of the calcaneus; insertion: the proximal phalanges
(c) Origin: the medial tubercle of the calcaneus; insertion: the proximal phalanges
(d) Origin: the plantar fascia; insertion: the middle phalanges
(e) Origin: the lateral tubercle of the calcaneus; insertion: the flexor digitorum longus tendon

16. What nerve innervates the extensor digitorum brevis?
(a) The superficial peroneal nerve
(b) The deep peroneal nerve
(c) The lateral plantar nerve
(d) The saphenous nerve
(e) The sural nerve

17. A 38-year-old woman complains of lateral forefoot pain that is most severe when she walks to work. The discomfort is aggravated by high heels. She has also noted paresthesias in her third and fourth toes. Based on these symptoms, which of the following tests would be the most effective in confirming the diagnosis?
(a) Magnetic resonance imaging of the tarsal tunnel
(b) Electromyogram and nerve conduction studies
(c) Injection of local anesthetic and steroid into the tarsal tunnel
(d) Injection of local anesthetic and steroid into the third webspace
(e) Symes filament testing

18. What structure passes through the space marked by the arrow in Fig. 7.3?
(a) None
(b) The artery of the tarsal tunnel
(c) The flexor hallucis longus tendon
(d) The artery of the sinus tarsi
(e) The artery of the tarsal canal

19. What is the most common malignant tumor in the foot?
(a) Malignant fibrous histiocytoma
(b) Squamous cell carcinoma
(c) Malignant melanoma
(d) Epithelioid sarcoma
(e) Osteosarcoma

20. What is the most common sarcoma in the foot?
(a) Ewing sarcoma

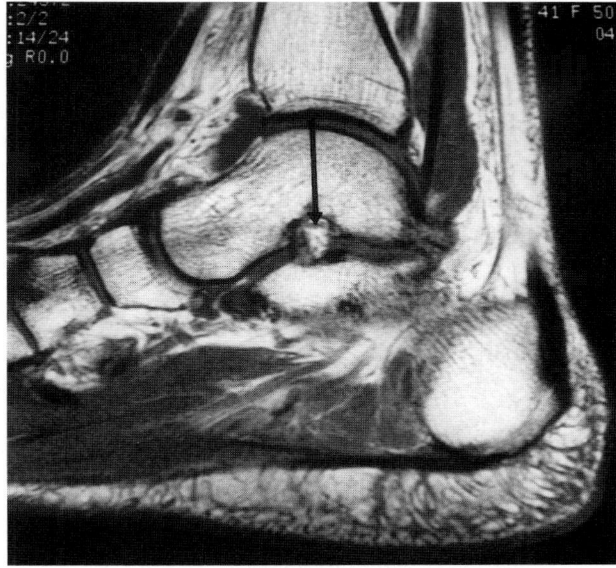

FIGURE 7.3

(b) Epithelioid sarcoma
(c) Synovial cell sarcoma
(d) Fibrosarcoma
(e) Liposarcoma

21. The most appropriate surgical treatment for a flexible clawtoe deformity is
(a) Extensor tendon lengthening
(b) Girdlestone-Taylor transfer
(c) Resection of the distal aspect of the proximal phalanx
(d) Proximal interphalangeal joint arthrodesis
(e) Tenotomy of the flexor digitorum longus tendon

22. The Coleman block test is used to determine whether a deformity is flexible or fixed by
(a) Confirming normal heel varus in toe rise
(b) Eliminating the effect of first ray plantar flexion
(c) Elevating the medial arch in a cavovarus foot
(d) Locking the transverse tarsal joint to form a rigid lever
(e) Placing the hindfoot into an equinus posture

23. A 48-year-old woman presents with right heel pain that is greatest early in the morning and when she rises from her desk. She cannot recall a specific traumatic event, but she estimates that she has gained approximately 20 pounds since her most recent promotion. Based on this history, what physical finding would you anticipate?
(a) Increased pain with passive dorsiflexion of the toes
(b) Localized tenderness over the medial aspect of the calcaneal tuberosity
(c) Reproduction of symptoms with percussion posterior to the medial malleolus
(d) Inability to perform a single toe rise on the right foot

(e) Pain with compression of the metatarsal heads

24. A concerned mother presents with her 2-month-old son because she has noted that "his toes turn in." Examination reveals bilateral metatarsus adductus and normal hindfeet. The heel bisector passes through the third toe. No medial crease is present, and the deformity passively corrects to neutral. Recommended treatment at this time should be
    (a) Passive stretching
    (b) Reverse-last shoes
    (c) Transmetatarsal osteotomies before 1 year of age
    (d) Serial casting
    (e) Heyman-Herndon tarsometatarsal capsulotomies before 6 months of age
25. A calcaneocavus foot deformity would most likely be associated with which of the following diseases?
    (a) Poliomyelitis
    (b) Ledderhose disease
    (c) Charcot-Marie-Tooth disease
    (d) Friedreich ataxia
    (e) Arthrogryposis
26. The primary fracture line of a typical intraarticular calcaneus fracture propagates
    (a) From posterolateral to anteromedial through the middle facet
    (b) From posteromedial to anterolateral through the middle facet
    (c) From posterolateral to anteromedial through the posterior facet
    (d) In the sagittal plane through the middle facet
    (e) From posteromedial to anterolateral through the posterior facet
27. A 40-year-old recreational basketball player ruptures his Achilles tendon. Which of the following statements regarding operative versus nonoperative management of his injury is most accurate?
    (a) The risk of recurrent rupture is higher with nonoperative management.
    (b) The costs of the two treatment options are comparable.
    (c) Surgical complications are rare.
    (d) Plantar flexion strength is greater after nonoperative management.
    (e) Patients treated operatively return to work more rapidly.
28. What is the most common deformity after an untreated compartment syndrome of the foot?
    (a) Pes planovalgus
    (b) Clawtoes
    (c) Calcaneocavus
    (d) Equinocavovarus
    (e) Mallet toes
29. A 55-year-old man with diabetes presents with a 1-cm diameter, painful mass on the medial plantar aspect of his right foot. The mass is fixed, and the overlying skin is intact. He denies trauma, fevers, or chills. Examination reveals flexion contractures of the fourth and fifth proximal interphalangeal joints of his left hand. Plain radiographs of the foot reveal no bony lesion or soft tissue mineral deposition. Review of his health maintenance organization chart reveals that he was seen by a urologist earlier in the year for evaluation of painful fibrous cords along his corpora cavernosa. What is the most appropriate treatment for this patient's foot lesion?
    (a) Low-dose radiation therapy
    (b) Systemic glucocorticoids
    (c) Topical glucocorticoids
    (d) Excision of the nodule
    (e) Complete excision of the plantar aponeurosis
30. What is the most common cause of intractable plantar keratoses?
    (a) Viral infection
    (b) Proliferation of fibrous tissue from the plantar aponeurosis
    (c) Rheumatoid arthritis
    (d) Prominent bony anatomy
    (e) Fungal infection
31. A 24-year-old man presents with recalcitrant pain at the insertion of his right Achilles tendon. There is no history of trauma, and he denies any form of recent exercise. Examination reveals focal tenderness and swelling at his Achilles insertion. Inspection of his right shoe confirms that it fits well, and there is no irregularity at the heel counter. Plain films of his right ankle are unremarkable. He has no other complaints. He states that he is otherwise perfectly healthy. He is sexually active, and he denies recent illness. What is the most appropriate next step in the management of this patient?
    (a) Computed tomography scan of the calcaneus
    (b) Magnetic resonance imaging scan of the Achilles and calcaneus
    (c) Bone scan
    (d) Glucocorticoid injection into the Achilles insertion
    (e) Urethral culture
32. A 19-year-old lifeguard presents with pain on the plantar aspect of his left heel. Examination reveals a discrete area of tender callus formation. On shaving the lesion, you note punctate bleeding from the base. What is the most appropriate next step for this patient?
    (a) Obtaining of foot radiographs
    (b) Serologic studies to establish HLA type
    (c) Marginal excision of the base of the lesion
    (d) Salicylic acid treatment
    (e) Topical steroids
33. What bone is affected by Köhler disease?
    (a) The first metatarsal
    (b) The second metatarsal
    (c) The tarsal navicular

(d) The cuboid
(e) The second cuneiform

34. A 14-year-old boy presents with hindfoot pain and recurrent ankle sprains. His examination demonstrates limited subtalar motion. Plain films reveal no abnormality. The most appropriate next radiographic study would be
(a) Bone scan
(b) Computed tomography scan
(c) Magnetic resonance imaging scan
(d) Stress radiographs
(e) Gallium scan

35. The two components of the bifurcate ligament are
(a) The calcaneonavicular and talonavicular ligaments
(b) The calcaneofibular and interosseous ligaments
(c) The calcaneocuboid and calcaneofibular ligaments
(d) The calcaneonavicular and calcaneocuboid ligaments
(e) The calcaneofibular and talofibular ligaments

36. What is the most accurate description of a metatarsal bar?
(a) A rigid pad applied to the sole of the shoe beneath the metatarsal diaphyses that provides a rocker-bottom effect
(b) An interior shoe pad that provides elevation just proximal to the metatarsal heads
(c) An interior shoe pad that provides elevation directly beneath the metatarsal heads
(d) An interior shoe pad that provides elevation just distal to the metatarsal heads
(e) An osseous coalition between the proximal metaphyses of the first and second metatarsals

37. A 64-year-old woman presents with pain in her great toe and difficulty with shoe wear. A radiograph is shown in Fig. 7.4. Her intermetatarsal angle measures 18 degrees. Her hallux valgus angle measures 42 degrees. If conservative treatment fails, what operation would be most appropriate?
(a) Keller procedure
(b) Distal chevron osteotomy
(c) Proximal crescentic osteotomy with a distal soft tissue procedure
(d) Akin procedure with a distal soft tissue procedure
(e) Metatarsophalangeal joint arthrodesis

38. A 34-year-old woman with sickle cell anemia is referred to you because of progressive, refractory ankle pain that severely limits her ambulation. Radiographs show multiple sclerotic areas with tibiotalar joint destruction and sclerosis of the distal tibia and fibula. What is the most likely cause of the abnormality seen?
(a) Acute infection
(b) Repetitive microtrauma
(c) Neuropathic osteoarthropathy
(d) Bone infarction
(e) Regional osteopenia

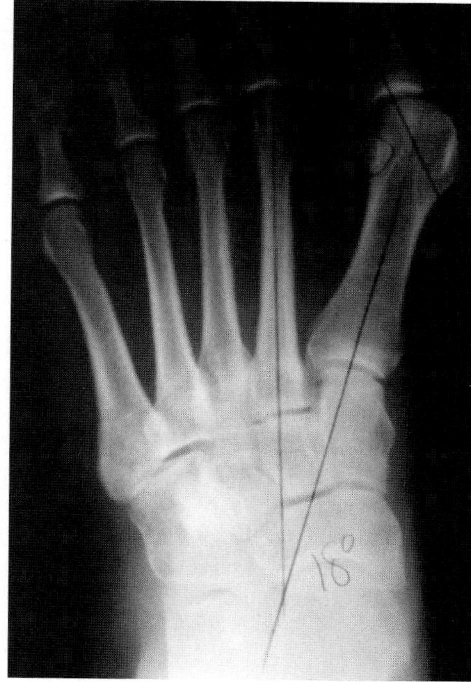

FIGURE 7.4

39. What surgical treatment should you offer the patient in question 38?
(a) Arthroscopic débridement
(b) Supramalleolar osteotomy
(c) Cheilectomy
(d) Tibiotalar arthrodesis
(e) Pantalar arthrodesis

40. A 34-year-old recreational jogger presents with increasing pain in her forefoot that is occasionally accompanied by numbness in her second and third toes. On examination, mild swelling and focal tenderness are present over the second metatarsophalangeal joint. There is no deformity, but passive dorsal translation of the proximal phalanx is significantly increased. The most likely diagnosis is
(a) Synovitis of the second metatarsophalangeal joint
(b) Interdigital neuroma
(c) Turf toe
(d) Stress fracture of the metatarsal head
(e) Dislocation of the second metatarsophalangeal joint

41. Despite compliance with conservative treatment, the patient described in question 40 continues to be symptomatic. What would be the most appropriate form of surgical intervention?
(a) Partial second proximal phalangectomy with syndactilization to the third toe
(b) Dorsiflexion osteotomy of the second metatarsal
(c) Second metatarsophalangeal synovectomy and possible flexor tendon transfer

(d) Extensor tendon lengthening, dorsal capsulotomy, and collateral ligament release with a Girdlestone-Taylor flexor to extensor tendon transfer
(e) Second metatarsophalangeal arthrodesis

42. Which of the following muscles demonstrates the greatest activity during the heel strike phase of gait?
(a) The tibialis anterior
(b) The tibialis posterior
(c) The gastrocnemius-soleus complex
(d) The peroneus brevis
(e) The peroneus longus

43. A 54-year-old man with diabetes slips on an icy sidewalk and sustains a bimalleolar ankle fracture that is treated with open reduction and internal fixation (Fig. 7.5A). His postoperative course is uneventful. He returns 6 months after his initial injury because he has noted persistent swelling of his ankle. Examination confirms moderate swelling, erythema, and deformity. There is minimal associated tenderness. All wounds are well healed without drainage. A follow-up radiograph is shown in Fig. 7.5B. Optimal treatment at this time should consist of
(a) Revision open reduction and internal fixation, adding a syndesmosis screw
(b) Primary arthrodesis of the ankle joint
(c) Removal of all hardware, wide débridement, and 6 weeks of culture-specific antibiotics
(d) Removal of all hardware, application of an external fixator, and delayed fusion after 6 weeks of culture-specific antibiotics
(e) Immobilization, elevation, and observation

44. Which of the following statements is most accurate regarding the anatomy of the Achilles tendon?
(a) The Achilles tendon is surrounded by a synovial sheath.
(b) The Achilles fibers spiral approximately 90 degrees around one another such that the gastrocnemius fibers insert medially to the soleus fibers.
(c) Stretching with knee flexed and ankle dorsiflexed will preferentially stretch the gastrocnemius fibers rather than the soleus.
(d) Most of the tendon's blood supply arises from its muscular origin and osseous insertion.
(e) Hyperpronation is believed to contribute to Achilles inflammation and degeneration.

45. What is the correct treatment for a symptomatic subungual exostosis?
(a) Excision of the associated granulation tissue and the adjacent nail plate
(b) Periodic soaks in half-strength hydrogen peroxide until symptoms subside
(c) Ablation of the affected nail matrix
(d) Excision of the exostosis
(e) Distal tuft amputation

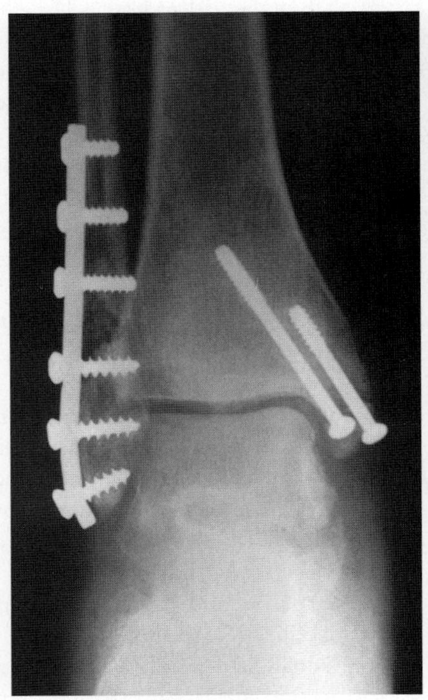
A

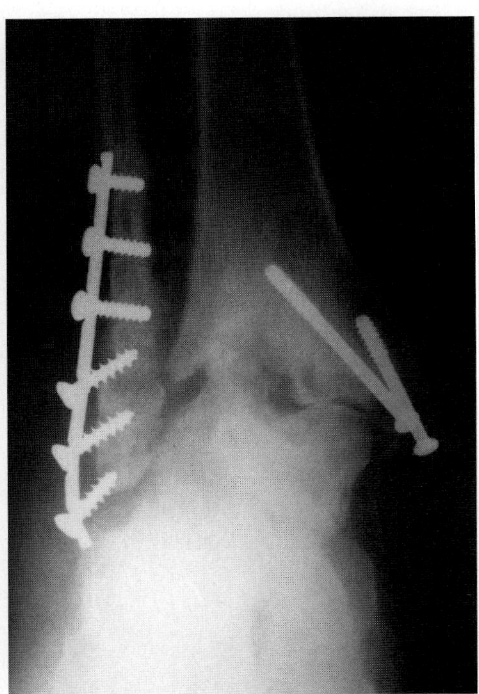
B

FIGURE 7.5A and B

46. The correct term for the thickened, darkened, curved "ram's horn" type of toenail that is seen most often in the great toe of elderly patients with poor hygiene is
    (a) Onychogryphosis
    (b) Onychotrophy
    (c) Onychomalacia
    (d) Onychocryptosis
    (e) Onycholysis
47. Which of the following statements about ankle biomechanics is false?
    (a) Plantar flexion of the ankle is coupled to internal deviation of the forefoot.
    (b) Osteotomy of the fibula at the level of the ankle joint and sectioning of the anterior inferior tibiofibular ligament will permit significant lateral talar subluxation.
    (c) Approximately 17% of the joint reaction force across the ankle is transmitted through the fibula.
    (d) The first structure to fail in a pronation-external rotation injury is either the deltoid or the medial malleolus itself.
    (e) The first structure to fail in a supination-external rotation injury is the anterior inferior tibiofibular ligament.
48. A 28-year-old attending dermatologist is involved in a head-on motor vehicle accident en route to morning rounds. Radiographs reveal a fracture of the talar neck. The talar body is displaced at both the ankle and the subtalar joints. Her injury is repaired anatomically and rigidly on the day of injury. Based on this information, what is the most accurate estimation of her risk of developing avascular necrosis of the talus?
    (a) Less than 10%
    (b) Less than 40%
    (c) More than 90%
    (d) 100%
    (e) 0%
49. What is the desired alignment for a tibiotalar arthrodesis?
    (a) Neutral varus and valgus; 5 degrees of plantar flexion
    (b) Neutral varus and valgus; neutral flexion
    (c) 5 degrees of valgus; 5 degrees of plantar flexion
    (d) 5 degrees of valgus; neutral flexion
    (e) 5 degrees of varus; neutral flexion
50. An 83-year-old retired postal worker presents with great toe pain and difficulty with shoe wear that limits her ability to ambulate. In fact, she has used a cane since her myocardial infarction 3 months ago. A radiograph is shown in Fig. 7.6. The intermetatarsal angle measures 17 degrees, and the hallux valgus angle is 41 degrees. The most appropriate recommendation would be
    (a) Modified McBride procedure
    (b) Arthrodesis of the first metatarsophalangeal joint
    (c) Keller procedure

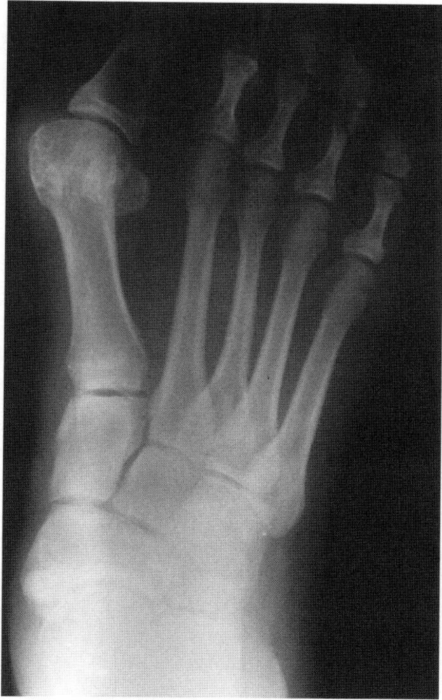

FIGURE 7.6

    (d) Wide toe-box shoes
    (e) A full-length orthotic with metatarsal pad
51. A 14-year-old girl complains of medial foot pain. Dress shoes are particularly uncomfortable. Examination reveals a normal longitudinal arch. There is a tender prominence at the medial midfoot in the region of the insertion of the posterior tibial tendon. She is able to perform a unilateral heel rise without difficulty. Standing anteroposterior and lateral radiographs reveal an accessory navicular. If conservative treatment fails, what would be the most appropriate form of intervention?
    (a) Posterior tibial tenosynovectomy
    (b) Simple excision
    (c) Flexor digitorum longus tendon transfer
    (d) Kidner procedure
    (e) Talonavicular arthrodesis
52. A 72-year-old woman with rheumatoid arthritis complains of diffuse right forefoot pain. She lives alone, and her foot pain limits her ability to ambulate in the community. Shoe wear modifications have not provided significant relief. There is no skin breakdown. A radiograph is shown in Fig. 7.7. Recommended surgical intervention should be
    (a) Akin procedure combined with resection arthroplasty of the lesser toes
    (b) Distal chevron osteotomy of the first metatarsal with metatarsophalangeal arthrodesis of the lesser toes

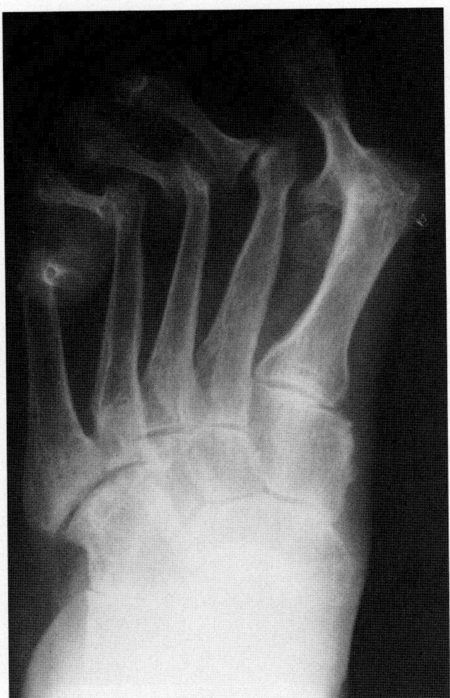

FIGURE 7.7

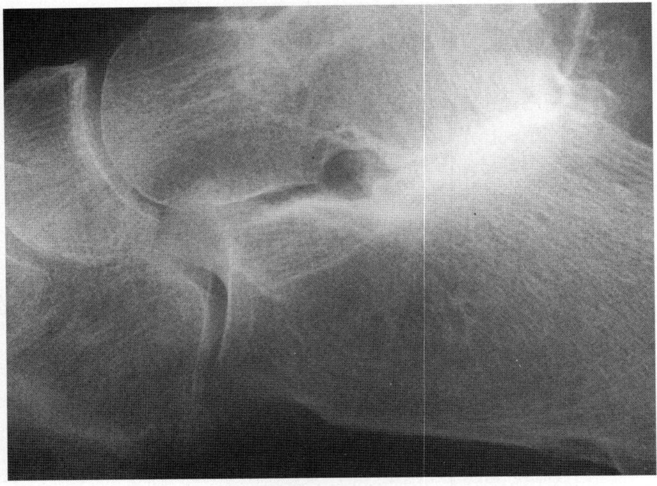

FIGURE 7.8

(c) Keller resection arthroplasty of the first metatarsophalangeal with metatarsophalangeal arthrodesis of the lesser toes
(d) Arthrodesis of the first metatarsophalangeal joint with resection arthroplasty of the lesser toes
(e) Transmetatarsal amputation

53. Which of the following is not an insertion site of the posterior tibial tendon?
(a) The first metatarsal
(b) The second metatarsal
(c) The medial cuneiform
(d) The middle cuneiform
(e) The navicular

54. An 17-year-old boy presents with hindfoot pain of insidious onset. A radiograph is shown in Fig. 7.8. What would be the most appropriate initial form of treatment for this condition?
(a) Short-leg cast
(b) Resection with interposition of an autogenous fat graft
(c) Resection with interposition of the extensor digitorum brevis
(d) Split anterior tibial tendon transfer
(e) Triple arthrodesis

55. Which of the following statements regarding the stance phase of gait is false?
(a) At midstance, the rate of tibial progression is decelerated by the soleus muscle.
(b) Prolonged heel contact in terminal stance is a potential sign of soleus weakness.
(c) Knee hyperextension and posterior trunk lean are midstance compensatory mechanisms for the compromised tibial progression associated with a rigid ankle plantar flexion deformity.
(d) Sustained knee flexion during late stance is a potential sign of soleus weakness.
(e) A rigid ankle plantar flexion deformity is a potential cause of premature heel rise.

56. A 54-year-old plumber with diabetes is referred to you because of idiopathic midfoot swelling. Examination demonstrates marked midfoot warmth and edema. You obtain the radiographs shown in Fig. 7.9. Your initial treatment should be
(a) Irrigation, débridement, and intravenous antibiotics
(b) Rest, elevation, and casting
(c) Open reduction and internal fixation
(d) Midfoot fusion
(e) Chopart amputation

57. A 13-year-old girl complains of 2 months of unilateral ankle pain. The pain intermittently causes her to limp and wakes her from sleep. Ibuprofen completely relieves her discomfort. An anteroposterior radiograph and a sagittal magnetic resonance imaging scan are shown in Fig. 7.10. What is the most likely diagnosis?
(a) Osteomyelitis with sequestrum
(b) Osteoid osteoma
(c) Avascular necrosis
(d) Enostosis
(e) Köhler disease

58. A 38-year-old construction worker presents with chronic pain in his great toe. Examination reveals mild tenderness with painful, restricted dorsiflexion of the

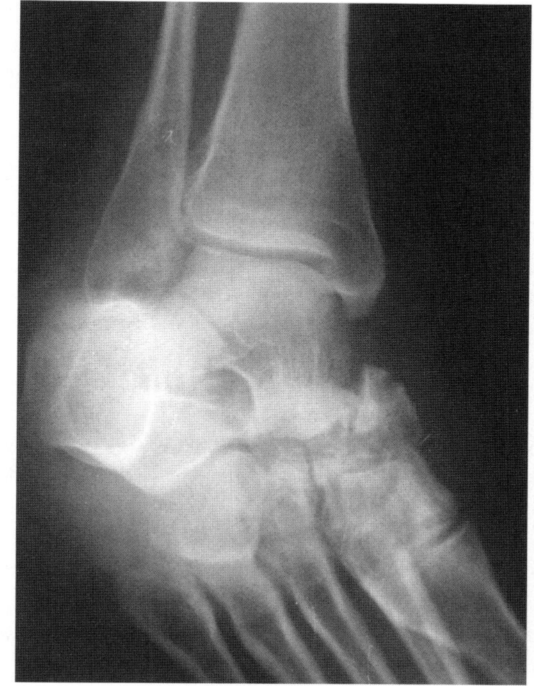

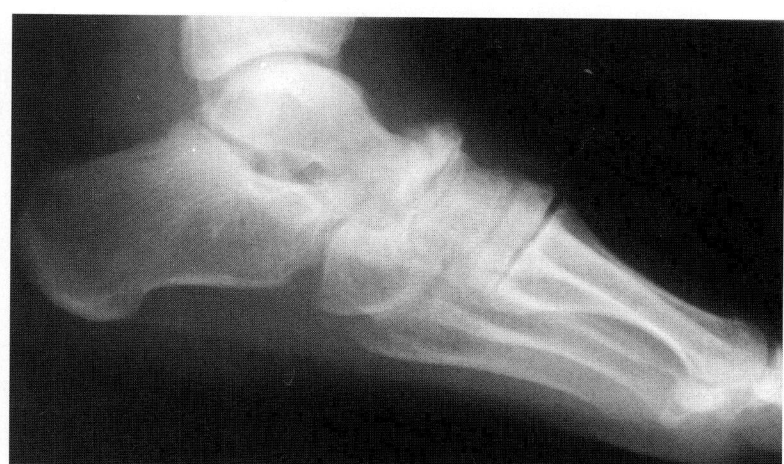

A B

FIGURE 7.9A and B

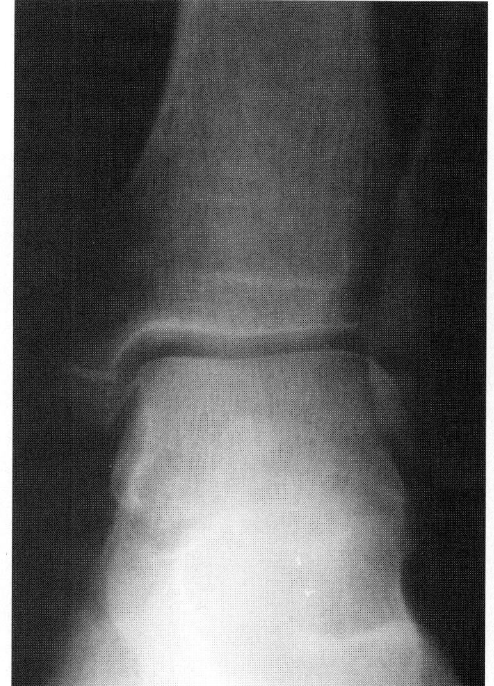

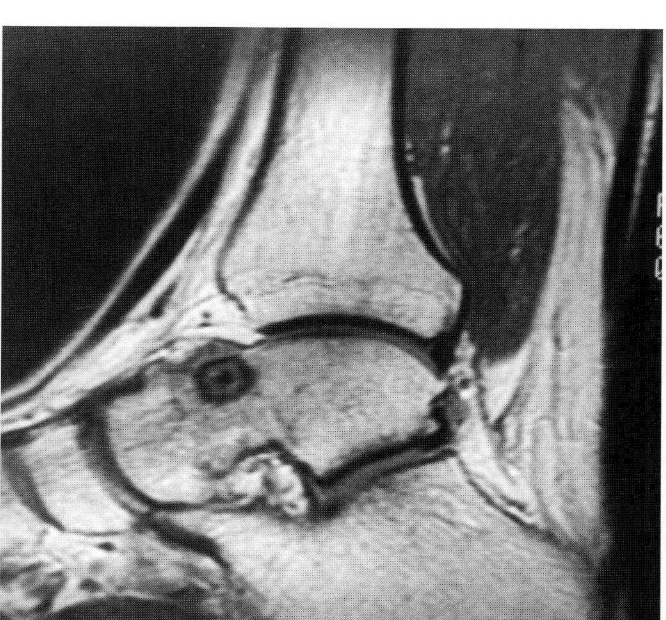

A B

FIGURE 7.10A and B

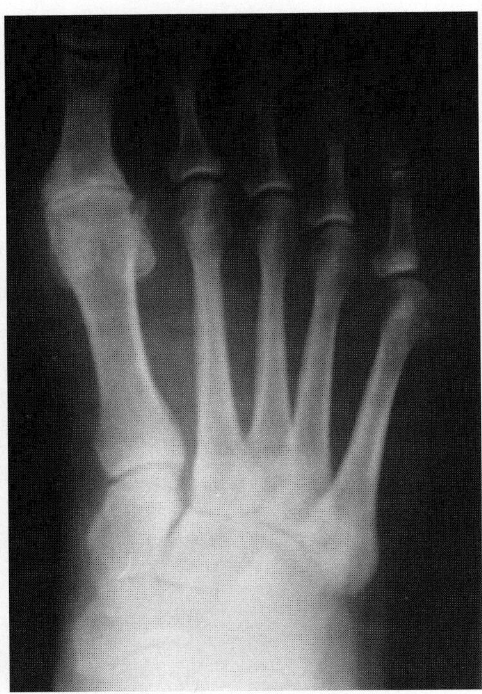

FIGURE 7.11

first metatarsophalangeal. An anteroposterior radiograph is shown in Fig. 7.11. Which of the following are the most appropriate diagnosis and initial treatment (respectively) for this patient?
(a) Gout; colchicine
(b) Subacute pyogenic arthritis; intravenous antibiotics
(c) Turf toe; indomethacin
(d) Gout; allopurinol
(e) Hallux rigidus; stiff-soled shoe

59. If nonoperative treatment fails, what would be the most appropriate treatment for the patient in question 58?
(a) Keller arthroplasty
(b) Cheilectomy
(c) Extension osteotomy of the base of the proximal phalanx
(d) Silastic implant arthroplasty
(e) First metatarsophalangeal joint fusion

60. A 23-year-old man is brought to the emergency room after a high-speed collision with a tree. A radiograph of his swollen right foot is shown in Fig. 7.12. What are the origin and insertion of the disrupted ligament?
(a) The medial cuneiform to the base of the first metatarsal
(b) The base of second metatarsal to the base of the first metatarsal
(c) The medial cuneiform to the base of the second metatarsal

A 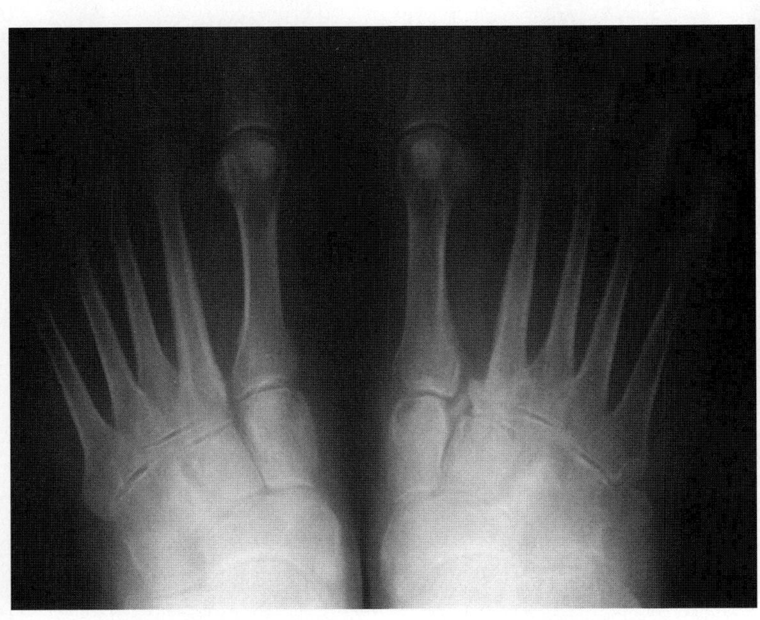

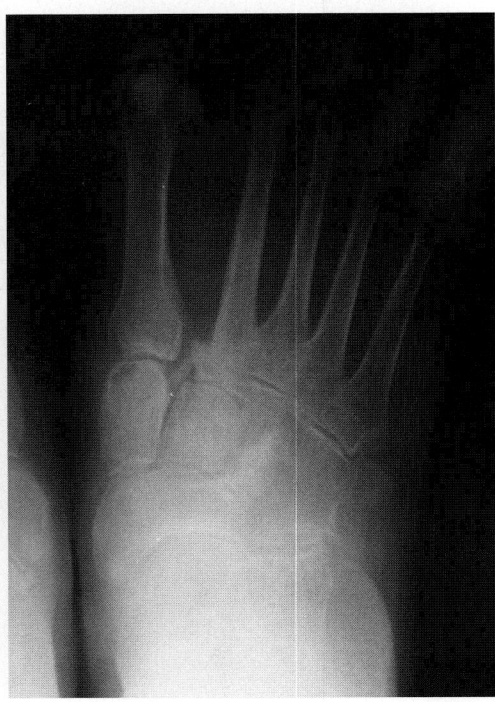 B

FIGURE 7.12A and B

(d) The base of first metatarsal to the middle cuneiform
(e) The middle cuneiform to the base of the second metatarsal

61. A 54-year-old postal worker presents with several months of intermittent acute pain and swelling in his right third toe. He is otherwise healthy, except for hypertension for which he takes furosemide. The distal interphalangeal joint of the third toe is swollen, tender, and erythematous. Anteroposterior and lateral radiographs are shown in Fig. 7.13. Aspiration of the joint would most likely reveal
(a) Inflammatory cells with a predominance of lymphocytes
(b) Negatively birefringent crystals
(c) Acid-fast bacilli
(d) Perivascular granuloma formation
(e) Positively birefringent crystals

62. A 26-year-old professional long-distance runner complains of 2 weeks of progressive foot pain while training. The pain has progressed to the point of precluding running for more than half a mile at a time. She denies pain with ambulation, and she has a nonantalgic gait. She states that she is otherwise perfectly healthy. Review of systems reveals that she has been amenorrheic for 2 years. A radiograph is reportedly normal, and a bone scan is shown in Fig. 7.14. You should recommend
(a) Incisional biopsy
(b) Nonsteroidal antiinflammatory drugs, calcium supplementation, and continued training
(c) Cross training, a hard-soled shoe, and referral to a gynecologist to consider hormone replacement therapy
(d) A short-leg walking cast, transvaginal ultrasound, and magnetic resonance imaging of the foot
(e) Percutaneous needle biopsy and culture

63. A 35-year-old woman has complaints of pain and deformity of the great toe. A standing anteroposterior radiograph is shown in Fig. 7.15. The hallux valgus angle measures 20 degrees, and the intermetatarsal angle measures 12 degrees. Which of the following operative procedures should be recommended if conservative measures fail?
(a) Mitchell procedure
(b) Distal chevron osteotomy
(c) Akin osteotomy
(d) Proximal crescentic osteotomy
(e) Metatarsophalangeal joint arthrodesis

64. A 32-year-old lawyer presents with acute pain on the lateral border of her foot after tripping at the office. Radiographs reveal an avulsion fracture of the tuberosity of the base of the fifth metatarsal with extension into the metatarsocuboid joint and 2 mm of articular step-off. What musculotendinous unit is implicated as the cause of this injury?

A
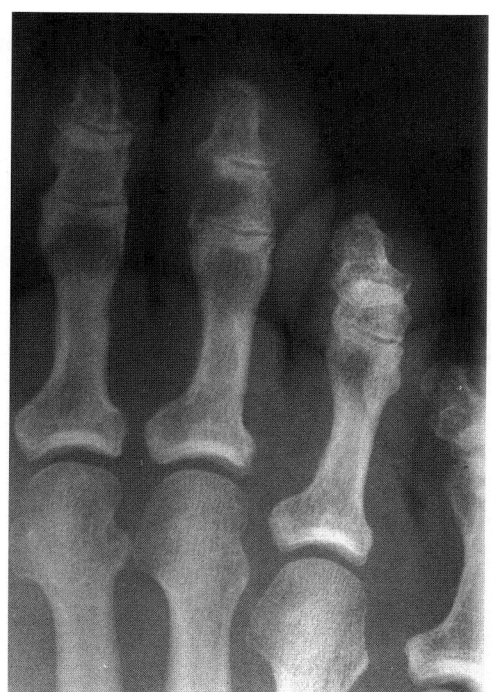

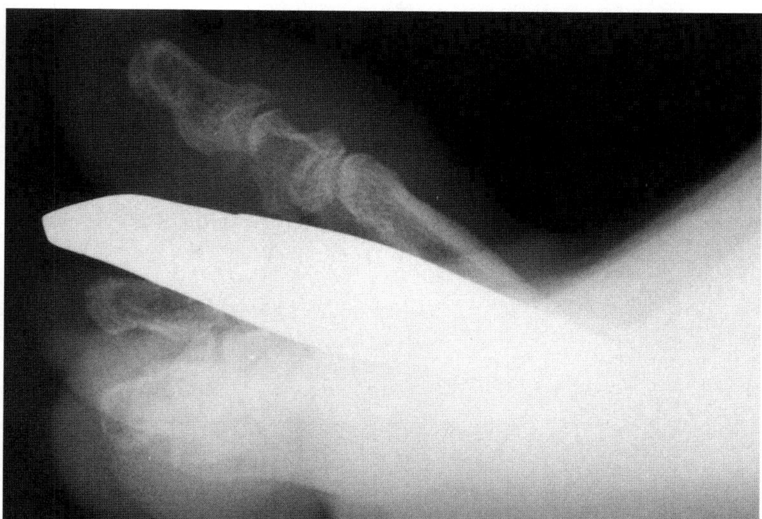
B

FIGURE 7.13A and B

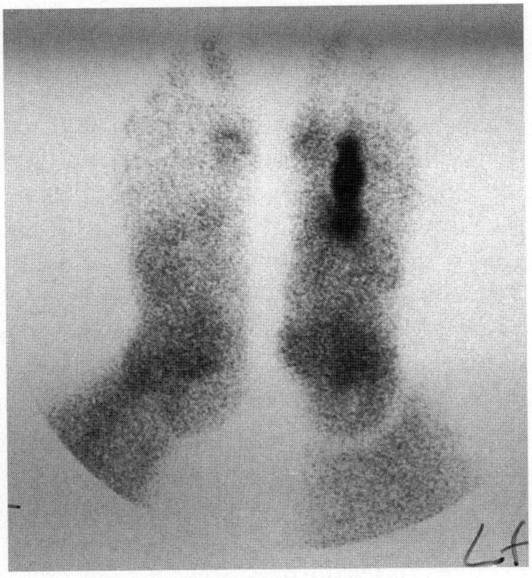

FIGURE 7.14

(a) The peroneus brevis
(b) The tibialis posterior
(c) The peroneus tertius
(d) The tibialis anterior
(e) The peroneus longus

65. What is the most appropriate treatment for the fracture in question 64?

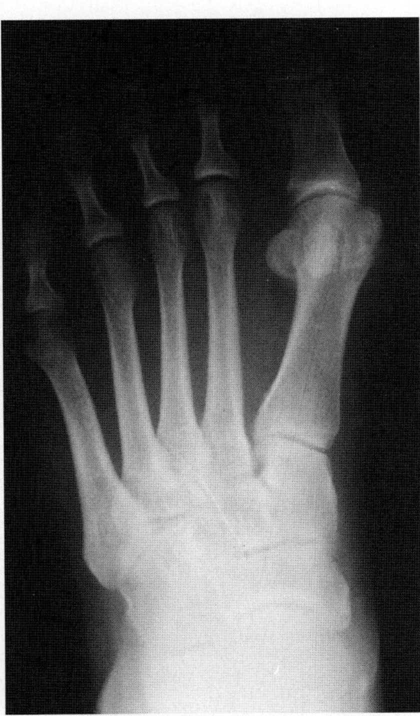

FIGURE 7.15

(a) Nonsteroidal antiinflammatory agents and a long-leg cast
(b) Weight bearing as tolerated in a hard-sole shoe
(c) Excision of the fragment and tendon advancement
(d) Short-leg cast (non–weight-bearing)
(e) Open reduction and internal fixation with an intramedullary screw

66. Which of the following statements is most accurate regarding the load transmitted by the Achilles tendon?
(a) During static single-leg toe rise, it transmits a force approximately equal to one-third body weight.
(b) During static single-leg toe rise, it transmits a force approximately equal to body weight.
(c) During static single-leg toe rise, it transmits a force approximately equal to three times body weight.
(d) During toe-off while running, it transmits a force approximately equal to two times body weight.
(e) During toe-off while running, it transmits a force approximately equal to three times body weight.

67. A 52-year-old waitress is concerned regarding her right fifth toe deformity. She experiences frequent pain, and she is unable to find shoes that fit comfortably. Examination reveals a 90-degree fixed flexion contracture of the proximal interphalangeal joint with a 60-degree fixed extension deformity of the metatarsophalangeal joint and dorsal subluxation of the proximal phalanx. The most appropriate surgical option would be
(a) Lengthening of the extensor digitorum longus
(b) Tenotomy of the flexor digitorum longus
(c) Syndactylization of the fourth and fifth toes
(d) Ruiz-Mora procedure
(e) Amputation of the fifth toe

68. Nonunion after an attempted triple arthrodesis is most commonly associated with what joint?
(a) The tibiotalar
(b) The calcaneocuboid
(c) The talonavicular
(d) The subtalar (middle facet)
(e) The subtalar (posterior facet)

69. What pathological findings characterize a Morton's neuroma?
(a) Vascular proliferation with noncaseating granuloma formation
(b) Fusiform enlargement at the proximal edge of the intermetatarsal ligament
(c) Perineural fibrosis with Renaut bodies
(d) Bulb neuroma
(e) Perineural fibrinous necrosis and an acute inflammatory infiltrate

70. A 58-year-old slender woman complains of a progressive flatfoot deformity with intermittent associated lateral ankle pain. She reports a history of long-standing medial ankle pain that resolved 2 months ago. Examination confirms a unilateral planovalgus deformity. She is unable to perform a heel rise on the affected side. She

has full passive range of motion of her subtalar and transverse talar joints. Based on this history and physical examination, what stage is the patient's disorder?
(a) I
(b) II
(c) III
(d) IV
(e) V

71. The treatment of the patient in question 70 should include
(a) Pantalar arthrodesis
(b) Tenosynovectomy of the posterior tibial tendon sheath
(c) Reconstruction with flexor digitorum longus tendon transfer
(d) Triple arthrodesis
(e) Primary tendon débridement and repair

72. Which of the following ligaments would you expect to be attenuated in this patient?
(a) The anterior talofibular ligament
(b) The deep deltoid ligament
(c) The long plantar ligament
(d) The spring ligament
(e) The talocalcaneal (interosseous) ligament

73. A 23-year-old semiprofessional skier presents with ankle pain after his ski tip straddled a gate on a slalom run. He has acute lateral ankle joint line tenderness anteriorly and posteriorly to the fibula. An external rotation stress on the foot causes pain. Compression of the midshaft of the fibula also reproduces his ankle discomfort. He has no medial ankle tenderness and no fibular head tenderness. Anteroposterior, lateral, and mortise views are normal and symmetric with comparison views of the contralateral ankle. The patient is taken to the operating room, where stress radiographs obtained while the patient is under anesthesia demonstrate no syndesmotic widening. The most appropriate next step would be
(a) Advise the patient to commence aggressive physical therapy and to anticipate a return to full activity within 1 to 2 weeks.
(b) Apply a short-leg cast and advise the patient to limit weight bearing and return for follow-up examination in 1 to 2 weeks.
(c) Perform open repair of the syndesmotic ligaments.
(d) Perform surgical stabilization of the syndesmosis with two fully threaded screws (three cortices each).
(e) Perform surgical stabilization of the syndesmosis with a single fully threaded screw (four cortices).

74. A 22-year-old professional ballerina presents with pain in her posteromedial ankle when she is *en pointe*. She denies a specific traumatic event. There is focal tenderness at the posteromedial aspect of her ankle. Symptoms are elicited when active ankle plantar flexion is resisted by pressure beneath her great toe. The most likely diagnosis is
(a) Achilles tendinitis
(b) Flexor hallucis longus tenosynovitis
(c) Posterior tibial tenosynovitis
(d) Fracture of the os trigonum
(e) Stress fracture of the sustentaculum tali

75. What is the knot of Henry?
(a) A fusiform thickening that characteristically occurs within the flexor hallucis longus tendon and results from tendinosis
(b) An accessory sesamoid bone within the flexor digitorum longus tendon
(c) A normal anatomic landmark where the flexor hallucis longus and flexor digitorum longus cross
(d) A fusiform thickening that characteristically occurs in the posterior tibial tendon and results from tendinosis
(e) A normal anatomic landmark where the peroneus longus tendon crosses beneath the flexor hallucis longus tendon

76. Use of fluoroquinolone antibiotics has been associated with which of the following foot and ankle disorders?
(a) Idiopathic fibrosis of the common peroneal tendon sheath
(b) Idiopathic synovitis of the second metatarsophalangeal joint
(c) Osteonecrosis of the talus
(d) Rupture of the Achilles tendon
(e) Idiopathic synovitis of the ankle joint

77. Which of the following is true regarding the sesamoid bones of the great toe?
(a) Approximately 80% of bipartite sesamoids occur in the tibial sesamoid.
(b) The fibular sesamoid receives a partial insertion from the abductor hallucis tendon.
(c) The sesamoids are contained within the flexor digitorum longus tendon.
(d) If one sesamoid requires excision, then both should be excised.
(e) Acute sesamoid fractures more commonly involve the fibular sesamoid.

78. A 20-year-old gymnast complains of recalcitrant posterior ankle pain that is exacerbated when she is on the balance beam and during her tumbling routine. On physical examination, mild swelling and tenderness are noted anterolateral to the Achilles tendon. Pain is reproduced with extreme ankle plantar flexion, but neither resisted flexion of the great toe nor resisted eversion causes appreciable discomfort. A radiograph is shown in Fig. 7.16. Injection of the flexor hallucis longus and peroneal tendon sheaths with local anesthetic provides minimal relief. What would be the most appropriate intervention after failure of conservative treatment?

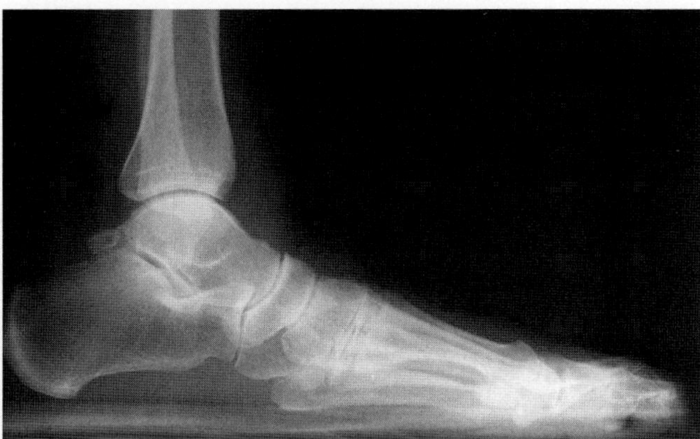

FIGURE 7.16

(a) Peroneal tenosynovectomy
(b) Excision of the os trigonum
(c) Open reduction and internal fixation of the avulsion fracture of the posterior process of the talus
(d) Haglund procedure (débridement of bone and bursa with Achilles reattachment if necessary)
(e) Resection of the calcaneal exostosis

79. A 19-year-old college student complains of persistent ankle pain 3 months after twisting her ankle while dancing in high-heeled shoes. Several doctors have assured her that her radiographs are normal and have advised her to bear weight progressively as tolerated in an ankle splint. Nonsteroidal antiiflammatory drugs have not effectively alleviated the discomfort. On physical examination, moderate ankle swelling and warmth are noted. There is severe, generalized, exquisite tenderness to light touch at the ankle and hindfoot with associated decreased ankle and subtalar range of motion (active and passive). There is no change in skin color or texture. Plain films are normal, but the delayed phase of a bone scan reveals diffuse increased periarticular uptake in the distal tibia and talus. What would be the most appropriate treatment?
(a) Aspiration of the distal tibia to rule out occult tumor or infection
(b) Physical therapy for motion exercises, whirlpool, and contrast baths
(c) Magnetic resonance imaging to rule out occult tumor or infection
(d) Aspiration of the ankle joint to rule out occult tumor or infection
(e) A narcotic pain medication to facilitate return to normal activities

80. What is the most common type of malunion after a type II fracture of the talar neck treated by closed reduction?
(a) Varus
(b) Valgus
(c) Dorsal displacement
(d) Plantar displacement
(e) Extension

81. A 52-year-old librarian with rheumatoid arthritis complains of forefoot pain. She has pain with walking and at rest. Her custom orthotic no longer controls her pain with ambulation. Examination reveals tenderness and minimal motion at the first metatarsophalangeal joint. A radiograph is shown in Fig. 7.17. You should recommend
(a) Keller resection
(b) Arthrodesis of the first metatarsophalangeal joint
(c) Forefoot reconstruction with arthrodesis of the first metatarsophalangeal joint and resection arthroplasties of the lesser metatarsal heads
(d) Flexion osteotomy of the first metatarsal
(e) Synovectomy of the first metatarsophalangeal joint

82. Compression of which of the following nerves should be considered in the differential diagnosis of plantar fasciitis?
(a) The sural nerve
(b) The medial plantar nerve
(c) The lateral plantar nerve
(d) The nerve to the abductor hallucis
(e) The nerve to the abductor digiti minimi

83. A 69-year-old man had suffered a stroke with resultant left hemiparesis. He has made considerable progress with his therapy, but he has developed painful calluses along the lateral border of his left foot in association

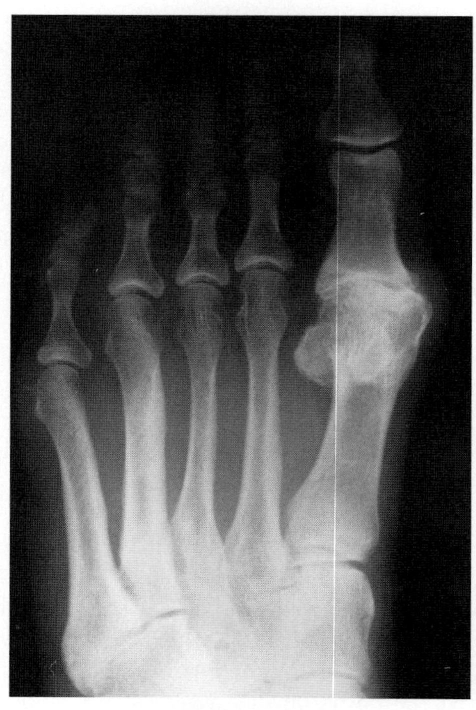

FIGURE 7.17

with a progressive flexible varus deformity. An ankle-foot orthosis has not provided relief. Electromyograms reveal continuous overactivity of the tibialis anterior. The most appropriate recommendation would be
(a) Split anterior tibial tendon transfer
(b) Peroneal tendon imbrication
(c) Triple arthrodesis in 5 degrees of hindfoot valgus
(d) Anterolateral transfer of the posterior tibial tendon
(e) Anterior tibial tendon release

84. Which of the following patients would be the best candidate for a total ankle replacement?
(a) A 48-year-old woman with rheumatoid arthritis who wants to retain choice of heel height
(b) A 60-year-old woman with posttraumatic arthritis after a tibial plafond fracture treated with internal fixation
(c) A 70-year-old woman with rheumatoid arthritis who is a household ambulator
(d) A 45-year-old man with osteonecrosis after a talar fracture
(e) A 66-year-old man with degenerative arthritis who has a nonunion of an attempted tibiotalar fusion

85. The most appropriate orthotic prescription to treat acute Achilles tendinitis in a patient with 10 degrees of hindfoot valgus alignment would be
(a) A 5-degree medial hindfoot wedge with a 9-mm heel lift
(b) A 5-degree lateral hindfoot wedge with a 9-mm heel lift
(c) A 5-degree medial hindfoot wedge with a 3-mm recessed heel cup
(d) A 5-degree lateral hindfoot wedge with a 3-mm recessed heel cup
(e) An ankle-foot orthosis with a hinged ankle

86. A 32-year-old marathoner presents with a 1-month history of vague midfoot pain. A bone scan reveals increased uptake in the tarsal navicular. A computed tomography scan demonstrates a nondisplaced linear sagittal defect in the middle third of the navicular. Recommended treatment should be
(a) A short-leg walking cast for 6 weeks
(b) Progressive weight bearing as tolerated in a hard-soled shoe
(c) A short-leg walking cast for 3 weeks followed by progressive weight bearing as tolerated in a hard-soled shoe
(d) Short-leg nonwalking cast for 6 to 8 weeks
(e) Internal fixation followed by a short-leg nonwalking cast for 6 to 8 weeks

87. Which of the following statements is most accurate regarding traumatic osteochondral lesions of the talar dome?
(a) The Berndt and Harty classification is predicated on the appearance of the lesion at the time of arthroscopy.
(b) Medial fragments are typically more accessible for screw fixation than lateral lesions.
(c) Lateral lesions are often wafer shaped, whereas medial lesions are often cup shaped.
(d) Most lateral lesions stem from an eversion mechanism, whereas most medial lesions result from inversion.
(e) All displaced fragments should be excised.

88. A professional basketball player presents at the end of the preseason with lateral forefoot pain. He states that it has been aching intermittently since the end of last season. Radiographs reveal a complete, nondisplaced fracture of the base of his fifth metatarsal 2 mm distal to the metaphyseal-diaphyseal junction with mild intermedullary sclerosis. What treatment should you recommend?
(a) Weight bearing as tolerated in a hard-soled shoe until symptoms subside
(b) Internal fixation with an intramedullary compression screw
(c) Short-leg cast (non–weight-bearing) for 3 months
(d) Internal fixation with a compression plate
(e) Short-leg walking cast for 3 months

89. A 48-year-old postal worker develops posttraumatic tibiotalar arthritis after a talar neck fracture. He is successfully treated by ankle arthrodesis. However, at 1-year follow-up, he complains of new ankle pain that limits his walking. He denies fever, chills, or rest pain. On physical examination, no tenderness, warmth, or perceptible motion is noted over the incision or fusion site. His symptoms are reproduced with inversion and eversion. Follow-up radiographs are shown in Fig. 7.18. Complete blood count and erythrocyte sedimentation rate are normal. Your next procedure should be
(a) Irrigation and débridement
(b) Talonavicular arthrodesis
(c) Triple arthrodesis
(d) Subtalar arthrodesis
(e) Wedge osteotomy through the fusion mass to optimize alignment

90. A 24-year-old woman "sprained" her ankle when she caught the tip of her ski and fell forward 4 months ago. Radiographs taken at the time were reportedly "negative." She now complains of intermittent painful "snapping" at the lateral aspect of her ankle during athletic activities. Examination reveals tenderness and mild swelling posterior to the lateral malleolus. Resisted dorsiflexion of the everted foot reproduces her pain and increases the fullness over the lateral malleolus. Repeat stress radiographs are normal. If conservative treatment fails, what would be the most appropriate form of intervention?
(a) Repair of the superficial peroneal retinaculum
(b) Débridement and reconstruction of the peroneus brevis tendon

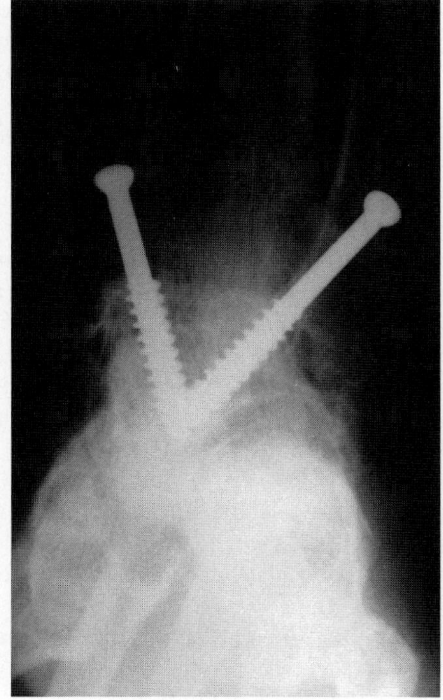

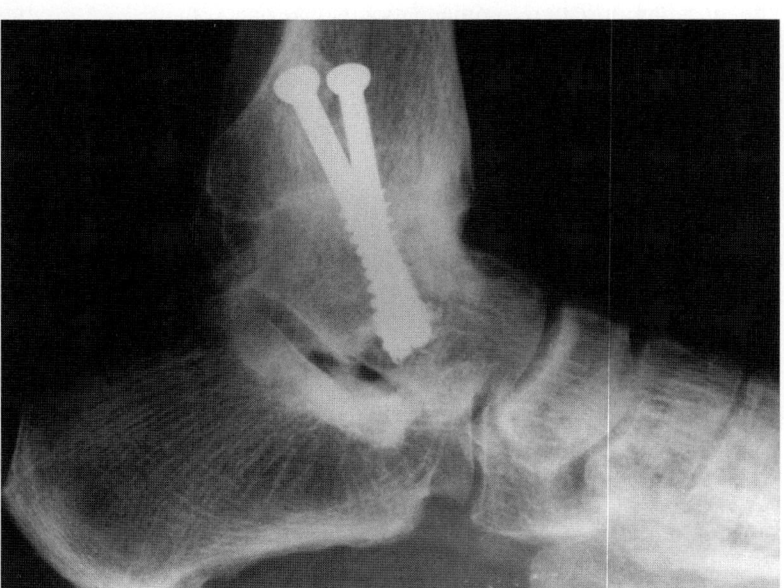

FIGURE 7.18A and B

(c) Chrisman-Snook procedure
(d) Sliding distal fibular bone block
(e) Tenodesis of the peroneus longus to the peroneus brevis

91. Which of the following associated injuries would be least anticipated in a patient presenting for evaluation of a lateral ankle "sprain" sustained by an inversion mechanism?
(a) Fracture of the lateral process of the talus
(b) Fracture of the base of the fifth metatarsal
(c) Lateral osteochondral fracture of the talar dome
(d) Avulsion of the calcaneal tuberosity
(e) Medial osteochondral fracture of the talar dome

92. Which of the following ligaments is the principal restraint to translation in the anterior drawer test?
(a) The calcaneofibular
(b) The posterior talofibular
(c) The posterior tibiofibular
(d) The deltoid
(e) The anterior talofibular

93. In a supination external rotation stage IV (SER-IV) trimalleolar ankle fracture, which of the following is responsible for the posterior malleolus fragment?
(a) The posterior tibiofibular ligament
(b) The posterior ankle capsule
(c) Axial compression by the talus
(d) Internal talar rotation
(e) Extreme ankle dorsiflexion

94. A 32-year-old anatomy professor presents with unilateral ankle pain and swelling. Plain radiographs and magnetic resonance images manifest two significant lesions: (1) a large medullary infarct in the distal tibia and (2) osteonecrosis of the medial talar dome with an associated subchondral fracture and a mild joint effusion. There is no periostitis. Given these images (and no history), what would be the most likely unifying diagnosis?
(a) Osteomyelitis
(b) Chondrosarcoma
(c) Lupus erythematosus
(d) Traumatic osteochondral fracture of the talus with reciprocal bone contusion
(e) Osteochondritis dissecans

95. A 1-mm lateral talar shift reduces tibiotalar surface contact area by what amount?
(a) 5%
(b) 10%
(c) 25%
(d) 40%
(e) 75%

96. Which of the following is least useful in contemporary management of high-energy pilon fractures?
(a) The 3.5-mm clover-leaf plate
(b) Immediate open reduction and internal fixation of the fibula
(c) External fixation
(d) The spoon plate

(e) Metaphyseal bone grafting

97. A 19-year-old woman sustains a lateral dislocation of her subtalar joint when she jumps off a balcony at a grunge rock concert. Which of the following is the most common obstruction to closed reduction of this injury?
   (a) The spring ligament
   (b) An interlocked impaction fracture of articular surfaces of the talus and navicular
   (c) The flexor hallucis longus tendon
   (d) The extensor digitorum brevis muscle
   (e) The posterior tibial tendon

ANSWERS

1. **b** Hypermobile metatarsus primus varus. First metatarsocuneiform fusion corrects metatarsus primus varus at the apex of the deformity. It is indicated for a hypermobile joint, metatarsocuneiform arthritis, and occasionally in revision situations. The procedure can be technically demanding, given the irregular contour of the joint. Fusion may require a long time (4 to 6 months).

   The presence of an open physis is a contraindication to this procedure. An intermetatarsal angle of 13 degrees is a moderate deformity, and fusion would be inappropriate unless accompanied by hypermobility. This procedure is contraindicated in patients with normal metatarsocuneiform stability. Because this procedure stiffens the foot, it should be avoided in athletic patients. Transfer metatarsalgia can be a complication of the procedure if the joint is not fused in slight plantar flexion.

Reference

Molden DM, et al.: Correction of Hallux Valgus with Metatarsocuneiform Stabilization. Foot Ankle, 11:59–66, 1990.

2. **a** Proximal metatarsal osteotomy for hallux valgus fixed in 20 degrees of dorsiflexion. A transfer lesion is a painful condition that results from a redistribution of force to the lesser metatarsals (usually the second). This is seen in deformities or postsurgical situations in which the first metatarsophalangeal joint is unloaded. When a proximal metatarsal osteotomy is performed, care must be taken to avoid excessive plantar flexion or dorsiflexion of the first ray. With increased dorsiflexion, the first metatarsophalangeal is unloaded, and the load is shifted to the second metatarsal. This can cause pain and hyperkeratosis beneath the second metatarsal head.

   Arthrodesis of the first metatarsophalangeal in plantar flexion would be disabling, but this would increase the load on the first interphalangeal joint, rather than transfer the load to the lesser metatarsophalangeal joints. The listed tendon transfer procedures are not associated with transfer lesions.

3. **b** Grade II. The Wagner classification remains a widely accepted system for diabetic foot ulcers. Grade 0 lesions have intact skin. Grade I ulcers are superficial, with only subcutaneous tissue exposed. Grade II lesions expose deeper structures, such as tendon and muscle, but they do not involve bone. Grade III lesions are characterized by periosteal reaction (indicating bone involvement) or extension of infection beyond the borders of the ulcer. Grade IV and V lesions both involve dysvascular feet with partial (IV) or total (V) gangrene of the foot.

Reference

Wagner FW: The Dysvascular Foot: A System for Diagnosis and Treatment. Foot Ankle, 2:64–122, 1981.

4. **b** Total contact cast. Total contact casting has been shown to be 90% effective for Wagner grade II diabetic ulcers. Antibiotics are not a necessary part of the treatment of grade II lesions. Grade I lesions should be addressed conservatively with elevation, restricted weight bearing, custom-molded shoes, or total contact casting. Grade III ulcers require surgical débridement and antibiotics. Grade IV wounds require local amputation, and grade V wounds necessitate regional amputation.

Reference

McDermott JE: The Diabetic Foot: Evolving Techniques. Instr Course Lect 42:169–171, 1993

5. **e** Dorsiflexion. Violent dorsiflexion causes impaction of the dorsum of the neck of the talus against the anterior tibia. Such extreme dorsiflexion is most commonly associated with motor vehicle accidents and falls. This injury was classically described to stem from aviation crashes (as the rudder bar drove the pilot's foot into hyperdorsiflexion). Hence the eponym *aviator's astralagus.*

Reference

Coltart WD: Aviators Astralagus. J Bone Joint Surg Br, 34:545–566, 1952.

6. **b** Tibiotalar dorsiflexion is coupled with proximal migration and external rotation of the fibula. With tibiotalar dorsiflexion, the lateral facet of the talus contacts the lateral malleolus and induces proximal migration and external rotation of the fibula.

   Dorsiflexion of the metatarsophalangeal joints raises the longitudinal arch by contraction of the plantar aponeurosis by the "windlass" mechanism (Fig. 7.19).

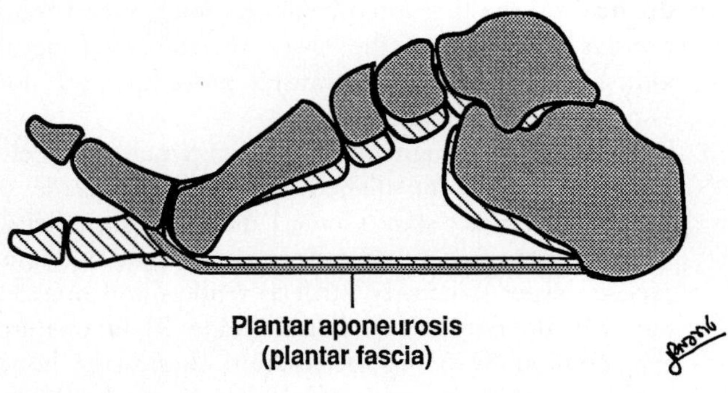

FIGURE 7.19

With foot pronation (subtalar eversion/hindfoot valgus), the axes of the talonavicular and calcaneocuboid joints become more parallel. Thus, the midfoot (transverse tarsal joint) becomes more flexible (for shock absorption) from heel strike through midstance. From midstance through toe-off, the foot supinates (subtalar inversion/hindfoot varus). This is coupled with divergence of the talonavicular and calcaneocuboid joint axes, thereby "locking" transverse tarsal motion.

Because of the inclined obliquity of the subtalar joint axis, this joint functions as a mitered hinge. Thus, subtalar eversion is coupled with internal rotation of the talus. The internal rotation of the talus is transmitted to the tibia through the ankle mortise. During terminal stance, the subtalar joint inverts. Subtalar inversion is coupled with external rotation of the talus. External talar rotation is, in turn, transmitted to the tibia by the talus.

7. **d** Modified Brostrom. The stress radiographs reveal 3+ (greater than 15 degrees) of talar tilt in the left ankle. This is consistent with a grade III injury, indicating disruption of both the anterior talofibular ligament and the calcaneofibular ligament.

The *modified Brostrom technique* (Fig. 7.20) has emerged as a popular technique for ankle stabilization because it is an anatomic repair (imbrication) of the elongated anterior talofibular ligament and calcaneofibular ligament. The modification incorporates suturing the extensor retinaculum to the tip of the lateral malleolus to reinforce the repair and to provide additional resistance to inversion. A major advantage of this procedure is that it does not sacrifice the peroneal tendons, which are dynamic stabilizers of the lateral ankle. Restoring the lateral ankle ligaments to their appropriate lengths may reestablish the proprioceptive function of these static stabilizers.

Numerous nonanatomic procedures have been described. These checkrein techniques recruit local tendons to replace the attenuated lateral ankle ligaments. Most of these procedures use the peroneus brevis tendon. The *Chrisman-Snook procedure* is the most anatomic of the tenodesis procedures. This technique uses half of the peroneus brevis tendon to reconstitute the anterior talofibular ligament and calcaneofibular ligament. It limits talar tilt, but it also compromises subtalar motion.

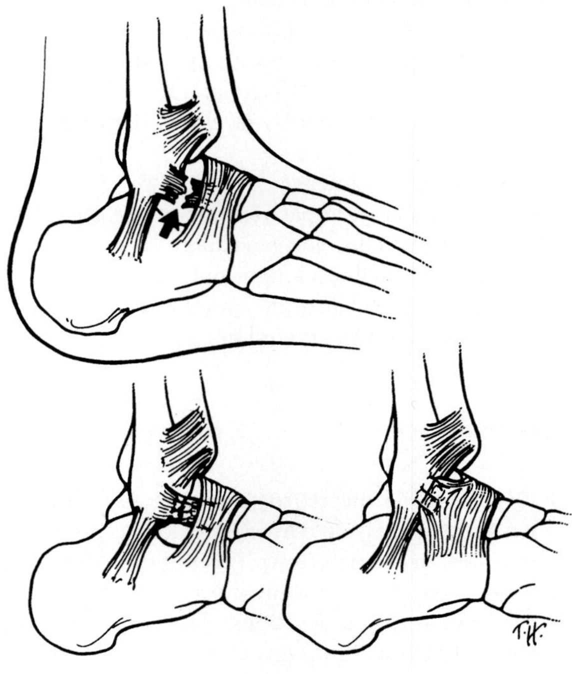

FIGURE 7.20

The *Watson-Jones procedure* also compromises subtalar motion. This procedure reconstructs only the anterior talofibular ligament. Thus, it provides the most stability in plantar flexion. This technique limits anterior talar translation more effectively than the Chrisman-Snook procedure, but it is less effective at limiting talar tilt.

The *Evans procedure* does not anatomically reconstitute either the anterior talofibular ligament or the calcaneofibular ligament. Advantages of this procedure include its relative simplicity and few complications. The *Lapidus procedure* refers to fusion of the first metatarsocuneiform joint and is irrelevant to the subject of lateral ankle instability.

Reference

Lutter LD et al., eds: Orthopaedic Knowledge Update: Foot and Ankle. Rosemont, IL, American Academy of Orthopedic Surgeons, pp. 241–251, 1994.

8. **b** Gradual return to play over the next 2 weeks with taping to restrict extension. The history and physical examination are classic for turf toe. This is a hyperextension injury of the first metatarsophalangeal joint

with variable damage to plantar structures. This injury has been encountered with increased frequency in association with artificial turf and the use of lightweight (flexible-soled) shoes.

A grade I injury is a mild sprain with local pain. There is minimal swelling or ecchymosis. These patients can usually return to play immediately, with ice, elevation, and nonsteroidal antiinflammatory drugs to control symptoms.

Grade II injuries are associated with a partial tear of the plantar capsule. This is associated with significant tenderness, swelling ecchymosis, and decreased motion. Typically, 1 to 2 weeks are required before return to play with taping and stiff-soled shoes to restrict metatarsophalangeal joint extension.

Grade III injuries represent complete tearing of the capsuloligamentous structures. This includes disruption of the plantar plate and injury to the metatarsal head. Sometimes this injury pattern represents a spontaneously reduced dorsal dislocation. Patients present with marked pain, swelling, ecchymosis, and greatly limited motion. Sesamoid fractures or avulsion fragments may be seen on radiographs. Return to play is usually not possible for 3 to 6 weeks. Surgical removal of loose bodies or repair of the plantar plate may be required.

The flexor hallucis brevis tendon is one of the components of the plantar plate. Disruption of the flexor hallucis brevis would present as a grade III injury, and radiographs would reveal displacement of the sesamoids.

References

Lutter LD, et al., eds: Orthopaedic Knowledge Update: Foot and Ankle. Rosemont, IL, American Academy of Orthopedic Surgeons, pp. 154–155, 1994.

Rodeo SA, et al.: Turf Toe. Am J Sports Med, 18:280–285, 1990.

9. **c** The dorsal intermediate cutaneous nerve. The anterolateral portal is made immediately lateral to the peroneus tertius tendon, and, thus, this tendon should not be injured. The dorsal intermediate cutaneous nerve (a branch of the superficial peroneal nerve) is subcutaneous in this vicinity. This nerve can often be palpated before one places the portal. To avoid injury to this structure, the skin should be incised with subsequent blunt dissection to the ankle capsule.

The sural nerve is at risk with the posterolateral portal. This portal is usually placed under arthroscopic visualization at the lateral border of the Achilles tendon. The artery of the sinus tarsi is distal to the joint line and, thus, it is at less risk. The saphenous nerve and vein are at risk during establishment of the anteromedial portal, which is made at the medial border of the tibialis anterior tendon.

Reference

Ferkel RD, Fischer SP: Progress in Ankle Arthroscopy. Clin Orthop, 240:210–220, 1989.

10. **b** Use of a lag screw to ensure adequate compression of the syndesmosis. It is crucial to avoid overcompression of the syndesmosis. The syndesmosis screw is a neutralization device. Lag screw technique should not be used. Overcompression will restrict ankle dorsiflexion because the anterior articular surface of the talus is wider than the posterior articular surface. Overcompression is avoided by positioning the ankle in 10 to 15 degrees of dorsiflexion during syndesmosis screw placement. This brings the wider (anterior) portion of the talus into the mortise to ensure that full range of ankle motion is preserved.

Because the fibula lies posterolaterally to the tibia, syndesmosis screws should be angulated from posterolateral to anteromedial (approximately 30 degrees anterior to the coronal plane). Screws should be placed 2 to 3 cm proximal to the plafond and parallel to the articular surface. Proximal or distal screw angulation can lead to shortening or lengthening of the fibula (when there is an associated proximal fibular fracture).

Note: Even if the syndesmosis ligaments are completely disrupted, a syndesmosis screw is not required if the fibula is anatomically reduced and the medial structures (deltoid ligament and medial malleolus) are intact. When there is medial stability, a nondisplaced syndesmosis disruption does not significantly alter tibiotalar biomechanics.

Reference

Boden SD, et al.: Mechanical Considerations for the Syndesmosis Screw: A Cadaver Study. J Bone Joint Surg Am, 69:1346–1352, 1989.

11. **d** Revascularization of the talus. Fractures of the neck of the talus have a high complication rate. Avascular necrosis is a common sequela because of the tenuous blood supply of the talus. For this reason, displaced fractures of the talar neck should be anatomically reduced and rigidly stabilized promptly. Serial radiographs can be used to assess the viability of the talar body.

Hawkins sign is the appearance of subchondral lucency in the dome of the talus (seen on the anteroposterior ankle radiograph). This sign signifies preserved vascularity to the talar body. Blood flow is necessary for this resorption to occur. Hawkins sign typically appears 6 to 8 weeks after injury. It indicates the absence of osteonecrosis.

Note: Osteonecrosis produces increased radiographic density, but this sclerosis may take several months to appear.

Reference

Hawkins LG: Fractures of the Neck of the Talus. J Bone Joint Surg Am, 52:991–1002, 1970.

12. **a** Antiinflammatory drugs, heel lift, and activity modification. *Haglund syndrome* consists of pain and swelling in the region of the retrocalcaneal bursa in association with a prominence of the posterosuperior margin of the calcaneus. Impingement of the bony prominence on the Achilles causes insertional tendinitis and inflammation of the intervening retrocalcaneal bursa.

    Initial treatment should be conservative. This includes nonsteroidal antiinflammatory drugs, ice, shoe modification (use of a heel lift and avoiding a hard heel counter), and activity modification (avoiding running on hilly terrain). If symptoms persist, immobilization in a walking cast (for 4 to 6 weeks) should be tried. If these measures fail to quell the inflammation, surgical excision of the bursa and bony prominence may be undertaken.

    Note: Retrocalcaneal steroid injection should be performed with caution because of the risk of Achilles tendon weakening.

Reference

Jones DC, James SL: Partial Calcaneal Ostectomy for Retrocalcaneal Bursitis. Am J Sports Med, 12:72–73, 1984.

13. **e** Flexor digitorum longus. The cross-sectional shape of the tibia and fibula localizes this image to the supramalleolar region of the ankle. Note the paucity of muscle in this cross section. Note the robust anterior tibiofibular syndesmotic ligament. The only significant muscle belly present in this image is the flexor hallucis longus (directly posterior to the tibia). The Achilles tendon is seen in its subcutaneous position posterior to the flexor hallucis longus. Two distinct structures lie directly posterior to the fibula in this image: (1) the peroneus longus tendon laterally and (2) the peroneus brevis musculotendinous junction medially.

    Note: The peroneus brevis passes closer to the lateral malleolus and its muscle belly extends further distally than that of the peroneus longus.

    The single arrow marks the tibialis posterior musculotendinous junction. The double arrow marks the flexor digitorum longus musculotendinous junction. Directly posterolateral to the flexor digitorum longus are the posterior tibial artery and paired posterior tibial veins. (The water molecules in the veins yield a higher signal because they are moving more slowly.) The structure that resembles a *bunch of grapes* between these vessels and the flexor hallucis longus is the tibial nerve.

    Note: A useful pneumonic for remembering the order in which these structures pass posterior to the medial malleolus is "Tom, Dick, And Very Nervous Harry."

14. **c** 15 degrees of valgus and 15 degrees of dorsiflexion in relation to the floor. The optimal position for a first metatarsophalangeal fusion is approximately 15 degrees of valgus and approximately 15 degrees of dorsiflexion in relation to the floor (which typically equals approximately 30 degrees of dorsiflexion in relation to the metatarsal shaft). Insufficient dorsiflexion can cause the patient to have to vault over the great toe during gait. Malalignment of the fusion (e.g., insufficient valgus) can lead to difficulty with shoe wear and excessive stress across the interphalangeal joint with accelerated interphalangeal degeneration. Indications for first metatarsophalangeal arthrodesis include advanced rheumatoid or degenerative arthritis, spasticity, or as a salvage procedure.

References

Coughlin MJ: Arthrodesis of the First Metatarsophalangeal Joint With Minifragment Plate Fixation. Orthopaedics, 13:1037–1044, 1990.
Fitzgerald J: A Review of the Longterm Results of Fusion of the First Metatarsophalangeal Joint. J Bone Joint Surg Br, 51:488–493, 1969.

15. **a** Origin: the medial tubercle of the calcaneus; insertion: the middle phalanges. The flexor digitorum brevis is an intrinsic muscle that flexes the proximal interphalangeal joints. It originates from the medial tubercle of the calcaneus and inserts on the middle phalanges. The flexor digitorum longus inserts on the distal phalanges. The metatarsophalangeal joint is flexed primarily by the lumbricals and the interossei.

    The lack of an extrinsic flexor insertion on the proximal phalanx helps to explain the origin of clawtoes, which result from an imbalance between intrinsic and extrinsic muscles. When extrinsic muscles overpower the intrinsics, the metatarsophalangeal joints hyperextend (because of the extrinsic extensor insertion onto the proximal phalanx), and the distal interphalangeal joints are flexed by the flexor digitorum longus *(intrinsic minus position)*.

    Note: Clawtoes are typically associated with an underlying neuromuscular disorder and tend to involve all the lesser toes. Hammer toes and mallet toes are the sequelae of extrinsic pressure, rather than an underlying neurologic disorder, and may affect only a single toe, usually the second (Table 7.1).

16. **b** Deep peroneal nerve. The deep peroneal nerve innervates the extensor digitorum brevis. The superficial peroneal nerve provides sensory innervation to the entire dorsum of the foot (except the first webspace), but it provides no motor innervation to the foot. The sural and saphenous nerves are purely sensory, inner-

TABLE 7.1. MALLET TOES, CLAWTOES, AND HAMMER TOES

Joint	Mallet	Claw	Hammer
Distal interphalangeal	Flexed	Flexed	Neutral
Proximal interphalangeal	Neutral	Flexed	Flexed
Metacarpophalangeal	Neutral	Hyperextended	Extended

vating the lateral and medial borders of the hindfoot, respectively.

17. **d** Injection of local anesthetic and steroid into the third webspace. The symptoms described are classic for an interdigital (Morton) neuroma. This condition is caused by tethering of the interdigital nerve beneath the distal edge of the transverse metatarsal ligament during metatarsophalangeal dorsiflexion. The third webspace is most commonly involved, followed by the second. Injection of local anesthetic and corticosteroid into the affected webspace (dorsal approach) can be both diagnostic and therapeutic. Conservative treatment includes low heels, a wide toe box, metatarsal pads, antiinflammatory medication, and ice. Excision can be performed for recalcitrant lesions.

    Electromyography and nerve conduction studies are useful in the diagnosis of tarsal tunnel syndrome but not in the diagnosis of Morton neuroma. The distribution of the dysesthesias in tarsal tunnel syndrome is typically broader and more proximal than those described in the question. Magnetic resonance imaging is useful for preoperatively identifying lesions causing compression of the posterior tibial nerve within the tarsal tunnel.

18. **e** The artery of the tarsal canal. The arrow marks the tarsal canal. The medial entrance to the tarsal canal lies directly caudal to the medial malleolus. The sagittal magnetic resonance image in Fig. 7.3 can be localized to the medial half of the foot based on (1) the presence of the talonavicular articulation and (2) the presence of the sustentaculum tali (directly below the space marked by the arrow). The medial side of the calcaneus is concave. Thus, only the most medial portions of the calcaneus (the sustentaculum tali and the medial portion of the tuberosity) are present on this image.

    The tarsal canal is continuous with the sinus tarsi on the lateral undersurface of the talus. The tarsal canal transmits the artery of the tarsal canal (a branch of the posterior tibial artery), which merges with the artery to the sinus tarsi to form an anastomotic sling beneath the talar neck. The canal runs obliquely from posteromedial to anterolateral between the posterior and middle articular facets of the calcaneus.

    The tarsal tunnel lies further medially than the image in Fig. 7.3. The flexor retinaculum or laciniate ligament forms the roof of the tarsal tunnel. Its contents are the tibial nerve (Fig. 7.21), the posterior tibial artery, the flexor digitorum longus tendon, the posterior tibial tendon, and the flexor hallucis longus tendon. The flexor hallucis longus tendon can be seen descending behind the talus in Fig. 7.3 before it passes beneath the sustentaculum tali in a more medial plane.

Reference

Mulfinger GL, Truetta J: The Blood Supply of the Talus. J Bone Joint Surg Br, 52:160–167, 1970.

19. **c** Malignant melanoma. (Please refer to the discussion for question 20.)
20. **c** Synovial cell sarcoma. *Malignant melanoma* is the most common malignant tumor in the foot. It is more common in women. Treatment typically consists of wide excision. Prognosis depends on the depth of invasion.

    Synovial cell sarcoma is the most common sarcoma in the foot. It accounts for approximately 50% of all foot sarcomas. Most specimens reveal a biphasic histologic pattern (pseudoglandular epithelial cells and fibroblas-

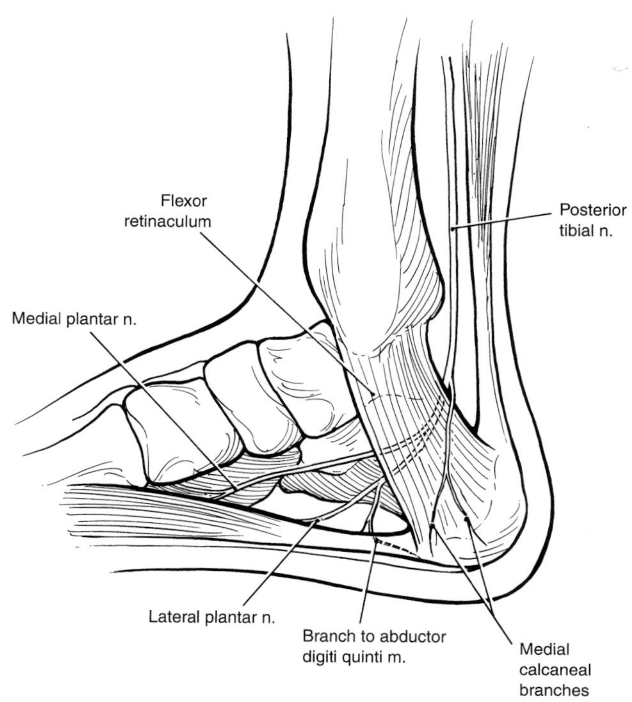

FIGURE 7.21

tic spindle cells). Some specimens reveal a monophasic (purely fibroblastic) population, and these lesions are associated with a worse prognosis. Approximately one-third of synovial cell sarcomas mineralize; those that mineralize carry a better prognosis.

Squamous cell carcinoma is the most common malignant tumor in the hand, but it is encountered less frequently in the foot. *Epithelioid sarcoma* is the most common sarcoma in the hand, but it occurs in less commonly in the foot.

Note: The most common location of melanoma in the foot is the plantar surface.

21. **b** Girdlestone-Taylor transfer. The *Girdlestone-Taylor tendon transfer* involves releasing the flexor digitorum longus from the distal phalanx, dividing it longitudinally, and suturing the ends to the extensor hood over the dorsum of the proximal phalanx. Thus, the deforming flexion force of the flexor digitorum longus at the distal interphalangeal joint is converted into a dynamic balancing force at the metatarsophalangeal. (Please refer to the discussion of question 15.)

    The Girdlestone-Taylor procedure is not effective for inflexible deformities. Rigid proximal interphalangeal deformities require excision of the distal aspect of the proximal phalanx. Lengthening of the extensor tendon and dorsal capsulotomy may also be necessary to achieve correction. Proximal interphalangeal joint arthrodesis is another alternative for rigid clawtoes. Isolated flexor digitorum longus tenotomy is the appropriate intervention for a flexible mallet toe.

22. **b** Eliminating the effect of first ray plantar flexion. The *Coleman block test* is used in the physical examination of the cavovarus foot to assess whether the hindfoot varus is fixed or flexible. First ray plantar flexion is believed to be the principal abnormality in the cavovarus foot. Because of the tripod effect, the forefoot supinates and the hindfoot inverts to bring the fifth ray into contact with the floor. This leads to elevation of the medial arch and heel varus.

    In the Coleman block test, the patient stands with the lateral border of the foot on a 1-inch block. This eliminates the tripod effect from first ray plantar flexion. If the heel varus is inflexible (no correction with the Coleman block test), then a valgus calcaneal osteotomy may be necessary to achieve full correction.

Reference

Paulos L, Coleman SS, Samuelson KM: Pes Cavovarus. J Bone Joint Surg Am, 62:942–953, 1980.

23. **b** Localized tenderness over the medial aspect of the calcaneal tuberosity. *Plantar fasciitis* occurs most often in middle-aged women, and it is often associated with weight gain. It is the most common cause of plantar heel pain. Classic symptoms include pain that is worse with the first steps in the morning or after a period of inactivity.

    The most reliable and most common physical finding is localized tenderness at the insertion of the plantar fascia on the medial tubercle of the calcaneus. Passive dorsiflexion of the toes will place the plantar fascia under tension (by the windlass mechanism), but this is not a sensitive provocative maneuver.

    Reproduction of symptoms with percussion posterior to the medial malleolus suggests the diagnosis of tarsal tunnel syndrome. Inability to perform a single toe rise would be anticipated in a patient with posterior tibial tendon insufficiency. Pain with compression of the metatarsal heads is a provocative maneuver for suspected cases of Morton neuroma.

24. **a** Passive stretching. *Metatarsus adductus* is common in infants, and 85% to 90% of cases resolve spontaneously. Approximately 60% of cases are bilateral. For flexible deformities, the mainstay of treatment is parental reassurance and stretching exercises. The heel bisector ordinarily passes between the second and third toes. A deformity in which the heel bisector bisects the third toe would be classified as mild.

    Findings that suggest that a case of metatarsus adductus is less likely to resolve spontaneously include (1) a medial crease and (2) a foot that does not passively correct to neutral. In these instances, serial casting should be initiated. Reverse-last shoes are used once correction has been obtained to prevent recurrence.

    Note: All children with metatarsus adductus should be conscientiously evaluated for concomitant developmental hip dysplasia because of the high association between the two conditions.

Reference

Bleck EE: Metatarsus Adductus: Classification and Relationship to Outcomes of Treatment. J Pediatr Orthop, 3:(2) 149–59, 1983.

25. **a** Poliomyelitis. The key features of this deformity are (1) an abnormally high longitudinal (sagittal) arch, (2) exaggerated dorsiflexion pitch angle of the calcaneus, and (3) excessive plantar flexion of the forefoot. This condition results from a muscular imbalance between a relatively weak triceps surae and a relative overpull by the tibialis anterior and peroneals. In addition, as the calcaneus becomes more vertical (increased dorsal pitch), the lever arm of the triceps surae becomes shorter. The shortened lever arm, in turn, exacerbates plantar flexion weakness. Conditions associated with calcaneocavus feet include poliomyelitis, cerebral palsy, and myelomeningocele.

    The calcaneocavus type of pes cavus should be distinguished from the more common cavovarus type.

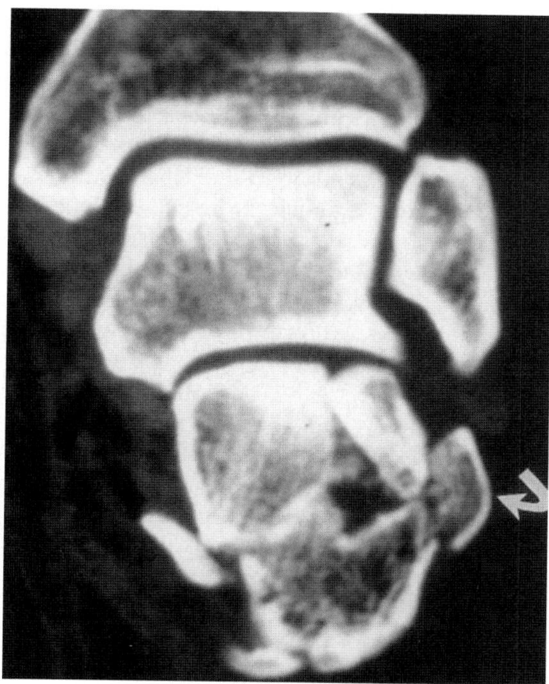

FIGURE 7.22

The cavovarus deformity consists of first ray plantar flexion and secondary hindfoot varus. The two most common underlying diseases are Charcot-Marie-Tooth and Friedreich ataxia. Ledderhose disease is a proliferative fibromatosis of the plantar fascia akin to Dupuytren contracture of the palm.

26. **e** From posteromedial to anterolateral through the posterior facet. The primary fracture line of an intraarticular calcaneus fracture runs from posteromedial to anterolateral through the posterior facet (Fig. 7.22). This fracture line is produced by axial compression of the calcaneus by the talus. The resultant medial fragment contains the sustentaculum tali and is referred to as the *constant fragment.* The constant fragment typically remains linked to the talus by the interosseous ligament. There is variable comminution of the bone posterolateral to the primary fracture line. Sanders, using orthogonal computed tomography evaluation, described a classification of calcaneus fractures based on the number of posterior facet fragments.

Reference

Sanders RW: Intraarticular Fractures of the Calcaneus. J Orthop Trauma, 6:252–265, 1992.

27. **a** The risk of recurrent rupture is higher with nonoperative management. Management of Achilles tendon ruptures remains controversial. However, most studies agree that there is a higher rate of recurrent rupture after nonoperative treatment. Wound complications (e.g., infection, adhesions, and skin necrosis) are not uncommon after surgical intervention because of the tenuous quality of the overlying skin.

Some studies report superior strength after operative treatment, whereas other studies report equivalent strength among operative and nonoperative groups. However, no studies report superior strength after conservative treatment.

Non-operative treatment classically involves casting in equinus with gradual correction to neutral over 8 to 10 weeks. A similar period of immobilization is typically employed after surgical management, and operative treatment does not ensure an earlier return to work. In fact, in Nistor's study, the nonoperative group returned to work more rapidly. The cost of nonoperative management is less.

References

Inglis AE et al.: Ruptures of the Tendo-Achilles: An Objective Assessment of Surgical and Non-surgical Treatment. J Bone Joint Surg Am, 58:990–993, 1976.

Nistor L: Surgical and Nonsurgical Treatment of Achilles Tendon Rupture: A Prospective Randomized Study. J Bone Joint Surg Am, 63:394–399, 1981.

28. **b** Clawtoes. Compartment syndrome of the foot is not common. However, the diagnosis should be considered in all cases of severe foot trauma, particularly crush injuries. Untreated foot compartment syndrome can result in sensory disturbances, loss of intrinsic muscle function, and intrinsic contractures. The most common resultant deformity is clawing of the toes.

Note: Nine fascial compartments have been documented in the foot, but only five compartments are considered functionally significant: (1) the interosseous compartment, (2) the medial compartment, (3) the lateral compartment, (4) the central (plantar) compartment, and (5) the calcaneal compartment. Double dorsal longitudinal incisions can be used to release compartments 1 to 4. Alternatively, these four compartments can be accessed through a single medial incision that can be extended posteriorly to reach compartment 5 and the tarsal tunnel.

Reference

Shereff MJ: Compartment Syndromes of the Foot. Instr Course Lect, 39: 127–132, 1990.

29. **e** Complete excision of the plantar aponeurosis. Given the associated conditions (Dupuytren contracture and Peyronie disease), the most likely cause of this patient's discomfort is Ledderhose disease (plantar fibromatosis). Because of the high rate of recurrence with local

excision (approximately 60%), complete fascial excision is advised when conservative treatment fails.

Reference

Kirby EJ, et al.: Soft Tissue Tumors and Tumor-Like Conditions of the Foot. J Bone Joint Surg Am, 71:621–626, 1989.

30. **d** Prominent bony anatomy. *Intractable plantar keratoses* are symptomatic, well-localized, hyperkeratotic skin lesions on the plantar surface of the foot. They are produced by excessive pressure, and, thus, they arise under bony prominences (e.g., metatarsal heads or sesamoids).

    Rheumatoid arthritis may indirectly produce intractable plantar keratoses (as bony deformities develop), but it is not a direct cause. Ledderhose disease may produce painful plantar nodules, but it is not commonly associated with intractable plantar keratoses.
31. **e** Urethral culture. Achilles enthesopathy (so-called "lover's heel") can be the presenting symptom of *Reiter syndrome.* Reiter syndrome is a reactive process that is initiated by a genital or gastrointestinal infection. Classic Reiter syndrome consists of the following triad of symptoms: (1) urethritis (or cervicitis), (2) arthritis, and (3) conjunctivitis. Associated mucocutaneous lesions (e.g., keratoderma blennorrhagica, hyperkeratosis of the nails, and balanitis circinata) can also be encountered. These multisystemic complaints typically develop between 1 and 6 weeks after the precipitating infection.

    An "incomplete" form of Reiter syndrome (reactive arthritis without other systemic features) is commonly encountered, as demonstrated by this case. Because the precipitating genitourinary infection *(Chlamydia trachomatis)* is often clinically silent, sexually active patients with clinical histories that are suggestive of Reiter syndrome should have cultures obtained and should be treated accordingly. Sexual contacts should also be treated. Unfortunately, treatment of the precipitating infection has not been proven to affect the course of the arthritis.

    Musculoskeletal manifestations of Reiter syndrome include sacroiliitis (asymmetric), enthesopathy, dactylitis ("sausage digits"), and oligoarthritis of the lower extremities (knees and ankles). Seventy-five percent of patients with Reiter syndrome are HLA-B27 positive. Nonsteroidal antiinflammatory drugs are the primary agents for alleviating the musculoskeletal symptoms. Glucocorticoid injections into the Achilles tendon are universally contraindicated because of their potential contribution to iatrogenic tendon rupture.
32. **d** Salicylic acid treatment. Punctate bleeding after paring is characteristic of plantar warts. Radiographs are not useful in establishing this diagnosis. These warts are caused by papillomavirus. Plantar warts typically occur in children and young adults, and they commonly produce significant discomfort with weight bearing. The initial treatment of painful warts consists of shoe modification for pressure relief (orthotics, pads) and keratolytics (e.g., salicylic acid). Surgical excision is a last resort for recalcitrant symptomatic lesions.

    Intractable plantar keratoses do not exhibit punctate bleeding. Heel pain, but not warts, can be produced by the seronegative arthropathies (e.g., ankylosing spondylitis and Reiter syndrome), which are commonly associated with HLA-B27 (see discussion of question 31).
33. **c** The tarsal navicular. *Köhler disease* is an eponym for osteochondrosis of the tarsal navicular. Other eponyms for osteochondroses are given in Table 7.2.
34. **b** Computed tomography scan. Hindfoot pain with associated compromised subtalar motion in this age group strongly suggests the diagnosis of tarsal coalition. The two most common forms of tarsal coalition are calcaneonavicular and talocalcaneal. Talocalcaneal coalitions tend to become symptomatic at a slightly later age (12 to 16 years) than calcaneonavicular coalitions (8 to 12 years). Although oblique radiographs often detect calcaneonavicular bars, computed tomography scanning is currently the imaging modality of choice for demonstrating talocalcaneal coalitions. A bone scan may be positive, but it is nonspecific. The utility of magnetic resonance imaging remains undefined, but it may assist in defining the composition of a coalition (bony versus fibrous versus cartilaginous).
35. **d** The calcaneonavicular and calcaneocuboid ligaments. The bifurcate ligament is one of the strongest connections between the first and second tarsal rows. Its two components are the calcaneocuboid and the calcaneonavicular bands. The interosseous ligament connects the talus and the calcaneus. The calcaneofibular ligament is part of the lateral collateral ligament complex.
36. **b** An interior shoe pad that provides elevation just proximal to the metatarsal heads. A metatarsal bar is

TABLE 7.2. EPONYMS FOR OSTEOCHONDROSES

Eponym	Affected Bone
Freiberg infraction	Second metatarsal head
Köhler disease	Tarsal navicular
Sever disease	Calcaneal apophysis
Panner disease	Capitellum (humerus)
Keinböck disease	Carpal navicular
Legg-Perthes disease	Femoral head
Scheuermann disease	Vertebral end plate

used to relieve pressure on the metatarsal heads. An elevation immediately proximal to the heads transfers the weight to the distal metatarsal diaphysis. Metatarsal bars can be used in the treatment of metatarsalgia, intractable plantar keratoses, or Morton neuroma.

37. **c** Proximal crescentic osteotomy with a distal soft tissue procedure. This patient has a moderate bunion deformity and an incongruent joint (lateral subluxation of the proximal phalanx). A proximal crescentic osteotomy combined with a distal soft tissue procedure is the most appropriate option in this setting because it could provide adequate correction of the incongruence, the intermetatarsal angle, and the hallux valgus angle.

A chevron osteotomy would be appropriate for a milder deformity, but it would not provide sufficient reduction of the intermetatarsal angle in this situation. A distal soft tissue procedure (alone) is also contraindicated when the intermetatarsal angle is greater than 15 degrees. The Akin procedure (proximal phalangeal osteotomy) is indicated for correction of hallux valgus interphalangeus. A Keller resection arthroplasty should be reserved for patients with minimal demands or as a salvage procedure. Metatarsophalangeal arthrodesis is indicated in the setting of severe deformity or metatarsophalangeal arthritis (or as a salvage procedure). An algorithm for hallux valgus treatment is shown in Fig. 7.23.

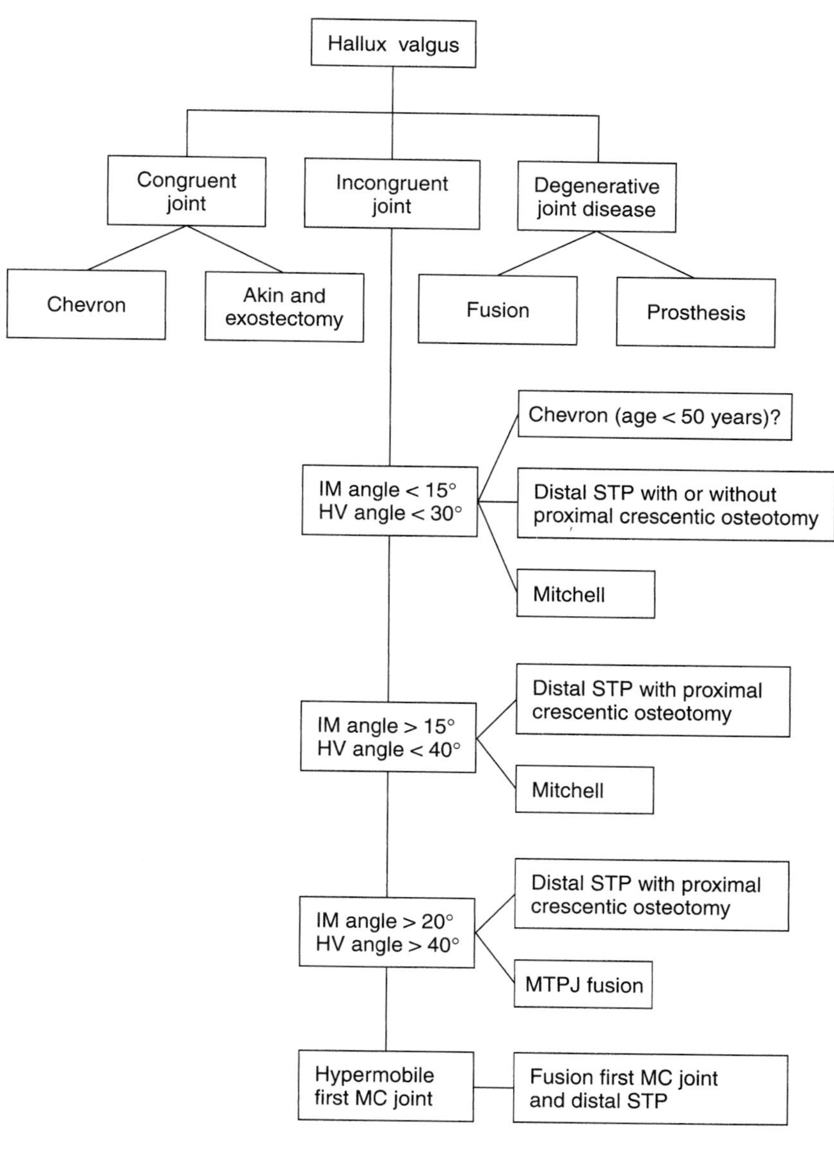

FIGURE 7.23

TABLE 7.3. HALLUX-VALGUS ANGLE AND INTERMETATARSAL ANGLE

Deformity	Mild	Moderate	Severe
Hallux-valgus angle	<30	<40	>40
Intermetatarsal angle	<13	>13	>20

Note: A normal intermetatarsal angle is less than 9 degrees. A normal hallux valgus angle is less than 15 degrees (Table 7.3).

Reference

Mann RA: Disorders of the First Metatarsophalangeal Joint. J Am Acad Orthop Surg, 3(1):34–43, 1995.

38. **d** Bone infarction. Radiographs demonstrating tibiotalar joint destruction and sclerosis of the distal tibia and fibula are characteristic of bone infarction, a common sequelae of *sickle cell anemia.* In sickle cell anemia, multifocal bone infarction is caused when sickled erythrocytes occlude vascular channels. Involvement of subchondral bone can cause secondary degenerative joint disease.

    Infection is also common in patients with sickle cell disease, and it can be difficult to distinguish from an acute infarct. However, the presentation of this case is not consistent with an acute infection. Furthermore, the radiographs show no periosteal reaction.
39. **d** Tibiotalar arthrodesis. Given the advanced joint destruction, a tibiotalar arthrodesis would be the only form of surgical intervention capable of providing significant, predictable, enduring relief. Other procedures (e.g., débridement, cheilectomy, or osteotomy) would be unlikely to provide significant benefit. With preserved subtalar, calcaneocuboid, and talonavicular joint spaces, a pantalar arthrodesis would not be appropriate.
40. **a** Synovitis of the second metatarsophalangeal joint. This is a classic description of *second metatarsophalangeal synovitis.* It typically arises insidiously in athletes as a result of recurrent microtrauma. Local inflammation can affect the adjacent digital nerves and mimic the signs of an interdigital neuroma. However, metatarsophalangeal synovitis is accompanied by laxity of the plantar capsule, as demonstrated by the positive drawer test described in this patient. Turf toe characteristically affects the first metatarsophalangeal joint and is associated with a specific precipitating traumatic event.

Reference

Thompson FM, Hamilton WG: Problems of the Second Metatarsophalangeal joint. Orthopaedics, 10:83–89, 1987.

41. **c** Second metatarsophalangeal synovectomy and possible flexor tendon transfer. The surgical treatment for synovitis without fixed deformity is synovectomy with flexor to extensor transfer if the joint is unstable. If a fixed deformity is present, then a more extensive procedure may be necessary (such as those described in options a and d). Conservative management of this condition includes a stiff-soled shoe, nonsteroidal anti-inflammatory drugs, activity modification, and metatarsal pads to unload the joint.

Reference

Coughlin MJ: Subluxation and Dislocation of the Second Metatarsophalangeal Joint. Orthop Clin North Am, 20:535–551, 1989.

42. **a** Tibialis anterior. During heel strike and early stance, the tibialis anterior demonstrates the greatest electromyographic activity. The eccentric contraction of the tibialis anterior during this phase of gait prevents a slap-foot gait. After ensuring a smooth transition to footflat, the tibialis anterior remains relatively inactive through the remainder of stance phase. Concentric tibialis anterior contraction during swing phase allows the forefoot to clear the ground.
43. **e** Immobilization, elevation, and observation. This is an example of a *Charcot joint.* The amount of destruction present is inconsistent with the minimal discomfort experienced by the patient. The most common cause of Charcot joints in the lower extremity is diabetes. Differentiating a Charcot joint from infection can sometimes be difficult, but infection is typically more painful. Initial treatment of an acutely inflamed Charcot joint consists of rest and elevation to allow the soft tissue inflammation to subside. This will also allow the fragmented bone to coalesce. Delayed arthrodesis may subsequently be performed through more hospitable soft tissues.
44. **e** Hyperpronation is believed to contribute to Achilles inflammation and degeneration. The Achilles tendon has no true investing synovium. Rather, it is enveloped by paratenon that provides a mucopolysaccharide-rich surface to facilitate gliding between the tendon and the surrounding pseudosheath (epitenon). The gastrocnemius crosses the knee as well as the ankle. Therefore, it will be preferentially stretched when the knee is extended and the ankle is dorsiflexed. Stretching with the knee flexed and ankle dorsiflexed preferentially stretches the soleus fibers. Most of the tendon's blood supply stems from its ventral paratenon, although it also receives contributions from its muscular origin and osseous insertion.

    The Achilles fibers spiral approximately 90 degrees around one another such that the gastrocnemius fibers insert lateral to the soleus fibers. Pronation exacerbates this twisting and theoretically produces a form of dynamic ischemia within the tendon through a "wringing" effect. Pronation also causes medial to lateral excursion of the tendon relative to the calcaneus (causing shear on the tendon). Because of the role of the Achilles tendon as an accessory hindfoot inverter, its medial half is eccentrically loaded during early stance because of foot pronation. Hyperpronation exacerbates all the effects of pronation and thus is thought to contribute to tendon inflammation and degeneration.

Note: Injection studies have demonstrated a region of relative avascularity 2 to 6 cm proximal to the Achilles insertion that corresponds to the region where the tendon most commonly fails.

References

Carr AJ, Norris SH: The Blood Supply to the Calcaneal Tendon. J Bone Joint Surg Br, 71:100–101, 1989.
Clement DB: Achilles Tendinitis and Peritendinitis. Am J Sports Med, 12:179–184, 1984.
Lagergen C, Lindholm A: Vascular Distribution in Achilles Tendon. Acta Chir Scand, 116:491–495, 1958.

45. **d** Excision of the exostosis. *Subungal exostoses* most commonly affect the great toe. They represent an overgrowth of normal bone from the distal phalangeal tuft that impinges on the overlying nail. Excision of the exostosis is the only effective treatment.
46. **a** Onychogryphosis. *Onychogryphosis* is affectionately known as a "ram's horn nail." Onychomycosis refers to fungal infection of the nail, one of many potential causes of nail thickening. Onychotrophy refers to atrophy of the nail plate. Onychocryptosis refers to an ingrown nail. Onychia refers to inflammation of the nail matrix. Onychomalacia is a term for softening of the nail plate. Onycholysis refers to loosening of the nail plate.
47. **b** Osteotomy of the fibula at the level of the ankle joint and sectioning of the anterior inferior tibiofibular ligament will permit significant lateral talar subluxation. Isolated fibular osteotomy and sectioning of the anterior inferior tibiofibular ligament will not allow significant lateral subluxation of the talus. The deep deltoid ligament must also be divided. These facts serve as the rationale for treating SER-II ankle fractures nonoperatively. If the deltoid and medial malleolus remain intact, then the proper anatomic relationship between the talus and the tibia will be preserved by the deltoid.

Because of the varus obliquity of the ankle joint axis (approximately 8 degrees), plantar flexion of the ankle is associated with approximately 4 to 8 degrees of internal foot rotation. Most axial force across the ankle is transmitted through the tibial plafond; only approximately 17% is transmitted through the fibula.

In the *Lauge-Hansen Classification,* the first word refers to the foot position at the time of impact, and the second word refers to the direction of the deforming force. Thus, when the foot is supinated and an external rotation force is applied to the foot, the first structure to come under tension (and, hence, to fail) is the anterior inferior tibiofibular ligament. The first structure to fail in the supination-adduction type of injury is either the lateral talofibular ligament or the lateral malleolus itself (Fig. 7.24). The first structure to fail in both the pronation-external rotation and pronation-abduction types is either the deltoid or the medial malleolus itself.

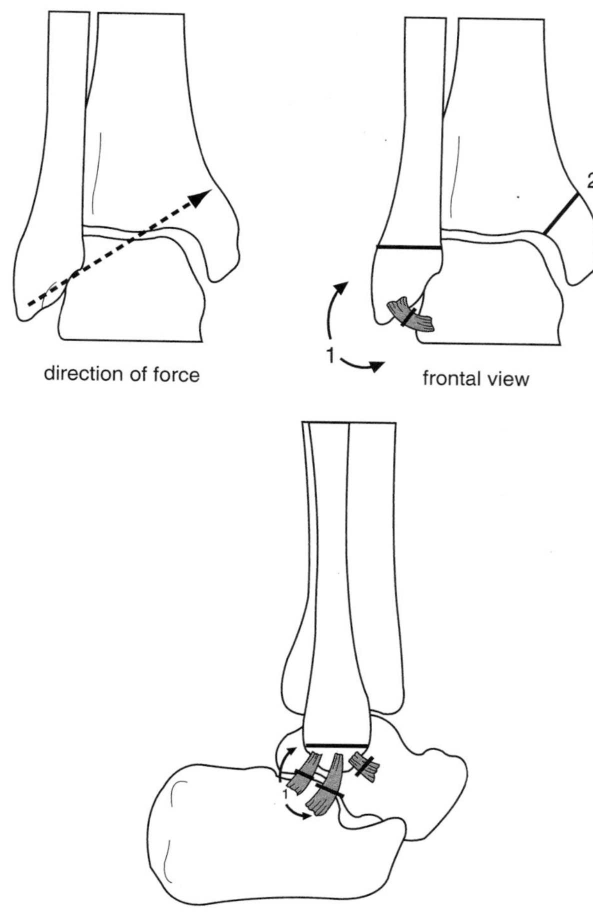

FIGURE 7.24

48. **c** >90%. The talus is at risk for avascular necrosis because of its precarious blood supply. Approximately 60% of the surface area of the talus is articular cartilage. No tendons or muscles attach to the talus.

The Hawkins Classification for talar neck fractures is useful for predicting the risk of avascular necrosis. According to this classification, this patient has a type III injury (Table 7.4).

Reference

Browner BD, et al.: Skeletal Trauma. Philadelphia WB Saunders, 1992.

TABLE 7.4. HAWKINS CLASSIFICATION OF TALAR NECK FRACTURES

Type	Description	Risk of Avascular Necrosis
I	Nondisplaced	<10%
II	Body displaced in the ankle or subtalar joint	<40%
III	Body displaced in the ankle and subtalar joints	>90%
IV	Extrusion of the body	~100%

49. **d** 5 degrees of valgus; neutral flexion. Tibiotalar (ankle) arthrodesis should be placed in 5 to 10 degrees of valgus with neutral flexion. Rotation should be matched to the contralateral side (approximately 5 to 10 degrees). It is crucial to avoid varus alignment because hindfoot inversion will lock the transverse tarsal joint and render the foot excessively stiff.

Additionally, the talus should be fixed in a slightly (approximately 1 cm) posteriorly translated position under the tibia. Posterior translation shortens the lever arm of foot, and this, in turn, reduces the forces on the midtarsal joints.

50. **d** Wide toe-box shoes. Although this patient has a severe symptomatic hallux valgus deformity, a trial of conservative treatment should not be omitted. A wide toe-box shoe should be prescribed for this patient. Metatarsal pads do not relieve the medial eminence pressure and pain associated with hallux valgus deformity.

A modified McBride procedure alone (distal soft tissue procedure) would be inappropriate for a deformity of this magnitude. If conservative treatment fails, arthrodesis or resection arthroplasty (Keller) can be considered to treat severe hallux valgus in a patient with minimal demands.

Note: This patient is a poor candidate for elective surgery, given her recent myocardial infarction.

51. **b** Simple excision. An *accessory navicular* is an anatomic variant present in approximately 15% of females and 8% of males. Many are asymptomatic. Symptomatic children often present with pes planus or posterior tibial tendinitis in association with the painful prominence. Symptoms usually resolve with use of a medial arch support. Temporary use of a walking cast may also be beneficial.

Excision of the ossicle provides relief in most patients in whom conservative management fails. The *Kidner procedure* involves excision of the accessory navicular plus advancement of the posterior tibial tendon to a more plantar location. The theoretic advantage of advancing the posterior tibial tendon is that it may help to rectify the pes planus that is commonly associated with the accessory navicular. However, many patients, including the patient described in this question, have a normal longitudinal arch. Furthermore, the Kidner procedure has not been proven to provide effective long-term arch correction.

Flexor digitorum longus and flexor hallucis longus tendon transfers are used for early posterior tibial tendon insufficiency, but neither of these procedures is indicated in the treatment of an isolated accessory navicular.

References

Bennett GL, et al.: Surgical Treatment of Symptomatic Accessory Talar Navicular. J Pediatr Orthop, 10:445–449, 1990.

MacNicol MF, Voutsinas S: Surgical Treatment of the Symptomatic Accessory Navicular. J Bone Joint Surg Br, 66:218, 1984.

52. **d** Arthrodesis of the first metatarsophalangeal joint with resection arthroplasty of the lesser toes. The films demonstrate severe hallux valgus with subluxations of all the lesser toes. This is a classic rheumatoid forefoot deformity. The foot is affected in approximately 90% of patients with rheumatoid arthritis. The forefoot is involved more often than the hindfoot.

The goals of reconstruction of this deformity are (1) to create a stable medial post (by fusion of the first metatarsophalangeal joint) and (2) to reduce the subluxated proximal phalanges of the lesser toes (by resection of the lesser metatarsal heads in a Hoffman-type procedure).

For a severe deformity in an elderly patient with limited demands, metatarsophalangeal arthrodesis provides reliable pain relief without significantly hampering ambulation. The desired position for fusion is 10 to 15 degrees of dorsiflexion and 15 degrees of valgus.

An *Akin procedure* (medial closing wedge osteotomy of the proximal phalanx) is indicated for hallux valgus interphalangeus. This would not restore first ray alignment for the deformity in this question, nor would it provide a stable medial post to prevent recurrent deformity of the lesser toes.

The *Keller procedure* (resection arthroplasty of the base of the proximal phalanx) is a salvage procedure for severe hallux valgus. This operation does not provide a stable medial post, but it may sometimes be appropriate for an elderly patient with minimal ambulatory demands and negligible lesser toe involvement.

53. **a** The first metatarsal. The posterior tibial tendon passes posterior to the medial malleolus and anterior to the sustentaculum tali. The tendon subdivides proximal to the tuberosity of the navicular and ultimately

gives rise to extensions that insert on the navicular, the three cuneiforms, the cuboid, and metatarsals 2 to 5. There is no posterior tibial tendon insertion onto the first metatarsal.

Reference

MacNicol MF, Voutsinas S: Surgical Treatment of the Symptomatic Accessory Navicular. J Bone Joint Surg Br, 66:218, 1984.

54. **a** Short-leg cast. This patient has a talocalcaneal coalition with sclerosis and loss of the subtalar joint. The other type of coalition is the calcaneonavicular coalition, best seen on a 45-degree internal oblique radiograph *(Sloman view).* Calcaneonavicular coalitions typically become symptomatic between the ages of 8 and 12 years. This period corresponds to the time frame when the calcaneonavicular bar characteristically ossifies.

Many coalitions are asymptomatic, and many patients who become symptomatic will respond to nonoperative treatment. Conservative measures include activity modification, orthotic inserts, intraarticular steroids, and short-term casting.

Surgery is indicated when symptoms fail to respond to nonoperative modalities. Operative management of calcaneonavicular coalitions consists of bar excision with interposition of the origin of the extensor digitorum brevis muscle. Operative management of talocalcaneal coalitions consists of bar excision with interposition of an autogenous fat graft.

Triple arthrodesis is indicated in the presence of failed resection or extensive associated articular degeneration. Scranton recommended triple arthrodesis for talocalcaneal coalitions that affect more than 50% of the subtalar joint surface area.

Note: Talar beaking (a dorsal talonavicular traction spur) is commonly associated with tarsal coalition. This finding is typically demonstrated on the lateral radiograph. It does not necessarily imply that significant articular degeneration is present.

References

Devriese L, et al.: Surgical Treatment of Tarsal Coalitions. J Pediatr Orthop, 3:96–101, 1994.

Gonzalez P, Kumar SJ: Calcaneonavicular Coalition Treated by Resection and Interposition of the Extensor Digitorum Brevis Muscle. J Bone Joint Surg Am, 72:71–77, 1990.

Scranton PE: Treatment of Symptomatic Talocalcaneal Coalition. J Bone Joint Surg Am, 69:533–539, 1987.

55. **c** Knee hyperextension and posterior trunk lean are midstance compensatory mechanisms for the compromised tibial progression associated with a rigid ankle plantar flexion deformity. During normal gait, the ankle plantar flexes immediately after heel strike. However, the ankle dorsiflexes throughout the midstance phase as the body progresses over the planted foot. During midstance, the rate of tibial progression is decelerated by eccentric soleus contraction. During terminal stance, the soleus and gastrocnemius continue to prevent excessive ankle dorsiflexion and permit heel rise to occur. Thus, a weak soleus may produce prolonged heel contact by failing to limit ankle dorsiflexion effectively.

Another manifestation of soleus weakness is sustained knee flexion in late stance. Under normal circumstances, the knee extends between midstance and toe-off. However, the quadriceps mechanism requires a stable base to extend the knee. If the soleus does not effectively stabilize the ankle, then the quadriceps cannot function appropriately.

If the ankle is fixed in plantar flexion, then the normal mechanism of controlled tibial progression by dampened ankle dorsiflexion "ankle rocker" is prevented. Therefore, for the body to progress over the foot, the heel must rise prematurely. Other compensatory mechanisms to help the body progress over the foot in this situation include (1) knee hyperextension and (2) anterior trunk lean. These two mechanisms represent attempts to keep the body's center of gravity anterior to the rigid equinus deformity to maintain anterior momentum. Posterior trunk lean would worsen the situation.

Reference

Perry J: Gait Analysis. Thorofare, NJ, Slack, pp. 185–220, 1992.

56. **b** Rest, elevation, and casting. The history and radiographs support a diagnosis of *Charcot arthropathy.* Diabetic peripheral neuropathy is the most common cause of Charcot arthropathy in the lower extremity. Figure 7.9 demonstrates early midfoot involvement with navicular fragmentation and sclerosis. If permitted to evolve, this process will typically lead to arch collapse and a rocker-bottom deformity. The altered architecture and the underlying compromised nociception and proprioception can produce neuropathic ulceration.

The *Eichenholtz classification* describes the three stages of Charcot arthropathy progression: stage I, fragmentation; stage II, coalescence; and stage III, consolidation. Treatment of the Charcot joint depends on the stage of disease. The principal goals of treatment in the acute phase (stage I) include controlling of swelling, preventing of skin breakdown, and preserving of bony architecture. This is accomplished by rest, non–weight bearing, elevation, and splinting. Total contact casting can subsequently be employed for swelling reduction, support, and protection. Once coalescence occurs, long-term orthosis use may be required to accommodate residual deformity. If these measures fail to prevent recurrent ulcerations, arthrodesis may be cautiously considered. However, operative intervention of any type is contraindicated in the acute phase, except when débridement of associated ulcers is required.

Note: The characteristic radiographic findings that are associated with advanced Charcot arthropathy include the so-called "5-Ds": joint distention, bony debris, dislocation, disorganization, and increased bone density.

57. **b** Osteoid osteoma. The anteroposterior radiograph reveals a approximately 1-cm sclerotic lesion in the talus. Night pain and relief with nonsteroidal antiinflammatory drugs are the classic features of *osteoid osteoma.* This lesion is most commonly encountered during the second decade. It can occur in any bone in the foot, but the tarsal bones are most commonly affected. Sclerotic reactive bone is formed in response to the central lucent nidus. This produces a characteristic target appearance on magnetic resonance imaging. A sequestrum could have a similar appearance. However, more surrounding edema and bone erosion would be expected. Additionally, such dramatic relief with antiinflammatory medication would not be expected.

Enostoses (bone islands) can present with similar symptoms, and they can mimic osteoid osteomas on plain radiographs. However, they do not produce a similar magnetic resonance imaging appearance. Furthermore, an enostosis does not produce the characteristic focal intense signal that is produced by osteoid osteoma on bone scan.

Avascular necrosis can affect the talus, but it is typically a posttraumatic phenomenon. Although avascular necrosis also produces sclerosis, avascular necrosis of the talus does not occur in the focal distribution demonstrated in this question. Köhler disease affects the navicular bone (not the talus).

Note: The diameter of the reactive sclerotic bone surrounding an osteoid osteoma may significantly exceed 1 cm, but the diameter of the central radiolucent nidus is characteristically less than 1 cm.

58. **e** Hallux rigidus; stiff-soled shoe. The radiograph demonstrates metatarsophalangeal joint space obliteration, metatarsal head flattening, and dorsal osteophyte formation. These films and history suggest a diagnosis of hallux rigidus.

Acute gout would present with extreme tenderness and restricted motion in all planes. Gout flares should be treated with indomethacin or colchicine to quell the acute inflammation. Allopurinol is indicated to reduce hyperuricemia and thereby to minimize the likelihood of an acute gout flare, but it does not treat the inflammation associated with an acute attack.

Chronic, recurrent gout may produce sharply marginated periarticular erosions, but it does not tend to produce the joint space obliteration demonstrated in Fig. 7.11.

Hallux rigidus does not typically demonstrate signs and symptoms of acute inflammation. Dorsiflexion is compromised disproportionately in hallux rigidus because of the tendency for dorsal metatarsal head osteophyte formation.

Turf toe stems from an acute traumatic event. A grade III injury is associated with articular cartilage injury and may ultimately produce hallux rigidus as a late sequela.

59. **e** First metatarsophalangeal joint fusion. The initial treatment of *hallux rigidus* should be conservative. Methods include nonsteroidal antiinflammatory drugs, periodic intraarticular steroids, and shoe modifications to minimize metatarsophalangeal motion (e.g., a stiff-sole or rocker-bottom shoe). Affected women should avoid wearing high heels.

Surgical treatment should be contemplated if the foregoing measures fail. Cheilectomy is appropriate when more than 50% of the plantar metatarsophalangeal joint space remains intact. However, it is inappropriate for more extensive joint destruction, such as in this case.

If excision of the dorsal osteophyte fails to restore sufficient metatarsophalangeal dorsiflexion, an extension osteotomy of the proximal phalanx may be added to the cheilectomy, but this procedure is also contraindicated in the presence of advanced, diffuse metatarsophalangeal degeneration.

Silastic implant arthroplasty is associated with a high incidence of synovitis and implant loosening. It should not be considered for a young patient with significant functional demands. Likewise, the Keller resection arthroplasty would be inappropriate for a young, active patient because of the potential for deformation, transfer lesions, and compromised function. Metatarsophalangeal fusion provides the most predictable and durable pain relief for young, active patients with advanced hallux rigidus.

Reference

Hattrup SJ, Johnson KA: Subjective Results of Hallux Rigidus Following Treatment by Cheilectomy. Clin. Orthop, 226:182–191, 1988.

60. **c** Medial cuneiform to base of second metatarsal. The radiograph demonstrates a fracture of the base of the second metatarsal and disruption of the tarsometatarsal joint *(Lisfranc joint).* The base of the second metatarsal serves as the keystone to this joint. The Lisfranc ligament runs on the dorsal aspect of the foot from the medial cuneiform to the base of the second metatarsal. The ligament itself can be torn, or it may be disrupted by avulsion of a portion of the second metatarsal base (as demonstrated in Fig. 7.12).

Because of the poor long-term prognosis of displaced Lisfranc fracture-dislocations, this injury mandates anatomic reduction and stabilization.

Note: The medial border of the middle cuneiform should be colinear with the medial border of the base of the second metatarsal base. Lateral subluxation of the second metatarsal base in relation to the middle cuneiform is pathognomonic for disruption of Lisfranc ligament.

Reference

Arntz CT, et al.: Fractures and Fracture-Dislocations of the Tarsometatarsal Joint. J Bone Joint Surg Am, 70:173–181, 1988.

61. **b** Negatively birefringent crystals. The radiograph reveals a sharply demarcated, periarticular erosion in the middle phalanx of the third ray. This is a potential manifestation of long-standing *gout.* Radiographic findings initially reveal only soft tissue swelling, but after repeated episodes, this type of osseous lesion may develop.

    Although gout most commonly affects the first metatarsophalangeal joint, 25% to 50% of cases involve other joints. Monosodium urate crystals exhibit negative birefringence under polarized light. Precipitation of monosodium urate provokes the characteristic acute inflammatory response, and recovery of these crystals by arthrocentesis is pathognomonic for gout.

    Any disease or medication that produces hyperuricemia can render someone susceptible to secondary gout. Furosemide (Lasix) decreases urate excretion by increasing urate resorption in the distal nephron. Other factors that contribute to secondary gout include myeloproliferative disorders, psoriasis, hemolytic anemias, and ethanol use.

    Pseudogout is caused by calcium pyrophosphate dihydrate crystals, which are positively birefringent. It most commonly affects the knee, and affected joints typically demonstrate chondrocalcinosis radiographically. Unlike true gout, pseudogout is not associated with the type of periarticular erosion seen in Fig. 7.13.

    Acid-fast bacilli would be seen in the setting of tuberculosis. The history does not support this diagnosis, and isolated involvement of a small joint would be atypical.

62. **c** Cross training, a hard-soled shoe, and referral to a gynecologist to consider hormone replacement therapy. There is marked increased uptake in the second metatarsal on the bone scan with no corresponding abnormality on the plain radiograph. These findings (combined with the classic history of increasing pain with activity) are characteristic of a metatarsal stress fracture. The second metatarsal is most commonly involved. Plain radiographs may take 2 to 4 weeks to demonstrate abnormality (Fig. 7.25). Treatment for this lesion includes cessation of running for 4 to 8 weeks. Symptomatic therapy includes a firm arch support and a stiff-soled shoe. Immobilization in a short-leg walking cast is recommended only when there is significant pain with ambulation or when the stress fracture evolves into a true fracture. Inappropriate immobilization will produce unnecessary muscle atrophy and osteopenia. Low-impact cross training (water training or biking) is permissible as long as it does not reproduce the metatarsal pain. Maintenance of aerobic conditioning will facilitate the patient's return to running after the fracture has healed. Use of nonsteroidal anti-inflammatory drugs or other analgesics to "train through" the discomfort is destined to fail and to delay ultimate recovery.

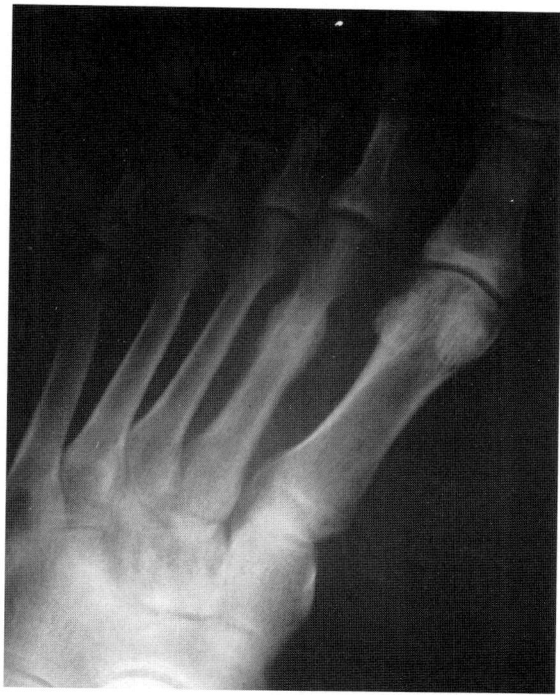

FIGURE 7.25

    Female athletes with stress fractures and exercise-associated amenorrhea should be referred for gynecologic evaluation to consider hormone replacement therapy. The associated hypoestrogenemic state may predispose the athlete to recurrent stress fractures and premature osteoporosis. The patient should also be screened for eating disorders to exclude "the female athlete triad" (osteoporosis, disordered eating, and amenorrhea).

    Procedures to rule out a more insidious process such as tumor or infection are not warranted at this time given the characteristic history and normal plain films.

References

Barrow GW, Saha S: Menstrual Irregularity and Stress Fractures in Collegiate Female Distance Runners. Am J Sports Med, 16:209–216, 1988.

Eisele SA, Sammarco GJ: Fatigue Fractures of the Foot and Ankle in the Athlete. Instr Course Lect, 42:175–183, 1993.

63. **b** Distal chevron osteotomy. The radiograph demonstrates a mild hallux valgus deformity associated with a congruent metatarsophalangeal joint. (Please refer to the discussion of question 37.) A *chevron osteotomy* is ideal for this type of deformity, particularly in a younger patient.

A *Mitchell procedure* is a biplane, step-cut osteotomy through the metatarsal neck that shortens and laterally displaces the first metatarsal. It is indicated for moderate deformities with subluxation of the metatarsophalangeal joint. It is not indicated for a congruent joint. This procedure is more technically demanding than the chevron osteotomy. Furthermore, it shortens the first metatarsal and can result in a transfer lesion.

A *proximal crescentic osteotomy* is indicted for moderate to severe deformity. It is usually performed with a distal soft tissue procedure.

Once again, the *Akin procedure* is indicated for hallux valgus interphalangeus. The principal indication for metatarsophalangeal joint arthrodesis is degeneration of the metatarsophalangeal joint.

Reference

Leventen EO: The Chevron Procedure. Orthopaedics, 13:973–976, 1990.

64. **a** The peroneus brevis. The mechanism of avulsion fractures involving the metaphysis of the base of the fifth metatarsal (also known as metatarsal styloid fractures) is sudden inversion. The peroneus brevis tendon inserts on the tuberosity. Avulsion putatively occurs as this muscle contracts in an effort to resist abrupt inversion.

The peroneus tertius inserts further distally on the shaft of the fifth metatarsal. The peroneus longus tendon lies posterolaterally to the brevis as the two tendons pass behind the lateral malleolus. The peroneus longus subsequently inserts on the plantar aspect of the base of the first metatarsal.

Reference

Lawrence SJ, Botte MJ: Jones Fractures and Related Fractures of the Base of the Fifth Metatarsal. Foot Ankle, 14:358–365, 1993.

65. **b** Weight bearing as tolerated in a hard-soled shoe. Avulsion fractures through the base of the fifth metatarsal generally heal readily with symptomatic management. The cancellous bone of the metaphysis has ample vascular supply, in contrast to the cortical bone of the fifth metatarsal diaphysis.

Symptomatic management typically consists of progressive weight bearing as tolerated with a compressive dressing or a hard-soled shoe. Temporary use of a short-leg walking cast may benefit the subset of patients who experience severe discomfort, but rigid immobilization is generally unnecessary.

Nonunions are very rare, even when there is significant displacement. The rare symptomatic nonunion can be treated with fragment excision and peroneus brevis tendon advancement. Open reduction and internal fixation of significantly displaced fractures are sometimes considered in highly competitive athletes. This fracture should be distinguished from fractures of the proximal fifth metatarsal diaphysis because the treatments and prognoses for the two injuries are quite different.

Reference

Dameron TB: Fractures of the Base of the Fifth Metatarsal: Selecting the Best Treatment Option. J Am Acad Orthop Surg, 3(2):110–114, 1995.

66. **c** During static single-leg toe rise, it transmits a force approximately equal to three times body weight. The distance from the ankle center of rotation to the first metatarsal head is approximately three times the distance from the ankle center of rotation to the Achilles insertion. This 3:1 moment arm ratio explains why the Achilles transmits a force of approximately three times body weight during static single-leg toe rise. During running and jumping, this force increases to six to eight times body weight.

Reference

Scott S, et al.: Internal Forces at Chronic Running Injury Sites. Semin Sci Sports Exerc, 22:357–369, 1990.

67. **d** Ruiz-Mora procedure. The situation describes a fifth toe "cock-up" deformity. If the deformity is mild and flexible, a soft tissue procedure such as extensor digitorum longus lengthening can be performed. However, for a fixed, severe cock-up deformity, soft tissue procedures would be ineffective.

Proximal phalangectomy *(Ruiz-Mora procedure)* would be appropriate in this situation. Duvries arthroplasty combined with syndactylization of the fourth and fifth toes is another effective option, but syndactylization alone would not correct the deformity.

Amputation of the fifth toe is not cosmetically pleasing, but it may be a valid salvage option.

Note: Despite its effectiveness in correcting hammer toe deformities of the fifth ray, high incidences of subsequent fourth hammer toes and painful prominent fifth metatarsal heads (32% and 23%, respectively) have been reported after the Ruiz-Mora procedure. This complication has been attributed to the excessive shortening caused by total proximal phalangectomy. Thus, a modified procedure has been proposed (resection of only the head and neck of the proximal phalanx).

Reference

Janecki CJ, Wilde AH: Results of Phalangectomy of the Fifth Toe for Hammertoe: The Ruiz-Mora Procedure. J Bone Joint Surg Am, 58:1005–1007, 1976.

68. **c** The talonavicular. The talonavicular joint is classically reportedly to be most commonly involved in nonunion after attempted triple arthrodesis. Suboptimal exposure is commonly implicated as the source of nonunion of this articulation. Talonavicular nonunion is more likely when a single (lateral) incision approach is used. The tibiotalar joint is incorporated in a pantalar arthrodesis, but it is not fused in a triple arthrodesis.
69. **c** Perineural fibrosis with Renaut bodies. Morton's neuroma occurs secondary to entrapment of the interdigital nerve beneath the intermetatarsal ligament. Grossly, the involved nerve manifests fusiform swelling immediately distal to the edge of intermetatarsal ligament. This is the region that becomes entrapped with metatarsophalangeal dorsiflexion.

    The most predominant histologic feature is perineural fibrosis with Renaut bodies. Limited inflammatory infiltrates may also be encountered, but this is an inconsistent finding. Granuloma formation, vascular proliferation, and necrosis are not characteristic features.

    A *Morton's neuroma* is a neuroma in continuity. This type of neuroma should be distinguished from a bulb neuroma. A Morton's neuroma is a response to extrinsic pressure, whereas a bulb (or "stump") neuroma results from axon proliferation at the end of a severed nerve.

    Note: Renaut bodies are dense whorls of collagen that are found in the subperineural region of Morton's neuromas.

Reference

Alexander IJ, et al.: Morton's Neuroma: A Review of Recent Concepts. Orthopedics, 10:103–106, 1987.

70. **b** II. The history and examination given describe a patient with posterior tibial tendon insufficiency. This entity is most commonly encountered in middle-aged women. Posterior tibial tendon dysfunction is a degenerative process that encompasses a broad spectrum of disease. Johnson and Myerson classified this disorder into stages I to IV (Table 7.5).

Reference

Myerson MS: Adult Acquired Flatfoot Deformity: Treatment of Dysfunction of the Posterior Tibial Tendon. Instr Course Lect, 46:393–405, 1997.

71. **c** Reconstruction with flexor digitorum longus tendon sheath. Treatment of posterior tibial tendon dysfunction is predicated on the stage of disease (Table 7.6).

    Results of reconstruction with tendon transfer alone deteriorate with time. Negative prognostic factors include obesity and fixed forefoot varus. The addition of osseous procedures has been advocated to improve the long-term success of tendon reconstruction.

References

Mann RA, Thompson FM: Rupture of the Posterior Tendon Causing Flatfoot: Surgical Treatment. J Bone Joint Surg Am, 67:556–561, 1985.
Myerson MS: Adult Acquired Flatfoot Deformity: Treatment of Dysfunction of the Posterior Tibial Tendon. Instr Course Lect, 46:393–405, 1997.

72. **d** The spring ligament. The progressive planovalgus deformity leads to laxity in the plantar medial structures. The *spring ligament* (also known as the plantar calcaneonavicular ligament) becomes secondarily attenuated in cases of posterior tibial tendon dysfunction. Reconstruction of the spring ligament has been proposed as a potential means of improving the outcome of surgical reconstruction for stage II disease because of its crucial role in maintaining the static architecture of the longitudinal arch.

    Acute traumatic rupture of the spring ligament can produce a rapidly progressive planovalgus deformity, even in the presence of an intact posterior tibial tendon. The deep deltoid ligament (which connects the medial malleolus to the medial wall of the talus) becomes attenuated in cases of stage IV posterior tibial tendon dysfunction in association with the onset of valgus talar tilt.

TABLE 7.5. JOHNSON AND MYERSON CLASSIFICATION OF POSTERIOR TIBIAL TENDON DYSFUNCTION

Stage	Findings
I	Inflammation with mild inversion weakness but without significant deformity; can perform single heel rise
II	Advanced tendon degeneration, attenuation, or rupture with secondary flexible planovalgus deformity and lateral impingement; cannot perform single heel rise
III	Rigid planovalgus deformity (from long-standing tendon insufficiency)
IV	Valgus angulation of talus with secondary degenerative changes in the tibiotalar joint

TABLE 7.6. TREATMENT OF POSTERIOR TIBIAL TENDON DYSFUNCTION

Stage	Treatment
I	Rest, nonsteroidal antiinflammatory drugs, immobilization, arch supports (tenosynovectomy +/– tendon débridement if above fails)
II	Reconstruction with tendon transfer (flexor digitorum longus) +/– calcaneal osteotomy or lateral column lengthening
III	Rigid ankle-foot orthosis or arthrodesis: Isolated subtalar fusion (if forefoot supple); triple (if transverse tarsal arthritis).
IV	Rigid ankle-foot orthosis or tibiotalocalcaneal arthrodesis

Reference

Myerson MS: Adult Acquired Flatfoot Deformity: Treatment of Dysfunction of the Posterior Tibial Tendon. Instr Course Lect, 46:393–405, 1997.

73. **b** Apply a short-leg cast and advise the patient to limit weight bearing and return for follow-up examination in 1 to 2 weeks. This is a classic history for a stable sprain of the distal tibiofibular syndesmosis. This injury is commonly confused with a simple lateral ankle sprain. Key physical findings include pain with an external rotation stress and a positive squeeze test of the midshaft of the fibula.

The goal of treatment of syndesmosis injuries is to obtain and maintain anatomic reduction. When there is instability (syndesmotic widening), then syndesmosis screw placement is indicated.

Surgical stabilization is not indicated in the absence of demonstrable diastasis, as in this case. This subset of patients should be immobilized (non–weight bearing) and informed to anticipate a considerably longer recovery time compared with that for a simple lateral ankle sprain. Many authorities recommend a non–weight-bearing cast for 4 to 6 weeks. Follow-up radiographs are important to document the absence of late syndesmotic widening.

Treatment of the subset syndesmotic sprains that are anatomically reduced but unstable when stressed is controversial. It is important to ascertain whether there is a concomitant medial ligament injury because some authorities recommend syndesmotic screw placement in this situation, even in the absence of static widening of the syndesmosis.

References

Amendola A: Controversies in Diagnosis and Management of Syndesmotic injuries of the Ankle. Foot Ankle, 13:44–50, 1992.

Burns WC et al.: Tibiotalar Joint Dynamics: Indications for the Syndesmotic Screw. A Cadaver Study. Foot Ankle, 14:153–158, 1993.

74. **b** Flexor hallucis longus tenosynovitis. The *en pointe* ballet position places an extraordinary demand on the flexor hallucis longus tendon. This is a common cause of stenosing tenosynovitis of the flexor hallucis longus. Affected patients often present with concomitant posterior impingement in extreme plantar flexion. Exacerbated pain with resisted flexion of the hallux is a key feature that assists in differentiating this diagnosis from disease in the Achilles or posterior tibial tendons. Flexor hallucis longus tenolysis with excision of the os trigonum (if present) is an effective treatment for recalcitrant cases.

Stress fractures of the sustentaculum tali or os trigonum could conceivably mimic flexor hallucis longus tendinitis. However, these diagnoses would be less likely.

Reference

Hamilton WG: Stenosing Tenosynovitis of the Flexor Hallucis Longus Tendon and Posterior Impingement upon the Os Trigonum in Ballet Dancers. Foot Ankle, 3:74–80, 1982.

75. **c** A normal anatomic landmark where the flexor hallucis longus and flexor digitorum longus tendon cross. The *knot of Henry* is the anatomic landmark where the flexor digitorum longus crosses superficial the flexor hallucis longus. In the leg, the flexor digitorum longus originates and travels medially to the flexor hallucis longus and subsequently crosses to its lateral side at the knot of Henry.

76. **d** Rupture of the Achilles tendon. Numerous case reports have associated tendon disorders (most commonly the Achilles) with use of fluoroquinolones. Both tendinitis and tendon rupture have been reported. The mechanism is unknown. Histologic studies have revealed edema, inflammatory infiltrates, and collagen changes.

Reference

Ribard P, et al.: Seven Achilles Tendinitis Including Three Complicated by Rupture During Fluoroquinolone Therapy. J Rheumatol, 19:1479–1481, 1992.

77. **a** Approximately 80% of bipartite sesamoids occur in the tibial sesamoid. Most (approximately 80%) of bipartite sesamoids occur in the tibial (medial) sesamoid. This is a normal finding that has been reported to occur in up to approximately 25% of the population. The increased frequency of multipartite sesamoids on the tibial side has been attributed to the finding that it transmits more weight than the fibular (lateral)

sesamoid. The same rationale is invoked to account for the higher incidence of acute fractures in the tibial sesamoid.

The sesamoids are contained within the flexor hallucis brevis tendon. Concomitant excision of both sesamoids should be avoided because of the associated risk of developing a clawtoe deformity.

The fibular sesamoid receives a partial insertion from the adductor hallucis tendon. The tibial sesamoid receives a partial insertion from the abductor hallucis tendon.

Note: Virtually all sesamoid disease is more common in the tibial sesamoid.

Reference

McBryde AM: Sesamoid Foot Problems in the Athlete. Clin Sports Med, 7:51–60, 1988.

78. **b** Excision of the os trigonum. The radiograph reveals an *os trigonum.* This normal anatomic variant is present in approximately 7% of the population. It is formed when the lateral tubercle ossification center fails to fuse with the posterior process of the talus.

The os trigonum may be an asymptomatic finding, but it can play a significant contributory role in patients who develop symptomatic posterior impingement, such as the patient described in this question. Excision of the os trigonum provides effective relief when this syndrome fails to respond to conservative therapy.

Posterior impingement symptoms tend to localize to the lateral hindfoot where they can be mistaken for inflammation of the peroneal tendons. The flexor hallucis longus runs in a groove between the medial and lateral tubercles of the posterior process of the talus. Thus, coexistent flexor hallucis longus tenosynovitis may be encountered, in which case concomitant tenosynovectomy would be indicated (see question 74). The lack of response to the local anesthetic injections suggests that neither the flexor hallucis longus nor the peroneal tendons is the principal cause of this patient's discomfort.

Reference

Hamilton WG: Stenosing Tenosynovitis of the Flexor Hallucis Longus Tendon and Posterior Impingement upon the Os Trigonum in Ballet Dancers. Foot Ankle, 3:74–80, 1982.

79. **b** Physical therapy for motion exercises, whirlpool, and contrast baths. The described situation is characteristic of reflex sympathetic dystrophy. Minor trauma is a common precipitant of this syndrome. Common early findings (within the first 3 months) include pain out of proportion to the initial injury, edema, allodynia (pain with nonpainful stimuli), and loss of motion. Later findings include alterations in skin color and texture with marked joint stiffness.

Decreased bone density on plain radiographs *(Sudeck atrophy)* is also a late finding, but bone scans may reveal diffuse periarticular uptake at an earlier stage. Regional uptake in the third phase of the bone scan has been reported to correlate with reflex sympathetic dystrophy.

Treatment of reflex sympathetic dystrophy focuses on early recognition. The goals of intervention are to (1) control pain (by desensitization modalities such as contrast baths and whirlpools or pharmacologic means) and (2) restore motion (through supervised physical therapy). Sympathetic blocks can be both diagnostic and therapeutic.

Reference

Seale KS: Reflex Sympathetic Dystrophy of the Lower Extremity. Clin Orthop, 243:80–85, 1989.

80. **a** Varus. Anatomic reduction of talar neck fractures not only is significant from the standpoint of minimizing the risk of osteonecrosis, but also it is important because small amounts of malalignment can significantly compromise function.

Varus malunion significantly limits subtalar motion and serves as a diathesis for joint degeneration. The associated forefoot adduction also redistributes weight to the lateral border of the foot with resultant calluses and painful gait. Varus malunion is attributed to two principal factors: (1) failure to obtain anatomic reduction and (2) failure to maintain anatomic reduction. Both these factors are less likely with open management. The most reasonable explanation for the finding that varus malunion is more common after type II fractures (versus after type III fractures) is that closed management is less commonly attempted in type III injuries. Dorsal malunion of the head fragment is less common and can compromise dorsiflexion.

Reference

Daniels T, Smith JW: Talar Neck Fractures. Foot Ankle, 14:225–234, 1993.

81. **b** Arthrodesis of the first metatarsophalangeal joint. Although the patient has rheumatoid arthritis, she does not manifest classic diffuse rheumatoid forefoot involvement (refer to question 52). Rather, she has an isolated hallux valgus deformity with associated metatarsophalangeal joint degeneration.

Given the advanced metatarsophalangeal degenerative changes, synovectomy and cheilectomy would be inappropriate. Flexion osteotomy of the first metatarsal would not treat the hallux valgus or the metatarsophalangeal arthritis, and it carries the risk of creating a transfer lesion to the second toe. A forefoot reconstruction is indicated for the classic rheumatoid forefoot with a hallux valgus and subluxated lesser metatarsophalangeal joints.

The *Keller procedure* (resection of the base of the proximal phalanx) is most appropriate for elderly, low-demand patients with hallux valgus and joint destruction or as a salvage procedure. It is associated with concerns for subsequent deformity, transfer metatarsalgia, and compromised toe-off strength. The Keller procedure does not provide a stable medial post to help prevent potential future lesser toe deformities. Metatarsophalangeal arthrodesis would be a superior option for this middle-aged, active patient with rheumatoid arthritis who may develop lesser toe disease in the future.

82. **e** Nerve to the abductor digiti minimi. The origin of heel pain can be elusive. Entrapment of the first branch of the lateral plantar nerve (the nerve to the abductor digiti minimi) may be difficult to distinguish from plantar fasciitis by history or physical examination. The point of maximal tenderness with nerve entrapment is classically described to be slightly more medial than is seen with plantar fasciitis, and the pain may radiate proximally and distally along the course of the nerve. The nerve to the abductor digiti minimi may be compressed by a hypertrophied abductor hallucis muscle belly, the margin of the quadratus plantae muscle, local inflammation, or a calcaneal spur.

Reference

Baxter DE, Thigpen CM: Heel Pain: Operative Results. Foot Ankle, 5:16–25, 1984.

83. **a** Split anterior tibial tendon transfer. Hindfoot varus in patients with acquired spasticity often results from continuous activity of the tibialis anterior. The indications for surgery include painful calluses, an inability to control the foot with an ankle-foot orthosis, and a desire to eliminate brace use in an ambulatory patient. The split anterior tibial tendon transfer is an effective means of correcting this type of varus deformity. In a split anterior tibial tendon transfer, the lateral portion of the tibialis anterior is released from its insertion and is rerouted to a bone tunnel in either the lateral cuneiform or the cuboid. Inflexibility of the varus deformity would preclude this procedure. A concomitant Achilles tendon lengthening may be indicated if there is a significant equinus component to the deformity.

Note: Neuromuscular hindfoot varus deformity typically results from overactivity of the tibialis anterior in cases of stroke or brain injury, whereas overactivity of the tibialis posterior is more commonly responsible in cases of cerebral palsy.

References

Edwards P, Hsu J: SPLATT combined with Tendo-Achilles Lengthening for Spastic Equinovarus in Adults. Foot Ankle, 14:335–338, 1993.
Waters, et al.: Surgical Correction of Gait Abnormalities after Stroke. Clin Orthop, 131:54–63, 1978.

84. **c** A 70-year-old woman with rheumatoid arthritis who is a household ambulator. Total ankle replacements are controversial. Most authors report poor results and suggest limited (if any) indications. However, some centers continue to use ankle replacements. The best results are seen in patients with rheumatoid arthritis who are more than 60 years old and who have not had prior surgical treatment. Patients with other types of arthrosis (avascular necrosis, posttraumatic arthrosis, failed arthrodesis) do not fare as well. Patients with severe associated osteopenia and deficient bone stock are not optimal candidates for total ankle arthroplasty, either. Salvage arthrodesis after a failed ankle replacement can be complicated by severe bone loss.

References

Unger AS, et al.: Total Ankle Arthroplasty in Rheumatoid Arthritis: A Long-Term Follow-Up Study. Foot Ankle, 8:173–179, 1988.
Wynn AH, Wilde AH: Long-term Follow-Up of the Conaxial Total Ankle Arthroplasty. Foot Ankle, 13:303–306, 1992.

85. **a** A 5-degree medial hindfoot wedge with a 9-mm heel lift. Elevation of the heel reduces tension on the Achilles tendon and can provide symptomatic relief. Correction of excessive valgus alignment (with a medial post or wedge) will alleviate the associated excessive tension in the medial Achilles fibers (see question 44 discussion).

86. **d** Short-leg nonwalking cast for 6 to 8 weeks. The history and radiographs are characteristic of a navicular stress fracture. Plain radiographs may be negative for 1 to 2 months. Supination of the forefoot will permit superior imaging of the full width of the navicular.

Early unprotected weight bearing has been implicated as a cause of displacement. Displacement has been associated with an increased risk of delayed union and nonunion. Nonunion, in turn, is a cause of chronic pain and degenerative arthritis.

Recommended treatment is given in Table 7.7.

TABLE 7.7. NAVICULAR STRESS FRACTURE TREATMENT

Navicular Stress Fracture	Treatment
Nondisplaced (acute)	SLC (NWB) for 6–8 wk
Displaced (acute)	ORIF + SLC (NWB) for 6–8 wk
Nonunion or delayed union	ORIF + inlay bone graft + SLC (NWB) for 6–8 wk

NWB, non–weight bearing; ORIF, open reduction and internal fixation; SLC, short leg cast.

Reference

Eisele SA, Sammarco GJ: Fatigue Fractures of the Foot and Ankle in the Athlete. J Bone Joint Surg Am, 75:290–298, 1993.

87. **c** Lateral lesions are often wafer shaped, whereas medial lesions are often cup shaped. In the past, lateral osteochondral lesions were thought to have a traumatic origin, but medial lesions were not. However, trauma is now considered to be responsible for most medial and lateral osteochondral lesions of the talar dome. An inversion mechanism is common to both medial and lateral lesions. Combined inversion and dorsiflexion creates impact between the anterolateral articular surface and the fibula. The classic posteromedial lesion stems from compression against the tibia with combined inversion and plantar flexion.

Lateral lesions are characteristically wafer shaped, whereas medial lesions are often cup shaped. An anterolateral arthrotomy provides adequate access to most lateral lesions. However, access to medial lesions is typically more difficult because of their more posterior location, and a medial malleolar osteotomy may be required for sufficient exposure.

The *Berndt and Harty classification* is based on the plain radiographic appearance of the lesion. It was originally described in 1959 (Table 7.8). This classification system has been criticized because of suboptimal correlation with arthroscopic findings, and alternative classification systems (based on magnetic resonance imaging or arthroscopy) have been proposed. However, the Berndt and Harty classification remains widely used.

Treatment options remain controversial. An initial course of nonoperative treatment is appropriate for most nondisplaced lesions. Small, displaced fragments should be excised, but larger fragments may be amenable to reduction and internal fixation.

Reference

Stone JW: Osteochondral Lesions of the Talar Dome. J Am Acad Orthop Surg, 4(2):63–73, 1996.

88. **b** Internal fixation with an intramedullary compression screw. Stress fractures of the base of the fifth metatarsal diaphysis (*Jones fractures*) are associated with a high rate of delayed union because of the suboptimal regional vascular supply. Nonoperative treatment (by immobilization and activity modification) will ultimately lead to union in most cases. However, healing may require several months to a year.

Intramedullary screw fixation is considered to be the most predictable and expedient means of facilitating the earliest possible return to full activity. Operative management is also favored in the presence of established nonunion, as suggested by the presence of intramedullary sclerosis in this case.

TABLE 7.8. BERNDT AND HARTY CLASSIFICATION OF MEDIAL LESIONS

Stage	Radiographic Appearance
I	Small subchondral compression fracture
II	Partially detached fragment
III	Completely detached fragment (nondisplaced from crater)
IV	Displaced fragment

References

Dameron TB: Fractures of the Proximal Fifth Metatarsal: Selecting the Best Treatment Option. J Am Acad Orthop Surg, 3(2):110–114, 1995.
Jones R: Fracture of the Base of the Fifth Metatarsal by Indirect Violence. Ann Surg, 35:697–700, 1902.
Sammarco GJ: The Jones Fracture. Instr Course Lect, 42:201–205, 1993.

89. **d** Subtalar arthrodesis. The radiographs demonstrate degenerative change in the subtalar joint (particularly the posterior facet) with no evidence of tibiotalar nonunion or hindfoot malalignment. Accelerated subtalar arthrosis is not an uncommon occurrence after ankle fusion because of the transmitted loads that result from lost ankle motion. Talar neck malunion is another diathesis for subtalar degeneration (see question 80).

Conservative management for this condition would include a rigid ankle-foot orthosis to restrict subtalar motion. If operative intervention had been required, the fusion would be extended to include only the involved joints, to preserve maximal motion. This patient's talonavicular joint appears normal, and, thus, it should not be fused.

Infection should always be considered in the setting of postoperative pain, but this clinical situation does not suggest it. Osteotomy would not be indicated in the absence of malalignment, but it could be considered if the ankle were fused in varus or excessive valgus.

Note: The ankle should be fused to produce 5 to 10 degrees of hindfoot valgus so transverse tarsal motion is not compromised. Remember: hindfoot varus "locks" Chopart joint by causing divergence of the talonavicular and calcaneocuboid joint axes.

90. **a** Repair of the superficial peroneal retinaculum. Posttraumatic subluxation of the peroneal tendons results from detachment of the superficial peroneal retinaculum from the distal fibula. The question describes the classic mechanism and physical findings.

The tendons typically reduce spontaneously after the acute dislocation, and, thus, the injury is often initially misconstrued as a simple ankle sprain. Controversy exists over optimal management in the acute setting. When the injury is recognized in the acute setting, immobilization in plantar flexion has yielded good results. Surgical repair of the retinaculum has also been advocated for acute dislocations.

Treatment for recurrent dislocations is less controversial. Direct repair of the superficial peroneal retinaculum has proven to be extremely effective with minimal morbidity. Reconstruction of the retinaculum with free tendon tissue (e.g., plantaris sling, Achilles slip, palmaris) may be necessary if residual retinacular tissues are insufficient. Tendon rerouting and fibular bone block procedures have relatively high morbidity rates. The Chrisman-Snook procedure may be applicable when there is associated chronic lateral ankle instability.

Reference

Das-De S, Balasubramaniam P: A Repair Operation for Recurrent Dislocation of Peroneal Tendons. J Bone Joint Surg Br, 67:585–587, 1985.

91. **d** Avulsion of the calcaneal tuberosity. Traumatic ankle inversion most commonly produces classic lateral ankle ligamentous injury. However, a similar mechanism of injury can produce various other injuries that should not be overlooked. These include avulsion fractures of the lateral process of the talus, the dorsal lip of the navicular, the base of the fifth metatarsal, and the cuboid. In addition, an inversion mechanism can account for both medial and lateral osteochondral fractures of the talar dome (see discussion of question 87).

Although combined inversion and plantar flexion can produce calcaneal avulsion fractures at the insertion of the bifurcate ligament, avulsions of the calcaneal tuberosity are typically produced by axial loading combined with sudden eccentric loading of the Achilles tendon.

Note: The treatment of most avulsion fractures that are associated with lateral ankle sprains does not differ significantly from the management of severe isolated ankle sprains themselves. However, a displaced avulsion of the lateral process of the talus requires open reduction and internal fixation (or fragment excision if the fragment is too small for fixation). Delayed recognition and management of this injury are associated with poor outcomes.

Reference

Mukherjee SK, et al.: Fracture of the Lateral Process of the Talus. J Bone Joint Surg Br, 56:263–273, 1974.

92. **e** The anterior talofibular. The anterior talofibular ligament runs anteromedially from the fibula to the body of the talus. Hence, it becomes taught when an anterior translation stress (the anterior drawer test) is applied to the talus. It also becomes taut with inversion and plantar flexion, and it is the most vulnerable component of the lateral ankle ligament complex.

The calcaneofibular ligament crosses both the ankle and the subtalar joint. It becomes taught with inversion and neutral flexion. The posterior talofibular ligament runs from the fibular fossa to the trigonal tubercle. It serves as a restraint to posterior talar translation and to external talar rotation. The posterior tibiofibular ligament is a component of the syndesmotic ligament complex. The spring ligament is a plantar link between the navicular and the calcaneus which helps to support the longitudinal arch.

Reference

Bulucu C, et al.: Biomechanical Evaluation of the Anterior Drawer Test: The Contribution of the Lateral Ligaments. Foot Ankle, 11:389–393, 1991.

93. **a** The posterior tibiofibular ligament. Because the talus imparts a posterior external rotation force to the fibula, the anterior tibiofibular ligament is first structure to fail. As additional deformation occurs, the fibula fractures and the posterior tibiofibular ligament comes under tension. Because of the strength of the posterior tibiofibular ligament and its attachments, an avulsion fracture of the posterior malleolus commonly occurs, rather than failure of the ligament itself. The final event in the SER-IV trimalleolar injury sequence is failure of the medial malleolus (or deltoid ligament). Axial compression by the talus is the mechanism for pilon fractures.

94. **c** Lupus erythematosus. Given these two significant lesions (a large medullary infarct in the distal tibia and osteonecrosis of the medial talar dome with an associated subchondral fracture and a mild joint effusion), the diagnosis of *lupus erythematosus* could account for both. Rheumatoid arthritis is also often associated with avascular necrosis and bone infarcts (from steroid exposure). Sickle cell disease is another potential unifying diagnosis.

The distal tibial lesion is not consistent with a diagnosis of osteomyelitis. A Brodie abscess would manifest higher signal intensity on T2-weighted magnetic resonance images. Neither the plain radiographs nor the magnetic resonance images manifest evidence of periostitis. Furthermore, osteomyelitis rarely crosses a joint space to involve an adjacent muscle.

Radiographically, talar osteonecrosis may be difficult to distinguish from a traumatic osteochondral lesion. However, the intramedullary tibial lesion in this case is not consistent with a bone contusion or any other sequela of trauma.

Chondrosarcoma typically demonstrates high signal intensity on T2-weighted magnetic resonance sequences because of the high water content of cartilage. Osteochondritis dissecans may produce a similar lesion of the talar dome, but this diagnosis could not account for the intramedullary tibial lesion. Although rheumatoid arthritis is often associated with avascular necrosis and bone infarcts (from steroid exposure), the absence of intrasynovial disease and the intact articular cartilage render rheumatoid arthritis an unlikely diagnosis in this case.

95. **d** 40%. According to the classic biomechanical study by Ramsey and Hamilton, 1 mm of static, experimentally induced lateral talar shift reduced ankle contact area by 42%. That study has been commonly invoked to justify open reduction and internal fixation of isolated lateral malleolar fractures. However, such a justification is based on the false assumption that an isolated lateral malleolar fracture will permit lateral talar shift. In fact, lateral talar subluxation is prevented in this setting by the intact deltoid ligament. Further biomechanical research (Michelson) in which isolated lateral malleolar fracture specimens were loaded dynamically (without extrinsically induced lateral talar shift) failed to corroborate altered ankle loading characteristics. Clinical research has demonstrated that surgical management offers no significant benefit over nonoperative treatment of these injuries.

    Note: This information is irrelevant when there is a concomitant medial injury (medial malleolus or deltoid).

References

Bauer M, et al.: Malleolar Fractures: Nonoperative Versus Operative Treatment. A Controlled Study. Clin Orthop, 199:17–27, 1985.
Michelson JD, Helgemo SL: Kinematics of the Axially Loaded Ankle. Foot Ankle, 16:577–582, 1995.
Ramsey PL, Hamilton W: Changes in Tibiotalar Area of Contact Caused by Lateral Talar Shift. J Bone Joint Surg Am, 58:356–357, 1976.

96. **d** The spoon plate. The paramount concern in managing high-energy pilon fractures is the tenuous state of the overlying soft tissues. Bulky tibial plates such as the spoon plate are no longer indicated because of their recognized propensity to compromise the surrounding soft tissue envelope. Low-profile buttress plates (such as the 3.5-mm clover-leaf plate) are preferable.

    The recommended reconstruction sequence is as follows: (1) restoration of length, by fibular reduction and stabilization; (2) restoration of tibial plafond articular congruity; (3) grafting of metaphyseal cancellous defects; and (4) tibial stabilization with buttress plate.

    Soft tissue concerns may limit early internal fixation to the fibula. In such cases, open reduction and internal fixation of the fibula and a spanning external fixator allow the soft tissues time to recover. In rare instances, swelling may also preclude internal fibular fixation. When open reduction and internal fixation are not feasible, indirect reduction by external fixation is necessary to restore and maintain length and alignment. External fixation will optimize the milieu for soft tissue recovery. Delayed open reduction and internal fixation and bone grafting can then be performed at 7 to 10 days or when the soft tissue swelling has subsided.

97. **e** The posterior tibial tendon. When the foot recoils from its laterally displaced position, the posterior tibial tendon may become entrapped along the lateral side of the talar neck. This interposition necessitates open reduction. Other potential obstructions to closed reduction include articular impaction fractures and capsular interposition. The extensor digitorum brevis muscle is a common obstacle to closed reduction of medial subtalar dislocations but does not commonly prevent reduction of lateral dislocations.

Reference

Leitner B: Obstacle to Reduction in Subtalar Dislocations. J Bone Joint Surg Am, 36:299, 1954.

FIGURE CREDITS

Figure 7.19. From Rockwood CA, Green DP, eds: Fractures in Adults, 4th Ed., vol 2. Philadelphia, Lippincott–Raven, p. 2278, 1996, with permission.
Figure 7.20. From Lutter LD, et al.: Orthopaedic Knowledge Update: Foot and Ankle. Rosemont, IL, American Academy of Orthopedic Surgeons, p. 249, 1994, with permission.
Figure 7.21. From Rockwood CA, Green DP, eds: Fractures in Adults, 4th Ed., vol 2. Philadelphia, Lippincott–Raven, p. 2293, 1996, with permission.
Figure 7.22. From Crim JR: Imaging of the Foot and Ankle, Philadelphia, PA, Lippincott–Raven, p. 70, 1996, with permission.
Figure 7.23. Adapted from Mann RA: Decision-making in bunion surgery. Instr Course Lect, 39:3–13, 1990, with permission.
Figure 7.24A and B. From Browner BD, et al., eds: Skeletal Trauma, vol 2. Philadelphia, WB Saunders, pp. 1878, 1891, 1992, with permission.

8

TUMOR AND METABOLIC BONE DISEASE

QUESTIONS

1. A 24-year-old man complains of a 3-month history of right-sided neck pain. His discomfort worsens at night. He has no neurologic symptoms or deficit. Although aspirin effectively eliminated his pain, he has now developed gastritis. A plain lateral radiograph and bone scan image are shown in Fig. 8.1. What is the most likely diagnosis?
   (a) Degenerative disc disease
   (b) Intracortical metastasis
   (c) Osteoid osteoma
   (d) Osteomyelitis
   (e) Osteogenic sarcoma
2. A 13-year-old girl undergoes a limb-sparing resection of an osteogenic sarcoma of her distal femur. A preoperative metastatic workup (including bone scan and computed tomography scans of the brain, chest, and abdomen) was completely negative. Pathologic examination of the resected specimen reveals a low-grade lesion that had violated the medial intermuscular septum. According to the Enneking system, how should this tumor be classified?
   (a) IA
   (b) IB
   (c) IIA
   (d) IIB
   (e) III
3. An 8-year-old boy presents with a low-grade Ewing sarcoma of the humerus and undergoes a limb-sparing resection. The lesion is confined to a single compartment. A single pulmonary metastasis is detected and resected. According to the Enneking system, how should this tumor be classified?
   (a) IA
   (b) IB
   (c) IIA
   (d) IIB
   (e) IIIA
4. Adamantinoma most commonly occurs in which of the following locations?
   (a) The metacarpals
   (b) The metatarsals
   (c) The forearm (radius or ulna)
   (d) The tibia
   (e) The humerus
5. A 66-year-old retired plumber presents for evaluation of a painless "lump" beneath his right scapula. He recently retired to Florida, and his wife incidentally noticed the mass while she was applying suntan lotion to his back. He is otherwise perfectly healthy with the exception of a 40-pack-year smoking history. On physical examination, you palpate a grape-sized, firm, nontender nodule at the inferior angle of the scapula. The mass seems to be fixed to the chest wall. Scapulothoracic motion is painless and unrestricted. Plain radiographs of the right shoulder, thoracic spine, chest, and ribs are unremarkable. A biopsy is performed, and the specimen stains heavily with elastin. What is the most likely diagnosis?
   (a) Mesothelioma with extrathoracic extension
   (b) Pancoast tumor
   (c) Elastofibroma
   (d) Liposarcoma
   (e) Fibrosarcoma
6. Which of the following conditions is most commonly associated with a low urine specific gravity?
   (a) Larsen syndrome
   (b) Hand-Schüller-Christian disease
   (c) Spondyloepiphyseal dysplasia
   (d) Maffucci syndrome
   (e) Prader-Willi syndrome
7. All the following statements regarding parosteal osteogenic sarcoma are true except
   (a) It occurs in an older population than standard osteogenic sarcoma.
   (b) Its typical histologic appearance consists of well-differentiated trabecular bone within a background of low-grade fibrous stroma.
   (c) In general, it is associated with a better prognosis than standard osteogenic sarcoma.

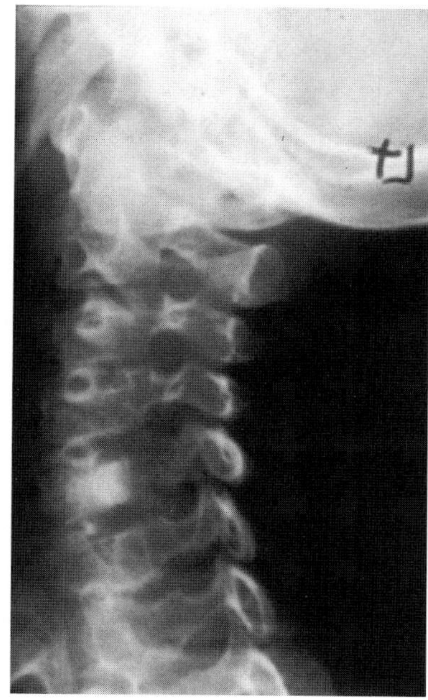
A

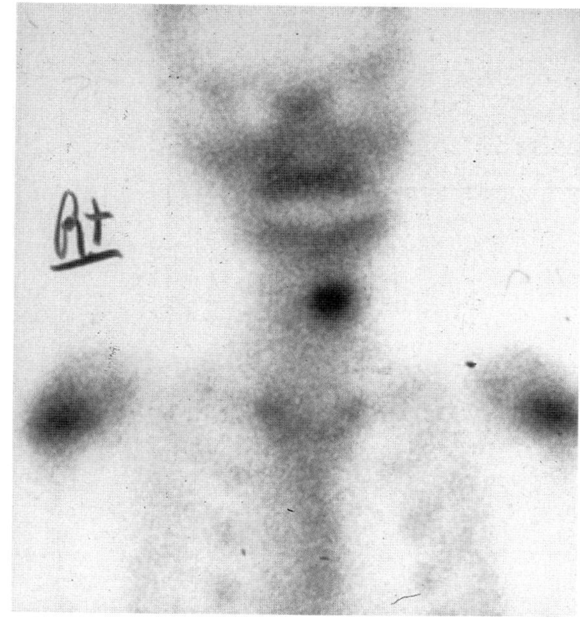

B

FIGURE 8.1A and B

(d) It has a tendency to grow around the surface of the affected bone without penetrating the cortex.
(e) The most common site of occurrence is the tibial shaft.

8. Chondrosarcoma most commonly occurs at what location?
   (a) The distal femur
   (b) The proximal humerus
   (c) The pelvis
   (d) The proximal femur
   (e) The proximal tibia
9. A 25-year-old snowboarder complains of medial left knee pain during a mandatory work physical. Examination reveals mild swelling and tenderness at the medial femur. A radiograph is shown in Fig. 8.2A. Histologic features from an incisional biopsy are shown in Fig. 8.2B. What is the most likely diagnosis?
   (a) Aneurysmal bone cyst
   (b) Fibrous dysplasia
   (c) Telangiectatic osteogenic sarcoma
   (d) Cavernous hemangioma
   (e) Giant cell tumor
10. What is the physiologic defect responsible for hypophosphatasia?
   (a) Decreased renal resorption of phosphate
   (b) Decreased alkaline phosphatase activity
   (c) Decreased gastrointestinal absorption of phosphate
   (d) Increased parathyroid hormone activity
   (e) Decreased parathyroid hormone activity
11. Physaliferous cells are associated with which of the following tumors?
   (a) Giant cell tumor
   (b) Chordoma
   (c) Hemangiopericytoma
   (d) Liposarcoma
   (e) Desmoplastic fibroma
12. Which of the following conditions is associated with an Erlenmeyer flask deformity of the distal femur?
   (a) Vitamin D–deficient rickets
   (b) Hypophosphatemic rickets
   (c) Hypophosphatasia
   (d) Gaucher disease
   (e) Kneist syndrome
13. Which of the following histologic features is associated with malignant fibrous histiocytoma?
   (a) "Herringbone" pattern
   (b) "Chinese letter" pattern
   (c) "Storiform" pattern
   (d) "Chicken wire" calcification
   (e) "Racquet-shaped" cells
14. A 59-year-old woman with metastatic breast carcinoma presents with acute, symptomatic hypercalcemia (calcium level higher than 15 mg/dL). Which of the following is not a potential symptom or sign of hypercalcemia?
   (a) Coma
   (b) Chvostek sign
   (c) Shortened QT interval
   (d) Hyporeflexia
   (e) Polydipsia
15. Which of the following is the most important first step in the management of the patient in question 14?

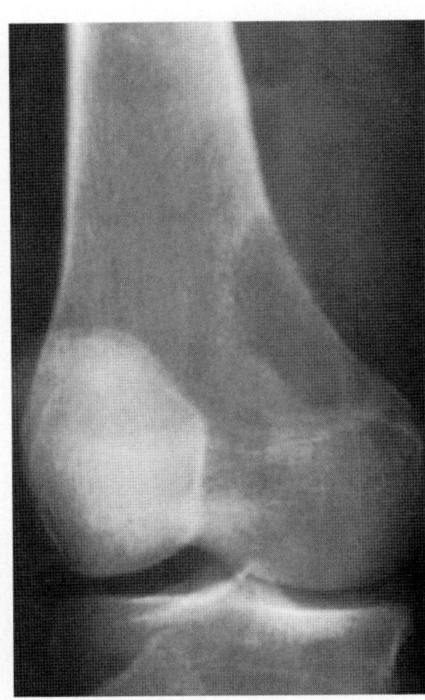

A

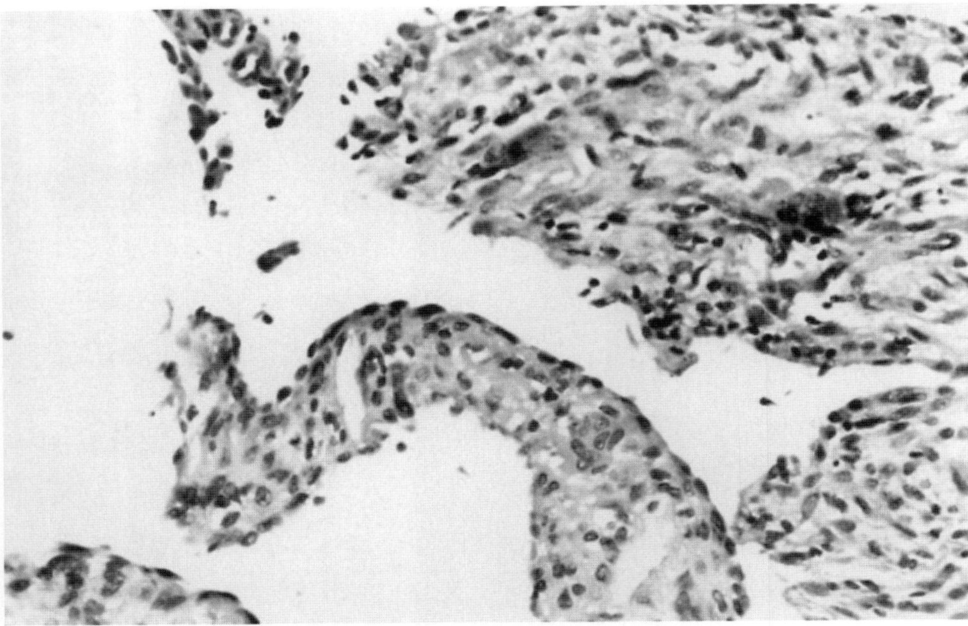

B

FIGURE 8.2A and B

(a) Intravenous furosemide administration
(b) Oral prednisone administration
(c) Intravenous mithramycin administration
(d) Subcutaneous calcitonin administration
(e) Intravenous fluid administration

16. Which of the following statements regarding hypophosphatemic vitamin D–resistant rickets is true?
 (a) It is inherited as an autosomal recessive trait.
 (b) The disease produces secondary hyperparathyroidism.
 (c) Supplementary 1-25 vitamin D is a component of the treatment.
 (d) Stunted growth and lower extremity deformities are prominent features during the first year of life.
 (e) Renal phosphate wasting is no longer considered to be the fundamental defect in the disease.
17. Which of the following tumors is associated with high glycogen content?
 (a) Malignant fibrous histiocytoma
 (b) Ewing sarcoma
 (c) Fibrosarcoma
 (d) Liposarcoma
 (e) Telangiectatic osteogenic sarcoma
18. Disproportionately short fourth and fifth metacarpals are associated with which of the following?
 (a) Hemochromatosis
 (b) Pseudohypoparathyroidism
 (c) Wilson disease
 (d) Acromegaly
 (e) Hypothyroidism
19. A 17-year-old girl presents with progressive right hip pain and difficulty with ambulation. Examination reveals a coxalgic gait. A plain radiograph of the right hip is shown in Fig. 8.3A. A histologic specimen from curettage of the lesion is shown in Fig. 8.3B. What is the most likely diagnosis?
 (a) Osteomyelitis
 (b) Fibrous dysplasia
 (c) Chondromyxoid fibroma
 (d) Chondroblastoma
 (e) Giant cell tumor
20. An 18-year-old woman presents with a myelophthisic anemia and a radiograph that demonstrates a well-defined "rugger jersey" spine. What is the most likely diagnosis?
 (a) Fanconi anemia
 (b) Albright syndrome
 (c) Osteopetrosis
 (d) Renal osteodystrophy
 (e) Juvenile Paget disease
21. Which of the following statements regarding the effects of glucocorticoids on bone mineral metabolism is false?
 (a) Supraphysiologic glucocorticoid levels do not cause secondary hyperparathyroidism.
 (b) Glucocorticoids inhibit gastrointestinal absorption of calcium.
 (c) Glucocorticoids increase renal excretion of calcium.
 (d) Glucocorticoids inhibit osteoblastic bone formation.

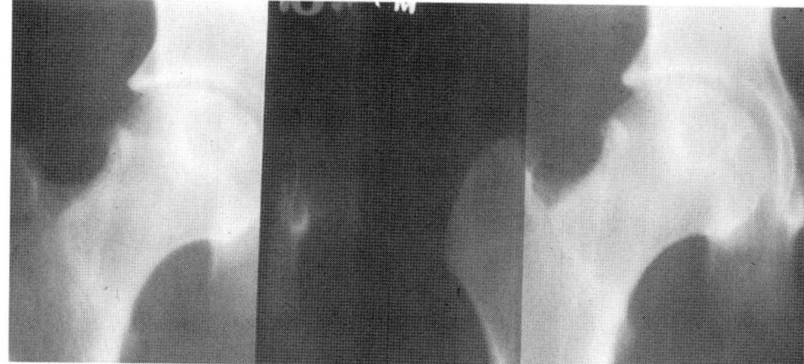

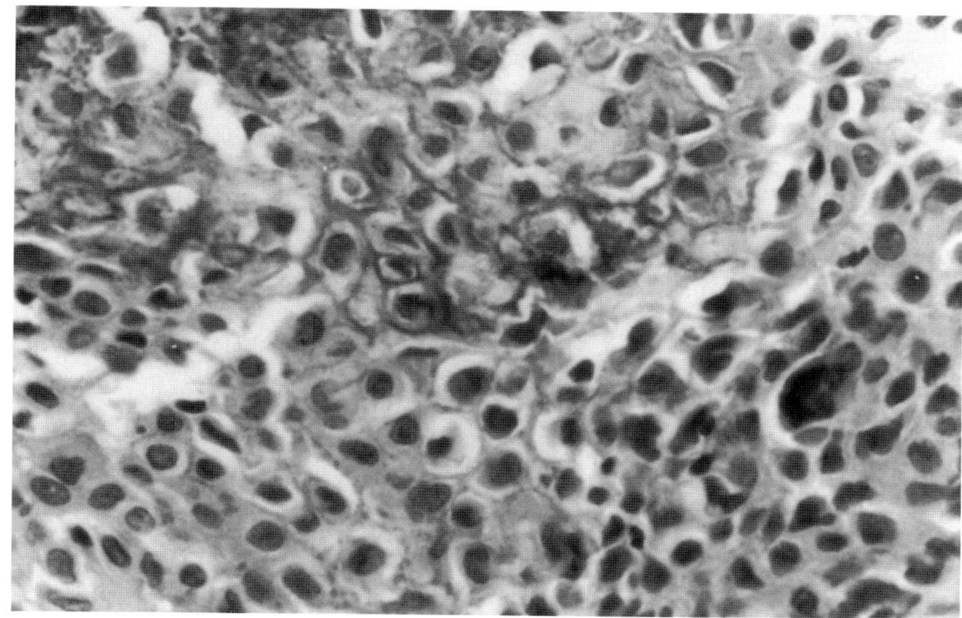

FIGURE 8.3A and B

(e) Glucocorticoids increase bone resorption by inhibiting pituitary secretion of gonadotropins.

22. A 13-year-old girl presents to her dermatologist because she is concerned over the cosmetic appearance of a "birthmark" on her arm. Examination reveals a 3 × 2-cm hyperpigmented lesion with a jagged border. Review of systems reveals premature menarche. She has been treated in the past for a pathologic fracture through a lytic lesion in her femur (at which time a skeletal survey revealed similar lesions in several other bones). What is the most likely diagnosis?
    (a) Letterer-Siwe disease
    (b) Maffucci syndrome
    (c) Neurofibromatosis
    (d) Enchondromatosis
    (e) Albright syndrome
23. Which of the following factors is not characteristic of giant cell tumor of bone?
    (a) It has an eccentric location.
    (b) It has a well-defined border.
    (c) It abuts the subchondral bone of the articular surface.
    (d) It has a sclerotic border.
    (e) It occurs in the epiphyseal region.
24. Which of the following is not associated with Paget disease?
    (a) High-output cardiac failure
    (b) Hearing impairment by otosclerosis
    (c) Spinal stenosis
    (d) Hearing impairment by nerve entrapment
    (e) High serum calcium
25. A 40-year-old man visiting New York City from the Dominican Republic was brought to the emergency room with a 2-week history of right knee pain. Examination revealed an antalgic gait. A radiograph of the right proximal tibia was obtained (Fig. 8.4A). An orthopaedic consultant in the emergency room recommended further workup which included a magnetic resonance imaging scan (Fig. 8.4B) and a biopsy. The patient and his family refused the biopsy, and the patient was lost to follow-up. Two weeks later, the man was brought back to the emergency room with severe

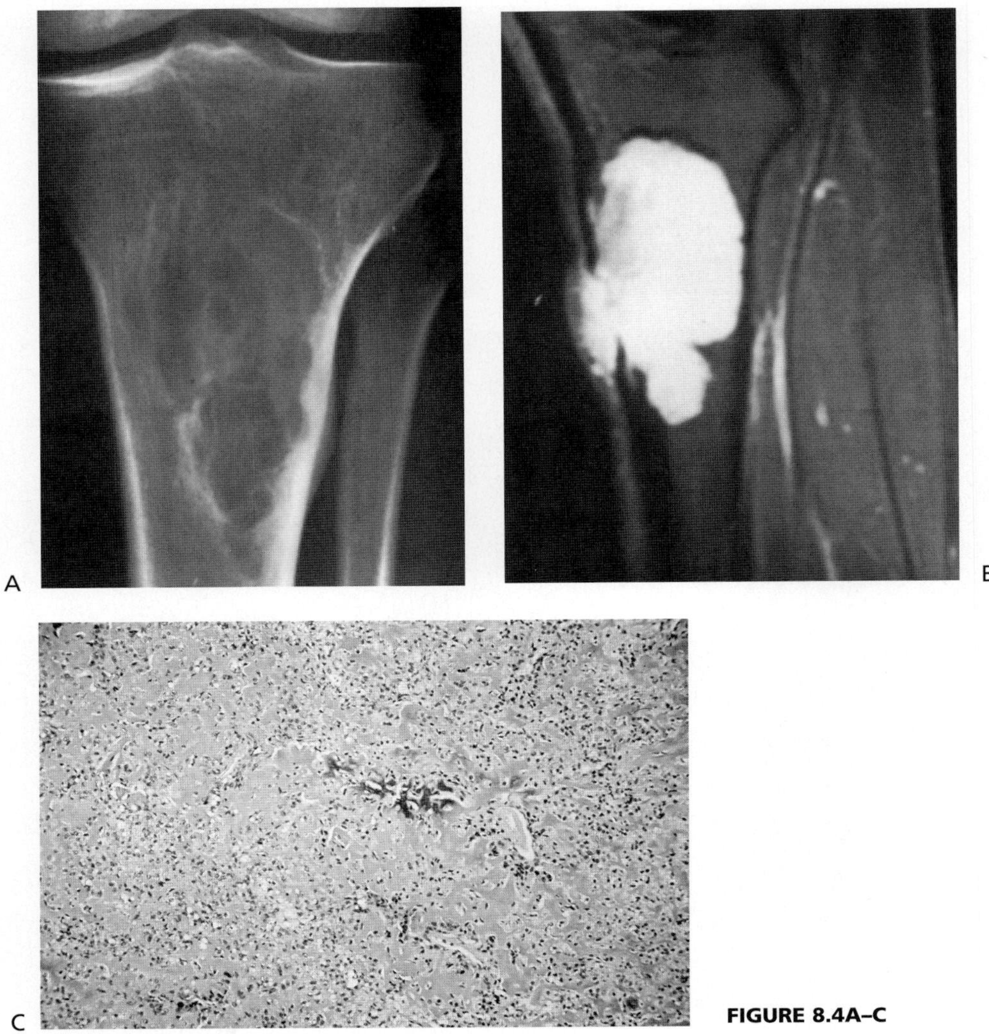

FIGURE 8.4A–C

right knee pain and an inability to ambulate. Histologic features from an incisional biopsy are shown in Fig. 8.4C. What is the diagnosis?
(a) Chondrosarcoma
(b) Central osteogenic sarcoma
(c) Osteomyelitis
(d) Ewing sarcoma
(e) Malignant fibrous histiocytoma

26. Which of the following bony lesions is most commonly associated with Gardner syndrome?
(a) Multiple osteomas
(b) Multiple enchondromas
(c) Multiple osteochondromas
(d) Multiple giant cell tumors of bone
(e) Neurofibromatosis

27. What is the mode of inheritance of Ollier disease?
(a) Autosomal dominant
(b) Sex-linked dominant
(c) Autosomal recessive
(d) Sex-linked recessive
(e) Nonhereditary

28. Which of the following statements is true regarding chondrosarcoma?
(a) The peak incidence is in persons older than 65 years.
(b) Maffucci syndrome is associated with a higher incidence of secondary malignancy than Ollier disease.
(c) Chemotherapy is the mainstay of treatment.
(d) Females are affected approximately twice as often as males.
(e) Pain is a rare presenting complaint.

29. A 55-year-old attorney presents with insidious pain and deformity of his right leg. His ambulation is limited to two blocks with a cane. Examination reveals marked bowing of the patient's right tibia. A plain radiograph is shown in Fig. 8.5A. A photomicrograph from a biopsy of the lesion is shown in Fig. 8.5B. The most likely diagnosis for this patient's condition is

A

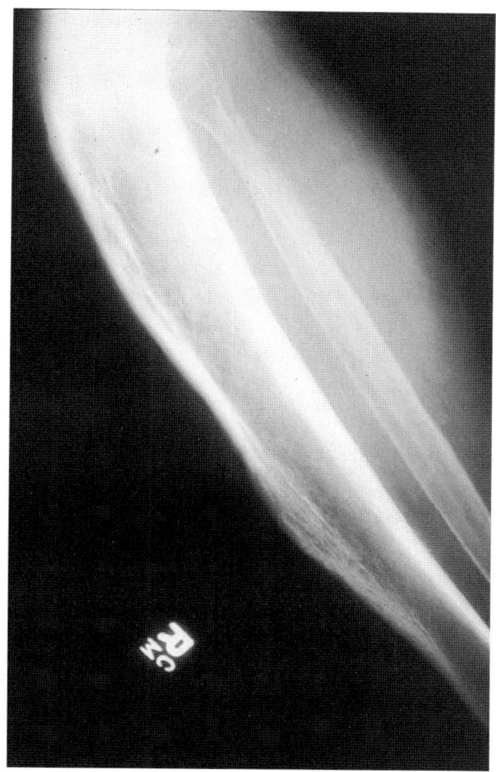

B

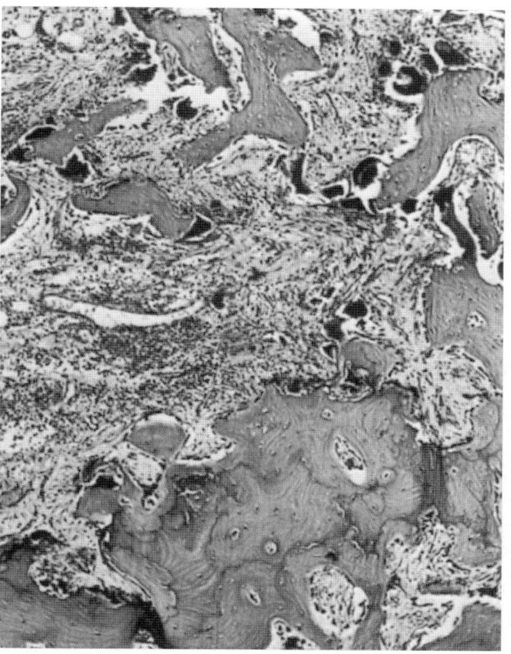

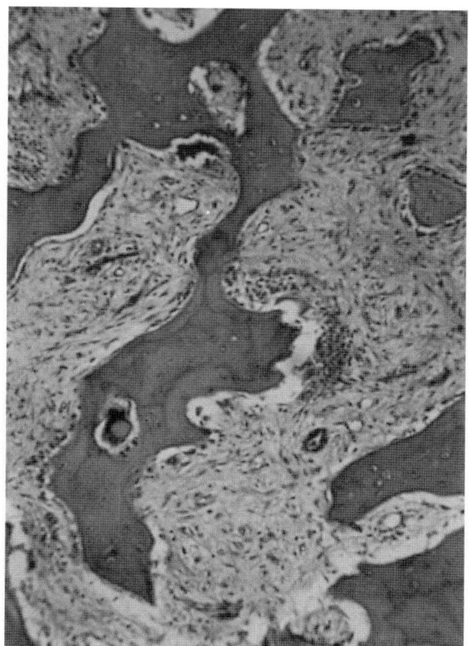

FIGURE 8.5A and B

(a) Hyperparathyroidism
(b) Renal osteodystrophy
(c) Paget disease
(d) Fibrous dysplasia
(e) Neurofibromatosis

30. Which of the following tumors tends to affect the vertebral body more commonly than the posterior elements of the spine?
    (a) Eosinophilic granuloma
    (b) Osteoid osteoma

(c) Osteoblastoma
(d) Aneurysmal bone cyst

31. The embryologic origin of the parathyroid glands is
    (a) The foramen cecum
    (b) The third and fourth pharyngeal pouches
    (c) The neural crest
    (d) The mesoderm from the urogenital ridge
    (e) Rathke pouch
32. When performing an incisional biopsy of a suspected malignant musculoskeletal neoplasm, the surgeon should adhere to all the following guidelines except
    (a) The biopsy should be performed through muscle rather than through intermuscular planes.
    (b) Neurovascular bundles should not be exposed during the procedure.
    (c) The incision should be transverse.
    (d) The biopsy should be performed at the institution where the definitive operation will be performed rather than at a referral center.
    (e) The approach should not violate a compartment that is not already occupied by the lesion.
33. The 11:22 translocation is a marker for which of the following neoplasms?
    (a) Osteogenic sarcoma
    (b) Osteoblastoma
    (c) Fibrosarcoma
    (d) Ewing sarcoma
    (e) Malignant fibrous histiocytoma
34. Which of the following statements regarding Ewing sarcoma is false?
    (a) An elevated lactate dehydrogenase level is a poor prognostic sign.
    (b) Survival is greater than 50% at 5 years.
    (c) Males are affected more commonly than females.
    (d) The bone lesion is usually associated with an extraosseous soft tissue mass.
    (e) The tibia is the most common site of origin.
35. When evaluating a bone tumor, bone scintigraphy is most effective for which of the following purposes?
    (a) To determine whether the lesion is benign or malignant
    (b) To assess whether the lesion is intracompartmental or extracompartmental
    (c) To detect the presence of other osseous disease foci
    (d) To define the tissue of origin for metastasis of unknown origin
    (e) To assess the grade of the lesion
36. The initial evaluation of a suspected bone neoplasm should consist of which of the following imaging studies?
    (a) Magnetic resonance imaging
    (b) Computed tomography
    (c) Plain radiography
    (d) Bone scintigraphy
    (e) Tomography
37. Which of the following should be the initial imaging study of a suspected soft tissue tumor?
    (a) Magnetic resonance imaging
    (b) Computed tomography
    (c) Plain radiography
    (d) Bone scintigraphy
    (e) Tomography
38. When magnetic resonance imaging is used to evaluate an osseous neoplasm, it is important to remember that when shifting from T1-weighted images to T2-weighted images,
    (a) Fat signal intensity decreases, and water signal intensity decreases.
    (b) Fat signal intensity increases, and water signal intensity decreases.
    (c) Fat signal intensity decreases, and water signal intensity increases.
    (d) Fat signal intensity increases, and water signal intensity increases.
    (e) Muscle signal intensity decreases, and water signal intensity decreases.
39. Which of the following is the most accurate statement regarding the radiographic features of spondyloarthropathies?
    (a) In psoriatic arthritis, syndesmophytes tend to be thin, marginal, and symmetric.
    (b) In ankylosing spondylitis, syndesmophytes tend to be thick, asymmetric, and nonmarginal.
    (c) Ankylosing spondylitis and inflammatory bowel disease are associated with bilaterally symmetric sacroiliac disease.
    (d) Syndesmophytes do not occur in association with inflammatory bowel disease.
    (e) Psoriatic arthritis does not affect the sacroiliac joints.
40. Ledderhose disease is also known as which of the following?
    (a) Extraabdominal desmoid
    (b) Plantar fibromatosis
    (c) Nodular fasciitis
    (d) Palmar fibromatosis
    (e) Neurofibromatosis
41. A 17-year-old computer maven presents with a painless, slow-growing mass on the dorsal aspect of his right hand. It is firm, mobile, and nontender to palpation. Plain radiographs demonstrate intralesional calcific stippling. The mass appears to be confined to the soft tissues with no effect on the adjacent bones. Histologic examination from an excisional biopsy reveals a fibrous stroma with centrally located regions of cartilage. What is the most likely diagnosis?
    (a) Nodular fasciitis
    (b) Calcifying aponeurotic fibroma
    (c) Malignant fibrous histiocytoma
    (d) Dermatofibrosarcoma protuberans

(e) Fibrosarcoma

42. A patient with a long-standing radiographic diagnosis of Paget disease presents with recent onset of groin pain. He relates the onset of pain to "bumping" into a door. An anteroposterior radiograph of his hip is shown in Fig. 8.6. What is the most appropriate next step?
    (a) Bone scan
    (b) Long-arm cast at 90 degrees for 4 weeks
    (c) Cast brace permitting a controlled 90-degree arc of elbow motion until the pain has resolved
    (d) Initiation of bisphosphonate therapy and a removable splint for comfort
    (e) Open biopsy for definitive diagnosis
43. Osteoclasts are derived from what cells?
    (a) Osteoblasts
    (b) Osteocytes
    (c) Hematopoietic stem cell precursors
    (d) Inducible osteoprogenitor cells
    (e) Fibroblast precursors
44. Which of the following statements about diphosphonates is incorrect?
    (a) They enhance bone mineral deposition at high doses.
    (b) They are useful in managing hypercalcemia of malignant disease.
    (c) They inhibit bone resorption.
    (d) They are pyrophosphate analogs.
    (e) They can cause osteomalacia.
45. Which of the following statements is least accurate with regard to Paget disease?

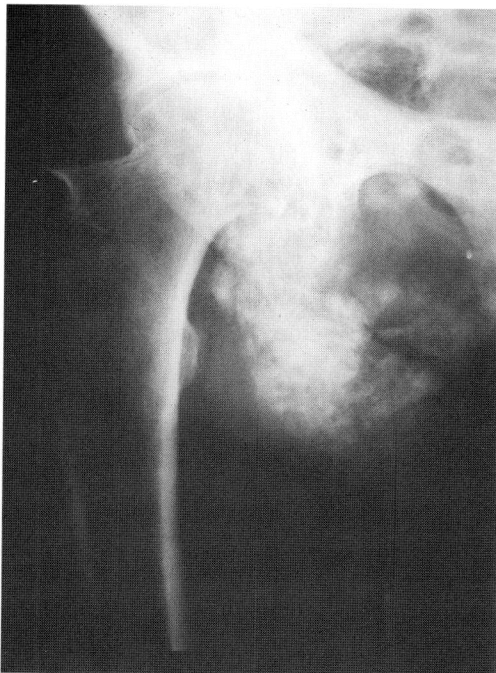

FIGURE 8.6

    (a) Serum calcium levels are characteristically normal.
    (b) It is most commonly diagnosed in patients in their 50s.
    (c) Most affected patients have elevated serum levels of alkaline phosphatase.
    (d) Bone biopsy should be performed routinely to confirm the diagnosis.
    (e) Facial bones, scapulae, ribs, clavicles, and forearm bones are uncommonly affected.
46. Calcitonin is produced by which of the following cell types?
    (a) Parafollicular cells of the thyroid
    (b) Chief cells of the parathyroid
    (c) Osteoclasts
    (d) Oxyphil cells of the parathyroid
    (e) Zona fasciculata cells of the adrenal cortex
47. Which of the following statements is true regarding vitamin D?
    (a) It is a protein.
    (b) $1,25(OH)_2$ vitamin D is synthesized by the liver.
    (c) Increased skin melanin does not decrease the rate of photosynthesis of vitamin D.
    (d) $1,25(OH)_2$ vitamin D decreases the production of parathyroid hormone.
    (e) Parathyroid hormone increases the synthesis of 25(OH)vitamin D.
48. All the following decrease gastrointestinal calcium reabsorption (directly or indirectly) except
    (a) Glucocorticoids
    (b) Gluten enteropathy
    (c) Excess thyroid hormone
    (d) Phosphate depletion
    (e) Metabolic acidosis
49. All the following drugs cause osteomalacia by affecting vitamin D except
    (a) Phenytoin
    (b) Aluminum-containing antacids
    (c) Rifampin
    (d) Cholestyramine
    (e) Phenobarbital
50. The risk of osseous metastasis is greatest with which of the following types of thyroid cancer?
    (a) Medullary
    (b) Papillary
    (c) Follicular
    (d) Mixed papillary and follicular
    (e) Anaplastic
51. A 43-year-old man presented to his primary care physician with "dull pain" in the right groin. A diagnosis of "transient synovitis" was made, and nonsteroidal anti-inflammatory drugs were prescribed. Progressive pain and limping over the subsequent month prompted the radiograph shown in Fig. 8.7A. A biopsy of the lesion yielded the histologic features shown in Fig. 8.7B. What is the most likely diagnosis?

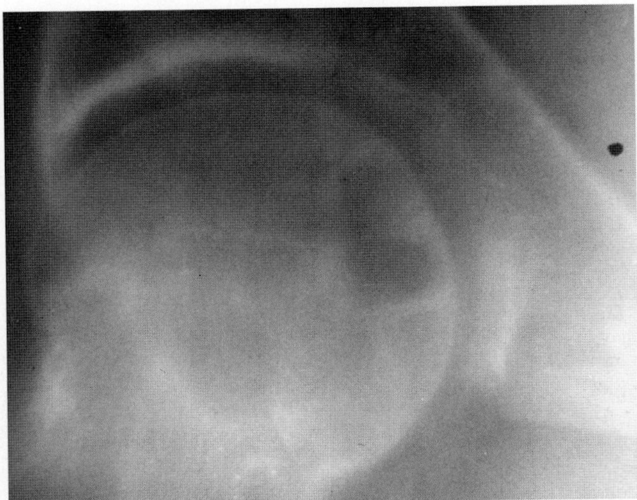
A

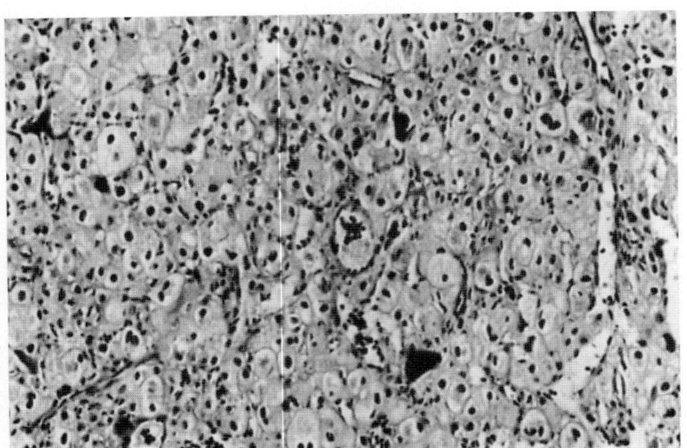
B

FIGURE 8.7A and B

(a) Clear cell chondrosarcoma
(b) Giant cell tumor
(c) Aneurysmal bone cyst
(d) Chondroblastoma
(e) Avascular necrosis

52. Which of the following lesions is least likely to produce a lytic defect in an epiphyseal region?
(a) Giant cell tumor
(b) Chondroblastoma
(c) Eosinophilic granuloma
(d) Nonossifying fibroma
(e) Osteomyelitis

53. Which of the following laboratory findings is not consistent with type II vitamin D–dependent rickets?
(a) Low serum calcium
(b) Low serum phosphate
(c) Elevated parathyroid hormone
(d) Elevated alkaline phosphatase
(e) Low 1,25-$(OH)_2$ vitamin D_3

54. Patients with hereditary retinoblastoma are genetically predisposed to which of the following lesions?
(a) Ewing sarcoma
(b) Neuroblastoma
(c) Rhabdomyosarcoma
(d) Malignant fibrous histiocytoma
(e) Osteogenic sarcoma

55. Which of the following statements regarding fibrous dysplasia is false?
(a) It is a nonhereditary condition.
(b) The polyostotic form exhibits bilateral symmetry.
(c) It may produce cortical erosion.
(d) Lesions often contain cartilage tissue.
(e) Osseous spicules within the lesion are composed of woven bone.

56. Which of the following statements regarding osteoid osteoma of the thoracic spine is false?
(a) The level of the lesion typically corresponds to the level of the apex of the resultant scoliosis.
(b) The most common location is the posterior elements.
(c) It is the most common cause of painful scoliosis.
(d) The curvature of the associated scoliosis is concave toward the side of the lesion.
(e) Surgical excision ensures complete resolution of the associated scoliosis.

57. All the following are significant prognostic factors for disease-free survival after limb-salvage surgery for stage II conventional osteogenic sarcoma except
(a) The presence of a skip metastasis
(b) Preoperative serum lactate dehydrogenase level
(c) The status of surgical margins
(d) The extent of neoadjuvant chemotherapy-induced tumor necrosis
(e) None of the above

58. A 65-year-old stockbroker presents with pain and swelling of the shoulder. She cannot pinpoint a precipitating event for the pain. The discomfort interferes with sleep. Examination reveals a firm, nodular mass in the axilla. Range of motion of the shoulder is limited by pain. A plain anteroposterior radiograph is shown in Fig. 8.8A. Biopsy specimens are shown in Fig. 8.8B and C. Based on the information given, what is the most likely diagnosis?
(a) Fibrosarcoma
(b) Malignant fibrous histiocytoma
(c) Osteogenic sarcoma
(d) Liposarcoma
(e) Fibrous dysplasia

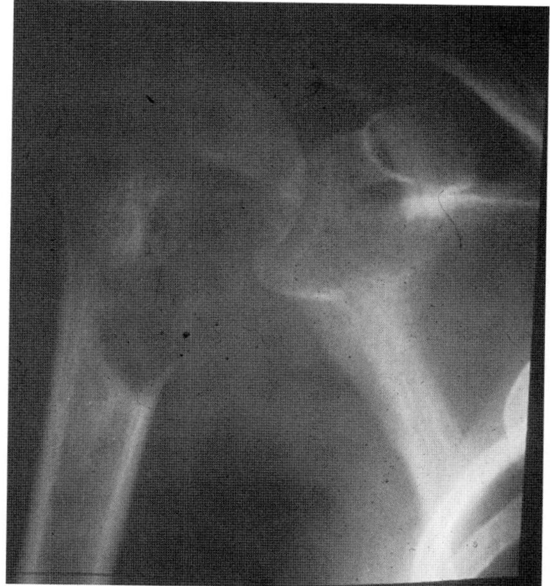

A

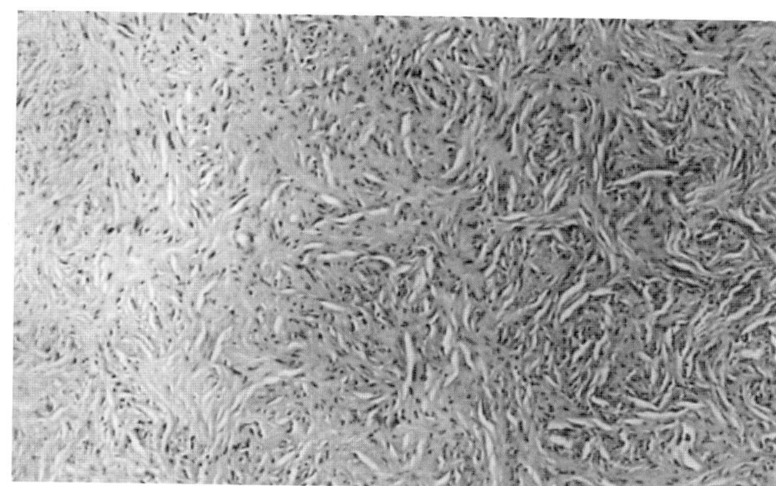

B

FIGURE 8.8A and B

59. What is the local recurrence rate when osteogenic sarcoma of the distal femur is treated with limb-salvage surgery and neoadjuvant chemotherapy?
    (a) 0%
    (b) 1%
    (c) 5% to 10%
    (d) 20% to 30%
    (e) 50%
60. Looser zones refer to
    (a) Regions of stippled mineral deposition within a chondrosarcoma
    (b) A lytic osseous defect in a patient with hyperparathyroidism that contains multiple giant cells within a cellular fibrous stroma
    (c) Cortical lucent lines oriented perpendicularly to the long axis of the bones of a patient with osteomalacia
    (d) Regions of cartilage hypertrophy at the costochondral junction of a child with rickets
    (e) A condensation of horizontally oriented trabeculae formed adjacent and parallel to the physis at times of decelerated skeletal growth
61. What is the pharmacologic mechanism of allopurinol?
    (a) It inhibits metabolism of pyrimidine ribonucleotides.
    (b) It inhibits leukocyte migration and phagocytosis by inhibiting polymerization of the microtubular protein tubulin.
    (c) It inhibits xanthine oxidase.
    (d) It increases renal excretion of uric acid.
    (e) It inhibits cyclooxygenase.
62. An 18-year-old child prodigy medical student noticed a fixed, painless mass on the medial aspect of his distal thigh while he was tracing the course of his sartorius muscle in preparation for an anatomy examination. He believed (after palpation by the entire first-year medical school class) that the mass had grown and had become painful. A plain radiograph was obtained (Fig. 8.9A). Excision was performed, yielding the specimen in Fig. 8.9B. What is the most appropriate diagnosis?
    (a) Parosteal osteogenic sarcoma
    (b) Osteochondroma
    (c) Chronic enthesitis of the adductor magnus insertion with formation of an accessory apophysis
    (d) Periosteal osteogenic sarcoma
    (e) Chondrosarcoma
63. Periosteal osteogenic sarcoma is distinguished from the other varieties of osteogenic sarcoma based on
    (a) Its predilection to arise in the metaphyseal region of long bones
    (b) The relative predominance of cartilage tissue within the tumor
    (c) The absence of new bone production by the tumor cells
    (d) The presence of large blood-filled channels
    (e) Its presence most commonly in the upper extremity
64. A 65-year-old man presents to his primary care physician with right hip pain. He has no significant past medical history but has a 20-pack-year history of smoking. The primary care physician is unsure of the diagnosis and prescribes nonsteroidal antiinflammatory

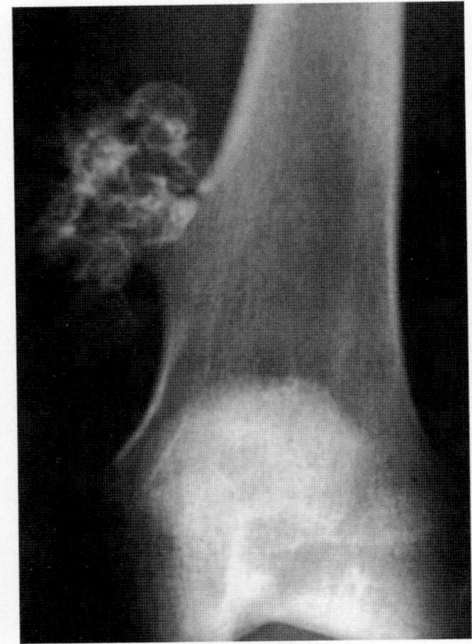

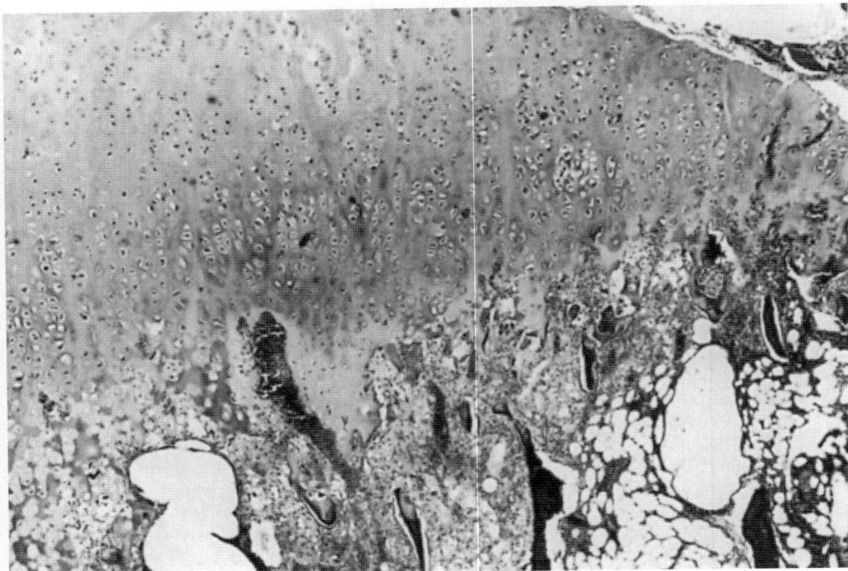

FIGURE 8.9A and B

drugs. After 6 months of failed nonsteroidal antiinflammatory drug therapy, a magnetic resonance imaging scan is obtained, which is read as "degenerative joint disease." A week later the patient develops acute pain and the inability to bear weight. Plain films are subsequently performed (Fig. 8.10). Before an incisional biopsy, what is the most likely diagnosis?
(a) Multiple myeloma
(b) Fibrosarcoma
(c) Osteomyelitis
(d) Metastatic carcinoma
(e) Avascular necrosis

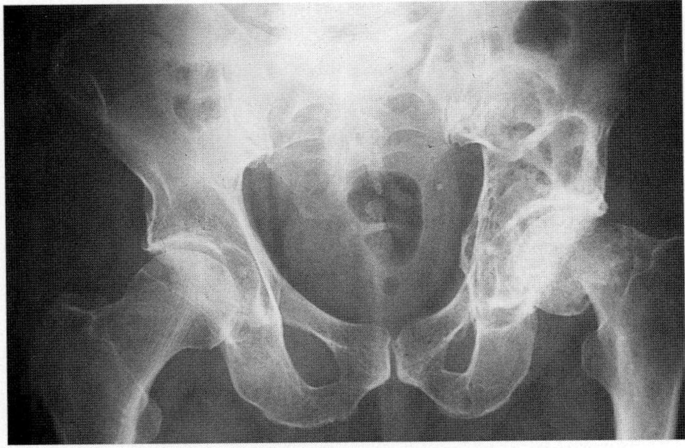

FIGURE 8.10

65. Which of the following statements regarding chondroblastoma is false?
(a) It may metastasize to the lung.
(b) It can be distinguished from giant cell tumor by differential immunohistochemical staining for the S-100 protein.
(c) It most commonly occurs in adults between 30 and 60 years of age.
(d) It typically originates in the epiphysis.
(e) There is approximately a 10% local recurrence rate after intralesional excision.
66. A 22-year-old basketball player presents with shoulder pain after an injury during a game. He states that he felt like his shoulder almost "popped out," although he denies a previous history of dislocation. Examination reveals mild tenderness, and apprehension, but no instability. Plain radiographs are obtained (Fig. 8.11A) and reveal the lesion in the humerus. The patient denies a history of arm pain. No soft tissue mass is palpable. A bone scan (Fig. 8.11B) and computed tomography scan (Fig. 8.11C) are obtained. A biopsy is performed (Fig. 8.11D). What is the most likely diagnosis?
(a) Osteochondroma
(b) Fibrous dysplasia
(c) Chondrosarcoma
(d) Enchondroma
(e) Osteomyelitis
67. Anticipated findings in a child with scurvy include all the following except
(a) Subperiosteal hemorrhage

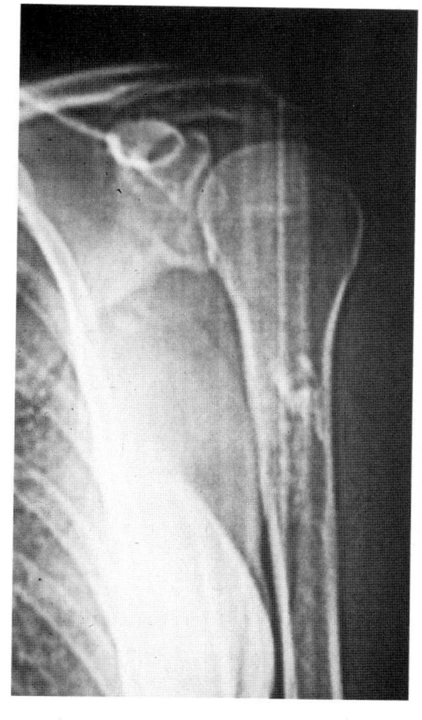

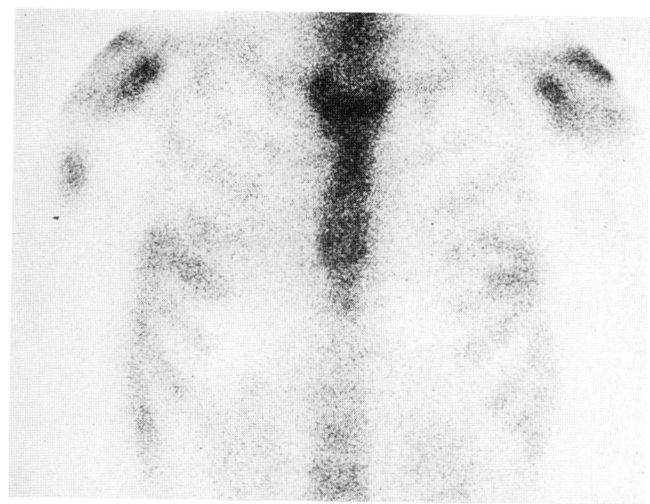

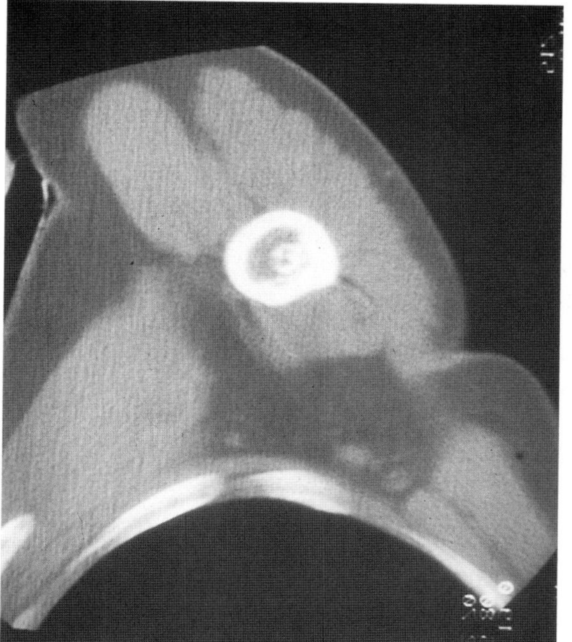

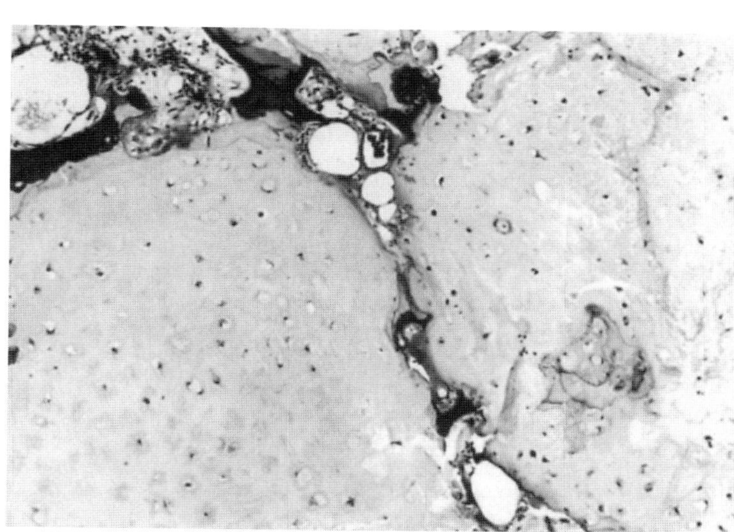

FIGURE 8.11A–D

(b) The Wimberger ring sign
(c) Metaphyseal compression fractures
(d) Periostitis
(e) Multiple cystic, extraosseous, calcium-containing masses adjacent to large joints

68. A 34-year-old flight attendant presents for evaluation of a posterior right knee mass. She had been told that it was a Baker cyst by a family practitioner who had examined her aboard a flight several months earlier. She is concerned because she believes that the mass has gradually enlarged. A radiograph is obtained (Fig. 8.12A). An open biopsy of the lesion yields the histologic features seen in Fig. 8.12B. What is the most likely diagnosis?

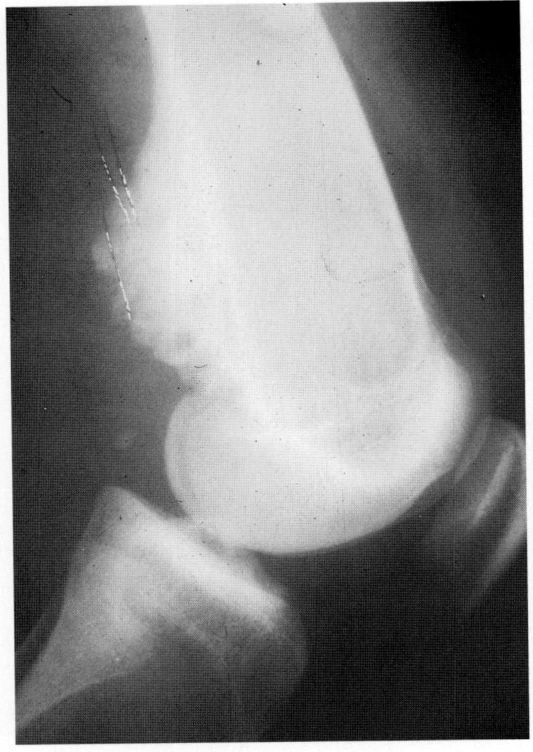

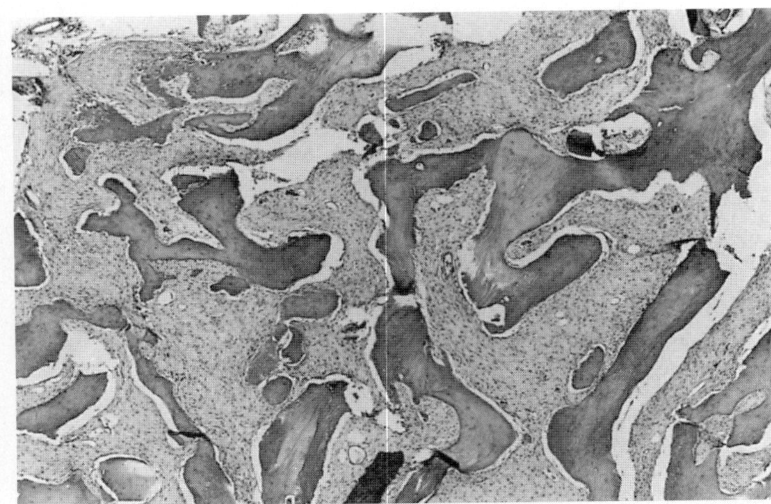

FIGURE 8.12A and B

(a) Osteochondroma
(b) Periosteal osteogenic sarcoma
(c) Myositis ossificans
(d) Parosteal osteogenic sarcoma
(e) Periosteal chondroma

69. All the following are radiographic features of Paget disease except
   (a) Cortical thickening and expansion
   (b) "Cotton-wool" skull
   (c) Initial involvement of the middiaphysis
   (d) Osteoporosis circumscripta
   (e) A "flame-shaped" leading edge

70. A 47-year-old competitive dressage rider presents with unilateral knee pain and swelling. Her past medical history is significant for breast cancer and smoking. Magnetic resonance images are shown in Fig. 8.13A and B. A biopsy of the lesion is obtained (Fig. 8.13C). What is the most likely diagnosis?
   (a) Chondroblastoma
   (b) Metastatic breast cancer
   (c) Giant cell tumor
   (d) Reparative granuloma
   (e) Fibrous dysplasia

71. A 19-year-old African-American violinist presents with painless soft tissue masses on the extensor surfaces of her wrists and elbows. Radiographs of the affected regions reveal extraarticular, multilobulated, mineralized masses. She denies trauma, and her past medical history is unremarkable. Her serum calcium level is normal. Biopsy reveals the presence of hydroxyapatite. What is the most likely diagnosis?
   (a) Gout
   (b) Sarcoidosis
   (c) Tumoral calcinosis
   (d) Metastatic calcification
   (e) Hypervitaminosis D

72. What is the most common site of skeletal metastasis?
   (a) The femur
   (b) The pelvis
   (c) The proximal humerus
   (d) The ribs
   (e) The spine

73. Which of the laboratory profiles in Fig. 8.14 would you anticipate in a patient with primary hyperparathyroidism?
   (a) A
   (b) B
   (c) C
   (d) D
   (e) E

74. Which of the laboratory profiles in Fig. 8.14 would you anticipate in a patient with pseudohypoparathyroidism?
   (a) A

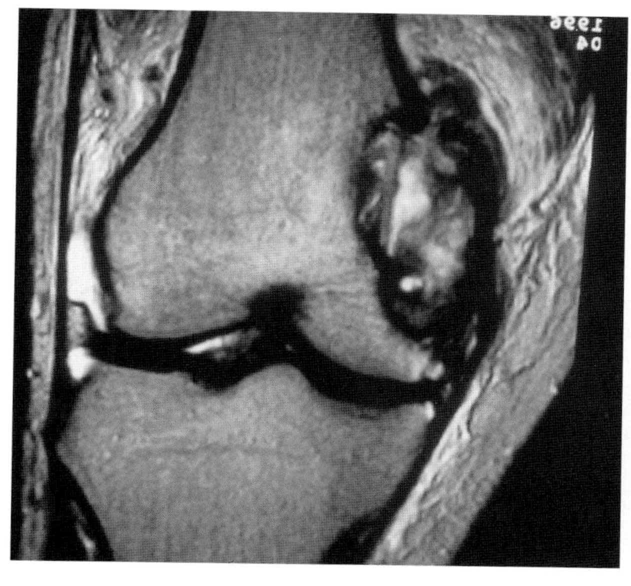

A

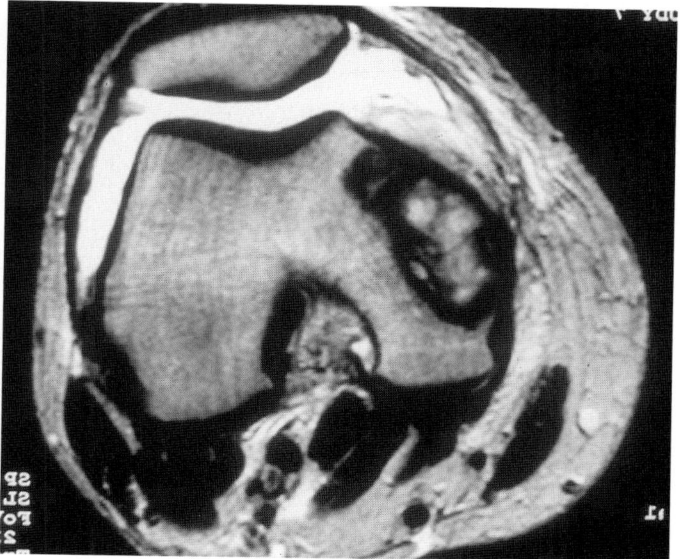

B

C

FIGURE 8.13A–C

	Calcium	Phosphate	PTH	25-Vitamin D	1-25-Vitamin D
A	N	N	L	N	H
B	L	L	H	L	L
C	H	L	H	N	H
D	H	N	H	L	H
E	L	H	H	N	L

("N" = normal ; "L" = low ; "H" = high)

FIGURE 8.14

(b) B
(c) C
(d) D
(e) E

75. Which of the laboratory profiles in Fig. 8.14 would you anticipate in a patient with secondary hyperparathyroidism associated with Crohn disease?
(a) A
(b) B
(c) C
(d) D
(e) E

76. A 32-year-old woman collides with a taxi while she is in-line skating. A plain radiograph is obtained as part of a routine trauma series (Fig. 8.15A). Her past medical history is unremarkable except for endometriosis, cervical dysplasia, and an isolated episode of pelvic inflammatory disease. A subsequent biopsy of her proximal femur yields the histologic specimen in Fig. 8.15B. What is the most likely diagnosis?
(a) Osteogenic sarcoma
(b) Ossifying fibroma
(c) Osteomyelitis
(d) Desmoplastic fibroma
(e) Fibrous dysplasia

77. A 54-year-old waitress presents with a nontender, mobile mass on the back of her knee. She reports that the lesion has been present for approximately 2 years. Magnetic resonance images and intraoperative photographs are shown in Fig. 8.16. Based on the magnetic resonance and gross appearance, what is the most likely diagnosis?
(a) Chordoma
(b) Hemangiopericytoma
(c) Schwannoma
(d) Reticulum cell sarcoma
(e) Liposarcoma

78. A 15-year-old gymnast is referred by her trainer because of recalcitrant "arm-splints" and malaise. Examination reveals tenderness over the humerus with focal swelling. Review of systems is significant for a recent history of fevers and anorexia. A radiograph is shown in Fig. 8.17A. A biopsy of the lesion is shown in Fig. 8.17B. What is the most likely diagnosis?
(a) Osteomyelitis
(b) Ewing sarcoma
(c) Osteogenic sarcoma
(d) Giant cell tumor
(e) Aneurysmal bone cyst

79. Birbeck granules are associated with electron microscopy of which of the following neoplasms?
(a) Telangiectatic osteogenic sarcoma
(b) Dedifferentiated chondrosarcoma
(c) Chondroblastoma
(d) Eosinophilic granuloma
(e) Desmoplastic fibroma

80. A 64-year-old retired postal carrier undergoes lumbar decompression for spinal stenosis. Preoperative imaging studies are shown in Fig. 8.18. What is the diagnosis?
(a) Telangiectatic osteogenic sarcoma
(b) Angiosarcoma
(c) Multiple myeloma
(d) Hemangioma
(e) Aneurysmal bone cyst

81. Which of the following lesions frequently arises within (or adjacent to) another benign primary lesion of bone?
(a) Unicameral bone cyst
(b) Giant cell tumor
(c) Chondromyxoid fibroma
(d) Aneurysmal bone cyst
(e) Nonossifying fibroma

82. A 15-year-old cross-country runner presents with a 6-month history of distal thigh pain. Physical examination

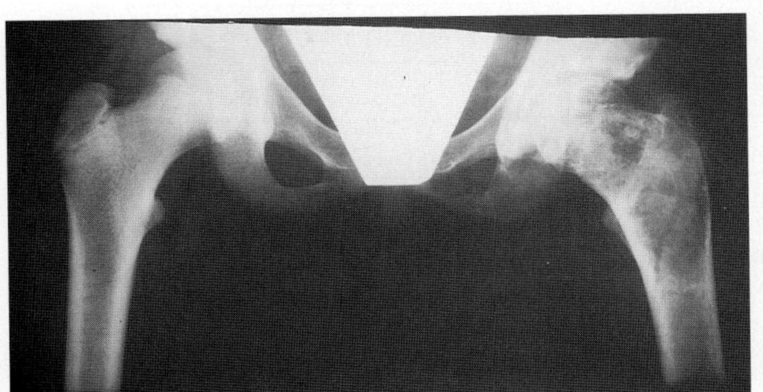
A

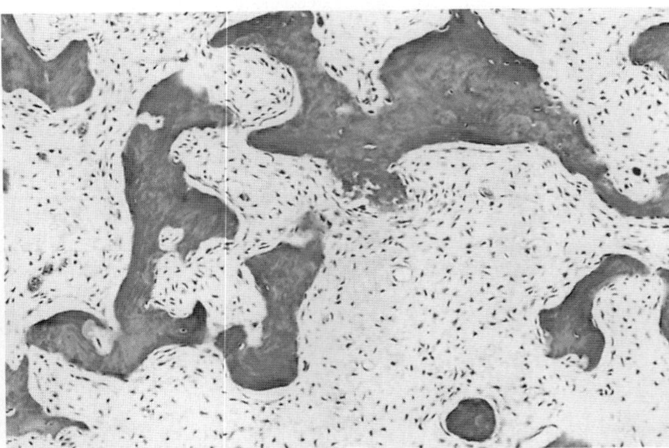

FIGURE 8.15A and B

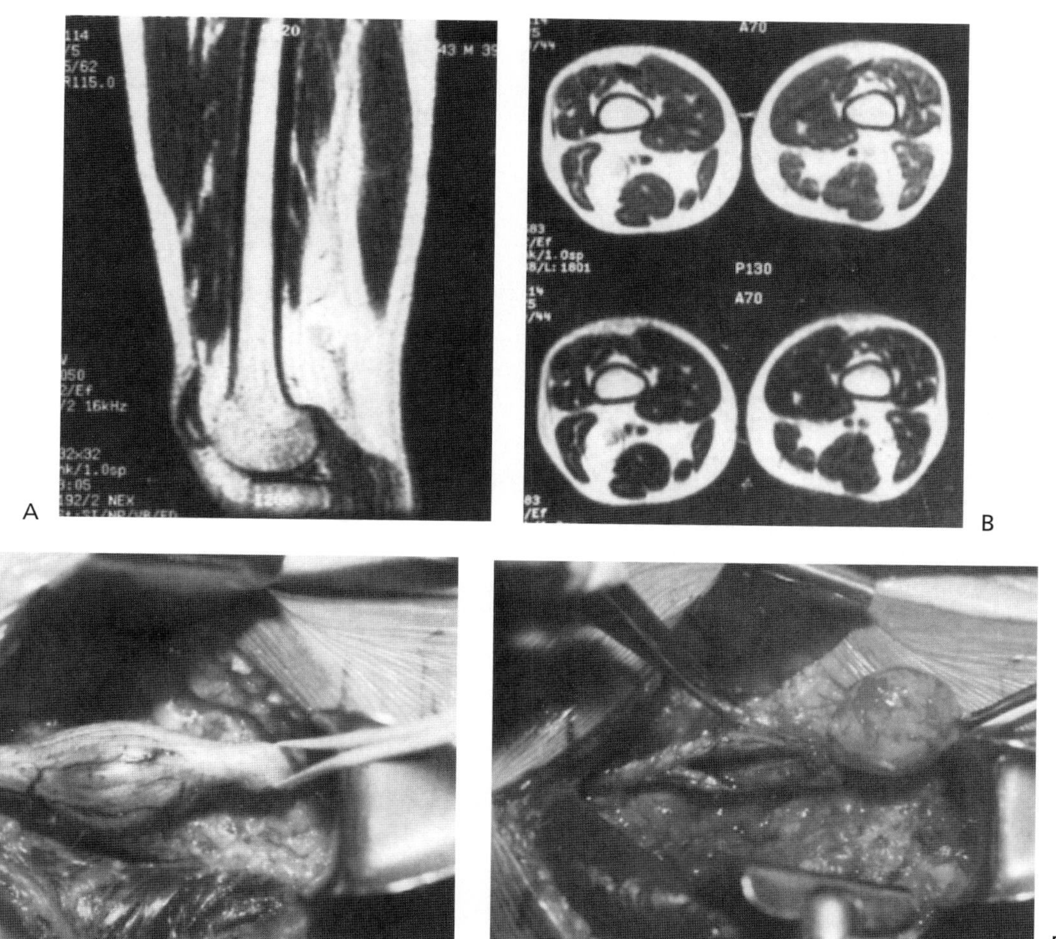

FIGURE 8.16A–D

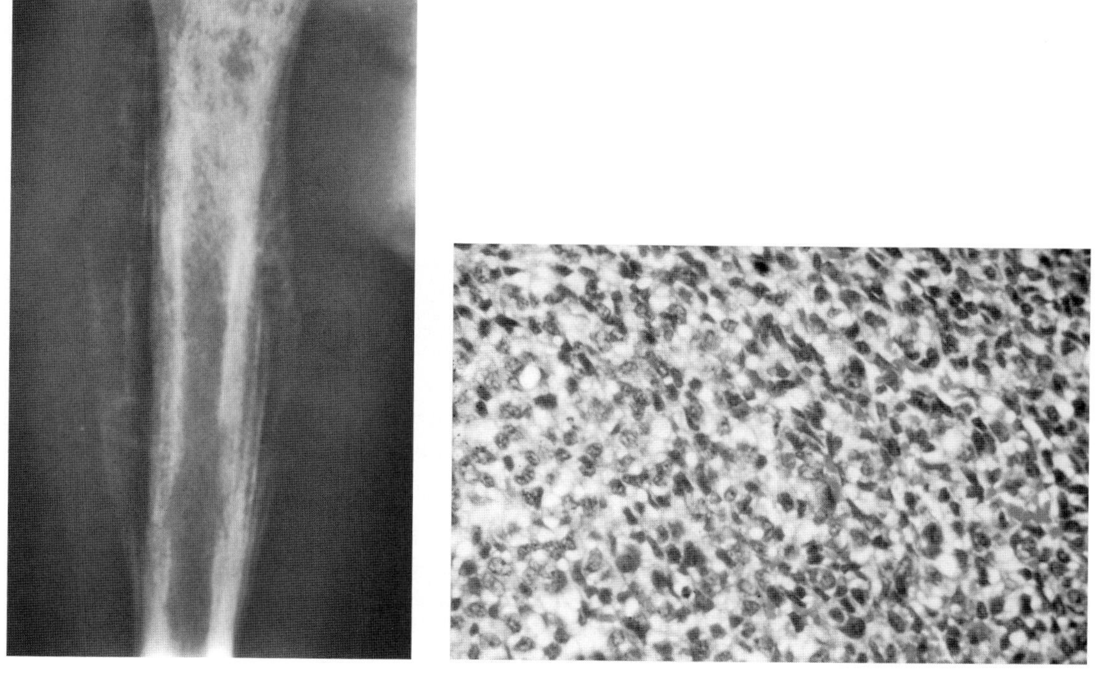

FIGURE 8.17A and B

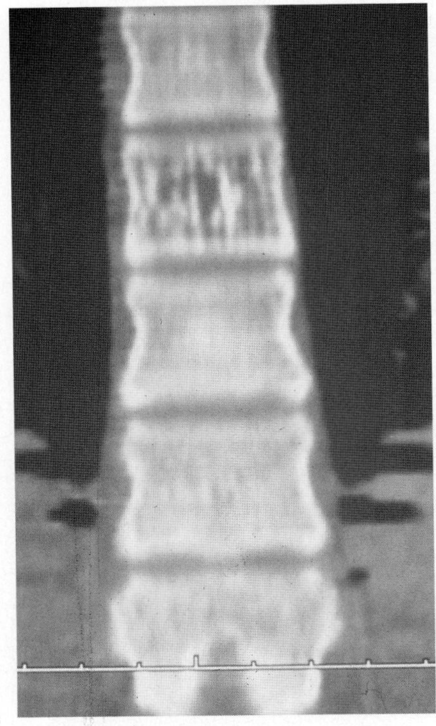

FIGURE 8.18A–C

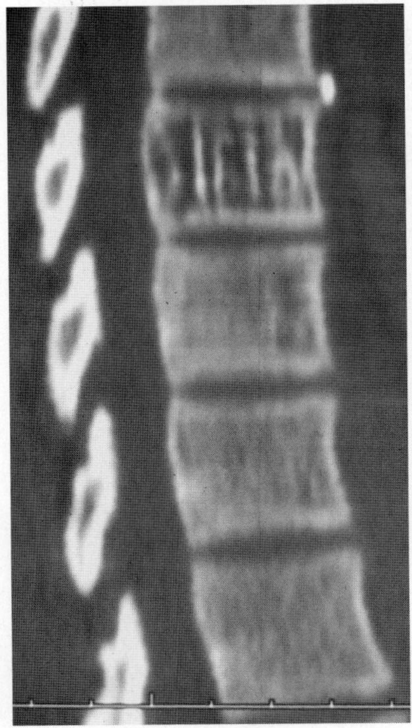

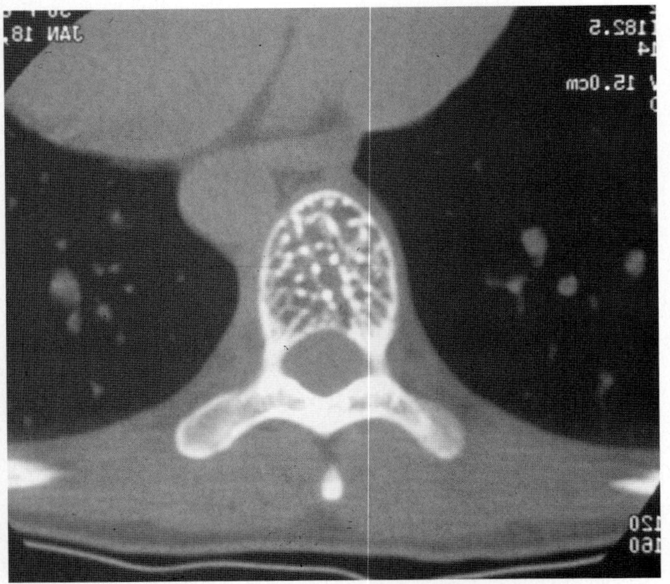

is unremarkable. A plain radiograph of the distal femur is shown in Fig. 8.19A and B. A bone scan reveals intense focal signal at the anterior femur. A low-magnification photomicrograph of the excisional biopsy is shown in Fig. 8.19C. What is the most likely diagnosis?
(a) Intraosseous ganglion
(b) Bone island
(c) Osteoid osteoma
(d) Aneurysmal bone cyst
(e) Stress fracture

83. The incidence of malignant transformation in patients with multiple hereditary exostoses is

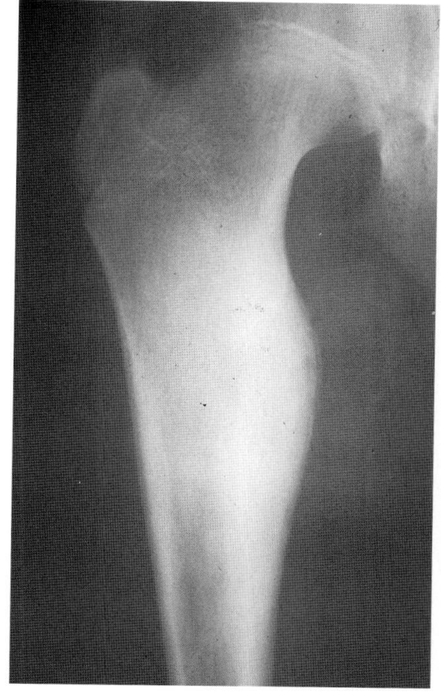

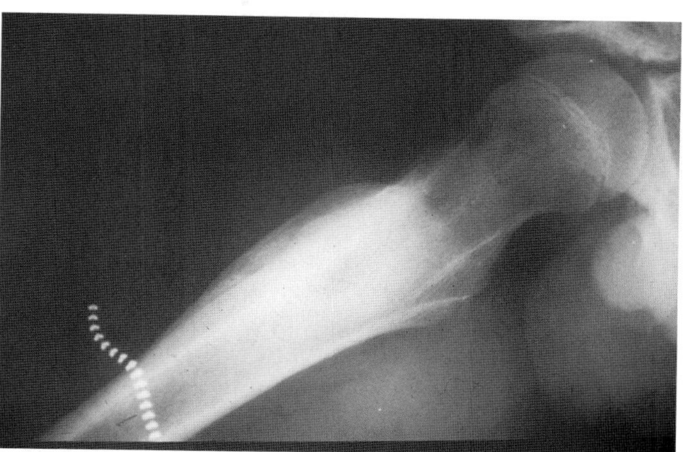

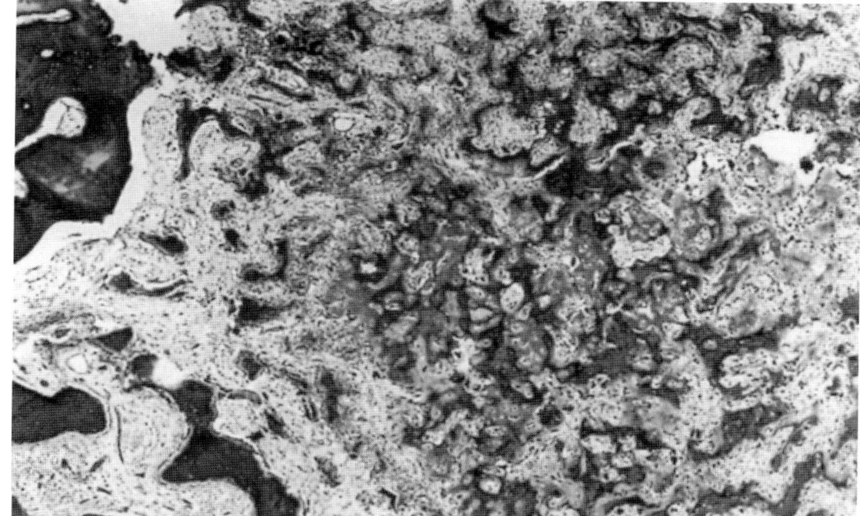

FIGURE 8.19A–C

(a) 0%
(b) 1%
(c) 10%
(d) 50%
(e) 100%

84. A 14-year-old boy scout complains of sudden onset of acute low back pain after he jumped over a log. A lateral radiograph of his lumbar spine is shown in Fig. 8.20A. The results of a computed tomography–guided needle biopsy of the lesion are shown in Fig. 8.20B and C. Based on the information given, the most likely diagnosis for this lesion is

(a) Langerhans histiocytosis
(b) Osteoporosis
(c) Vertebral osteomyelitis
(d) Ewing sarcoma
(e) Lymphoma

85. A 60-year-old man complains of foot pain and swelling. His past medical history is significant for gout (for which he had been treated 25 years earlier with an experimental radiation therapy protocol). A plain radiograph is shown in Fig. 8.21. Histologic features of the lesion are shown in Fig. 8.21B. What is the most likely diagnosis?

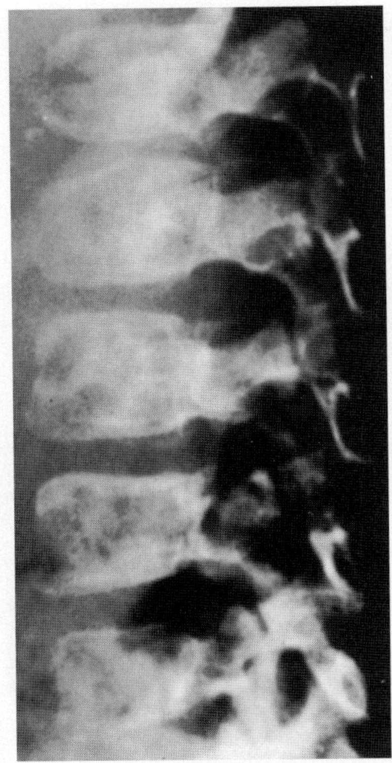
A

FIGURE 8.20A–C

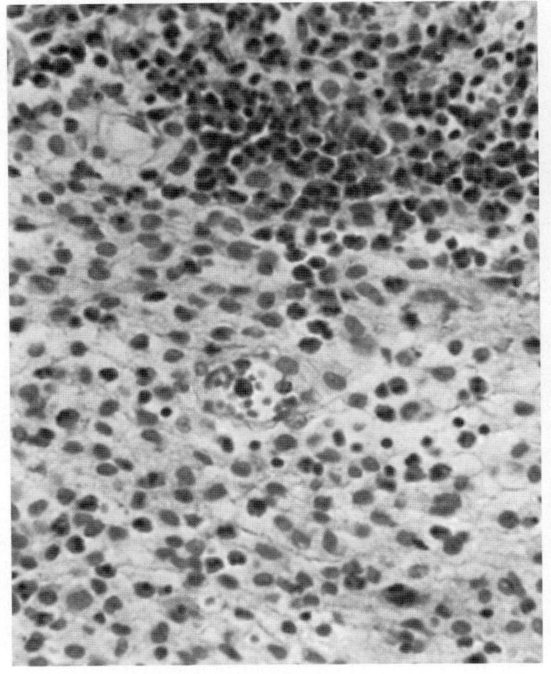
B

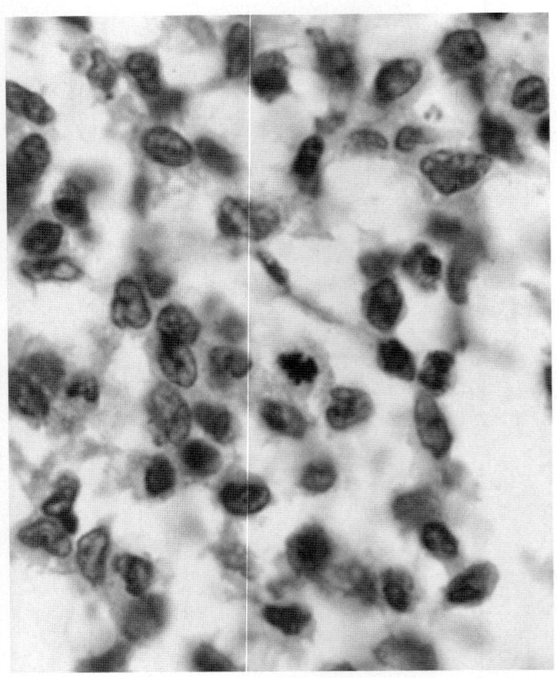
C

(a) Osteogenic sarcoma
(b) Pseudogout
(c) Chondrosarcoma
(d) Fibrosarcoma
(e) Malignant fibrous histiocytoma

86. Osseous metastases from which of the following primary carcinomas are noted for being hypervascular?
    (a) Breast
    (b) Thyroid
    (c) Lung

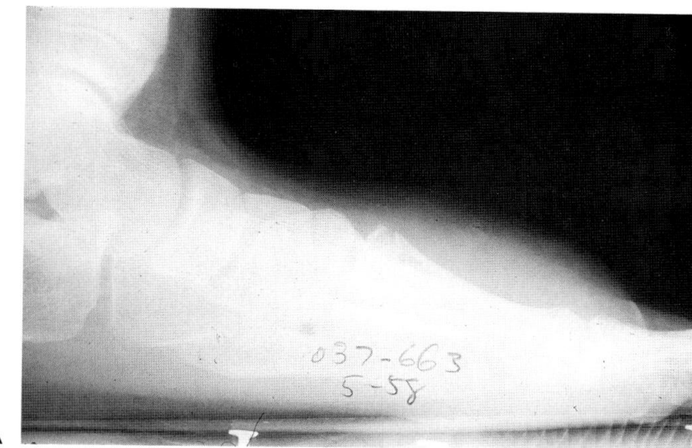

A

B

FIGURE 8.21A–C

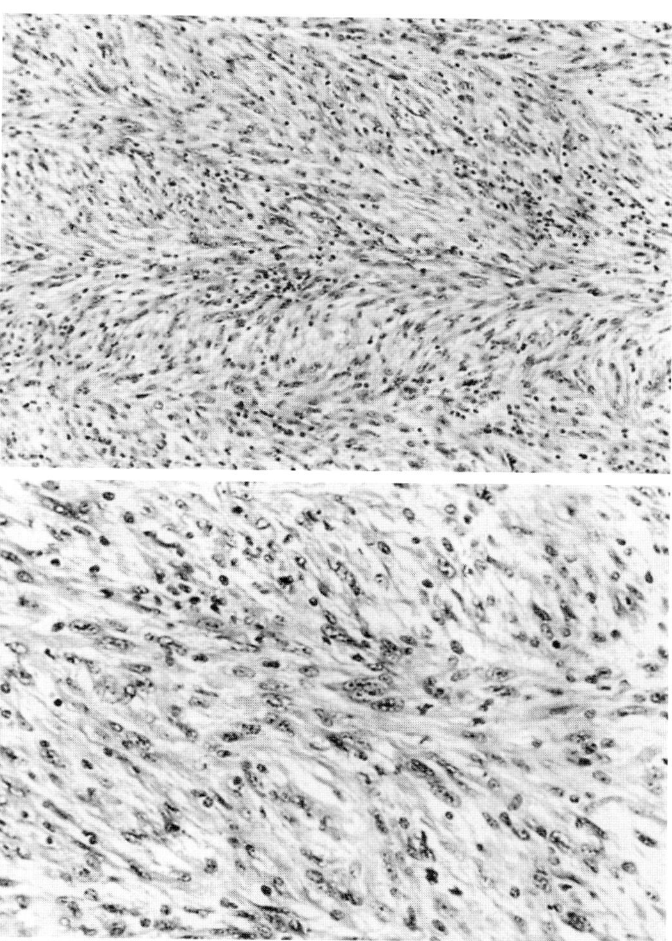

C

(d) Renal
(e) Prostate

87. A 62-year-old nurse complains of 3 months of progressive neck pain. Her past medical history is significant for a 50-pack-year smoking history and mild chronic obstructive pulmonary disease. A lateral radiograph is shown in Fig. 8.22A. Biopsy results are shown in Fig. 8.22B. What is the most likely diagnosis?
(a) Pyogenic osteomyelitis
(b) Osteoblastoma
(c) Tuberculosis
(d) Metastatic carcinoma
(e) Chordoma

88. Which of the following tumors is more common in females than males?
(a) Ewing sarcoma
(b) Chordoma
(c) Malignant lymphoma of bone
(d) Giant cell tumor
(e) Chondrosarcoma

89. The childhood constellation of adrenocortical carcinoma, brain tumors, soft tissue sarcomas, and early presentation of breast cancer is referred to as
(a) Li-Fraumeni syndrome
(b) Sipple syndrome
(c) Type I multiple endocrine neoplasia

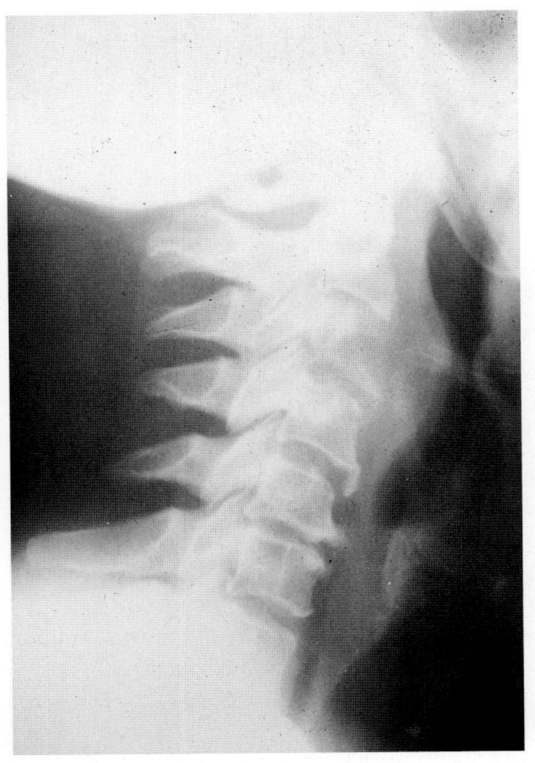
A

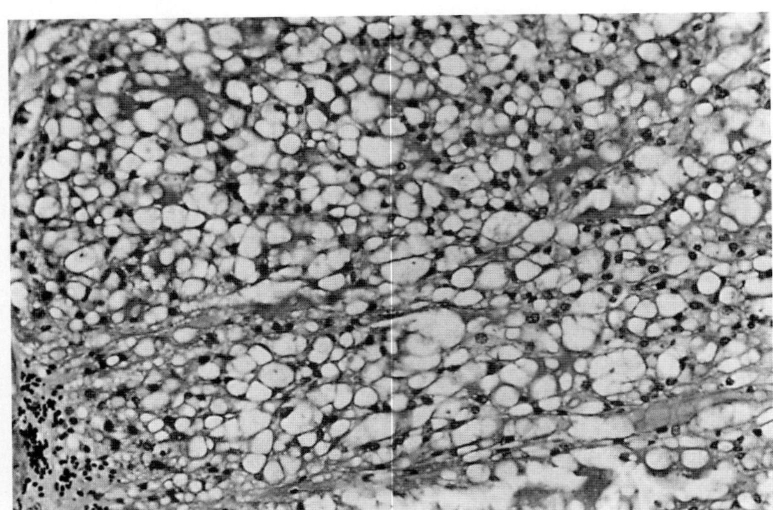
B

FIGURE 8.22A and B

(d) Peutz-Jeghers syndrome
(e) Von Recklinghausen disease

90. A 20-year-old man undergoes neoadjuvant chemotherapy and resection of a distal femoral osteogenic sarcoma. His distal femur is reconstructed with an osteochondral allograft. What is his risk of deep infection after this procedure?
(a) Approximately 1%
(b) Approximately 5%
(c) Approximately 10%
(d) Approximately 25%
(e) Approximately 50%

91. The t (X;18) (p11.;q11.) translocation is a characteristic cytogenetic finding in which of the following neoplasms?
(a) Dedifferentiated chondrosarcoma
(b) Periosteal osteogenic sarcoma
(c) Synovial sarcoma
(d) Hemangiopericytoma
(e) Malignant schwannoma

92. Which of the following lesions demonstrates the greatest tendency for metastasis to regional lymph nodes?
(a) Malignant fibrous histiocytoma
(b) Synovial sarcoma
(c) Chondrosarcoma
(d) Liposarcoma
(e) Ewing sarcoma

ANSWERS

1. c Osteoid osteoma. The patient has an *osteoid osteoma* involving the axis. The clinical history of night pain is typical of this lesion. Relief with nonsteroidal antiinflammatory drugs is another hallmark. The peak incidence of this lesion is in the second and third decades. Males are affected approximately twice as often as females. This particular osteoid osteoma is obscure on the plain radiographs but is not subtle on the bone scan. In addition, the radiograph reveals a well-demarcated nidus. The nidus in osteoid osteoma is a round or oval region that is composed of a rich capillary network with varying amounts of central woven bone production. The nidus is usually less than 1 cm in diameter but may be as large as 2 cm. The nidus, itself, is the osteoid osteoma. Radiographically, there may be varying amounts of surrounding reactive sclerotic host bone. The nidus is radiolucent with a central radiodensity. The size of the central radiodensity depends on the amount of blastic activity in the particular nidus. (This particular example reveals abundant blastic activity.) The femur and tibia are the two most common locations for osteoid osteoma. When the lesion occurs in the spine, it is virtually always situated in the neural arch in the vicinity of the pedicles. Osteoblastomas are similar-appearing lesions that also have a predilection

for the posterior (versus anterior) elements of the spine. However, osteoblastomas are typically larger than 2 cm.

The permeative radiographic appearance that typifies osteogenic sarcoma is distinctly absent with osteoid osteoma. The spine is the most common location for skeletal metastases. However, skeletal metastases rarely seed the posterior elements, and they are rare in this age group.

References

Levine AM, et al.: Benign Tumors of the Cervical Spine. Spine, 17:10 Suppl, S399-406, 1992.

Sim FH, et al.: Osteoid Osteoma: Diagnostic Problems. J Bone Joint Surg Am, 57:154, 1975.

2. **b** IB. The *Enneking classification* of malignant musculoskeletal tumors is based on three variables: (1) histologic grade, (2) whether the lesion is confined to a single compartment, and (3) the presence or absence of metastases. Thus, the tumor described in the question would be considered a IB lesion (low-grade, extracompartmental lesion with no metastases): I, low grade; II, high grade; III, metastasis; A, intracompartmental; B, extracompartmental.

Reference

Enneking WF, et al.: A System for the Surgical Staging of Musculoskeletal Sarcoma. Clin Orthop, 153:106–120, 1980.

3. **e** IIIA. Regardless of the grade or compartmental status of a tumor, all tumors with associated metastasis are stage III by the Enneking classification. (Please refer to the discussion of question 2.)
4. **d** The tibia. *Adamantinoma* is an extremely rare malignant tumor that occurs far more commonly on in-training and board examinations than in reality. The lesion typically presents during the second or third decade of life. Sex distribution is equivalent. The mandible is a common location. The most common extragnathic site is the tibia. Most appendicular adamantimomas arise at the anterior tibial cortex. With its mixed lytic-sclerotic, multiloculated "soap-bubble" appearance, the lesion is radiographically akin to monostotic fibrous dysplasia.

   Histologically, the lesion manifests islands of epithelium-like tissue superimposed on a background of dense fibrous stroma. This "pseudoglandular" histologic pattern, together with immunohistochemical and electron microscopic studies, suggests an epithelial origin. Recommended treatment is wide excision.

Reference

Campanacci M, et al.: Adamantinoma of the Long Bones. Am J Surg Pathol, 5:553, 1981.

5. **c** Elastofibroma. *Elastofibroma* is another rare lesion with a predilection for appearing on standardized tests. This tumorlike condition typically arises in elderly persons within the connective tissue between the chest wall and the caudal portion of the scapula. Bilateral involvement is uncommon (approximately 10% of cases). Other locations (greater trochanter and deltoid) are exceptionally unusual. The lesion has a putative posttraumatic origin, and an occupational history involving heavy, repetitive physical labor is commonly elicited. Histologic examination of the specimen reveals abundant strands of matrix (elastin fibers) interspersed within an interstitium of fibroadipose tissue. Use of an elastin-specific stain would manifest the plethora of beaded elastin strands within this lesion.

   A *Pancoast tumor* is an apical lung carcinoma that has infiltrated the chest wall and has invaded the brachial plexus and cervical sympathetic chain. These lesions characteristically produce upper extremity neurologic deficits and ipsilateral Horner syndrome.

   Mesothelioma is a pleural-based (or peritoneally based) tumor. Pancoast tumor and mesothelioma are ruled out in this case by the absence of chest wall penetration on the computed tomography scan. *Fibrosarcoma* has a far more cellular histologic appearance and lacks the abundant extracellular matrix seen in this lesion.

Reference

Renshaw TS, Simon MA: Elastofibroma. J Bone Joint Surg Am, 55:409, 1973.

6. **b** Hand-Schüller-Christian disease. *Hand-Schüller-Christian disease* is a form of eosinophilic granuloma that demonstrates a predilection for involvement of the sella turcica. Involvement of the sella turcica can disrupt the function of the neurohypophysis (posterior pituitary). The resultant decrease in antidiuretic hormone produces diabetes insipidus.

   Larsen syndrome is an arthrogrypotic syndrome consisting of multiple congenital dislocations and scoliosis. *Maffucci syndrome* is a subtype of enchondromatosis with associated hemangiomas and a high incidence of malignant transformation. *Prader-Willi syndrome* is a congenital disorder characterized by hypogonadism, insatiable appetite, mental retardation, and a rounded face with almond-shaped eyes.
7. **e** The most common site of occurrence is the tibial shaft. *Parosteal ("juxtacortical") osteogenic sarcoma* most commonly occurs at the posterior distal femur. An early parosteal osteogenic sarcoma in this region may be mistaken for a cortical desmoid. The tibial shaft is the most common site of occurrence of another osteogenic sarcoma variant, periosteal osteogenic sarcoma. Parosteal osteogenic sarcoma occurs in an older

population than conventional (central) osteogenic sarcoma and carries a more favorable prognosis (if treated appropriately with wide excision). It displays a tendency to grow around the surface of the affected bone and not to invade the medullary canal. Its typical histologic features include nonsinister trabecular bone formation intermixed with a background of low-grade fibrous stroma.

Reference

Campanacci M, et al.: Parosteal Osteogenic Sarcoma. J Bone Joint Surg Br, 66:313, 1984.

8. **c** The pelvis. Although *chondrosarcoma* may occur in a wide variety of locations, approximately 25% of these lesions arise from the pelvis. The second most commonly affected site is the proximal femur (approximately 16%).

Reference

Springfield DS, et al.: Chondrosarcoma: A Review. J Bone Joint Surg Am, 78:141–149, 1996.

9. **a** Aneurysmal bone cyst. *Aneurysmal bone cysts* are solitary, eccentric, expansile cystic lesions that typically occur in the second or third decades. They manifest a predilection for the posterior elements of the spine and the metaphyseal region of long bones.

   Figure 8.2A demonstrates an eccentric, lucent region at the medial aspect of the metaphysis of the distal femur. There is compromise of the adjacent femoral cortex. Magnetic resonance imaging often reveals a characteristic fluid-fluid level within the lesion. Although not evident in this particular case, the expansile portion of an aneurysmal bone cyst typically forms an "eggshell" neocortex at its margin.

   The histologic specimen (Fig. 8.2B) manifests septated cystic spaces that contain erythrocytes. The composition of the septa (giant cells, spindle cells, and fibrous stroma) is characteristic of an aneurysmal bone cyst. Ossification of the septa may be also be encountered.

   Mononuclear cells are condensed at the septal margins, where they form a pseudolining, but, unlike cavernous hemangiomas, these cysts lack a true vascular endothelium.

   The presence of giant cells in an aneurysmal bone cyst should not lead to a misdiagnosis of *giant cell tumor.* Distinguishing features of giant cell tumor include its characteristic epiphyseal location and its noncystic histologic features.

   Telangiectatic osteogenic sarcoma shares two principal histologic features with aneurysmal bone cysts (giant cells and large blood-filled spaces). However, it can be distinguished from an aneurysmal bone cyst based on its more cellular, anaplastic, sarcomatous stroma.

   The treatment of choice for aneurysmal bone cysts is curettage, but the local recurrence rate is approximately 50%. Adjuvant cryotherapy is advocated by some authorities. Local recurrence rates are increased in young children.

References

Biesecker JL, Marcove RC, Huvos AG: Aneurysmal Bone Cysts: A Clinicopathologic Study of 66 Cases. Cancer, 26:615–625, 1970.
Freiberg AA, Loder RT, Heidelberger KP: Aneurysmal Bone Cysts in Young Children. J Pediatr Orthop, 14(1):86–91, 1994.

10. **b** Decreased alkaline phosphatase activity. *Hypophosphatasia* is caused by a deficiency of alkaline phosphatase activity. Although this disease produces skeletal hypomineralization and rachitic bone deformities, it is not associated with decreased serum levels of inorganic phosphate or calcium. Serum vitamin D and parathyroid hormone levels are usually normal.

    Nonorganic pyrophosphate accumulates as a result of the lack of alkaline phosphatase activity. Nonorganic phosphate inhibits hydroxyapatite crystal growth.

Reference

Anderton JM: Orthopaedic Problems in Adult Hypophosphatasia. J Bone Joint Surg Br, 61:82, 1979.

11. **b** Chordoma. *Chordomas* arise from notochord remnants. Therefore, they occur in the axial skeleton (sacrum, coccyx, and base of skull). Their histologic appearance is marked by the presence of physaliferous cells. These cells contain characteristic "bull's-eye" nuclei and prominent cytoplasmic vacuoles.

Reference

Mindell ER: Chordomas. J Bone Joint Surg Am, 63:501, 1981.

12. **d** Gaucher disease. The *Erlenmeyer flask deformity* of *Gaucher disease* is produced by defective metaphyseal remodeling. Incomplete tubulation produces the characteristic fusiform enlargement of the metaphysis.

    Rickets produces flared, cupped metaphyses but not in an Erlenmeyer flask pattern. *Kneist syndrome* is a form of short-trunk disproportionate dwarfism. It is characterized by platyspondyly, dumbbell-shaped long bones, and an autosomal dominant mode of inheritance.

    Note: An Erlenmeyer flask deformity is also encountered in other conditions that involve defective remodeling, such as osteopetrosis and Pyle disease.

Reference

Goldblatt J, et al.: The Orthopaedic Aspects of Gaucher's Disease. Clin Orthop, 137:208, 1978.

13. **c** "Storiform" pattern. Certain catch phrases are commonly used to describe the characteristic histologic patterns of specific lesions. Some of the more common catch phrases are given in Table 8.1.
14. **b** Chvostek sign. Patients with malignant disease may develop *hypercalcemia* for various reasons including widespread bony metastases and various paraneoplastic syndromes. Symptoms of hypercalcemia include lethargy, polyuria, polydipsia, hyporeflexia, constipation, anorexia, nausea, abdominal pain, confusion, psychosis, and, ultimately, coma. The QT interval may be shortened on the electrocardiogram, and death may occur from dysrhythmia. *Chvostek sign* (spasm of the facial muscles from tapping on the facial nerve) is a sign of hypocalcemia.
15. **e** Intravenous fluid administration. All the agents listed in the question have a role in managing hypercalcemia. However, the initial step in the emergency management of hypercalcemia is intravenous hydration with thorough repletion of any preexisting volume deficit. Patients with acute hypercalcemia may be severely dehydrated at presentation. Hypercalcemia impairs the kidney's concentrating ability. Associated gastrointestinal symptoms can also contribute to dehydration. Hypovolemia decreases the glomerular filtration rate, which, in turn, exacerbates the hypercalcemia by promoting increased calcium reabsorption.

    Restitution of euvolemia will reestablish normal glomerular filtration rate, which, alone, will promote calciuria. Additional calciuria can be induced with continued extracellular volume expansion and furosemide administration. Fluid and electrolyte balance must be carefully monitored in this setting.
16. **c** Supplementary 1-25 vitamin D is a component of the treatment. *Vitamin D–resistant rickets* is inherited as an X-linked dominant (not autosomal recessive) trait. Renal phosphate wasting is believed to be the underlying defect, and a candidate mutant gene has been isolated in a murine model. Putatively, the normal gene plays a role in proximal renal tubule phosphate transport.

TABLE 8.1. "CATCH PHRASES" DESCRIBING SPECIFIC LESIONS

Pattern	Disease
"Storiform" (cartwheel) pattern	Malignant fibrous histiocytoma
"Chinese letter" pattern	Fibrodysplasia
"Herringbone" pattern	Fibrosarcoma
"Chicken wire" calcification	Chondroblastoma
"Racquet-shaped" cells	Rhabdomyosarcoma
"Physaliferous" cells	Chordoma
"Biphasic" pattern	Synovial sarcoma

Vitamin D–resistant rickets itself does not produce secondary hyperparathyroidism. However, treatment of the disease (phosphate supplementation) has a hypocalcemic effect that, in turn, does produce secondary hyperparathyroidism. 1-25 vitamin D supplementation is often used to prevent iatrogenic hyperparathyroidism (1-25 vitamin D inhibits parathyroid hormone secretion). Stunted growth and lower extremity deformities are not prominent features during the first year of life. These features are typically not detected until weight bearing commences. Low serum phosphate, conversely, can be detected early in life. Short stature and lower extremity deformity can be averted by early disease detection and early initiation of treatment.

17. **b** Ewing sarcoma. *Ewing sarcoma* is notable for its large intracellular glycogen stores. The presence of these deposits is detected on periodic acid-Schiff–stained histologic specimens. This feature can assist in differentiating Ewing sarcoma from other round cell lesions (in both reality as well as on standardized tests).

Reference

Schajowicz F: Ewing's Sarcoma and Reticulum Cell Sarcoma of Bone With Special Reference to the Histochemical Demonstration of Glycogen as an Aid to Differential Diagnosis. J Bone Joint Surg Am, 41:394, 1959.

18. **b** Pseudohypoparathyroidism. Short fourth and fifth metacarpal and metatarsal bones are distinctive features of *pseudohypoparathyroidism.*

    Hemochromatosis is associated with a noninflammatory arthropathy with a predilection for the metacarpophalangeal joints. *Hemosiderin deposition* within involved synovium produces brown discoloration. *Acromegaly* causes bony overgrowth, particularly in the hands, jaw, and feet. Characteristic radiographic findings include overgrowth of the metacarpal heads and the terminal tufts of the distal phalanges. Distinctive radiographic features of hypothyroidism include delayed skeletal maturation, dwarfism, and pseudofragmentation of secondary ossification centers.

    Note: Pseudofragmentation of the capital femoral epiphysis (secondary to hypothyroidism) may simulate Legg-Calvé-Perthes disease.

Reference

Spiegel AM, et al.: Pseudohypoparathyroidism: The Molecular Basis for Hormone Resistance. N Engl J Med, 307:679, 1982.

19. **d** Chondroblastoma. *Chondroblastoma* characteristically arises in the epiphysis of skeletally immature long bones. It manifests a predilection for the proximal humerus and the proximal and distal femoral epiphyses. The lesion produces a lytic defect with variable

degrees of internal mineral deposition. The lytic defect characteristically abuts the adjacent articular surface.

The lesion may expand from the epiphysis into the adjacent metaphysis. Although it is a "benign" neoplasm, chondroblastoma may produce considerable local destruction. This particular lesion has replaced 30% of the lateral femoral head.

The histologic appearance of chondroblastoma is distinctive. The photomicrograph in Fig. 8.4B demonstrates the characteristic "chicken wire" pattern of calcification superimposed on a field of polygonal cells with uniform nuclei and an intercellular chondroid matrix. The borders of individual chondroblasts are highlighted by the lacework of calcification that traces their perimeter. Scattered giant cells are often encountered in chondroblastoma.

Note: Because both lesions occur in the epiphysis and contain giant cells, chondroblastoma can be confused with giant cell tumor. The presence of chondroid matrix and the "chicken wire" calcification in chondroblastoma distinguish it from giant cell tumor.

Reference

Caterini R, Manili M, Spinelli M, et al.: Epiphyseal Chondroblastoma of Bone. Arch Orthop Trauma Surg, 111(6):327–332, 1992.

20. **c** Osteopetrosis. The radiograph reveals a "rugger-jersey" spine. This pattern of horizontal sclerotic bands adjacent to vertebral end plates can be produced by either osteopetrosis (Albers-Schönberg disease) or renal osteodystrophy (with secondary hyperparathyroidism). Furthermore, both osteopetrosis and renal osteodystrophy can be associated with anemia.

The anemia in *osteopetrosis* is a myelophthisic process. Failure of bone remodeling obliterates the marrow spaces, and the resultant decreased amount of functioning hematopoietic tissue leads to anemia.

The anemia of renal osteodystrophy is not a myelophthisic process. Rather, the anemia stems from a lack of erythropoietin production by the diseased renal parenchyma.

Furthermore, the stripes of the "rugger-jersey" spine of hyperparathyroidism are not as well defined as those in osteopetrosis. The sclerotic vertebral stripes in osteopetrosis may be so pronounced that they produce a "sandwich vertebrae" appearance.

Reference

Helms CA: Fundamentals of Skeletal Radiology, 2nd Ed. Philadelphia, WB Saunders, 1994.

21. **a** Supraphysiologic glucocorticoid levels do not cause secondary hyperparathyroidism. *Glucocorticoids* affect calcium homeostasis on multiple levels. In the gut, glu-

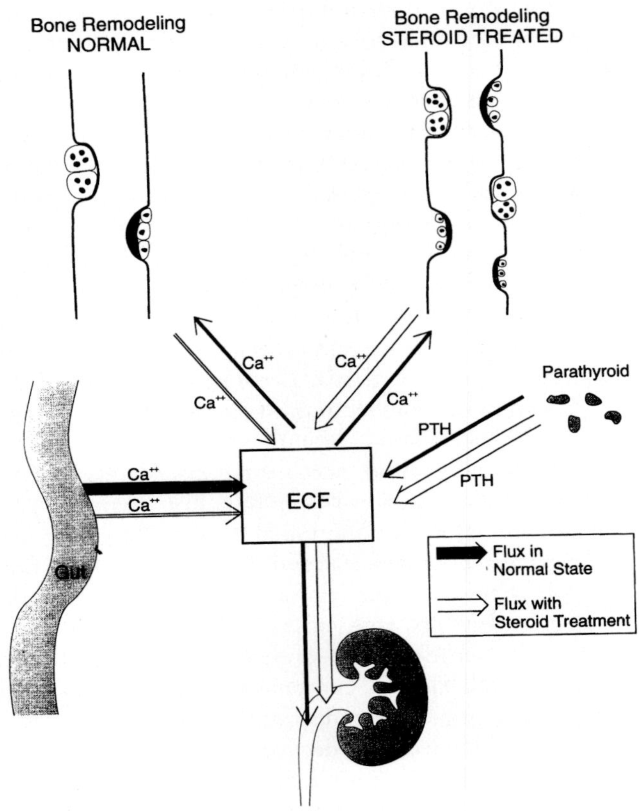

FIGURE 8.23

cocorticoids disrupt calcium absorption. This effect is believed to be mediated (at least in part) by an inhibitory effect on vitamin D. Glucocorticoids decrease renal tubular resorption of calcium. Supraphysiologic doses of glucocorticoids impair osteoblast collagen synthesis. Glucocorticoids increase bone resorption by inhibiting pituitary secretion of gonadotropins.

Secondary hyperparathyroidism develops as a result of impaired gastrointestinal calcium resorption and enhanced renal calcium excretion. Secondary hyperparathyroidism, in turn, accelerates bone resorption (Fig. 8.23).

Reference

Favus MJ, ed: Primer on the Metabolic Bone Diseases, 3rd Ed. Philadelphia, Lippincott–Raven, 1996.

22. **e** Albright syndrome. *Albright syndrome* consists of the triad of precocious puberty, polyostotic fibrous dysplasia, and café-au-lait spots. Café-au-lait spots are also seen in association with neurofibromatosis, but the peripheral contour of these hyperpigmented lesions differs between the two diseases. Café-au-lait spots in the context of neurofibromatosis have a smooth ("coast

of California") border. Café-au-lait spots in association with Albright syndrome have a jagged ("coast of Maine") perimeter.

Enchondromatosis (Ollier disease) may produce lesions in multiple bones with an associated predisposition to pathologic fracture. However, it is not associated with skin pigment change or endocrinopathy. *Maffucci syndrome* is a variant of enchondromatosis with associated soft tissue hemangiomas. *Letterer-Siwe disease* is a form of eosinophilic granuloma that typically leads to death in early childhood.

23. **d** It has a sclerotic border. Helms defined four useful radiographic criteria for the diagnosis of giant cell tumor of bone: (1) the epiphysis must be closed, (2) the lesion must be epiphyseal and abut the articular surface, (3) the lesion must be eccentric, and (4) the lesion must have a well-defined but nonsclerotic margin.

The characteristic absence of a sclerotic margin assists in distinguishing giant cell tumor from other lytic epiphyseal lesions (e.g., clear cell chondrosarcoma). The matrix of giant cell tumors does not mineralize (they are purely lytic lesions). On occasion, an aneurysmal bone cyst may arise within a giant cell tumor.

Reference

Helms CA: Fundamentals of Skeletal Radiology, 2nd Ed. Philadelphia, WB Saunders, 1994.

24. **e** High serum calcium. *Paget disease* is a disorder of bone remodeling characterized by excessive osteoclast activity and accelerated bone turnover. Even though bone resorption is increased, serum calcium levels are characteristically normal in this disease.

New bone formation occurs in a chaotic, expanded fashion. The distorted bone architecture can cause nerve compression. When the spine is affected, spinal stenosis may occur. When the skull is involved, sensorineural hearing loss may be produced by compression of the eighth cranial nerve. Alternatively, if the auditory ossicles are directly affected by Paget disease, a conductive form of deafness may ensue.

Because active pagetic bone is hypervascular, hip involvement may lead to increased hemorrhage during total hip arthroplasty, and diffuse disease may produce high-output cardiac failure in extreme cases. A predisposition to pathologic fracture has also been reported.

25. **b** Central osteogenic sarcoma. *Osteogenic sarcoma* is the most common primary bone malignancy in childhood. It affects boys more commonly than girls. Osteogenic sarcoma is characterized by a malignant spindle cell stroma that produces osteoid (hence the name). "Central" osteogenic sarcomas originate within the medullary canal. There is a 20% incidence of skip lesions.

The initial plain radiograph (Fig. 8.4A) reveals a sclerotic lesion at the proximal tibia with surrounding lucency. The findings include destruction of normal tibial architecture and copious new bone formation. The magnetic resonance image in Fig. 8.5B is shows how the tumor has broken through the cortex to form a soft tissue mass. The photomicrograph (Fig. 8.5B) shows sinister cells within a fibrillar matrix. Note the malignant cytologic features of the tumor cells: anaplasia, hyperchromatic nuclei, increased nucleus-to-cytoplasm ratio, and pleomorphism. The surrounding matrix *(tumor osteoid)* is produced by the malignant osteoblasts.

Ewing sarcoma has a distinctly different histologic appearance (copious, uniform, small round cells). New bone formation may be seen in association with Ewing sarcoma, but the new bone in Ewing sarcoma is reactive and not formed by the malignant cells. *Malignant fibrous histiocytoma* and *chondrosarcoma* do not characteristically affect children. Chondrosarcoma produces a chondroid matrix, which has a distinctly different ("glassy") appearance than osteoid.

Reference

Link MP, Eilber F: Osteogenic Sarcoma. In Pizzo PA, Poplack DG, eds: Principles and Practice of Pediatric Oncology, 3rd Ed. Philadelphia, Lippincott–Raven, 1997.

26. **a** Multiple osteomas. *Gardner syndrome* includes (1) adenomatous intestinal polyposis, (2) multiple osteomas, (3) supernumerary teeth, and (4) a variety of soft tissue lesions (including desmoids, fibromas, and epithelial cysts). The syndrome has an autosomal dominant inheritance pattern. The associated multiple osteomas typically present as painless masses. These lesions demonstrate a predilection for the facial bones and skull. The syndrome has also been associated with nonspecific thickening of long and short tubular bones.

References

Carl W: Dental and Bone Abnormalities in Patients with Familial Polyposis Coli. Semin Surg Oncol, 3:77–83, 1987.

Gardner EJ: A Genetic and Clinical Study of Intestinal Polyposis. Am J Hum Genet 3:167, 1951.

27. **e** Nonhereditary. *Ollier disease (multiple enchondromatosis)* is a nonhereditary phenomenon. Enchondromas have a predilection for the short tubular bones of the hand. Enchondromas adjacent to the physis of a long bone may disturb growth.

Note: The syndrome of multiple hereditary exostoses is an autosomal dominant condition.

Reference

Schwartz HS, et al.: The Management of Enchondromatosis. J Bone Joint Surg Am, 69:269, 1987.

28. **b** Maffucci syndrome is associated with a higher incidence of secondary malignancy than Ollier disease. *Maffucci syndrome* is associated with a higher rate of secondary malignant disease than Ollier disease. Secondary chondrosarcoma develops in approximately 25% of patients with Ollier disease. The incidence of secondary malignancy in the setting of Maffucci syndrome has been estimated to be as high as 100%.

Chondrosarcoma affects males more commonly than females (approximately 3:2). The peak incidence is between 40 and 60 years old. Pain is the most common presenting complaint. Resection is the treatment of choice for most cases. Chemotherapy is rarely indicated.

Note: Maffucci syndrome refers to multiple enchondromas occurring in association with soft tissue hemangiomas. Radiographs of hemangiomatous regions characteristically reveal phleboliths.

References

Springfield DS, et al.: Chondrosarcoma: A Review. J Bone Joint Surg Am, 78:141–149, 1996.

Lewis RJ, Ketcham AS: Maffucci's Syndrome: Functional and Neoplastic Significance. J Bone Joint Surg Am, 55:1465, 1973.

29. **c** Paget disease. *Paget disease* affects approximately 3% of the population. It is a disease of bone remodeling characterized by increased bone turnover. The radiographic and histologic features of Paget disease reflect the underlying disorder of bone remodeling.

Figure 8.5A demonstrates a bowing deformity of the tibia with coarsened trabeculae and a thickened posterior cortex. The photomicrograph (Fig. 8.5B) shows a section of trabecular bone undergoing surface resorption by several abnormally large osteoclasts. These osteoclasts contain more than the usual two to four nuclei. Multiple episodes alternating bone resorption and formation produce an increased number of bone-cement lines that impart a characteristic mosaic pattern. Paget disease is associated with elevated alkaline phosphatase, which is indicative of increased osteoblast activity, and elevated urine hydroxyproline, which is indicative of increased osteoclast activity.

Note: The scalloped lacunae (occupied by osteoclasts) at the leading edge of trabecular resorption are referred to as *Howship lacunae.*

Reference

Mirra JM, et al.: Paget's Disease of Bone: Review with Emphasis on Radiologic Features. Skeletal Radiol, 24(3):163–184, 1995.

30. **a** Eosinophilic granuloma. *Eosinophilic granuloma,* unlike most other benign tumors of the spine, demonstrates a predilection for the vertebral body rather than the posterior elements. The characteristic radiographic finding in affected children is *vertebra plana,* which represents collapse of the vertebral body. This lesion typically heals spontaneously without adverse sequelae. Bracing or decompression may be indicated (respectively) in the rare circumstances that kyphosis or neurologic compromise occur as a result of collapse. Biopsy is usually not recommended when the patient has a characteristic history and radiographic appearance.

Reference

Lauffenburger MD, et al.: Eosinophilic Granuloma of the Adult Spine. J Spinal Disord, 8(3):243–248, 1995.

31. **b** The third and fourth pharyngeal pouches. The two upper parathyroid glands originate from the endoderm of the fourth pharyngeal pouch. The two lower parathyroid glands originate from the endoderm of the third pharyngeal pouch.

The thyroid gland is derived from the foramen cecum, a tubular invagination from the base of the tongue. The anterior pituitary gland (adenohypophysis) originates from Rathke pouch, an invagination from the roof of the oral canal. The adrenal medulla is one of many structures derived from the neural crest; the adrenal cortex originates from mesoderm from the urogenital ridge.

32. **c** The incision should be transverse. When one performs a biopsy of a musculoskeletal neoplasm, incisions should always be longitudinal. This guideline facilitates longitudinal (extensile) exposure and excision of the biopsy tract during the subsequent definitive procedure. Other appropriate technical considerations include (1) avoiding contamination of intermuscular planes, (2) avoiding contamination of neurovascular bundles, (3) avoiding contamination of uninvolved compartments, (4) obtaining an adequate quantity of representative tissue, and (5) waiting for the results of the frozen section to confirm that diagnostic tissue has been obtained. The Musculoskeletal Tumor Society has reported that the incidence of errors, complications, and compromised outcomes is two to 12 times greater when the biopsy is performed in a referral institution rather than in a treatment center.

Reference

Mankin HJ, et al.: The Hazards of Biopsy in Patients with Malignant Primary Bone and Soft Tissue Tumors, J Bone Joint Surg Am, 64:1121–1127, 1982.

Mankin HJ, et al.: The Hazards of the Biopsy: Revisited. J Bone Joint Surg Am, 78:656–663, 1996.

33. **d** Ewing sarcoma. *Ewing sarcoma* and *peripheral neuroectodermal tumor* have both been associated with the t(11:22)(q24;q12) somatic mutation.

Reference

Morrissy RT, Weinstein SL: Lovell and Winter's Pediatric Orthopaedics, 4th Ed. Philadelphia, Lippincott–Raven, p. 453, 1996.

34. **e** The tibia is the most common site of origin. The femur is the most common location of Ewing sarcoma. Males are more commonly affected than females (approximately 3:2). Five-year survival has improved to more than 50% since the introduction of adjuvant chemotherapy. The lesion characteristically presents with an extraosseous soft tissue mass. An elevated lactate dehydrogenase level is a poor prognostic sign.

Reference

Morrissy RT, Weinstein SL: Lovell and Winter's Pediatric Orthopaedics, 4th Ed. Philadelphia, Lippincott–Raven, p. 453, 1996.

35. **c** To detect the presence of other osseous disease foci. Bone scintigraphy uses a radioactive tracer that is taken up by regions of osteoblastic activity. It is a sensitive means of detecting areas of increased bone turnover. Thus, it is an effective modality for detecting synchronous metastatic osseous loci or osseous skip lesions.

    Bone scintigraphy will also detect nonmalignant processes in which there is increased osteoblastic activity (e.g., osteoid osteoma, fractures, and osteomyelitis), and it is not useful for differentiating malignant processes from benign ones. The resolution of scintigraphy is poor, and it cannot define the specific shape of a lesion or the extent of associated soft tissue extension.

    Note: Multiple myeloma is notorious for its potential to produce a false-negative bone scan result. This can occur in situations of pure bone resorption and virtually no new bone deposition. (No tracer can be deposited unless there is at least some reactive new bone formation.)

Reference

Frank JA, et al.: Detection of Malignant Bone Tumors: MRI Versus Scintigraphy. AJR Am J Roentgenol, 155(5):1043–1048, 1990.

36. **c** Plain radiographs. Plain radiographs should always be the first radiographic study ordered in a bone tumor workup. In most cases, the plain radiograph can provide valuable information about the characteristics of a bone lesion including the location of the lesion, the quality of the lesion's margin, its effect on the adjacent bone, the extent of periosteal reaction, the presence of an associated soft tissue mass, and the presence of intralesional mineral deposition.

Reference

Simon MA, Finn HA: Diagnostic Strategy for Bone and Soft Tissue Tumors. J Bone Joint Surg Am, 75:622–623, 1993.

37. **c** Plain radiographs. Imaging of a suspected soft tissue tumor should begin with plain radiographs. Plain radiographs provide useful information regarding the presence of underlying osseous involvement (primary or secondary) and the presence of intralesional mineral deposition.

    A magnetic resonance imaging scan may subsequently be ordered to characterize a soft tissue tumor more fully. However, it should not be the first imaging study obtained.

Reference

Simon MA, Finn HA: Diagnostic Strategy for Bone and Soft Tissue Tumors. J Bone Joint Surg Am, 75:622–623, 1993.

38. **c** Fat signal intensity decreases, and water signal intensity increases. Magnetic resonance imaging uses a magnetic field to measure the response of tissue protons to radiofrequency. Water content influences proton behavior. Thus, tissues with different water contents have different magnetic resonance imaging signal characteristics. On T1-weighted images, water has a low signal intensity, and fat has a high signal intensity. On T2-weighted images, water has an increased signal intensity, and fat has a decreased signal intensity. Muscle has an intermediate signal on T1-weighted images and has a decreased signal on T2-weighted images.

    Most tumors have an intermediate signal on T1-weighted imaging, which contrasts with the higher signal of intermuscular fat planes. Most tumors have a high signal on T2-weighted imaging, a feature that is useful for differentiating tumor tissue from the lower signal of adjacent normal muscle tissue.

    Note: H_2O = water

39. **c** Ankylosing spondylitis and inflammatory bowel disease are associated with bilaterally symmetric sacroiliac disease. The syndesmophytes associated with *ankylosing spondylitis* tend to be thin, marginal, and symmetric. This yields a characteristic "bamboo spine" appearance. When syndesmophytes occur in association with the arthritis of *inflammatory bowel disease,* they tend to have an identical appearance. Conversely, the syndesmophytes that occur in association with psoriasis and Reiter syndrome tend to be thick, nonmarginal, and asymmetric.

    Sacroiliac involvement tends to be bilateral and symmetric in both ankylosing spondylitis and the arthritis of inflammatory bowel disease. In these two conditions, sacroiliac disease may progress to sacroiliac autofusion. The sacroiliac involvement that is seen in association with psoriasis and Reiter syndrome is unpredictable with regard to symmetry.

Reference

Helms C: Fundamentals of Skeletal Radiology. Philadelphia, WB Saunders, 1989.

40. **b** Plantar fibromatosis. *Ledderhose disease (plantar fibromatosis)* is characterized by nodular thickening of the

plantar fascia. It is the plantar equivalent of Dupuytren contracture of the palm.

Nodular fasciitis presents as a rapidly proliferating, tender subcutaneous nodule. It most commonly affects the volar surface of the forearm. It is a benign condition, but its histologic appearance is "pseudosarcomatous." *Extraabdominal desmoid,* despite a bland microscopic appearance, is an aggressive infiltrating lesion that can be associated with retroperitoneal and intrathoracic involvement and a high rate of morbidity and mortality.

41. **b** Calcifying aponeurotic fibroma. *Calcifying aponeurotic fibroma* is a slow-growing, benign fibrous tumor that occurs in the hands and feet of children and adolescents. Local excision carries a approximately 50% chance of recurrence. The described radiographic and histologic features are characteristic of this lesion.

Nodular fasciitis is another fibrous tumor that occurs in children and adolescents. However, unlike calcifying aponeurotic fibroma, it tends to grow rapidly and to produce pain. Histologically, nodular fasciitis contains areas of mature collagen surrounded by fragmented collagen bundles and a reticular network.

Dermatofibrosarcoma protuberans is a fibrous, nodular cutaneous tumor that occurs in the fourth and fifth decades. It arises on the extremities approximately 40% of the time. Malignant fibrous histiocytoma and fibrosarcoma are both rapidly growing tumors with highly cellular, malignant histologic appearances.

42. **e** Open biopsy for definitive diagnosis. The pelvis in Fig. 8.6 reveals characteristic pagetoid features (expanded cortex with obscured differentiation between the cortex and medullary cavity). However, the region around the ischial tuberosity demonstrates a superimposed phenomenon. Note the regional bone resorption, the discontinuity of the cortex, and the associated soft tissue mass.

Whenever pain occurs in a previously asymptomatic region of pagetoid bone, one must consider the possibility of sarcomatous degeneration. One should not be led astray by the vague history of trauma provided by this patient, particularly given the grave radiographic findings. A bone scan would serve little purpose in this setting given the background of pagetoid bone.

Note: Secondary osteogenic sarcoma occurs in approximately 1% of patients with Paget disease.

Reference

Wick MR, et al.: Sarcoma of Bone Complicating Osteitis Deformans. Am J Surg Pathol, 5:47, 1981.

43. **c** Hematopoietic stem cell precursors. *Osteoclasts* are derived from hematopoietic stem cell precursors (the same cell that gives rise to the monocyte/macrophage lineage). *Osteoblasts* stem from inducible osteoprogenitor cells, which, in turn, arise from undifferentiated mesenchymal cells. *Osteocytes* are derived directly from osteoblasts when the osteoblasts encase themselves in bony lacunae.

Reference

Favus MJ, ed: Primer on the Metabolic Bone Diseases, 3rd Ed. Philadelphia, Lippincott–Raven, 1996.

44. **a** They enhance bone mineral deposition at high doses. *Bisphosphonates* are pyrophosphate analogs. In diphosphonates, a nonhydrolyzable P-C-P bond replaces the normal pyrophosphate P-O-P bond. Pyrophosphate is a potent inhibitor of bone mineralization.

Bisphosphonates are able to retard hydroxyapatite formation and resorption. At high doses, the antideposition effect of bisphosphonates predominates. Therefore, high doses have been used in attempts to prevent ectopic calcification. High or prolonged doses of bisphosphonates are also capable of producing iatrogenic osteomalacia (without affecting calcium or vitamin D levels).

At lower or intermittent doses, the antiresorptive effect of bisphosphonates predominates, hence their application in the management of Paget disease, the hypercalcemia of malignancy, and (more recently) osteoporosis prophylaxis. They are also being used experimentally to prevent and treat particulate-induced osteolysis around total joint implants. Maintenance of a cyclic dosing regimen is important to avert iatrogenic bone pain, fracture, or osteomalacia.

References

Favus MJ, ed: Primer on the Metabolic Bone Diseases, 3rd Ed. Philadelphia, Lippincott–Raven, 1996.

Millett PJ, Allen MJ, Bostrom MPJ: Effects of Alendronate on Particulate-Induced Osteolysis in a Rat Model. J Bone Joint Surg.

45. **d** Bone biopsy should be performed routinely to confirm the diagnosis. *Paget disease* most commonly affects the skull, tibia, pelvis, femur, and spine. Facial bones, scapulae, ribs, clavicles, and forearm bones are less commonly affected. It is rarely diagnosed in patients less than 40 years old and is most commonly diagnosed in patients in their 50s.

Characteristic biochemical parameters include normal serum calcium and a markedly elevated alkaline phosphate level. The elevated alkaline phosphate level is not only a marker for the disease, but it can also be used to monitor the level of disease activity and the efficacy of therapy. The diagnosis is typically made based on the characteristic biochemical parameters and radiographic findings, and bone biopsy is not required in most instances.

Note: A biopsy should be considered in patients with new pain at sites of known Paget disease, particularly if there is new osteolytic change. (See question 42.)

Reference

Favus MJ, ed: Primer on the Metabolic Bone Diseases, 3rd Ed. Philadelphia, Lippincott–Raven, 1996.

46. **a** Parafollicular cells of the thyroid. Calcitonin is synthesized by the parafollicular cells of the thyroid gland. Chief cells of the parathyroid gland produce parathyroid hormone. Oxyphil cells of the parathyroid gland are less numerous and less synthetically active. The zona fasciculata cells of the adrenal cortex produce glucocorticoids.
47. **d** 1,25(OH)$_2$ vitamin D decreases the production of parathyroid hormone. Vitamin D is a steroid hormone and hence it has an intracellular (nuclear) receptor. 7-Dehydrocholesterol (provitamin D) is converted into previtamin D (in the skin) by ultraviolet B radiation. Previtamin D subsequently isomerizes into vitamin D and enters the circulation. Melanin competes with 7-dehydrocholesterol for photons, and people who are more heavily pigmented require longer periods of exposure to ultraviolet light to produce an equivalent quantity of vitamin D. Diet is an alternative sources of vitamin D. Although it is rare in most foods, certain foods such as fatty fish (e.g., salmon and codfish oil) and commercially vitamin D–fortified foods (e.g., some milk and cereals) are sources. The recommended dietary allowance of vitamin D is 200 IU for adults and 400 IU for children and pregnant or lactating women.

    Vitamin D$_3$ lacks significant biological activity. The liver converts vitamin D$_3$ to 25(OH)D, which also has no significant hormonal activity. The kidney subsequently converts 25(OH)D into its active form, 1,25(OH)$_2$D. Parathyroid hormone promotes 1,25(OH)$_2$D production by the kidney, but it does not affect 25(OH)D production by the liver. 1,25(OH)$_2$D, in turn, decreases parathyroid hormone production by an inhibitory feedback loop.

Reference

Favus MJ, ed: Primer on the Metabolic Bone Diseases, 3rd Ed. Philadelphia, Lippincott–Raven, 1996.

48. **d** Phosphate depletion. *Phosphate depletion* stimulates renal conversion of 25(OH)D to 1,25(OH)$_2$D (independently of parathyroid hormone) and thus increases gastrointestinal calcium absorption.

    Glucocorticoids suppress gastrointestinal calcium reabsorption by inhibiting calcium transport. Gluten enteropathy (celiac sprue) and other gastrointestinal malabsorption syndromes decrease calcium reabsorption both directly (by calcium binding to unabsorbed fatty acids) and indirectly (by decreasing vitamin D absorption). Hyperthyroidism increases calcium release from skeletal tissues; the resultant high serum calcium suppresses the formation of 1,25(OH)$_2$D. Metabolic acidosis decreases serum 1,25(OH)$_2$D by raising the ratio of ionized to unionized serum calcium.

Reference

Favus MJ, ed: Primer on the Metabolic Bone Diseases, 3rd Ed. Philadelphia, Lippincott–Raven, 1996.

49. **b** Aluminum-containing antacids. Phenytoin, rifampin, and phenobarbital all cause vitamin D deficiency by accelerating the metabolism and clearance of vitamin D and its metabolites (by inducing the hepatic P-450 system). Cholestyramine is a bile acid-binding resin used clinically to decrease cholesterol absorption from the gut. Not only does it bind intestinal cholesterol, but it also binds intestinal vitamin D and thereby decreases vitamin D absorption.

    Excessive intake of aluminum-based antacids is a cause of hypophosphatemic osteomalacia. Aluminum-hydroxide antacids inhibit intestinal phosphate absorption by binding to phosphate in the intestine. Thus, aluminum causes osteomalacia independently of vitamin D. In fact 1,25(OH)$_2$ vitamin D levels are often reflexively elevated in response to this condition.

    Osteomalacia does not necessarily stem from a deficiency of vitamin D or calcium, although it most commonly does. Osteomalacia may also be the result of deficient phosphate levels, as is the case with excessive aluminum ingestion.

    Note: Osteomalacia is a defect in bone mineralization that occurs after the cessation of growth, as opposed to rickets, which is a defect in bone mineralization that occurs before the cessation of growth.

Reference

Cotran RS, et al., eds: Robbins Pathologic Basis of Disease, 4th Ed. Philadelphia, WB Saunders, 1989.

50. **c** Follicular. *Papillary carcinoma* is the most common histologic type of thyroid carcinoma (approximately 70%). It commonly spreads to regional lymph nodes, but bone metastasis is uncommon. *Follicular carcinoma* is the second most common histologic type (approximately 20%). Metastases to regional lymph nodes are relatively rare, and hematogenous dissemination is far more common (particularly to bone). Mixed papillary-follicular carcinoma behaves similarly to papillary carcinoma. Medullary carcinoma arises from the parafol-

licular C cells (the cells that secrete calcitonin). This variant also demonstrates a tendency for spread to regional lymph nodes.

Even though papillary carcinoma is the most prevalent type of thyroid carcinoma, the risk of skeletal metastasis is highest with follicular cell tumors. The risk of skeletal metastasis by type of primary thyroid neoplasm is as follows: follicular cell, 17%; Hurthle cell, 12%; medullary carcinoma, 10%; anaplastic carcinoma, 5%; and papillary carcinoma, 2%.

Note: Serum calcitonin levels are a marker for medullary thyroid carcinoma.

Reference

Hay ID, et al. In Sim FH, et al., eds: Diagnosis and Management of Metastatic Bone Disease. New York, Raven, 1987.

51. **a** Clear cell chondrosarcoma. *Clear cell chondrosarcoma* is a slow-growing tumor that occurs in the epiphyseal regions of long bones with closed growth plates. It is the least common variety of chondrosarcoma. It typically arises in the third or fourth decades of life. It is approximately twice as frequent in males than females.

The plain radiograph (Fig. 8.8A) demonstrates a well-circumscribed lucent lesion in the femoral head. Although giant cell tumor also characteristically occurs in the epiphyseal region of long bones with closed physes, the sclerotic margin of this particular lesion renders the diagnosis of giant cell tumor unlikely.

The matrix in the histologic specimen can be identified as cartilaginous because of its smooth, "glassy" texture. This matrix has a characteristically blue hue on hematoxylin and eosin stain. The vast clear cytoplasm of these tumor cells gives this lesion its name (Fig. 8.8B), not the well-defined cytoplasmic borders and eccentrically placed nuclei. In some lesions, osseous tissue may be intermixed with the clear cells and the cartilaginous matrix.

Although it is slow growing, this tumor's malignant potential and propensity for local recurrence warrant *en bloc* resection. Definitive treatment carries a good prognosis.

Reference

Leggon RE Jr, Unni KK, Beabout JW, et al.: Clear Cell Chondrosarcoma. Orthopedics, 13(5):593–596, 1990.

52. **d** Nonossifying fibroma. According to Helms, the following differential diagnosis covers 99% of lytic epiphyseal lesions in patients less than 30 years of age: infection, chondroblastoma, giant cell tumor, aneurysmal bone cyst, and eosinophilic granuloma. In an older population, the differential diagnosis should include metastasis, geode, chondrosarcoma (clear cell variety), and myeloma. *Nonossifying fibroma* (fibrous cortical defect) characteristically occurs in the metaphyseal region.

Reference

Helms CA: Fundamentals of Skeletal Radiology, 2nd Ed. Philadelphia, WB Saunders, 1994.

53. **e** Low 1,25-$(OH)_2$ vitamin D_3. *Vitamin D–deficient rickets* refers to an inadequate endogenous synthesis or a dietary insufficiency of vitamin D. The two types of vitamin D–dependent rickets are distinguished by different biochemical defects. Type I involves an autosomal recessive defect in the renal enzyme (1-α-hydroxylase) that converts 25(OH) vitamin D to 1,25$(OH)_2$ vitamin D. In type II, there is sufficient 1,25$(OH)_2$ vitamin D production, but there is end-organ resistance to 1,25$(OH)_2$ vitamin D.

The clinical manifestations of the various types of rickets are indistinguishable from one another. Characteristic bony deformities include bowing of the lower extremities, widened osteoid seams, and physeal cupping. Comparative laboratory findings are given in Table 8.2.

Reference

Cotran RS, et al., eds: Robbins Pathologic Basis of Disease, 4th Ed. Philadelphia, WB Saunders, 1989.

54. **e** Osteosarcoma. Patients with the hereditary form of *retinoblastoma* are at markedly increased risk for developing osteogenic sarcoma compared with the general population. This risk is independent of exposure to radiation therapy. A genetic mutation at the q14 locus of chromosome 13 has been implicated in the genesis or both retinoblastoma and osteogenic sarcoma.

The retinoblastoma phenotype exhibits an autosomal recessive inheritance pattern. The *RB* gene is a prototype antioncogene. Inactivation of this gene product requires a homozygous defect at the RB locus.

TABLE 8.2. CLINICAL MANIFESTATIONS OF RICKETS

Disorder	Calcium	Phosphate	Alkaline Phosphatase	Parathyroid Hormone	25(OH) Vitamin D	1,25(OH)2 Vitamin D
Vitamin D–deficient rickets	Normal to low	Low	High	High	Low	Low
Vitamin D–dependent rickets type I	Low	Low	High	High	Normal	Very low
Vitamin D–dependent rickets type II	Low	Low	High	High	Normal	Very high

Note: Many osteogenic sarcoma cell lines express normal RB protein. A defect in the *RB* gene is not the only route of oncogenesis for osteogenic sarcoma.

Reference

Link MP, Eilber F: Osteogenic Sarcoma. In Pizzo PA, Poplack DG, eds: Principles and Practice of Pediatric Oncology, 3rd Ed. Philadelphia, Lippincott–Raven, 1997.

55. **b** The polyostotic form exhibits bilateral symmetry. *Fibrous dysplasia* is a benign, nonhereditary dysplastic condition characterized by replacement of normal bone by fibroosseous tissue. It may be either monostotic or polyostotic. The monostotic form commonly affects the ribs and the diaphyseal-metaphyseal regions of long bones. It most commonly occurs in the proximal femur, where it may produce a characteristic varus ("shepherd's crook") deformity. The polyostotic form tends to affect only one side of the body. Involvement of the craniofacial bones may produce *hemihypertrophy cranii* or cranial nerve dysfunction secondary to foraminal narrowing.

Lesions often produce expansion and thinning of the overlying cortex. Pathologic fracture is a common complication. The extent of sclerosis within these lesions varies widely, depending on the relative content of osseous and fibrous tissue. Bone spicules within the lesion are composed of woven bone. Lesions also often contain a significant amount of cartilage tissue.

Note: Fibrous dysplasia characteristically spares the epiphysis.

Reference

Stanton RP, Montgomery BE: Fibrous Dysplasia. Orthopedics, 19(8): 679–685, 1996.

56. **e** Surgical excision assures complete resolution of the associated scoliosis. In the spine, *osteoid osteoma* most commonly occurs in the posterior elements (laminae and pedicles). It is the most common cause of painful scoliosis. The level of the lesion typically corresponds to the level of the apex of the resultant scoliosis, except in the lower lumbar spine, where the apex may be above the lesion. The apex of the associated curve is typically concave toward the side of the lesion.

Prompt excision of the lesion typically results in spontaneous correction of the scoliosis. However, postoperative behavior of the curve depends on the duration of symptoms, the size of the curve, and the skeletal age of the patient. Cases of delayed excision of large curves in younger children have been associated with persistent structural deformity and curve progression.

References

Pettine KA, Klassen RA: Osteoid Osteoma and Osteoblastoma of the Spine. J Bone Joint Surg Am, 68:354–361, 1986.

Ransford AO, Pozo JL, Hutton P, Kirwan OG: The Behaviour Pattern of the Scoliosis Associated with Osteoid Osteoma or Osteoblastoma of the Spine. J Bone Joint Surg Br, 66:16–20, 1984.

57. **e** None of the above. *Osteogenic sarcoma* is the most common primary malignant tumor of bone. The conventional form of osteogenic sarcoma is more common in males than in females and typically occurs during in the second or third decade of life.

Significant prognostic factors include (1) stage, (2) the extent of neoadjuvant chemotherapy-induced tumor necrosis, (3) surgical margin status, (4) preoperative serum lactate dehydrogenase levels, and (5) the presence of skip metastases.

References

Picci P, Sangiorgi L, Rougraff BT, Neff JR, Casadei R, Campanacci M.: Relationship of Chemotherapy-Induced Necrosis and Surgical Margins to Local Recurrence in Osteogenic Sarcoma. J Clin Oncol, 12(12):2699–2705, 1994.

Taylor WF, Irvins JC, Unni KK, Beabout JW, Golenzer HJ, Black LE: Prognostic Variables in Osteogenic Sarcoma: A Multi-Institutional Study. J Natl Cancer Inst, 41:21–30, 1989.

Wuisman P, Enneking WF: Prognosis for Patients Who Have Osteogenic sarcoma With Skip Metastases. J Bone Joint Surg Am, 72:60–70, 1990.

58. **b** Malignant fibrous histiocytoma. *Malignant fibrous histiocytoma* is the most common soft tissue sarcoma of late adulthood. It is aggressive and typically presents with swelling and pain. The most common site of occurrence is in the thigh.

The plain radiograph (Fig. 8.9A) shows a lytic, poorly defined lesion in the proximal humerus with cortical destruction and an associated soft tissue mass. The photomicrographs in Fig. 8.9B and C show a cellular lesion composed of spindle cells in a fibrous stroma arranged in a vague storiform pattern. The spindle cells manifest atypia and pleomorphism. Atypical giant cells are also commonly encountered in malignant fibrous histiocytoma specimens. When present, these giant cells may resemble osteoclasts, but they tend to have a more bizarre, "ugly" appearance.

Note: "Storiform" refers to a tight swirling pattern of spindle cells. This pattern is also seen in association with a wide variety of benign fibrous lesions. However, the presence a storiform cellular pattern in association with atypical nuclei and bizarre giant cells is highly suggestive of the diagnosis of malignant fibrous histiocytoma.

Reference

Kumar RV, Mukherjee G, Bhargava MK, et al.: Malignant fibrous histiocytoma of bone. J Surg Oncol, 44(3):166–170, 1990.

59. **c** 5% to 10%. When limb-salvage surgery with neoadjuvant chemotherapy is performed for osteogenic sar-

coma of the distal femur, the reported local recurrence rate is 5% to 10%. This is approximately equivalent to the local recurrence rate when above-knee amputation is performed for such lesions. Patients with limb salvage have higher functional scores. There is no statistically significant difference in the disease-free survival rates for the two types of treatment.

References

Rougraff BT, et al.: Limb Salvage Compared to Amputation for Osteogenic Sarcoma of the Distal Femur. J Bone Joint Surg Am, 76:649–656, 1994.

Simon MA: Limb Salvage for Osteogenic Sarcoma. J Bone Joint Surg Am, 70:307–310, 1988.

60. **c** Cortical lucent lines oriented perpendicularly to the long axis of the bones of a patient with osteomalacia. *Looser zones* result from pathologic fractures that occur in the setting of osteomalacia. The pathologic fracture gap is bridged by fibrous tissue and suboptimally mineralized callus. This produces the characteristic linear radiolucency.

    A lytic defect containing multiple giant cells in a patient with hyperparathyroidism is referred to as a *brown tumor.* The horizontal condensations of trabeculae formed adjacent to the physis at times of decelerated skeletal growth are referred to as *transverse lines of Park* or *Harris growth arrest lines.* Costochondral cartilage hypertrophy in a child with rickets is known as *rachitic rosary.*

61. **c** It inhibits xanthine oxidase. *Allopurinol* is used to decrease urate production in patients with gout or hyperuricemia. Uric acid is a product of purine (not pyrimidine) ribonucleotide metabolism. The last step in purine breakdown is the conversion of xanthine and hypoxanthine to urate by the enzyme, xanthine oxidase. Allopurinol (an isomer of hypoxanthine) blocks xanthine oxidase.

    An alternative to decreasing urate production in cases of hyperuricemia is to increase urate excretion. Uricosuric agents (e.g., probenecid and sulfinpyrazone) increase renal excretion of uric acid by decreasing the net urate reabsorption in the proximal tubule.

    Colchicine exerts its antiinflammatory effect by inhibiting leukocyte phagocytosis and migration by preventing polymerization of tubulin. Nonsteroidal antiinflammatory drugs inhibit the enzyme, cyclooxygenase, which converts arachidonic acid to prostaglandins.

Reference

Katzung BG, ed: Basic and Clinical Pharmacology, 4th Ed. Norwalk, CT, Appleton & Lange, 1989.

62. **b** Osteochondroma. *Osteocartilaginous exostosis (osteochondroma)* is one of the most common benign tumors of bone. An osteochondroma may be either pedunculated (as seen in this case) or sessile. These osseous outgrowths typically originate from the metaphyseal cortex of a long bone. The pedunculated variety characteristically projects toward the diaphysis.

    Radiographic hallmarks of this lesion include cortical continuity with the bone of origin and a resultant continuous intramedullary space. Slow growth occurs until maturity, but it rarely causes a significant deformity.

    Histologic hallmarks of this lesion include (1) a thin fibrous layer (representing the attenuated periosteum/perichondrium) covering the surface, (2) a uniform cartilage cap; (3) endochondral ossification beneath the cartilage cap, and (4) osseous trabeculae at the base of the lesion. The cartilage cap can be distinguished from articular cartilage based on its fibrous coating. The fibrous tissue adjacent to an apophysis is typically perpendicular to its surface (forming an enthesis), in contrast to the parallel orientation of the overlying fibrous layer in this case.

    Exostoses may be either solitary or multiple. Malignant degeneration is rare (approximately 1%) in cases of solitary osteochondromas. The incidence of malignant degeneration is greater among persons with multiple hereditary exostosis *(Ehrenfried disease).* Computed tomography and magnetic resonance imaging can be helpful in determining the size of the cartilage cap in cases of suspected malignant transformation. A cartilage cap larger than 2 cm is suggestive of secondary chondrosarcoma. The absence of cytologic atypia in the chondrocytes in the cap of this exostosis excludes the diagnosis of secondary chondrosarcoma.

Reference

Greenspan A: Benign Bone Forming Lesions: Osteoma, Osteoid Osteoma, and Osteoblastoma. Skeletal Radiol, 22(7):485–500, 1993.

63. **b** The relative predominance of cartilage tissue within the tumor. The relative prevalence of cartilage production in *periosteal osteogenic sarcoma* specimens is a feature that distinguishes this tumor from other varieties of osteogenic sarcoma. By definition, all varieties of osteogenic sarcoma (including periosteal osteogenic sarcoma) produce new bone.

    Unlike conventional osteogenic sarcoma, periosteal osteogenic sarcoma tends to affect the middiaphyseal region of the long bones (rather than the metaphysis). It most commonly arises in the tibia. Telangiectatic osteogenic sarcoma is noted for its characteristic blood-filled cavities.

64. **d** Metastatic carcinoma. The radiograph reveals a pathologic femoral neck fracture with a lytic lesion in the acetabulum as well. Given the patient's age and

smoking history, the most likely diagnosis is *metastatic carcinoma.*

Although magnetic resonance imaging is an inappropriate screening test, it should have picked up the lesion and was probably misread. The radiograph reveals an infiltrative process in the acetabular dome with lysis and destruction of subchondral acetabular bone. Advanced avascular necrosis of the femoral head can lead to reciprocal degenerative changes of the acetabulum. However, the fracture and acetabular findings in the image are not consistent with degeneration. The other processes (fibrosarcoma, metastatic disease, osteomyelitis, and multiple myeloma) could all conceivably produce the radiographic findings; however, they are far less common than metastatic disease. The patient underwent excision of the tumor and reconstruction. The femur was reconstructed with a long-stem prosthesis, and the acetabulum was reconstructed with a Harrington-type reconstruction with threaded Steinmann pins and cement (Fig. 8.24).

65. **c** It most commonly occurs in adults between 30 and 60 years of age. *Chondroblastoma* is a rare tumor that is believed to arise from chondral precursor cells. Chondroblastoma characteristically arises in the epiphyseal (or apophyseal) portion of a bone. It occurs most commonly in the proximal humerus, distal femur, and proximal tibia. Radiographically, it appears as an oval, lytic lesion with a sclerotic rim of reactive bone. Associated cortical destruction and soft tissue extension may be encountered in advanced stages.

Chondroblastoma occurs most commonly in males 10 to 20 years old, in contrast to chondrosarcoma, which most commonly affects adults between 30 and 60 years of age.

Giant cell tumor may be confused with chondroblastoma radiographically and histologically. Furthermore, both lesions may metastasize to the lungs on rare occasions. A distinguishing radiographic factor is the lack of a sclerotic border in giant cell tumor. The two can be distinguished immunohistochemically based on reactivity to the S100 protein: chondroblastoma will be reactive, whereas giant cell tumor will not.

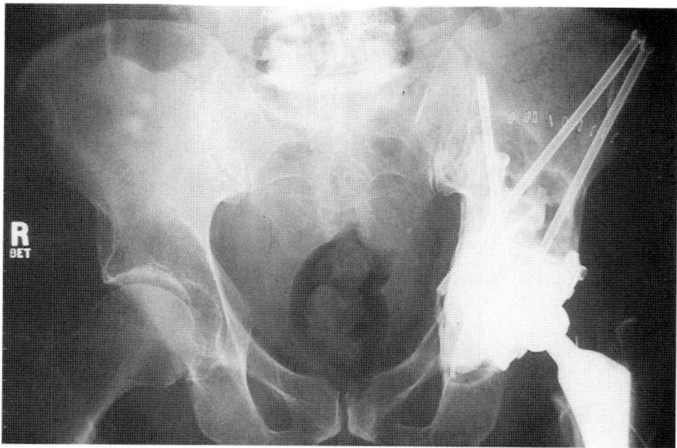

FIGURE 8.24

Reference

Scarborough MT, Moreau G: Benign Cartilage Tumors. Orthop Clin North Am, 27(3):583–589, 1996.

66. **d** Enchondroma. The radiographic and histologic features of this lesion indicate that it is an incidental benign intraosseous cartilaginous lesion. The lack of cortical destruction on the computed tomography is consistent with this benign lesion.

The photomicrograph of the lesion demonstrates a homogeneous glassy matrix, which acquires a characteristic pale blue hue on hematoxylin and eosin stain. Benign histologic features include the sparse cellularity and the lack of nuclear atypia, hyperchromatism, and pleomorphism.

It is theorized that *enchondromas* arise from epiphyseal plate remnants. Although enchondromas are most commonly located in the tubular bones of the hands and feet, these benign lesions can be located in any long bone.

Note: The stippled pattern of calcification in the humerus (Fig. 8.11A) is highly characteristic of cartilaginous neoplasms, but this pattern does not assist in differentiating a benign from a malignant process.

67. **e** Multiple cystic, extraosseous, calcium-containing masses adjacent to large joints. *Scurvy* produces several characteristic radiographic findings. Periosteal reaction results from subperiosteal hemorrhage. Metaphyseal collapse produce metaphyseal beaking *(Pelkan sign).* The *Wimberger ring sign* represents increased osseous density around the perimeter of secondary ossification centers. The regional increased density results from continued mineral deposition despite compromised osteoid formation. The same process produces linear condensations (growth arrest lines) adjacent to physes. These metaphyseal stripes are referred to as "white lines of scurvy." Soft tissue mineral deposition is not a characteristic feature of scurvy.

Reference

Hirsch M et al.: Neonatal Scurvy. Pediatr Radiol, 4:251, 1976.

68. **d** Parosteal osteosarcoma. The parosteal (juxtacortical) variant of osteogenic sarcoma is less aggressive than conventional (intramedullary) osteogenic sarcoma. It typically occurs in the third or fourth decade of life. The most common site for this tumor is the posterior aspect of the distal femur.

Imaging studies characteristically reveal a well-circumscribed, blastic, extraosseous mass directly adjacent to the cortex. Juxtacortical osteogenic sarcoma characteristically does not violate the cortex that it abuts.

Histologic examination reveals a fibrosarcomatous stroma with low-grade spindle cells and interspersed condensations of woven bone. The relatively bland histologic appearance of this lesion corresponds to its relatively benign behavior.

Figure 8.12B reveals no chondral tissue. Thus, alternative diagnoses such as osteochondroma and periosteal chondroma are unlikely. Periosteal osteogenic sarcoma also has a marked chondrogenic tendency. At first glance, this lesion's histologic features bear some resemblance to those of fibrous dysplasia. However, fibrous dysplasia is an intraosseous lesion with a less cellular stroma and many osteoclasts.

Note: The pattern of mineral deposition in Fig. 8.12A (decreased density toward the periphery) is opposite to the zonal pattern associated with myositis ossificans (radiolucent center with peripheral mature cortex).

Reference

Okada K, Frassica FJ, Sim FH, et al.: Parosteal Osteogenic Sarcoma: A Clinicopathological Study. J Bone Joint Surg Am, 76(3):366–378, 1994.

69. c Initial involvement of the middiaphysis. There are three defined radiographic stages of Paget disease: (1) lytic, (2) sclerotic, and (3) mixed. When Paget disease affects long bones, it typically commences at one end of the bone (not the middiaphysis). As the disease progresses along a bone, the leading edge has a characteristic lytic appearance that has been referred to as an "advancing flame" or a "blade of grass." Lytic involvement of the skull typically manifests a well-defined osteolytic parietooccipital lesion that has been referred to as *osteoporosis circumscripta.*

    The later stages of the disease are characterized by coarsened trabeculae with cortical thickening and expansion. The distinction between the cortex and the medullary cavity becomes obscured. Thickened, sclerotic skull involvement has a typical "cotton-wool" appearance. Sclerotic vertebral involvement yields a stereotypic "picture frame" pattern. Bowing deformities are commonly seen in affected long bones. Secondary degenerative joint disease is another common feature.

70. c Giant cell tumor. The magnetic resonance image of the knee (Fig. 8.13A and B) shows an eccentric, lytic lesion of the distal femoral epiphysis that extends to the juxtaarticular surface. These magnetic resonance imaging features are characteristic of *giant cell tumor.* (Please refer to question 23.)

    The photomicrograph in Fig. 8.13C reveals a field of closely packed giant cells with admixed mononuclear cells. No significant stroma is apparent. These histologic features are characteristic of giant cell tumor.

    Giant cell tumor is benign but locally aggressive. Treatment includes curettage plus various adjuvant modalities (e.g., phenol, cryosurgery, laser ablation, bone grafting, or polymethylmethacrylate). Local recurrence rates are high (up to 30%). Giant cell tumor is associated with approximately a 5% incidence of malignant degeneration and approximately a 1% incidence of metastasis (usually pulmonary).

Reference

Carrasco CH, Murray JA: Giant Cell Tumors. Orthop Clin North Am, 20:395, 1989.

71. c Tumoral calcinosis. *Tumoral calcinosis* is a rare condition that almost exclusively affects persons of African heritage. The multilobulated calcific deposits characteristically occur in periarticular locations over the extensor surfaces of the extremities. In contrast to other potential sources of soft tissue calcification (e.g., primary hyperparathyroidism, metastatic calcification, sarcoidosis, or hypervitaminosis D), serum calcium levels are not elevated. Another distinguishing feature of tumoral calcinosis is the presence of hydroxyapatite on ultrastructural analysis. Gout tophi also tend to occur in paraarticular regions, but tophaceous deposits are composed of urate crystals (not hydroxyapatite).

References

Boskey AL, et al.: Chemical, Microscopic, and Ultrastructural Characterization of the Mineral Deposits in Tumoral Calcinosis. Clin Orthop, 178:258–270, 1983.

Slavin RE, et al.: Familial Tumoral Calcinosis: A Clinical, Histopathological, and Ultrastructural Study. Am J Surg Pathol, 17:788, 1993.

72. e Spine. Bone is the third most common site of metastatic disease (pulmonary and hepatic metastases are more common). The most common site of osseous metastasis is the *spine.* The high incidence of metastasis to the axial skeleton has been attributed to presence of Batson plexus, a large network of valveless venous channels which provide a route from the pelvic viscera to the spine.

References

Batson OV: The Role of the Vertebral Veins in Metastatic Processes. Ann Intern Med, 16:38–45, 1942.

Harrington KD: Metastatic Disease of the Spine. J Bone Joint Surg Am, 68:1110–1115, 1986.

73. c C. Primary hypersecretion of parathyroid hormone may be produced by parathyroid gland hyperplasia

(most commonly), parathyroid adenoma, or parathyroid carcinoma (rarely). High serum parathyroid hormone concentration accompanied by high serum calcium concentration is the *sine qua non* of *primary hyperparathyroidism.*

Parathyroid hormone has four principal actions: (1) it increases osteoclastic bone resorption; (2) it increases renal calcium absorption; (3) it decreases renal phosphate resorption; and (4) it stimulates the renal enzyme, 1α-hydroxylase, to convert 25-vitamin D to its active form, 1-25-vitamin D.

Note: Parathyroid hormone does not stimulate osteoclasts directly. Rather, the hormone acts directly on osteoblasts, which, in turn, stimulate osteoclastic bone resorption.

74. **e** E. Pseudohypoparathyroidism is a rare hereditary disorder resulting from end-organ resistance to biologically active parathyroid hormone. Because of defective parathyroid hormone signal transduction, renal calcium resorption is decreased, renal phosphate excretion is decreased, and renal conversion of 25-vitamin D to 1-25-vitamin D is decreased.

Affected patients present with signs and symptoms of hypoparathyroidism (hypocalcemia, hyperphosphatemia) despite paradoxically elevated levels of parathyroid hormone. The elevated parathyroid hormone level is an appropriate (albeit ineffective) compensatory response.

Reference

Spiegel AM, et al.: Pseudohypoparathyroidism: The Molecular Basis for Hormone Resistance. N Engl J Med, 307:679, 1982.

75. **b** B. Secondary hyperparathyroidism consists of compensatory parathyroid hormone hypersecretion in response to hypocalcemia. The causes of *secondary hyperparathyroidism* include chronic renal insufficiency, pseudohypoparathyroidism, and vitamin D deficiency.

One source of vitamin D deficiency is intestinal malabsorption associated with Crohn disease. High parathyroid hormone results in decreased serum phosphate (phosphate diuresis).

76. **e** Fibrous dysplasia. *Fibrous dysplasia* is a benign hamartomatous lesion that is typically asymptomatic. Thus, incidental radiographic discovery is common. This lesion has a characteristic cystic "ground glass" appearance on radiographs. Commonly affected locations include the ribs, skull, and long bones. Recurrent pathologic fractures through a proximal femoral lesion may produce a characteristic "shepherd's crook" varus deformity.

The photomicrograph (Fig. 8.15B) displays the classic appearance of fibrous dysplasia. Irregular spicules of woven bone are interspersed within a loose homogeneous cellular background, imparting a characteristic "Chinese letters" or "alphabet soup" pattern. *Ossifying fibroma* is another benign fibrous lesion that contains scattered bony spicules. However, the surface of the spicules of ossifying fibroma is characteristically coated by a layer of osteoblasts. In contrast, minimal "osteoblastic rimming" is seen in fibrous dysplasia. Figure 8.16B lacks the inflammatory infiltrate and necrosis that characterize osteomyelitis.

Note: The architecture of the foci of immature bone formation in fibrous dysplasia is nonlamellar.

Reference

Enneking WF, Gearen PF: Fibrous Dysplasia of the Femoral Neck. J Bone Joint Surg Am, 68:1415, 1986.

77. **c** Schwannoma. *Neurilemoma (also known as schwannoma)* is a benign neoplasm that arises within peripheral nerve sheaths. It is encapsulated by epineurium and is slow growing. Neurilemomas are almost always solitary and usually appear as fusiform enlargements in continuity with the nerve (as demonstrated in Fig. 8.16C and D around the sciatic nerve). They manifest a predilection for the flexor surfaces of the extremity as well.

Microscopic examination demonstrates two distinct populations of cells (Antoni A and Antoni B). Antoni A regions are comprised of densely arranged spindle cells in a whirling, pallisading pattern. Salient features of Antoni B regions are their diminished cellularity and the presence of a myxoid matrix. Chordoma, hemangiopericytoma, reticulum cell sarcoma, and liposarcoma are all malignant neoplasms.

Reference

Weiss SW, Nickoloff BJ CD-34 is expressed by a distinctive cell population in peripheral nerve, nerve sheath tumors, and related lesions. Am J Surg Pathol, 17(10):1039–1045, 1993.

78. **b** Ewing sarcoma. *Ewing sarcoma* is the second most common malignant bone tumor in adolescents (after osteogenic sarcoma). It is a rapidly growing tumor that is thought to arise from neuroectodermal tissue. Common locations include the pelvis and the diaphyses of long bones. Ewing sarcoma often simulates osteomyelitis because of its propensity to present with local swelling, erythema, and constitutional symptoms.

Figure 8.17A demonstrates a poorly defined, lytic lesion in the humerus. Notice the pronounced new bone formation producing the characteristic "onion skin" appearance. The photomicrograph (Fig. 8.17B) demonstrates a solid field of uniform small cells. The cells contain prominent nuclei and scant cytoplasm. There is no evidence of matrix production. Immunohistochemical staining (for the presence of the O-13 marker) aids in distinguishing Ewing sarcoma from other small cell tumors such as eosinophilic granuloma and lymphoma.

79. **d** Eosinophilic granuloma. Photomicrographs of *eosinophilic granuloma* reveal multiple cell populations in addition to eosinophils. These include plasma cells, histiocytes, and giant cells. Electron microscopy of the associated Langerhans cells manifests characteristic racket-shaped cytoplasmic inclusion bodies. These are referred to as *Birbeck granules.*

80. **d** Hemangioma. *Hemangioma* is a benign vascular lesion that is typically asymptomatic and is discovered incidentally. Hemangioma of the vertebral body produces a characteristic imaging appearance. The distinctive "jailhouse vertebrae" (Fig. 8.18A and B) are caused by resorption of horizontal trabeculae with relative sparing of vertical trabeculae. The resultant vertically striated appearance resembles bars on a jailhouse door.

Reference

Gutierez RM, Spjut HJ: Skeletal Angiomatosis. Clin Orthop, 85:82, 1972.

81. **d** Aneurysmal bone cyst. Approximately 30% of *aneurysmal bone cysts* are noted to be secondary lesions. One theory for the pathogenesis of aneurysmal bone cysts is the arteriovenous fistula theory. This theory proposes that a preexisting benign osseous lesion (such as a giant cell tumor) precipitates the formation of an arteriovenous fistula. The pressure differential within the arteriovenous fistula, in turn, leads to the formation of the aneurysmal bone cyst.

Reference

Biesecker JL, Marcove RC, Huvos AG: Aneurysmal Bone Cysts: A Clinicopathologic Study of 66 Cases. Cancer, 26:615–625, 1970.

82. **c** Osteoid osteoma. The plain radiograph reveals a discrete radiolucent lesion within the sclerotic cortex of the proximal medial femur. The central radiolucency is the *nidus.* As shown in the low magnification photomicrograph, the nidus contains delicate, lacy, bony trabeculae. (The cytologic details within the nidus cannot be discerned at this magnification.) The surrounding host response is composed of robust, dense trabeculae. *Osteoid osteoma* is defined by the presence of the nidus. The extent of host reaction is variable.

    The diameter of the nidus must be less than 1.5 cm. Larger lesions are, by definition, *osteoblastomas.* The histologic features of the nidus of an osteoid osteoma are indistinguishable from those of the osteoblastoma. Osteoblastomas tend to provoke less reactive host sclerosis.

    Although the possibility of a stress fracture is suggested by the history and the bone scan, a stress fracture tends to produce a more linear radiolucency. Bone islands are rarely hot on bone scans. Intraosseous ganglia are purely lytic lesions. Unlike osteoid osteomas, they contain no intralesional mineral deposition. They are characteristically surrounded by a thin rim of sclerotic bone.

    Note: The pain associated with osteoid osteoma is characteristically exacerbated at night and is relieved by salicylates. However, the presence of these stereotypical features is variable.

Reference

Greenspan A: Benign Bone Forming Lesions: Osteoma, Osteoid Osteoma, and Osteoblastoma. Skeletal Radiol, 22(7):485—500, 1993.

83. **b** 1%. Transformation to secondary chondrosarcoma occurs in approximately 1% of patients with multiple hereditary exostoses. Central lesions (those involving the spine, ribs, scapula, and pelvis) demonstrate a greater propensity for malignant transformation than appendicular lesions.

Reference

Schmale GA, et al.: The Natural History of Hereditary Multiple Exostoses. J Bone Joint Surg Am, 76:986–992, 1994.

84. **a** Langerhans histiocytosis. The radiographic demonstrates a *vertebra plana* that should help with the diagnosis. Note that the disc space height is maintained and that there is no involvement of the posterior elements.

    The low- and high-power magnification photomicrographs (Fig. 8.20B and C) show a predominance of large cells (histiocytes) that have clear cytoplasm and single, large oval (or bean-shaped) nuclei. The eosinophils are the smaller cells with bilobed nuclei that are scattered throughout the image. The cytoplasm of these cells demonstrates characteristic eosinophilia on hematoxylin and eosin stains. Other cells, such as lymphocytes, giant cells, and plasma cells may also be present.

    Lymphoma and Ewing sarcoma demonstrate a more uniform small cell population. Pyogenic vertebral osteomyelitis originates in the disc space. Thus, disc height is characteristically lost. The predominant histologic features of pyogenic osteomyelitis are necrosis and abundant neutrophils (neither of which is present in Fig. 8.20B and C).

Reference

Seimon LP: Eosinophilic Granuloma of the Spine. J Pediatr Orthop, 1:371–376, 1981.

85. **d** Fibrosarcoma. The lateral radiograph of the foot demonstrates a prominent soft tissue mass in the third interspace. The photomicrograph reveals fascicles of spindle cells arranged in a "herringbone" pattern. This pattern is characteristic of *fibrosarcoma.* Intercellular collagen is produced by the tumor cells. However, unlike osteogenic sarcoma and chondrosarcoma, these cells produce no bone or cartilage matrix.

Fibrosarcoma typically arises in the metaphyses of long bones. The tumor may arise in the setting of chronic osteomyelitis, Paget disease, or radiation treatment.

Reference

Huvos AG : Primary Fibrosarcoma of Bone. Cancer, 35:837, 1975.

86. **d** Renal. Hypervascularity is a characteristic feature of metastatic *renal cell carcinoma.* When surgical intervention is contemplated for a renal metastasis, preoperative angiography is recommended. Preoperative embolization may curtail intraoperative hemorrhage in this setting.

Reference

Roscoe MW, et al.: Pre-operative Embolization in the Treatment of Osseous Metastases from Renal Cell Carcinoma. Clin Orthop, 238:303–307, 1989.

87. **e** Chordoma. *Chordoma* is malignant tumor that originates from remnants of the notochord. Thus, it occurs exclusively in the axial skeleton, most commonly in the sacrum. Chordoma typically presents during the sixth or seventh decade of life. The lesion causes a lytic osseous defect. It commonly gives rise to an associated soft tissue mass that may produce neurologic compromise.

Figure 8.22A reveals an osteolytic defect in the C2 vertebral body with an associated retropharyngeal soft tissue mass. The characteristic histologic appearance of a chordoma includes aggregates of large, extensively vacuolated cells *(physaliphorous cells)* within a background of loose mucoid material. (See question 11.)

Reference

Healey JH, Lane JM: Chordoma: A Critical Review of Diagnosis and Treatment. Orthop Clin North Am, 20:417, 1989.

88. **d** Giant cell tumor. As a general rule, none of the osseous neoplasms are more common in females except for (1) giant cell tumor and (2) parosteal osteogenic sarcoma.

89. **a** Li-Fraumeni syndrome. *Li-Fraumeni syndrome* is an autosomal dominant inherited condition that confers susceptibility to multiple childhood neoplasms. These include soft tissue sarcomas, adrenocortical carcinoma, osteogenic sarcoma, and brain tumors. When affected persons survive until puberty, they manifest a high incidence of premature breast cancer. The syndrome is associated with altered expression of the p53 tumor suppressor gene.

Peutz-Jeghers syndrome is an inherited form of intestinal polyposis. *Type I multiple endocrine neoplasia* consists of gastrinoma, parathyroid hyperplasia, and pituitary adenomas. *Sipple syndrome (multiple endocrine neoplasia type II)* includes medullary thyroid cancer and pheochromocytoma. *Von Recklinghausen disease* is another name for neurofibromatosis (type I).

Reference

Li FP, Fraumeni JF: Soft Tissue Sarcomas, Breast Cancer, and Other Neoplasms. Ann Intern Med, 71:747, 1969.

90. **c** Approximately 10%. Mankin et al. reported an 11% incidence of infection in their series of 718 allografts. Infection accounted for 43% of the allograft failures in this series. The incidence of fracture was 17% in this series; 16% of the patients with distal femoral or proximal tibial allografts ultimately required total joint replacement.

Reference

Mankin HJ, et al.: Long-Term Results of Allograft Replacement in the Management of Bone Tumors. Clin Orthop, 324:86–97, 1996.

91. **c** Synovial sarcoma. The t (X;18) (p11;q11) translocation is a useful cytogenetic marker for *synovial sarcoma.* This translocation is present in more than 90% of synovial sarcomas (both monophasic and biphasic subtypes). The translocation produces a fusion gene that is presumed to play a primary pathogenetic role in this tumor.

The fusion gene transcript can be detected by polymerase chain reaction. This reaction can therefore be used as a diagnostic test for synovial sarcoma. Subtle variations in the chimeric protein provide prognostic information.

Reference

Turc-Care C, et al.: Translocation X;18 in Synovial Sarcoma. Cancer Genet Cytogenet, 23:9, 1986.

92. **b** Synovial sarcoma. Whereas carcinomas tend to metastasize to regional lymph nodes, most sarcomas demonstrate a predilection for hematogenous dissemination. *Synovial sarcoma* demonstrates a greater tendency for lymphatic spread than most other sarcomas.

Note: Epithelioid sarcoma is another exception to the generalization that sarcomas do not disseminate by the lymphatic system.

FIGURE CREDITS

Figure 8.2. From Unni KK: Dahlin's Bone Tumors, 5th Ed. Philadelphia, Lippincott–Raven, pp. 384, 387, 1996, with permission.
Figure 8.3B. From Unni KK: Dahlin's Bone Tumors, 5th Ed. Philadelphia, Lippincott–Raven, p. 54, 1996, with permission.
Figure 8.4. From Unni KK: Dahlin's Bone Tumors, 5th Ed. Philadelphia, Lippincott–Raven, pp. 169, 171, 1996, with permission.
Figure 8.5B. From Unni KK: Dahlin's Bone Tumors, 5th Ed. Philadelphia, Lippincott–Raven, p. 417, 1996, with permission.
Figure 8.7B. From Unni KK: Dahlin's Bone Tumors, 5th Ed. Philadelphia, Lippincott–Raven, p. 105, 1996, with permission.
Figure 8.8B and C. From Unni KK: Dahlin's Bone Tumors, 5th Ed. Philadelphia, Lippincott–Raven, p. 222, 1996, with permission.
Figure 8.9. From Unni KK: Dahlin's Bone Tumors, 5th Ed. Philadelphia, Lippincott–Raven, pp. 13, 16, 1996, with permission.
Figure 8.11D. From Unni KK: Dahlin's Bone Tumors, 5th Ed. Philadelphia, Lippincott–Raven, p. 32, 1996, with permission.
Figure 8.12B. From Unni KK: Dahlin's Bone Tumors, 5th Ed. Philadelphia, Lippincott–Raven, p. 191, 1996, with permission.
Figure 8.15B. From Unni KK: Dahlin's Bone Tumors, 5th Ed. Philadelphia, Lippincott–Raven, p. 373, 1996, with permission.
Figure 8.16. From Craig EV: Clinical Orthopaedics. Philadelphia, Lippincott Williams & Wilkins, p. 1002, 1999, with permission.
Figure 8.17A. From Unni KK: Dahlin's Bone Tumors, 5th Ed. Philadelphia, Lippincott–Raven, p. 252, 1996, with permission.
Figure 8.19C. From Unni KK: Dahlin's Bone Tumors, 5th Ed. Philadelphia, Lippincott–Raven, p. 127, 1996, with permission.
Figure 8.20A. From Greenfield GB: Radiology of Bone Diseases. Philadelphia, J.B. Lippincott, p. 530, 1990, with permission.
Figure 8.20B and C. From Unni KK: Dahlin's Bone Tumors, 5th Ed. Philadelphia, , p. 410, 1996, with permission.
Figure 8.21C. From Unni KK: Dahlin's Bone Tumors, 5th Ed. Philadelphia, Lippincott–Raven, p. 202, 1996, with permission.
Figure 8.22B. From Unni KK: Dahlin's Bone Tumors, 5th Ed. Philadelphia, Lippincott–Raven, p. 298, 1996, with permission.
Figure 8.23. From Favus MJ, ed: Primer on the Metabolic Bone Diseases and Disorders of Mineral Metabolism, 3rd Ed. Philadelphia, Lippincott–Raven, p. 279, 1996, with permission.

9

PEDIATRICS

QUESTIONS

1. What type of collagen is associated with calcification of cartilage at the epiphyseal growth plate?
   (a) Type I
   (b) Type II
   (c) Type IX
   (d) Type IV
   (e) Type X
2. Which of the following is inaccurate regarding Morquio-Brailsford syndrome?
   (a) The disorder is transmitted in an autosomal recessive fashion.
   (b) At birth, weight and height are abnormally low.
   (c) Affected persons excrete both keratan sulfate and chondroitin sulfate at abnormally high levels in the urine.
   (d) Genu valgum is the most common associated knee deformity.
   (e) Surgical stabilization of the upper cervical spine is commonly required.
3. Which of the following is not a derivative of the neural crest?
   (a) Dorsal root ganglia cells
   (b) Melanocytes
   (c) Schwann cells
   (d) Sympathetic chain ganglia cells
   (e) Anterior horn cells
4. Which of the following ossification centers is the last to appear during normal elbow development?
   (a) The olecranon
   (b) The radial head
   (c) The medial epicondyle
   (d) The capitellum
   (e) The lateral epicondyle
5. Which of the following neoplasms is most commonly associated with hemihypertrophy?
   (a) Adrenal carcinoma
   (b) Retinoblastoma
   (c) Wilms tumor
   (d) Hepatoblastoma
   (e) Neuroblastoma
6. The concept that excessive compression across the physis retards growth is referred to as
   (a) Wolff law
   (b) Bischoff rule
   (c) Von Schwann law
   (d) Heuter-Volkman principle
   (e) Premise of Tolo
7. Which of the following statements regarding pediatric popliteal cysts is most accurate?
   (a) They rarely resolve spontaneously.
   (b) They are rarely associated with intraarticular disease.
   (c) Most arise from the posterolateral aspect of the joint.
   (d) Most communicate directly with meniscal lesions.
   (e) They are commonly associated with discoid lateral menisci.
8. Osteogenesis imperfecta results from a defect in the gene for
   (a) Type I collagen
   (b) Fibrillin
   (c) Insulinlike growth factor I
   (d) Bone morphogenetic protein
   (e) Osteocalcin
9. A 7-year-old boy complains of vague aching pains in both lower extremities. His past medical history is unremarkable. Physical examination reveals normal stature with mild atrophy of both calves. His mother was told that she had abnormal bones in her legs when she broke her ankle 10 years ago. Anteroposterior radiographs of the child's lower extremities are shown in Fig. 9.1. What is the most likely diagnosis?
   (a) Metatropic dysplasia
   (b) Hypophosphatasia
   (c) Camurati-Engelmann disease
   (d) Pyle dysplasia
   (e) Hurler disease
10. A 2-year-old girl is referred by her pediatrician because her toes "point in" when she walks. The foot progression angle is negative bilaterally (left to right). What is the most likely source of this child's in-toeing?
   (a) Excessive femoral retroversion

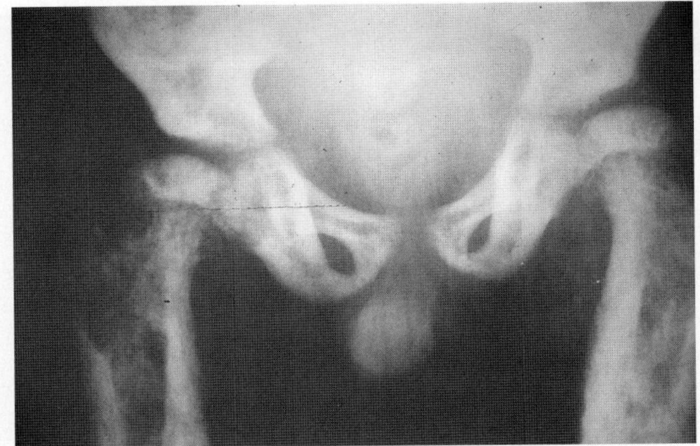

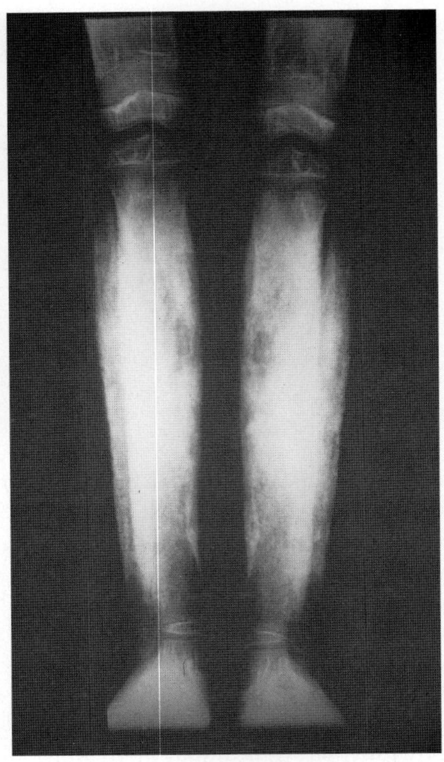

FIGURE 9.1A and B

(b) Internal tibial torsion
(c) Metatarsus adductus
(d) Internal rotation contracture of the hip
(e) Excessive femoral anteversion

11. Which of the following statements correctly describes infantile idiopathic scoliosis?
    (a) Right thoracic curves are more common than left thoracic curves.
    (b) Girls are affected more commonly than boys.
    (c) The rib-vertebra angle is more acute on the convex side of the curve than the rib-vertebra angle on the concave side.
    (d) It has traditionally been reported to be more common in North America than in England.
    (e) Most phase II curves with an apical rib-vertebra angle difference of less than 20 degrees will resolve.
12. Which of the following conditions is least likely to be associated with congenital radial deficiency (radial clubhand)?
    (a) Holt-Oram syndrome
    (b) Fanconi syndrome
    (c) VATER syndrome
    (d) Scheie syndrome
    (e) TAR syndrome
13. What is the likelihood of achondroplasia among the children of a man with achondroplasia and an unaffected woman? (You may assume 100% penetrance, and you may assume that there is no family history of achondroplasia on the maternal side.)
    (a) 50% if the child is male; 50% if the child is female
    (b) 100% if the child is male; 0% if the child is female
    (c) 0% if the child is male; 100% if the child is female
    (d) 25% if the child is male; 25% if the child is female
    (e) 0% if the child is male; 50% if the child is female
14. Which portion of the distal tibial physis fuses last?
    (a) The anteromedial
    (b) The posterolateral
    (c) The central
    (d) The posteromedial
    (e) The anterolateral
15. Erythroblastosis fetalis is most likely to produce which of the following forms of cerebral palsy?
    (a) Hemiplegia
    (b) Diplegia
    (c) Athetosis
    (d) Quadriplegia
    (e) Totally involved child
16. The "hitchhiker's thumb" deformity is a characteristic of which of the following conditions?
    (a) Arthrogryposis multiplex congenita
    (b) Sanfilippo syndrome
    (c) Diastrophic dysplasia
    (d) Trisomy 21
    (e) Klippel-Feil syndrome

17. A 16-year-old soccer player experiences acute left groin pain after being tackled while shooting. He holds his left hip flexed. An anteroposterior radiograph of the hip is shown in Fig. 9.2. Recommended treatment should be
    (a) Excision of the fragment
    (b) Lag screw fixation
    (c) Spica cast immobilization
    (d) Protected weight-bearing and progressive mobilization as tolerated
    (e) Fixation with a cerclage wire
18. McCune-Albright syndrome has been associated with a mutation of which of the following genes?
    (a) Keratin
    (b) G protein (α subunit).
    (c) Type III collagen
    (d) Fibroblast growth factor receptor 3
    (e) Osteonectin
19. Quinolone antibiotics work by which of the following mechanisms?
    (a) Inhibition of transcription
    (b) Inhibition of DNA polymerase
    (c) Disruption of ribosome function
    (d) Inhibition of DNA gyrase
    (e) Disruption of peptidoglycan synthesis
20. A child is referred for evaluation of a waddling gate. He demonstrates mildly short stature, frontal bossing, drooping shoulders, deformed teeth, and a high-arched palate. An anteroposterior pelvis film is shown in Fig. 9.3. What is the most likely diagnosis? (If you need a hint, look at Fig. 9.16, which may be found in the answer to this question).
    (a) Metaphyseal chondrodysplasia (Jansen type)
    (b) Stickler disease
    (c) Cleidocranial dysplasia
    (d) Metaphyseal chondrodysplasia (McKusick type)
    (e) Meyer dysplasia

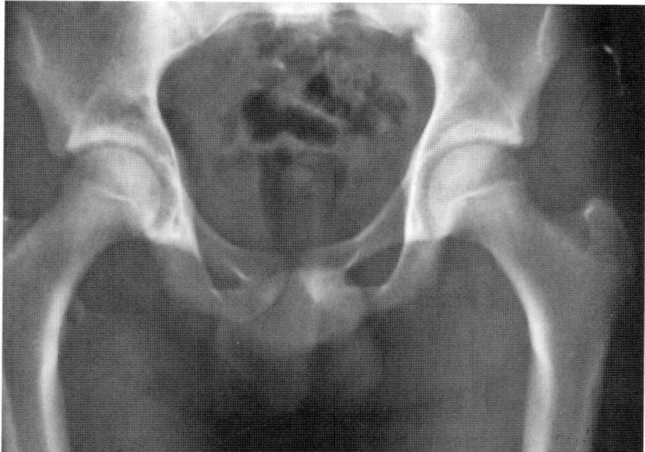

FIGURE 9.2

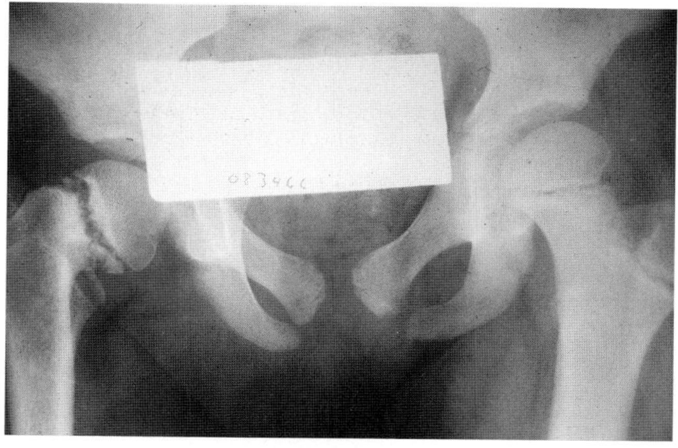

FIGURE 9.3

21. Which of the following is an adaptive response to quadriceps weakness in Duchenne muscular dystrophy?
    (a) Equinus contracture of the ankle
    (b) Meryon sign
    (c) Accelerated cadence
    (d) Knee flexion contracture
    (e) Increased lumbar lordosis
22. The limb buds appear during what period of gestation?
    (a) 2 to 3 weeks
    (b) 3 to 5 weeks
    (c) 5 to 7 weeks
    (d) 7 to 10 weeks
    (e) 10 to 12 weeks
23. A 21-year-old man requests evaluation of a painless, asymmetric gait. He underwent an unspecified procedure for developmental dysplasia of his left hip as an infant, after which he developed sepsis. Examination reveals a positive Trendelenburg sign. An anteroposterior pelvis film is shown in Fig. 9.4. Which of the following would be the most appropriate recommendation?
    (a) Valgus intertrochanteric osteotomy
    (b) Total hip arthroplasty
    (c) Varus intertrochanteric osteotomy
    (d) Right femoral lengthening
    (e) Trochanteric osteotomy
24. The distal radial physis accounts for what percentage of the longitudinal growth of the forearm?
    (a) 20%
    (b) 40%
    (c) 50%
    (d) 60%
    (e) 80%
25. The proximal femoral physis accounts for what percentage of the total longitudinal growth of the lower extremity?
    (a) 5%

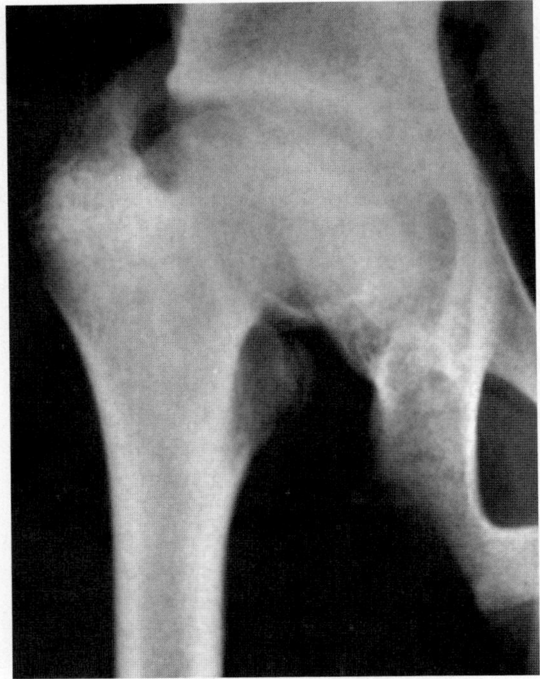

FIGURE 9.4

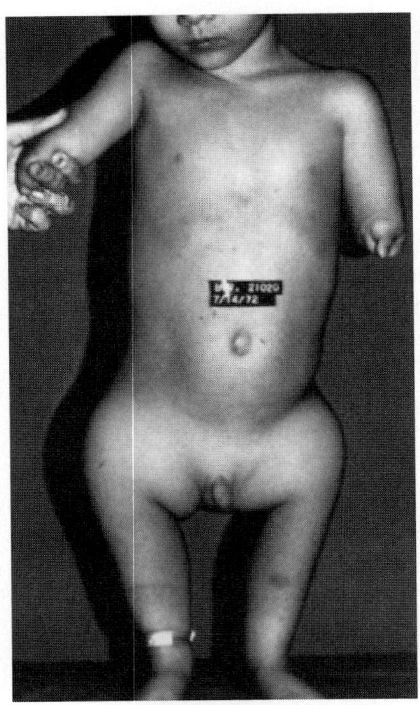

FIGURE 9.5

(b) 10%
(c) 15%
(d) 25%
(e) 35%

26. A 7-year-old girl sustains a Salter II fracture of her proximal humerus. After several attempts at closed reduction, the fracture remains angulated 35 degrees with 40% displacement. What is the most appropriate next course of action?
(a) Sling and swathe
(b) Open reduction and internal fixation with transphyseal smooth Kirschner wires
(c) Closed reduction under anesthesia and percutaneous pinning
(d) Open reduction and internal fixation with metaphyseal fixation through the Thurston-Holland fragment
(e) Olecranon pin traction for 2 weeks followed by spica cast application

27. Which of the following organisms is the most commonly isolated pathogen in neonatal septic arthritis of the hip?
(a) *Staphylococcus aureus*
(b) Group A *Streptococcus*
(c) *Haemophilus influenzae*
(d) *Neisseria gonorrhoeae*
(e) *Staphylococcus epidermidis*

28. What would be the most accurate description of the longitudinal deficiency demonstrated by the patient in Fig. 9.5?
(a) Rhizomelic shortening
(b) Mesomelic shortening
(c) Phocomelia
(d) Acromelic shortening
(e) Hemimelia

29. Which of the following types of tibial bowing is most commonly associated with neurofibromatosis?
(a) Posterolateral
(b) Anterolateral
(c) Posteromedial
(d) Anteromedial
(e) Complex

30. Which of the following organisms would be the most likely pathogen in a child with osteomyelitis and underlying sickle cell disease?
(a) *Salmonella*
(b) *Proteus mirabilis*
(c) *Pseudomonas*
(d) *Shigella*
(e) Group A *Streptococcus*

31. Which of the following forms of management would be most appropriate for a patient presenting with the radiograph in Fig. 9.6?
(a) Medial tibial hemiepiphysiodesis
(b) Closing lateral wedge osteotomy of the distal femur
(c) Hip-knee-ankle-foot orthosis and close observation
(d) Epiphysiodesis of the entire tibial physis
(e) Lateral closing wedge osteotomy of the proximal tibia

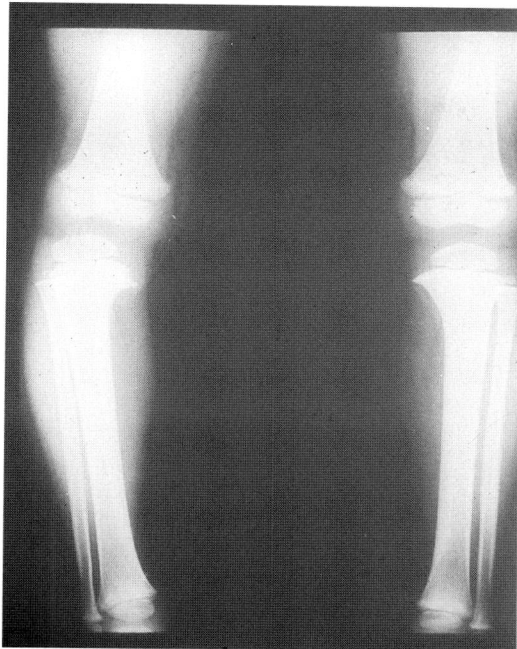

FIGURE 9.6

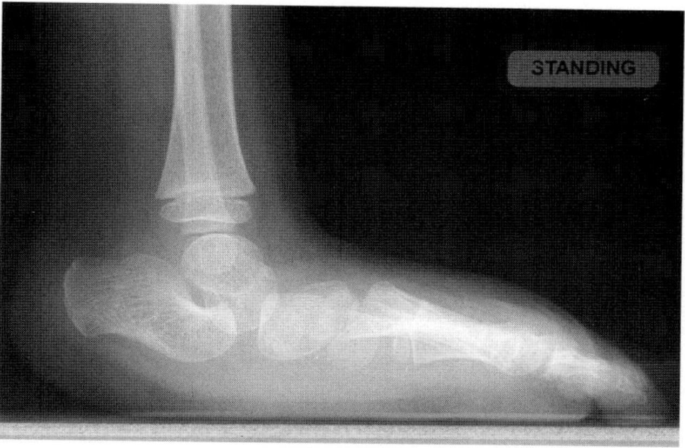

FIGURE 9.7

32. Physiologic genu valgum generally peaks at what age?
    (a) 12 months
    (b) 18 months
    (c) 2 years
    (d) 3 years
    (e) 4 years
33. How many discrete centers of ossification are typically present in the C2 vertebra at birth?
    (a) Two
    (b) Three
    (c) Four
    (d) Five
    (e) Six
34. Which of the following abnormalities is least characteristically associated with the Marfan phenotype?
    (a) Scoliosis
    (b) Inferior lens subluxation
    (c) Pectus excavatum
    (d) Mitral valve murmurs
    (e) Arm span–to-height ratio greater than 1
35. A toddler is brought in for evaluation because of a "flatfoot" and an awkward gait. Examination reveals a prominent callus on his plantar midfoot and a dorsal crease over his sinus tarsi. His past medical history is unremarkable. Radiographs are shown in Fig. 9.7. The deformity does not correct with maximal dorsiflexion or plantar flexion. What is the most appropriate diagnosis?
    (a) Idiopathic flatfoot
    (b) Congenital vertical talus
    (c) Diastematomyelia
    (d) Fibrous talocalcaneal coalition
    (e) Pes equinocavovarus
36. Deficiency of glucocerebrosidase produces which of the following diseases?
    (a) Ehlers-Danlos syndrome
    (b) Pseudoachondroplasia
    (c) Niemann-Pick disease (type A)
    (d) Gaucher disease
    (e) Sanfilippo syndrome
37. The pharmacologic mechanism of botulinum A toxin in the management of cerebral palsy is
    (a) Inhibition of postsynaptic acetylcholine endocytosis at the myoneural junction
    (b) Stimulation of acetylcholinesterase at the motor end plate
    (c) Inhibition of axonal transport of acetylcholine from the anterior horn cell body to the motor end plate
    (d) Inhibition of presynaptic acetylcholine exocytosis at the myoneural junction
    (e) Competitive inhibition of postsynaptic acetylcholine binding at the myoneural junction
38. An 11-year-old running back experiences acute left knee pain and swelling after being tackled. Examination of the knee reveals increased anterior tibial translation (2B Lachman test) and 2+ instability to valgus stress. Anteroposterior and lateral radiographs are seen in Fig. 9.8. What is the most appropriate form of management for this injury?
    (a) Primary repair of the medial collateral ligament and anterior cruciate ligament
    (b) Anterior cruciate ligament reconstruction using a hamstring tendon autograft
    (c) Hinged knee brace and progressive range of motion followed by hamstring and quadriceps strengthening

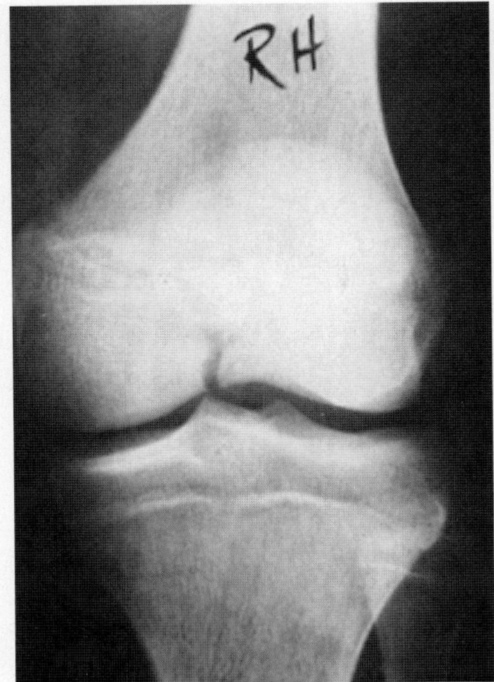

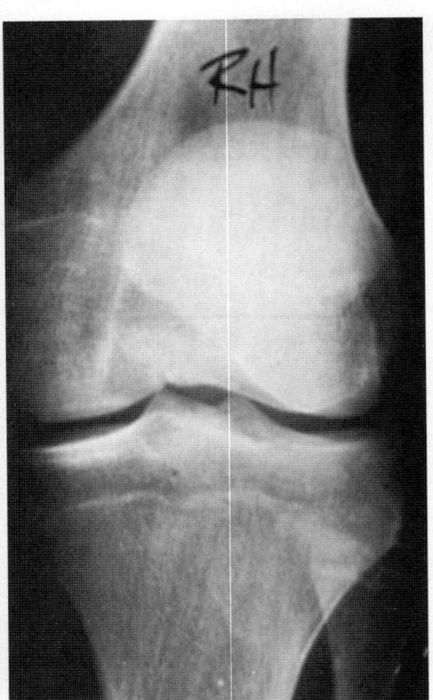

FIGURE 9.8A and B

(d) Primary repair of the medial collateral ligament and delayed anterior cruciate ligament reconstruction if instability persists at skeletal maturity
(e) Reduction and transphyseal fixation with crossed pins

39. Which of the following conditions is autosomal recessive?
(a) Cleidocranial dysplasia
(b) Diastrophic dysplasia
(c) Kneist syndrome
(d) Metaphyseal chondrodysplasia (Jansen type)
(e) Multiple epiphyseal dysplasia

40. Physeal fractures propagate primarily through what zone of the growth plate?
(a) The proliferative zone
(b) The resting zone
(c) The hypertrophic zone
(d) The maturation zone
(e) The primary spongiosa of the metaphysis

41. Which of the following is not a characteristic of familial dysautonomia?
(a) Absence of filiform papillae on the tongue
(b) Kyphoscoliosis
(c) Relative indifference to pain
(d) Hyperemesis
(e) Gastric reflux

42. A 5-year-old girl presents for routine orthopaedic follow-up 3 months after being diagnosed with pauciarticular juvenile rheumatoid arthritis. Her right knee is her only symptomatic joint. Examination reveals mild bogginess of the knee and a 5-degree flexion contracture. What is the most important component of management at this point?
(a) Knee aspiration
(b) Plain films of the cervical spine
(c) Lower extremity scanograms
(d) Physical therapy for active assisted range-of-motion exercises
(e) Ophthalmologic referral

43. Which of the following types of congenital scoliosis is associated with the worst prognosis?
(a) An incarcerated fully segmented hemivertebra
(b) Bilateral semisegmented hemivertebrae with a metameric shift
(c) A block vertebra
(d) A unilateral fully segmented hemivertebra with a contralateral bar
(e) Two consecutive convex hemivertebrae

44. Which of the following conditions is associated with juvenile hypothyroidism?
(a) Legg-Calvé-Perthes disease
(b) Early appearance of secondary ossification centers
(c) Slipped capital femoral epiphysis
(d) Premature physeal closure
(e) Arthrogryposis multiplex congenita

45. At what chronologic age does the ossification center of the femoral head epiphysis typically become radiographically detectable?

(a) During the third trimester
(b) At birth
(c) At 1 month
(d) At 4 months
(e) At 1 year

46. What is the most important form of management for a 7-year-old patient with the condition in Fig. 9.9?
(a) Green procedure
(b) Physical therapy
(c) Clavicular osteotomy and excision of the omovertebral bone
(d) Woodward procedure
(e) Flexion-extension views of the cervical spine

47. Arthrodesis of a paralytic shoulder in skeletally immature patients has been associated with which of the following postoperative radiographic changes?
(a) Progressive internal rotation
(b) Progressive abduction
(c) Progressive external rotation
(d) Progressive adduction
(e) Progressive forward flexion

48. Achondroplasia is associated with an aberration in which zone of the growth plate?
(a) The zone of provisional calcification.
(b) The resting zone
(c) The zone of hypertrophy
(d) The zone of proliferation
(e) The primary spongiosa of the metaphysis

49. The general surgery service consults you to evaluate a 16-year-old boy with pain in the region of his left sternoclavicular joint after a head-on motor vehicle accident. A splenectomy had been performed on the day of admission (3 days earlier). A computed tomography scan reveals a medial clavicular physeal injury with posterior clavicular displacement but no apparent compression of the mediastinal vessels, trachea, or esophagus. He denies dysphagia and dyspnea. His upper extremity neurovascular examination is normal. An attempted closed reduction while the patient is under general anesthesia is unsuccessful. What would be the most appropriate subsequent management of this patient?
(a) Figure-of-eight strap until the patient's discomfort resolves
(b) Open reduction with postoperative immobilization in a figure-of-eight strap for 6 weeks
(c) Open reduction and pin fixation of the sternoclavicular joint with Kirschner wires
(d) Open reduction and costoclavicular ligament reconstruction
(e) Open reduction and sternoclavicular capsular ligament reconstruction

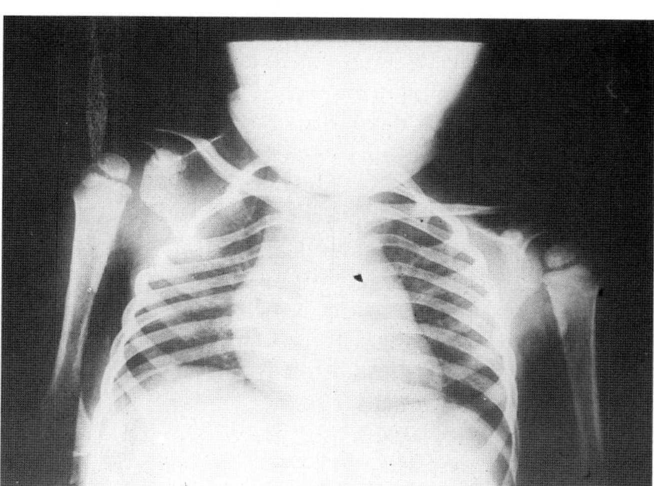

FIGURE 9.9

50. Which of the following statements correctly describes the Baumann angle?
(a) It is the angle subtended by the physeal line of the lateral condyle and the long axis of the humerus.
(b) It is synonymous with the "carrying angle."
(c) It is the angle subtended by the transepicondylar axis of the distal humerus and the physeal line of the lateral condyle.
(d) It is the angle subtended by the long axis of the humerus and the transepicondylar axis of the distal humerus.
(e) It is the angle subtended by the transepicondylar axis of the distal humerus and the physeal line of the trochlea.

51. Which of the following threshold values for the metaphyseal-diaphyseal angle provides the greatest accuracy for diagnosing infantile Blount disease?
(a) 5 degrees.
(b) 7 degrees.
(c) 9 degrees.
(d) 11 degrees.
(e) 16 degrees.

52. A 3-year-old child presents with a previously untreated dislocated hip. Pathoanatomic changes that may block reduction at this age are least likely to include
(a) Osteophyte formation at the margin of the pseudoacetabulum
(b) Hourglass capsular deformity
(c) Hypertrophy of the ligamentum teres and pulvinar
(d) Limbus formation
(e) Superior elongation of inferior capsule and transverse acetabular ligament

53. A 9-month-old child is brought to the emergency room by his mother, who states that the child is irritable and not moving his right leg after "slipping in the tub." Plain films reveal a displaced proximal femoral shaft fracture with 1 cm of shortening. In addition to notifying social services, what would be the most appropriate course of action?

(a) 90-90 femoral traction for 4 to 6 weeks
(b) Hip spica cast for 4 to 6 weeks
(c) External fixation
(d) Open reduction and internal fixation (compression plate)
(e) Delayed application of a hip spica cast after initial treatment with 90-90 femoral traction for 1 to 2 weeks

54. Which of the following is a correct description of skewfoot?
(a) Hindfoot valgus, forefoot abduction, and talar plantar flexion
(b) Hindfoot varus, absent navicular, and forefoot adduction
(c) Hindfoot valgus, abduction at the midtarsal joints, plantar flexion of the talus, and metatarsus adductus
(d) Hindfoot varus, absent talus, and forefoot adduction
(e) Hindfoot varus, forefoot equinus, and calcaneal dorsiflexion

55. A minimally displaced, two-part triplane fracture typically manifests which of the following appearances on plain radiographs?
(a) Salter-Harris I on anteroposterior view; Salter-Harris III on lateral view
(b) Salter-Harris III on anteroposterior view; Salter-Harris II on lateral view
(c) Salter-Harris IV on anteroposterior view; Salter-Harris III on lateral view
(d) Salter-Harris II on anteroposterior view; Salter-Harris III on lateral view
(e) Salter-Harris III on anteroposterior view; Salter-Harris IV on lateral view

56. Acute paralysis in an infant with achondroplasia is most likely to be the result of
(a) Intracranial hemorrhage
(b) C1-C2 instability
(c) Cardiac arrhythmia
(d) Foramen magnum stenosis
(e) Subaxial cervical instability

57. A 13-year-old gymnast presents with insidious low back pain and hamstring tightness. Her pain is precipitated by activity and is relieved by rest. A thorough neurologic examination is normal. A lateral radiograph of her lumbar spine is shown in Fig. 9.10. What form of motion is believed to be the principal mechanism responsible for this lesion?
(a) Repetitive axial loading
(b) Repetitive extension
(c) Acute hyperflexion
(d) Repetitive flexion with lateral rotation
(e) Acute flexion-distraction

58. What would be the most appropriate surgical treatment for the patient in question 57 if her symptoms and radiographs are unchanged after an adequate course of conservative treatment?
(a) Fusion *in situ*
(b) Laminectomy
(c) Gill procedure
(d) Instrumented fusion *in situ*
(e) Reduction and instrumented fusion

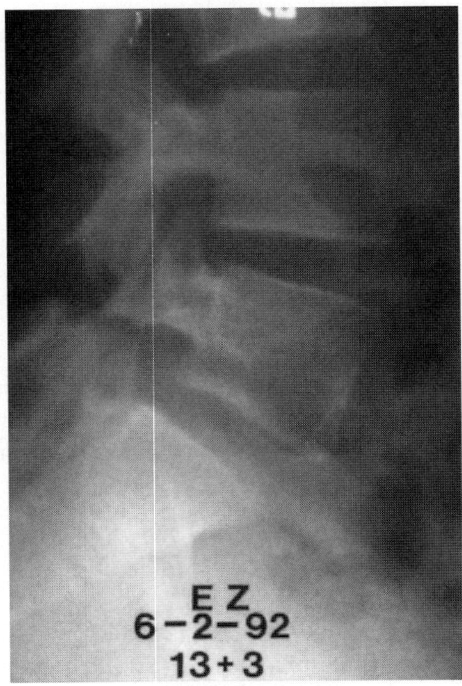

FIGURE 9.10

59. Which of the following characteristics is least commonly associated with Morquio-Brailsford syndrome?
(a) Ligamentous laxity
(b) Platyspondyly
(c) Thoracolumbar kyphosis
(d) Short stature
(e) Congenital fusion of the odontoid to the atlas

60. Which of the following disease is characterized by an Erlenmeyer flask deformity of the femoral metaphysis?
(a) Sprengel deformity
(b) Melorheostosis
(c) Osteogenesis imperfecta
(d) Dysplasia epiphysealis hemimelica
(e) Osteopoikilosis

61. Early-onset osteoarthritis of the hip is most commonly associated with which of the following conditions?
(a) Tetracycline administration before skeletal maturity
(b) Achondroplasia
(c) Meyer dysplasia
(d) Multiple epiphyseal dysplasia
(e) Down syndrome

62. Figure 9.11 represents the hip radiograph of a nonambulatory patient with spastic quadriplegia. The patient's caregiver has noted the patient's progressively compromised ability to sit upright and associated difficulty with feeding, perineal care, impending ischial and sacral skin breakdown, and compromised ability to clear pulmonary secretions. Range of motion of both hips is extremely limited, and left hip motion provokes significant discomfort. The child has had multiple soft tissue releases about the hips in the past. How should this patient be managed at this time?
    (a) Increased analgesic dosage
    (b) Left femoral shortening with varus left femoral derotational and pelvic osteotomies
    (c) Left hip arthrodesis in 90 degrees of flexion
    (d) Left subtrochanteric resection arthroplasty
    (e) Bilateral hip arthrodesis in full extension
63. A 4-year-old boy presents with multiple masses on his upper back. Physical examination reveals decreased cervical range of motion, multiple firm, nonmobile nodules on his back, and bilateral hallux valgus. Anteroposterior radiographs of the feet demonstrate bilateral delta-shaped proximal phalanges. The chest radiograph reveals mineral deposition within the paraspinal muscles. What is the most likely diagnosis?
    (a) Pseudohyperparathyroidism
    (b) Trichorhinophalangeal syndrome
    (c) Sarcoidosis
    (d) Behçet syndrome
    (e) Fibrodysplasia ossificans progressiva
64. A 16-year-old boy presents for evaluation of bilateral knee pain. A lateral radiograph is shown in Fig. 9.12. Which of the following childhood diseases is most compatible with these radiographic findings?
    (a) Hemophilia

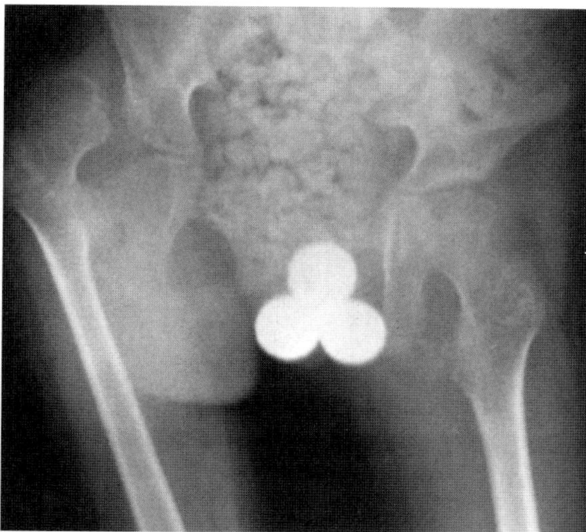

FIGURE 9.11

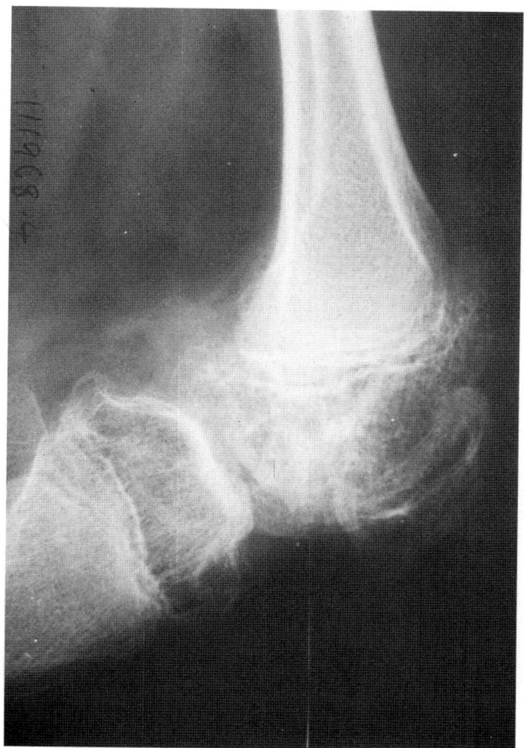

FIGURE 9.12

    (b) Congenital syphilis
    (c) Caffey disease
    (d) Fluorosis
    (e) Lead poisoning
65. A 15-year-old boy complains of thoracic back pain that is aggravated by standing, sitting, and physical activity. There is no history of trauma. He has no neurologic deficit. A lateral radiograph is shown in Fig. 9.13. What is the most likely diagnosis?
    (a) Slipped vertebral apophysis
    (b) Acute leukemia
    (c) Scheuermann disease
    (d) Thoracic disc herniation
    (e) Discitis
66. Which of the following is the most favorable prognostic factor for a patient with Legg-Calvé-Perthes disease?
    (a) Onset before 6 years of age
    (b) Maintenance of 30% of the normal height of the lateral pillar
    (c) Mild lateral subluxation with a positive Gage sign
    (d) Coxa magna
    (e) Hinge abduction
67. A 12-year-old girl scout presents with recurrent ankle "sprains" and progressive lateral hindfoot pain 3 months after an initial "twisting" injury playing volleyball. Subtalar motion is limited, and there is tenderness in the sinus tarsi. Radiographs are shown in Fig. 9.14.

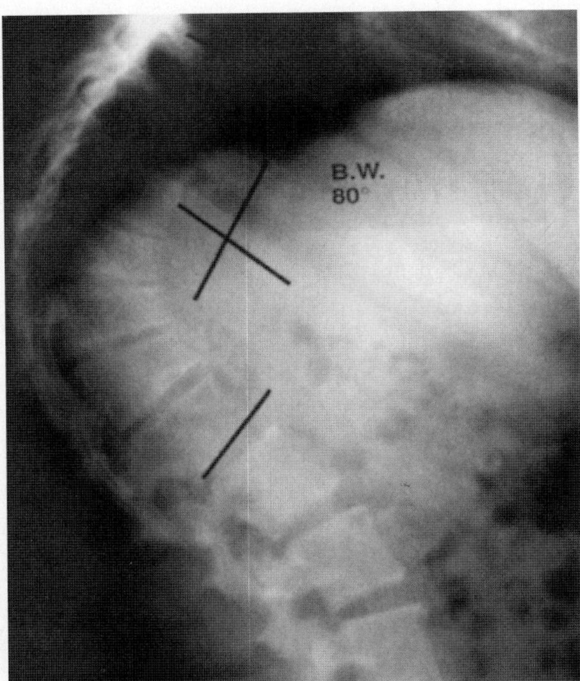

FIGURE 9.13

Her symptoms fail to resolve after 6 weeks in a short-leg walking cast. What would be the most appropriate form of intervention?
(a) Arthroscopic subtalar decompression
(b) Subtalar arthrodesis
(c) Excision with extensor digitorum brevis interposition
(d) Peroneal tenosynovectomy
(e) Triple arthrodesis

68. What type of disturbance in hip motion is most characteristic of a chronic slipped capital femoral epiphysis?
(a) Hyperextension and decreased external rotation
(b) Decreased flexion and decreased internal rotation
(c) Hyperextension and decreased adduction
(d) Decreased flexion and increased internal rotation
(e) Increased flexion and decreased internal rotation

69. Which of the following statements is true regarding pediatric cervical spine trauma?
(a) Most cervical spine trauma occurs distal to C3
(b) Atlantoaxial rotatory subluxation is associated with an identical pattern of sternocleidomastoid tightness as is encountered with congenital muscular torticollis.
(c) Spinal chord injury without radiographic abnormality is more common in skeletally immature persons than in adults.
(d) The upper limit of normal for the atlantodens interval is smaller for children than for skeletally mature persons.
(e) Anterior subluxation of the C2 vertebral body (relative to the C3 vertebral body) of 4 mm (on a lateral flexion view) mandates surgical stabilization.

70. An 8-year-old girl is brought in by her parents for evaluation because they have noticed that her knee "clunks" and "locks." There is no history of trauma. Magnetic resonance images are shown in Fig. 9.15. What is the most likely diagnosis?
(a) Osteochondritis dissecans (with an unstable fragment)
(b) Synovial chondromatosis
(c) Hypertrophic infrapatellar fat pad
(d) Congenital anterior cruciate ligament deficiency
(e) Discoid meniscus

A
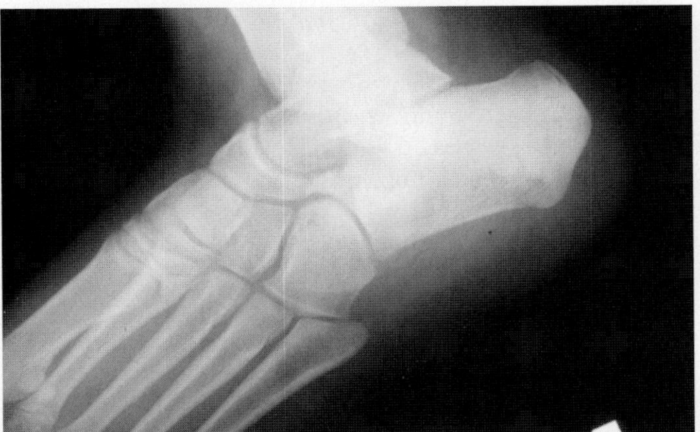

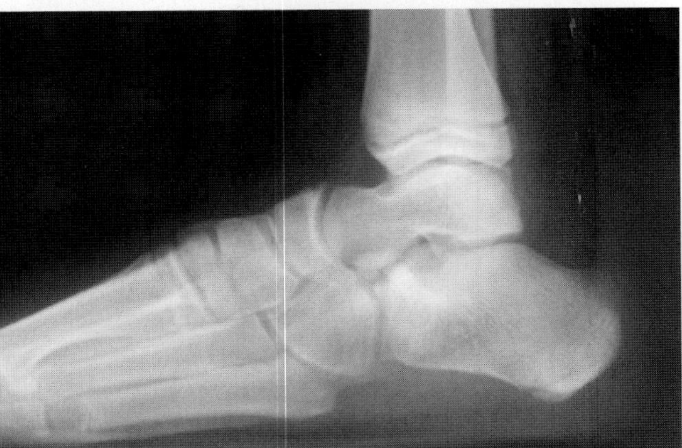
B

FIGURE 9.14A and B

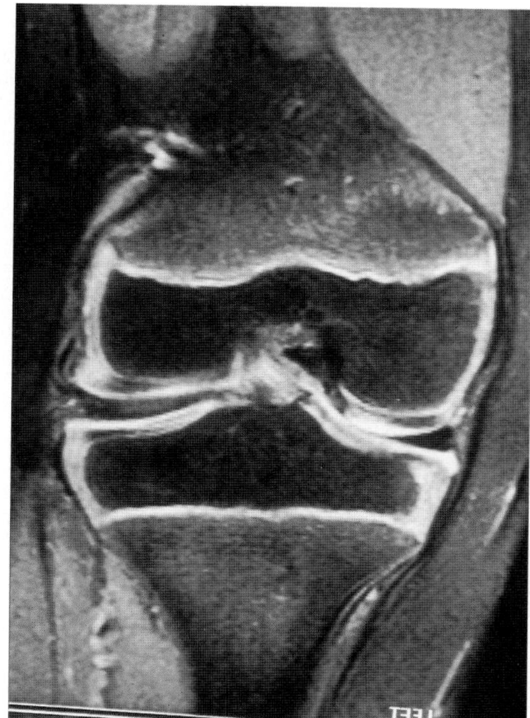

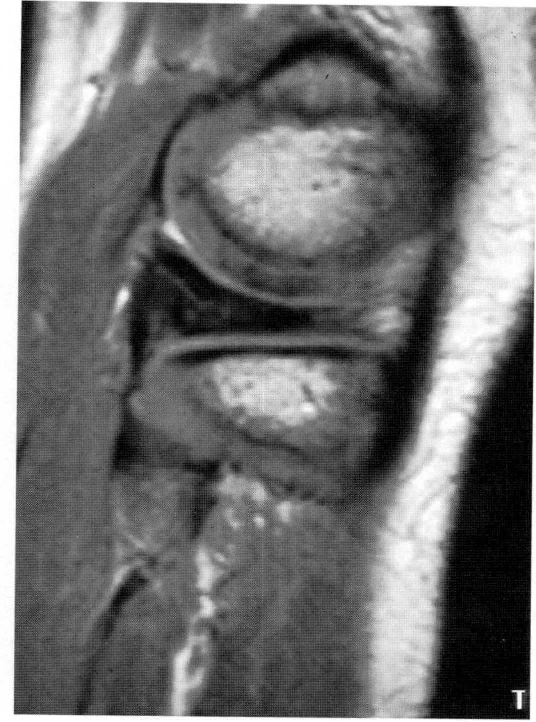

FIGURE 9.15A and B

ANSWERS

1. **e** Type X. *Collagen* is the most prevalent protein in the body. It accounts for more than 20% of total body weight, and multiple different forms exist.

   Types I to III are the *fibrillar collagens.* Type I collagen is the most prevalent form. It comprises approximately 90% of the body's collagen, and it is the principal component of bone, tendon, and skin. Type II collagen is the predominant form of collagen in cartilage, vitreous, and nucleus pulposus. Type III is common in fetal tissues, vascular wall, and intestinal tissue.

   Type IV collagen is nonfibrillar. It is associated with the lamina densa of basement membranes. Type X collagen *(short-chain collagen)* is produced by chondrocytes in the zone of hypertrophy of the growth plate. It is found exclusively in regions of active enchondral ossification, and it is believed to play a role in initiating mineralization.

   Note: Defective expression of type X collagen has been associated with metaphyseal chondrodysplasia (Schmid type).

Reference

Shumacher HR: Primer on the Rheumatic Diseases, 9th Ed. Atlanta, Arthritis Foundation, 1988.

2. **b** At birth, weight and height are abnormally low. *Morquio-Brailsford syndrome* is one of the mucopolysaccharidoses (type IV). It is an autosomal recessive disorder. Because of a lysosomal hydrolase defect, glycosaminoglycans accumulate. The enzymatic defect is different for the two subtypes of mucopolysaccharidosis type IV. Type A is produced by a lack of *N*-acetylgalactosamine-6-sulfatase activity; type B stems from decreased β-galactosidase activity. In both types, keratan sulfate and chondroitin sulfate are excreted at abnormally high levels in the urine.

   The intracellular accumulation of glycosaminoglycans disrupts connective tissue metabolism and causes abnormal skeletal formation and growth. However, at birth, weight and height are within normal limits.

   Genu valgum is the most common associated knee deformity. The genu valgum stems from irregular growth of the epiphyses of the proximal tibia and the distal femur. The most significant associated spinal abnormality is odontoid dysplasia. This is virtually a ubiquitous finding in Morquio syndrome, and the resulting C1-C2 instability commonly mandates surgical stabilization to prevent progressive myelopathy and death.

   Note: Elevated keratan sulfate excretion is unique to Morquio-Brailsford syndrome. Excretion of dermatan sulfate and heparan sulfate is elevated in Hurler syndrome (mucopolysaccharidosis type I) and Hunter syndrome (mucopolysaccharidosis type II).

Reference

Milkes M, Stanton RP: A Review of Morquio Syndrome. Am J Orthop, 26(8):533–540, 1997.

3. **e** Anterior horn cells. The neural crest gives rise to all the sensory cells of the peripheral nervous system (somatic and visceral). Additional neural crest derivatives include the adrenal medulla, sympathetic chain ganglia cells, Schwann cells, and melanocytes.

   The neural crest does not give rise to anterior horn cells. Anterior horn cells are derived from the basal plate of the neural tube.

   Note: The notochord induces overlying ectoderm to form the neural plate. The vertebral column subsequently forms around the notochord. The nucleus pulposus of each intervertebral disc is derived from notochord remnants.

Reference

Moore KL: The Developing Human: Clinically Oriented Embryology, 4th Ed. Philadelphia, WB Saunders, 1988.

4. **e** The lateral epicondyle. The approximate age of appearance for the epiphyseal ossification centers of the elbow is given in Table 9.1.

   Ossification of the respective epiphyses typically occurs earlier among girls than boys. Here are two useful mnemonics for recalling the order of appearance of the elbow ossification centers: Come Rod My Tibia On Lithium or Come Rub My Tummy Of Love.

   Note: This information has essentially no clinical relevance because most parents can tell you their child's age (without the assistance of an elbow film). However, it is precisely this lack of application to reality that renders these data relevant to board examinations. Thus, it may be worth remembering.

Reference

Rockwood CA, et al., eds: Fractures in Children, 3rd Ed. Philadelphia, JB Lippincott, p. 90, 1991.

TABLE 9.1. OSSIFICATION CENTER: AGE OF APPEARANCE

	Males	Females
Capitellum	1–2 mo	1–6 mo
Radial head	3–6 yr	3–6 yr
Medial epicondyle	5–7 yr	3–6 yr
Trochlea	8–10 yr	7–9 yr
Olecranon	8–10 yr	8–10 yr
Lateral epicondyle	12 yr	11 yr

5. **c** Wilms tumor. The neoplasm that is most commonly associated with hemihypertrophy is *Wilms tumor.* Adrenal carcinoma and hepatoblastoma are the next most frequently affiliated lesions. Because most of the neoplasms associated with hemihypertrophy occur in the abdomen, many authorities recommend that patients with hemihypertrophy should receive serial screening with abdominal ultrasound.

Reference

Ballock RT, et al.: Hemihypertrophy: Concepts and Controversies. J Bone Joint Surg Am, 79:1731–1738, 1997.

6. **d** The Heuter-Volkman principle. *Wolff law* states that bone will remodel according to the stress to which it is subjected. Bone will be deposited in regions of increased stress; bone will be resorbed in regions of decreased stress.

   The *Hueter-Volkman principle* states that excessive physeal compression will retard growth. This principle is often invoked to support the mechanical theory of the pathogenesis of Blount disease. The corollary to the Heuter-Volkman principle states that distraction across the physis will stimulate growth. The *law of Von Schwann* states that the contractile tension of a muscle diminishes as its muscle fibers shorten.

7. **b** They are rarely associated with intraarticular disease. Like their adult counterparts, most pediatric popliteal cysts occur at the posteromedial aspect of the joint. Unlike their adult counterparts, popliteal cysts in the pediatric population are rarely associated with intraarticular disease. Most cysts are asymptomatic and resolve spontaneously. Recommended treatment is observation.

   Note: Sarcomas may also produce popliteal masses in childhood. If there is any doubt regarding the diagnosis, magnetic resonance imaging is useful to differentiate a sarcoma from a popliteal cyst.

Reference

Dinham JM: Popliteal Cysts in Children: The Case Against Surgery. J Bone Joint Surg Br, 57:69–71, 1975.

8. **a** Type I collagen. *Osteogenesis imperfecta* is produced by defective expression of type I collagen. The defect may be either qualitative or quantitative. Osteogenesis imperfecta is typically transmitted in an autosomal dominant pattern. Characteristic phenotypic features include osseous fragility, ligamentous laxity, and blue sclerae.

   Note: Osteocalcin is a noncollagenous bone matrix protein. It is made by osteoblasts, and it is involved in regulating bone density.

Reference

Prockop DJ, Kivirikko KI: Heritable Diseases of Collagen. N Engl J Med, 311:376, 1984.

9. **c** Camurati-Engelmann disease. *Camurati-Engelmann* disease is an autosomal dominant dysplasia that affects the diaphyses of long bones in a symmetric fashion, with a predilection for the lower extremities. The involved diaphyses are expanded with thickened cortices and narrowed medullary cavities. These osseous findings may be associated with muscle atrophy and leg pain. The expression of this disease is quite variable.

   Hypophosphatasia is radiographically indistinguishable from rickets. Its radiographic hallmarks include flared metaphyses, bowing of long bones, and widening of the growth plates. The associated generalized osteopenia tends to be most marked in the metaphyseal regions. In addition, focal radiolucent "tongues" sometimes project into the metaphyses from affected physes.

   Pyle disease is a metaphyseal dysplasia which is characterized by *Erlenmeyer flask deformities* of the distal femora and proximal tibiae.

   Hurler disease is one of the mucopolysaccharidoses. It is associated with progressive mental retardation, hepatosplenomegaly, corneal clouding, frontal bossing, kyphoscoliosis, and generalized stunted growth. Its mode of inheritance is autosomal recessive.

Reference

Kumar B, et al.: Progressive Diaphyseal Dysplasia (Engelmann Disease). Radiology, 140:87, 1981.

10. **b** Internal tibial torsion. Metatarsus adductus, tibial torsion, and excessive femoral anteversion are all common causes of in-toeing in children. *Metatarsus adductus* is responsible for most cases of apparent in-toeing during the first year of life. This deformity is usually flexible, and it characteristically corrects spontaneously within the first few months of life.

    Among toddlers, in-toeing is most commonly caused by internal tibial torsion. *Tibial version* is defined by the angle subtended by the transcondylar axis of the distal femur and the transmalleolar axis of the ankle. *Tibial torsion* typically becomes evident when the child begins to walk. The transmalleolar axis progressively rotates laterally during growth.

    Excessive femoral anteversion is the most common source of in-toeing presenting in early childhood. Most cases of internal tibial torsion and excessive femoral anteversion correct spontaneously with growth. Corrective osteotomy is indicated on the rare occasion that severe deformity (with associated dysfunction) persists until late childhood.

    Note: Whereas excessive femoral anteversion is almost universally a bilateral phenomenon, internal tibial torsion has a greater tendency for asymmetry. Unilateral tibial torsion predominantly affects the left side.

Reference

Staheli LT: Rotational Problems in Children. J Bone Joint Surg Am, 75:939–949, 1993.

11. **c** The rib-vertebra angle is more acute on the convex side of the curve than the rib-vertebra angle on the concave side. On a posteroanterior radiograph of a scoliotic spine, the ribs on the convex side of the curve form a more acute angle with the vertebral body than those on the concave side. This occurs because the vertebral bodies are rotated toward the convexity.

    Unlike adolescent idiopathic scoliosis, *infantile idiopathic scoliosis* is more common in boys, and left thoracic curves predominate. Infantile idiopathic scoliosis has traditionally been reported to be more common in England than in North America.

    If untreated, all phase II curves (head of rib overlaps vertebra) will progress. The rib-vertebra angle difference is a useful means of predicting which phase I curves will progress. In Mehta's classic article, 83% of the nonprogressive phase I curves had an apical rib-vertebra angle difference of less than 20 degrees; 84% of the progressive phase I curves had an apical rib-vertebra angle difference of greater than 20 degrees.

    To summarize, infantile scoliosis is more common in boys, left thoracic curves predominate, it is more common in England, the rib-vertebra angle is more acute on the convex side of the curve, and all phase II curves progress. Of phase I curves with rib-vertebra angles of less than 20 degrees, only 17% progress; of phase I curves with rib-vertebra angles greater than 20 degrees, 84% progress.

Reference

Mehta MH: The Rib-Vertebra Angle in the Early Diagnosis Between Resolving and Progressive Infantile Idiopathic Scoliosis. J Bone Joint Surg Br, 54:230–243, 1972.

12. **d** Scheie syndrome. *Radial clubhand* is a preaxial deformity that is commonly associated with a variety of nonmusculoskeletal abnormalities. In contrast to radial clubhand, ulnar clubhand tends to occur without associated cardiovascular, genitourinary, gastrointestinal, or hematologic anomalies.

    Holt-Oram syndrome consists of radial clubhand with cardiac septal defects. *Fanconi syndrome* is an autosomal recessively transmitted form of aplastic pancytopenia. *TAR syndrome* refers to thrombocytopenia with absent radius. *VATER syndrome* consists of *v*entricular (or vertebral) abnormalities, imperforate *a*nus, *t*racheo*e*sophageal fistula, and *r*enal anomalies.

Scheie syndrome is a form of mucopolysaccharidosis that is associated with progressively compromised vision and digital stiffness. This syndrome has not been associated with radial clubhand.

Note: Preaxial refers to the radial side of the long finger; postaxial refers to the ulnar side of the long finger.

13. **a** 50% if the child is male; 50% if the child is female. Achondroplasia is transmitted in an autosomal dominant fashion. The chance of inheritance of an autosomal dominant trait when only one parent carries the trait is 50% regardless of sex. If both parents had the disease, the probability of the child's inheriting the condition would be 75%, assuming that both parents were heterozygotes.

Note: Approximately 85% of cases of achondroplasia arise from spontaneous mutation.

Reference

Lovell WW, Winter RB: Pediatric Orthopaedics, 2nd Ed. Philadelphia, JB Lippincott, p. 45, 1986.

14. **e** The anterolateral. Physiologic epiphysiodesis of the distal tibial physis occurs in a medial to lateral sequence. The anterolateral portion of the physis is the last to close. This sequence explains the phenomenon of the *juvenile Tillaux fracture,* which is a Salter III fracture involving the anterolateral portion of the epiphysis.

Note: The juvenile Tillaux fracture is typically produced by an external rotation mechanism. The anterolateral section of the epiphysis is displaced by the anterior tibiofibular ligament.

Reference

Von Laer L: Classification, Diagnosis and Treatment of Transitional Fractures of the Distal Part of the Tibia. J Bone Joint Surg Am, 67:687–698, 1985.

15. **c** Athetosis. Rh incompatibility (erythroblastosis fetalis) is a source of unconjugated hyperbilirubinemia. In the setting of kernicterus (severe bilirubin accumulation), bilirubin is deposited in the basal ganglia. This produces characteristic involuntary writhing (athetoid) motor dysfunction.

Note: Improvements in maternal-fetal medicine have dramatically reduced the incidence of athetoid cerebral palsy.

Reference

Lovell WW, Winter RB: Pediatric Orthopaedics, 2nd Ed. Philadelphia, JB Lippincott, p. 347, 1986.

16. **c** Diastrophic dysplasia. *Diastrophic dysplasia* is a form of short-limbed, disproportionate dwarfism. Characteristics include rigid kyphoscoliosis, multiple joint contractures, hip dislocation, "cauliflower" ear deformities, rigid clubfeet, and short digits. The *hitchhiker's thumb* deformity consists of increased carpometacarpal abduction and apparent proximal displacement of the base of the thumb (toward the wrist).

Note: Trident hands are characteristic features of achondroplasia. This refers to an inability to approximate the long and ring fingers when they are extended.

17. **d** Protected weight-bearing and progressive mobilization as tolerated. Figure 9.2 reveals an avulsion of the lesser trochanter apophysis. This injury characteristically responds favorably to conservative management.

Nonoperative management is recommended for almost all apophyseal avulsions in the pelvic region. One exception to this rule is an avulsion of the ischial apophysis in which the apophysis is displaced more than 1 to 2 cm. Some authorities recommend internal fixation of this injury to avoid weakness, ischial prominence, and resultant painful sitting.

Reference

Metzmaker JN, Pappas AM: Avulsion Fractures of the Pelvis. Am J Sports Med, 13:349–358, 1985.

18. **b** G protein (α subunit). *McCune-Albright syndrome* consists of the triad of (1) fibrous dysplasia, (2) café-au-lait spots, and (3) precocious puberty. This syndrome has been associated with a mutation in the α subunit of a G protein. The mutation produces a disturbance in signal transduction.

Note: Achondroplasia has been associated with a mutation in fibroblast growth factor receptor 3.

References

Lefkowitz RJ: G-Proteins in Medicine. N Engl J Med, 332:186, 1995.

Shiang R, et al.: Mutations in the Transmembrane Domain of FGFR3 Cause the Most Common Form of Genetic Dwarfism, Achondroplasia. Cell, 78:335–342, 1994.

19. **d** Inhibition of DNA gyrase. The quinolone antibiotics inhibit DNA gyrase. Aminoglycosides, erythromycin, and clindamycin disrupt ribosome function. The penicillins and cephalosporins inhibit peptidoglycan synthesis.

Note: Quinolone antibiotics are contraindicated in children.

20. **c** Cleidocranial dysplasia. The anteroposterior pelvis film demonstrates unilateral coxa vara and delayed ossification of the pubic bones. These findings (together with the specified clinical features) are all characteristic of *cleidocranial dysplasia.* The absence of clavicles in Fig. 9.16 confirms the diagnosis. Additional character-

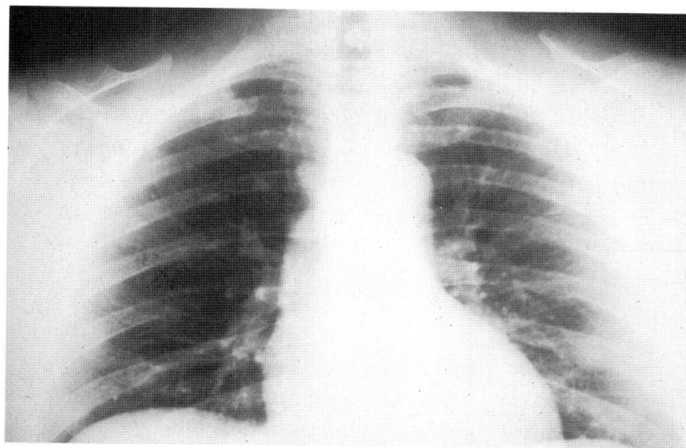

FIGURE 9.16

istics include hypoplastic scapulae, a bell-shaped thorax, wormian bone, and delayed closure of fontanelles and skull sutures. When only a portion of the clavicle is missing, it is usually the lateral segment.

Metaphyseal chondrodysplasia (Jansen type) is characterized by short-limbed dwarfism, joint contractures, osseous fragility, rachitic metaphyses (cupping and flaring), mental retardation, hypercalcemia, and a "monkeylike" stance.

Metaphyseal chondrodysplasia (McKusick type) is another form short-limbed dwarfism that resembles achondroplasia. It is characterized by light-colored attenuated hair, impaired intelligence, distal fibular overgrowth, increased susceptibility to chickenpox, rachitic metaphyses, and absence of trident hands (see question 16 discussion).

Stickler disease refers to hereditary arthroophthalmopathy. Its principal features include myopia, flattened vertebral bodies, and severe hip arthropathy.

Meyer dysplasia (dysplasia epiphysealis capitis femoris) may mimic Legg-Calvé-Perthes disease. It is characterized by delayed appearance and granularity of the femoral head ossification centers.

Reference

Jarvis JL, Keats TE: Cleidocranial Dysostosis. AJR Am J Roentgenol, 121:5, 1974.

21. **a** Equinus contracture of the ankle. Ordinarily, knee flexion is prevented by eccentric quadriceps contraction during early stance. As proximal muscle weakness evolves in *Duchenne dystrophy,* quadriceps weakness allows the knee to buckle. Ankle plantar flexion creates an extension moment at the knee and keeps the weight-bearing axis anterior to the knee center of rotation. This resists the tendency for the knee to flex.

The *Meryon sign* refers to the tendency for an affected child to slip through an examiner's hands when the child is lifted beneath the arms. It is a manifestation of shoulder girdle weakness.

The *Gower sign* describes an affected child's tendency to walk the hands up the front of the lower extremities to assist reaching a standing position. This maneuver compensates for weak hip and trunk extensors. In addition, the pressure from the hands resists knee flexion.

Increased lumbar lordosis compensates for weak hip extensors by moving the torso's center of gravity posteriorly. This is not an adaptive response for quadriceps weakness.

Note: Duchenne muscular dystrophy is an X-linked recessive disorder. Thus, it occurs almost exclusively in males, except on rare occasions when it is encountered in association with Turner syndrome.

Reference

Lovell WW, Winter RB: Pediatric Orthopaedics, 2nd Ed. Philadelphia, JB Lippincott, p. 264, 1986.

22. **b** 3 to 5 weeks. The upper extremity limb buds appear at the beginning of the fourth week (day 26 to 27), and the lower extremity limb buds appear a few days later. At each stage of development, the lower extremity lags slightly behind the upper extremity. Limb bud mesenchyme is derived from the somatic layer of the lateral mesoderm. Differentiation of the limb mesenchyme is induced according to the influence of the overlying apical ectodermal ridge. Mesenchymal condensations form the appendicular skeleton by day 33. This primordial skeleton is fully cartilaginous by the end of the sixth week. Primary ossification centers appear in the long bones during the seventh week.

Note: In contrast to trunk musculature, limb musculature is not derived from the myotomes of the somites. Rather, it forms from the limb bud mesenchyme.

Reference

Moore KL: The Developing Human: Clinically Oriented Embryology, 4th Ed. Philadelphia, WB Saunders, 1988.

23. **e** Trochanteric osteotomy. Figure 9.4 demonstrates that the patient developed iatrogenic osteonecrosis of the femoral head after a presumed open reduction. The displayed sequelae include relative overgrowth of the greater trochanter and a textbook *coxa breva* deformity with associated disturbance of abductor biomechanics. At an earlier stage, the trochanteric overgrowth could have been prevented by performing a trochanteric apophysiodesis. The best option at this point would be to improve the mechanics of the abductor mechanism by advancing the greater trochanter. Total hip arthro-

plasty may be required in the future, but it would be an inappropriate consideration given this patient's age and absence of pain.

Note: Under normal circumstances, the abductor insertion (tip of the greater trochanter) and the center of rotation of the femoral head should be at the same level.

Reference

Gage JR, Cary JM: The Effect of Trochanteric Epiphysiodesis on Growth of the Proximal End of the Femur Following Necrosis of the Capital Femoral Epiphysis. J Bone Joint Surg Am, 62:785–794, 1980.

24. **e** 80%. The distal radial physis accounts for 80% of the longitudinal growth of the radius and 40% of the longitudinal growth of the upper extremity. The contributions of the upper extremity physes to the growth of their respective bones and to the overall growth of the upper extremity are depicted in Fig. 9.17.

Reference

Rockwood CA, et al., eds: Fractures in Children, 3rd Ed. Philadelphia, JB Lippincott, p.50, 1991.

25. **c** 15%. The proximal femoral physis accounts for 30% of the longitudinal growth of the femur and 15% of the overall longitudinal growth of the lower extremity. The contributions of the lower extremity physes to the growth of their respective bones and to the overall growth of the lower extremity are depicted in Fig. 9.17.

Note: Approximately 67% of the longitudinal growth of the lower extremity occurs at the knee.

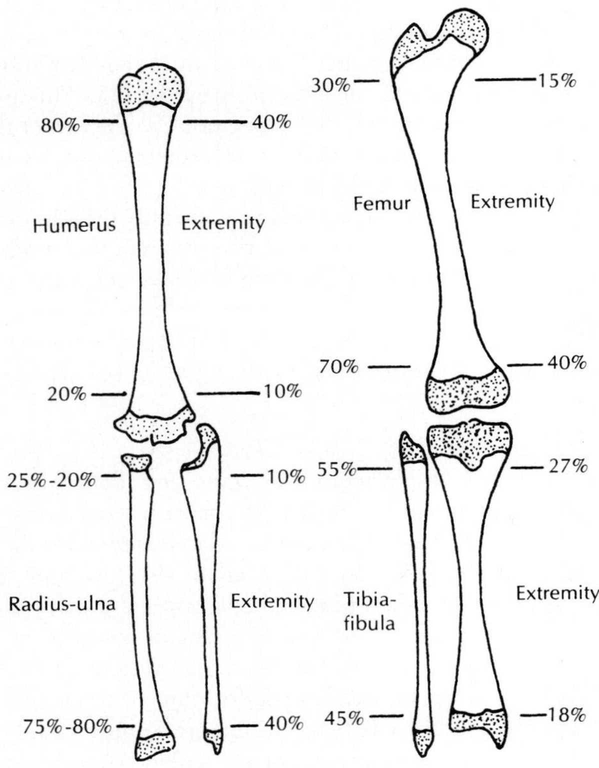

FIGURE 9.17

Reference

Rockwood CA, et al., eds: Fractures in Children, 3rd Ed. Philadelphia, JB Lippincott, p.50, 1991.

26. **a** Sling and swathe. The proximal humerus has tremendous remodeling potential in younger patients. Hence, considerable displacement and angulation may be accepted without risk of significant subsequent shortening or dysfunction. According to Beaty, up to 70-degree angulation and 100% displacement can be accepted in children younger than 5 years. Permissible displacement and angulation decrease with increasing patient age. Because of decreased remodeling potential, Beaty recommends reduction for fractures that are angulated 40 degrees or are displaced 50% in children older than 12 years. However, for the deformity specified in this question, an acceptable outcome would be expected after management with a sling and swathe.

References

Beaty JH: Fractures of the Proximal Humerus and Shaft in Children. Instr Course Lect 41:369–372, 1992.

Neer CS, Horwitz BS: Fractures of the Proximal Humeral Epiphyseal Plate. Clin Orthop, 41:24, 1965.

27. **a** *Staphylococcus aureus.* According to the 1996 pediatric *Orthopaedic Knowledge Update,* the most common pathogens in *neonatal septic arthritis* are group B *Streptococcus, S. aureus,* and gram-negative coliform bacteria. Group B *Streptococcus* is often mentioned to be the most frequent source of neonatal septic arthritis. However, in an article by Choi et al., *S. aureus* was isolated in 22 hips, gram-negative rods were found in one hip, and group B *Streptococcus* was isolated in no hips. According to Knudsen and Hoffman, *S. aureus* is the most common pathogen in neonatal osteomyelitis as well, and the hip was the most common locus for this infection.

Historically, the most commonly reported pathogen responsible for septic arthritis among young children has been *Haemophilus influenzae. S. aureus* is the most common agent in septic arthritis among older children. Gonococcus should be considered in the adolescent.

Common physical findings in neonatal septic arthritis include restricted spontaneous motion *(pseudoparalysis),* asymmetric posturing, warmth, and tenderness.

Prematurity is a risk factor. The erythrocyte sedimentation rate is an unreliable test in this age group. Blood cultures are positive in only approximately 50% of cases; joint cultures may also be negative. Arthrocentesis demonstrates a preponderance of polymorphonuclear leukocytes, but the white blood cell count may not exceed 50,000 in the neonate because of a limited inflammatory response. Technetium bone scan is often negative unless there is concomitant osteomyelitis.

Note: In the neonate, communications persist between metaphyseal and epiphyseal vessels. These serve as potential routes for the migration of pus. Thus, septic arthritis and metaphyseal osteomyelitis are more likely to coexist in the neonate than in older children and adults, in whom these vascular communications are no longer patent.

References

Choi IH, Pizzutillo PD, Bowen JR, et al: Sequelae and Reconstruction After Septic Arthritis of the Hip in Infants. J Bone Joint Surg Am, 72:1150–1165, 1990.

Knudsen CJ, Hoffman EB: Neonatal Osteomyelitis. J Bone Joint Surg Br, 72:846–851, 1990.

Richards B, ed.: Orthopaedic Knowledge Update: Pediatrics. Rosemont, Illinois, American Academy of Orthopedic Surgeons, 1996.

28. **c** Phocomelia. *Phocomelia* is a type of congenital longitudinal limb deficiency in which there is an absence of an intercalary portion of the limb (as demonstrated in Fig. 9.5). In its most extreme form, this type of deformity consists of a normal hand attached to a normal shoulder without any intervening segment *(seal limb).*

Rhizomelic shortening pertains to shortening of the proximal limb segments (arms or thighs). Achondroplasia (the most common cause of dwarfism) manifests a rhizomelic pattern. *Mesomelic shortening* pertains to shortening of the middle region of a limb (forearm or leg). *Acromelic shortening* pertains to shortening of the most distal aspect of a limb (hands or feet).

Note: The mutagenic effect of thalidomide is a notorious source of phocomelia.

29. **b** Anterolateral. Congenital anterolateral tibial bowing is often the earliest sign of *neurofibromatosis.* This type of bow is frequently associated with a congenital pseudarthrosis of the tibia. Although approximately 50% of patients with tibial pseudarthrosis will ultimately be diagnosed with neurofibromatosis, only approximately 10% of patients with neurofibromatosis develop congenital pseudarthrosis of the tibia.

Congenital posteromedial tibial bowing is a relatively benign phenomenon. Its natural history typically follows a pattern of spontaneous correction with subtotal resolution of the associated limb-length discrepancy. This type of bow is typically associated with a calcaneovalgus hindfoot deformity.

Anteromedial tibial bowing is characteristically associated with fibular hemimelia. *Fibular hemimelia* is the most common congenital long bone deficiency. An easy way to remember this association is *AM-FM* (*a*ntero*m*edial–*f*ibular hemi*m*elia).

Note: Anterolateral tibial bowing with congenital pseudarthrosis is often associated with ipsilateral limb shortening and a dorsiflexion deformity of the hindfoot.

References

Boyd HB: Pathology and Natural History of Congenital Pseudarthrosis of the Tibia. Clin Orthop, 166:5–13, 1982.

Epps CH, Schneider PL: Treatment of Hemimelias of the Lower Extremity: Long-Term Results. J Bone Joint Surg Am, 71:273–277, 1989

30. **a** *Salmonella.* Discerning the source of bone pain in patients with sickle cell disease may be perplexing because of the difficulty in differentiating acute bone infarction from osteomyelitis.

Salmonella has traditionally been cited as the principal organism responsible for osteomyelitis in this immunocompromised population. However, a study by Epps et al. questioned the validity of this generalization. The osseous cultures in this study isolated *Staphylococcus aureus* in eight of the 15 patients. *Salmonella* was isolated in six of the remaining seven cases.

In a subsequent review by Piehl et al., 15 of 16 cases were caused by *Salmonella,* a finding supporting the traditional concept that *Salmonella* is the most common infecting organism in the setting of sickle cell disease.

Do not be surprised if someday (on a standardized test that mattered more than this one) you are confronted with the nebulous task of having to choose between *S. aureus* and *Salmonella* as answers to this question.

Note: Pseudomonas is a commonly reported pathogen in cases of plantar puncture wounds. This situation typically involves a nail through a sneaker. *Pseudomonas* is often cultured from the penetrated sneaker.

References

Epps CH, et al.: Osteomyelitis in Patients Who Have Sickle-Cell Disease: Diagnosis and Management. J Bone Joint Surg Am, 73:1281–1292, 1991.

Jarvis JG, Skipper J: Pseudomonas Osteochondritis Complicating Puncture Wounds in Children. J Pediatr Orthop, 14:755–759, 1994.

Piehl FC, et al.: Osteomyelitis in Sickle-Cell Disease. J Pediatr Orthop, 13:225–227, 1993.

31. **e** Lateral closing wedge osteotomy of the proximal tibia. Figure 9.6 demonstrates a case of *Blount disease* in an adolescent. Management goals include (1) prevention of future deformity and (2) correction of existing deformity. A hip-knee-ankle-foot orthosis may be effi-

cacious for patients less than 4 years of age, but it has no role in Blount disease in adolescents.

Epiphysiodesis of the entire proximal tibial physis would prevent progression of the tibial deformity, but it would not correct the undesirable preexisting varus tibiofemoral alignment. A medial tibial hemiepiphysiodesis would cause progression of the varus deformity.

Kline and colleagues reported that varus alignment of the distal femur sometimes coexists with the tibia vara. However, no femoral varus is evident on this radiograph. A closing lateral wedge osteotomy of the distal femur could correct the overall varus tibiofemoral alignment, but there would be residual joint-line obliquity. A lateral tibial hemiepiphysiodesis may be a valid consideration for an adolescent with a significant amount of remaining growth, but correction by this method is less predictable than osteotomy.

The most appropriate intervention for this patient would be a valgus osteotomy of the proximal tibia. Oblique and dome osteotomies have been advocated (in place of a lateral closing wedge osteotomy) because of their respective abilities to provide multiplanar correction and to avoid limb shortening. Gradual correction with an external fixator has also been effectively employed.

Note: Significant recurrent deformity is sometimes encountered after adequate surgical correction of infantile Blount disease. The medial aspect of the proximal tibial physis is abnormal in both adolescent and infantile Blount disease. However, significant recurrent deformity is much less likely to be seen in the adolescent variety of this disease. The reason is that the adolescent has less growth remaining.

References

Kline SC, et al.: Femoral Varus: An Important Component in Late-Onset Blount's Disease. J Pediatr Orthop, 12:197–206, 1992.

Martin SD, et al.: Proximal Tibial Osteotomy with Compression Plate Fixation for Tibia Vara. J Pediatr Orthop, 14:619–622, 1994.

32. **d** 3 years. According to the work of Salenius and Vankka, normal tibiofemoral alignment is approximately 15 degrees varus at birth. This characteristically corrects to neutral by approximately 18 months. Maximum physiologic valgum is typically seen at age 3.

Reference

Salenius P, Vankka E: The Development of the Tibiofemoral Angle in Children. J Bone Joint Surg Am, 57:260, 1975.

33. **c** Four. The axis (C2) typically manifests four separate ossification centers at birth (one body, two neural arches, one dens). The atlas and the subaxial vertebrae manifest only three ossification centers at birth. The odontoid is believed to be phylogenetically derived from the C1 body.

At birth, the linear radiolucencies (synchondroses) between the four ossification centers of C2 form a radiographic H-shaped pattern on an open-mouth view. These radiolucencies should not be mistaken for fracture lines. The horizontal component of the H is formed by the vestigial C1-2 intervertebral disc space (at the base of the odontoid). The dens typically fuses with the C2 body when the child is 3 to 6 years old. The neural arches characteristically unite with the body and dens at the same age. However, a horizontal line may be radiographically evident at the base of the dens until the age of 11 years, and this may mimic a nondisplaced type III odontoid fracture.

Note: A fifth ossification center appears at the tip of the odontoid postnatally. This *summit ossification center* typically appears between 3 to 6 years and fuses with the rest of the dens by the age of 12 years.

Reference

Rockwood CA, Wilkins KE, Beaty JH, eds: Fractures in Children, 4th Ed. Philadelphia, Lippincott–Raven, 1996.

34. **b** Inferior lens subluxation. The type of lens subluxation *(ectopia lentis)* associated with Marfan syndrome occurs in a superior direction. This deformity occurs *in utero.* This should be distinguished from the inferior lens subluxation associated with homocystinuria.

References

Brenton DP, et al.: Homocystinuria and Marfan's Syndrome: A Comparison. J Bone Joint Surg Br, 54:277, 1972.

Keenan NJ, et al.: Orthopedic Aspects of the Marfan Phenotype. Clin Orthop, 277:251–261, 1992.

35. **b** Congenital vertical talus. This situation demonstrates characteristic findings of *congenital vertical talus.* These include hindfoot plantar flexion, medial deviation of the talar head, forefoot abduction, and dorsiflexion at the transverse tarsal joint with displacement of the navicular onto the dorsolateral aspect of the talar head. The longitudinal axis of the talus assumes a vertical orientation and becomes virtually parallel with the tibia. Contracture of the Achilles tendon is an integral component of this deformity, but the talocalcaneal angle will characteristically demonstrate that talar plantar flexion exceeds calcaneal plantar flexion. These abnormal relationships are rigid. Serial casting is unsuccessful. Surgical correction is required to achieve a plantigrade foot.

Although congenital vertical talus may occur as an isolated abnormality, it commonly occurs in association with developmental dysplasia of the hip (DDH) or underlying neuromuscular disease such as diastematomyelia or myelomeningocele.

Note: Overzealous manipulation of congenital clubfoot may produce an iatrogenic "rocker-bottom" foot that may simulate congenital vertical talus.

Reference

Drennan JC: Congenital Vertical Talus. J Bone Joint Surg Am, 77:1916–1923, 1995.

36. **d** Gaucher disease. *Gaucher disease* is an autosomal recessive disorder that is caused by a deficiency of glucocerebrosidase. The must significant orthopaedic sequela of Gaucher disease is avascular necrosis of the femoral head. Other orthopaedic manifestations of this disease include periostitis and widened distal femoral metaphyses producing an "Erlenmeyer flask" appearance. (An Erlenmeyer flask appearance is also observed in osteopetrosis.)

Niemann-Pick disease (type A) results from a sphingomyelinase deficiency. *Ehlers-Danlos syndrome* is a heterogeneous group of disorders, but certain subtypes have been associated with defective lysyl hydroxylase expression.

Hunter syndrome is a mucopolysaccharidosis that results from a deficiency in l-iduronosulfate sulfatase. *Sanfilippo syndrome* is a mucopolysaccharidosis that results from a deficiency in heparan-*N*-sulfatase.

Note: All the mucopolysaccharidoses are autosomal recessive except Hunter syndrome, which is X-linked recessive.

Reference

Evans CH, Robbins PD: Possible Orthopaedic Applications of Gene Therapy. J Bone Joint Surg Am, 77:1103–1114, 1995.

37. **d** Inhibition of presynaptic acetylcholine exocytosis at the myoneural junction. Selective muscle injections with *botulinum A toxin* have been used to reduce spasticity in cerebral palsy. The pharmacologic mechanism behind the paralyzing effect of botulinum A toxin is to inhibit the exocytosis of acetylcholine from the presynaptic side of the myoneural junction.

Reference

Koman LA, et al.: Management of Cerebral Palsy with Botulinum-A Toxin: Preliminary Investigation. J Pediatr Orthop, 13:489–495, 1993.

38. **e** Reduction and transphyseal fixation with crossed pins. Not all knee injuries in football players are anterior cruciate ligament or medial collateral ligament tears, particularly in the skeletally immature patient. Figure 9.8 demonstrates a Salter-Harris type III fracture of the distal femoral physis.

Collateral ligament injuries are rare in children. The collateral ligaments insert on the femoral epiphysis and transfer varus and valgus loads to the distal femoral physis.

The distal femoral physis is vulnerable to growth disturbance. Anatomic reduction must be achieved and maintained. Cast treatment may be considered for stable injuries. Transphyseal fixation with two crossed smooth Steinmann pins is recommended for unstable Salter-Harris type I injuries. Salter-Harris type II fractures may be fixed with a single metaphyseal screw parallel to the physis. However, if the size of the Thurston-Holland fragment is too small, then the treatment is the same as for unstable type I lesions.

Note: The presence of a bloody effusion suggests the possibility of an associated intraarticular injury. Fixation of the physeal injury would remain the priority in such a situation. However, subsequent arthroscopy or magnetic resonance imaging should be considered to evaluate the cruciate ligaments and menisci. Stanitski and associates reported their arthroscopic findings on a cohort of 70 children with acute knee hemarthroses: 47% had meniscal tears, and 47% had anterior cruciate ligament tears, many of which were partial.

References

Beaty JH, Kumar A: Fractures About the Knee on Children. J Bone Joint Surg Am, 76:1870–1880, 1994.
Stanitski CL, et al.: Observations on Acute Knee Hemarthrosis in Children and Adolescents. J Pediatr Orthop , 13:506–510, 1993.
Tolo V: Distal Femoral Metaphyseal and Physeal Fractures. In Green N, Swiotkowski M, eds: Skeletal Trauma in Children, 2nd Ed. Philadelphia, WB Saunders, 1998.

39. **b** Diastrophic dysplasia. Most of the dwarfing dysplasias that have defined inheritance patterns demonstrate autosomal dominant transmission. These include achondroplasia, cleidocranial dysplasia, chondrodysplasia punctata, Kneist syndrome, mesomelic dwarfism, metaphyseal chondrodysplasia (Jansen and Schmid types), and multiple epiphyseal dysplasia.

Exceptions to this generalization include McKusick type metaphyseal chondrodysplasia and diastrophic dysplasia, which are both autosomal recessive. Conversely, most of the dwarfing dystrophies (such as the mucopolysaccharidoses) are autosomal recessive.

Note: Dystrophy implies a systemic metabolic disturbance, frequently an enzymatic deficiency. *Dysplasia* implies an intrinsic alteration in skeletal tissue.

Reference

Stelling FH, Rothenberg D: Bone Dysplasias. In Lovell WW, Winter RB, eds: Pediatric Orthopaedics, 2nd Ed. Philadelphia, JB Lippincott, p. 45, 1986.

40. **c** The hypertrophic zone. The structure of the *zone of hypertrophy* compromises its ability to resist shearing, bending, and tension. This zone is composed of

enlarged chondrocytes and relatively sparse intercellular matrix. Provisional calcification occurs within the metaphyseal region of this zone. Failure of the physis typically occurs through this zone. Specifically, fracture lines propagate along the junction of provisionally calcified chondrocytes and those that are not yet calcified.

Reference

Salter RB, Harris WR: Injuries Involving the Epiphyseal Plate. J Bone Joint Surg Am, 45:587–682, 1963.

41. **a** Absence of filiform papillae on the tongue. *Familial dysautonomia (Riley-Day syndrome)* is an inherited (autosomal recessive) sensory and autonomic neuropathy. This disease occurs almost exclusively within the Ashkenazi Jewish population. Characteristics of the syndrome include the absence of fungiform papillae on the tongue (pathognomonic), postural hypotension, relative indifference to pain, labile blood pressure, decreased tearing, poor temperature modulation, dysphagia, gastric reflux, hyperemesis (with vomiting crises), recurrent aspiration pneumonia, emotional lability, apneic spells, absence of deep tendon reflexes, ataxia (with frequent falls), kyphosis or scoliosis (the primary orthopaedic complication), frequent fractures, and Charcot joints.

    Pathologic findings include decreased populations of sympathetic ganglion neurons and dorsal root ganglion cells. The number of myelinated neurons is normal, but the number of nonmyelinated neurons is decreased.

Reference

Albanese SA, Bobechko WP: Spine Deformity in Familial Dysautonomia. J Pediatr Orthop, 7:179–183, 1987.

42. **e** Ophthalmologic referral. Pauciarticular juvenile rheumatoid arthritis is commonly associated with *iridocyclitis* (approximately 30%). The consequences of iridocyclitis are often more devastating than those of the arthritis itself. In fact, it is a potential source of blindness. Ophthalmologic referral for periodic slit-lamp examination is mandatory. Polyarticular juvenile rheumatoid arthritis is less commonly associated with iridocyclitis.

    Most forms of childhood arthritis, including pauciarticular and polyarticular juvenile rheumatoid arthritis, occur more commonly in girls than boys. Childhood ankylosing spondylitis, like its adult counterpart, is more common in males. Rheumatoid factor is rarely positive in juvenile rheumatoid arthritis.

    Note: Still disease refers to an acute presentation of juvenile rheumatoid arthritis with severe systemic manifestations including fever, rash, and splenomegaly.

Reference

Schaller JG, et al.: The Association of Antinuclear antibodies with the Chronic Iridocyclitis of Juvenile Rheumatoid Arthritis. Arthritis Rheum, 17:409, 1974.

43. **d** A unilateral fully segmented hemivertebra with a contralateral bar. A unilateral unsegmented bar with a contralateral hemivertebra causes the most progressive type of congenital scoliosis. According to Winter and colleagues, this type of curve may progress at a rate of 10 to 12 degrees per year.

    The next most rapidly progressive types of congenital scoliosis are those caused by (1) an isolated unilateral unsegmented bar followed by (2) two convex hemivertebrae. A *block vertebra* refers to a balanced defect created by bilateral failure of segmentation.

    Note: In general, congenital scoliosis curves caused by defects in segmentation (bars) are associated with more rapid progression than those caused by defects in formation (hemivertebrae). In contrast, congenital kyphosis resulting from a defect of formation has a much worse prognosis than that caused by a defect in segmentation. Congenital kyphosis mandates surgical intervention. Prevention of paraplegia is the primary goal.

Reference

Winter RB, Lonstein JE, Boachie-Adjei O: Congenital Spinal Deformity. J Bone Joint Surg Am, 78:300–311, 1996.

44. **c** Slipped capital femoral epiphysis. In general, processes that increase the height of the hypertrophic zone of the physis (such as excess growth hormone) compromise its resistance to shear. The precise pathophysiology underlying the association between *slipped capital femoral epiphysis* and *hypothyroidism* remains to be determined. Hypothyroidism retards osseous development. Specifically, it delays the appearance of secondary ossification centers and delays physeal closure.

    Hypothyroidism may simulate Perthes disease because of its propensity to cause a fragmented ossification pattern in secondary ossification centers *(epiphyseal dysgenesis)*. However, in the setting of hypothyroidism, the multicentric ossification in the femoral head is not an avascular phenomenon. The cause of arthrogryposis multiplex congenita is unknown.

    Note: Calcium pyrophosphate dihydrate crystal deposition has been associated with hypothyroidism in adults.

References

Puri R, et al.: Slipped Upper Femoral Epiphysis and Primary Juvenile Hypothyroidism. J Bone Joint Surg Br, 67:14, 1985.
Wells D, et al: Review of Slipped Capital Femoral Epiphysis Associated With Endocrine Disease. J Pediatr Orthop, 13:610–614, 1993.

45. **d** At 4 months. The ossification center of the femoral capital epiphysis characteristically appears at 4 months of age. Absence of the ossific nucleus of the femoral head limits the utility of plain radiography in the neonate. Hence, ultrasonography has evolved into the imaging modality of choice for the detection and management of DDH in this population.

Note: Delayed ossification of the femoral capital epiphysis may herald avascular necrosis in the setting of DDH.

References

Garvey M, et al.: Radiographic Screening at Four Months of Infants at Risk for Congenital Hip Dislocation. J Bone Joint Surg Br, 74:704–707, 1992.
Harcke HT: Imaging in Congenital Dislocation and Dysplasia of the Hip. Clin Orthop, 281:22–28, 1992.

46. **e** Flexion-extension views of the cervical spine. The radiograph demonstrates a left-sided *Sprengel deformity.* The principal components of this congenital anomaly include scapular elevation, medial rotation of the inferior scapular pole, and varying degrees of atrophy of the scapula and parascapular musculature. It is commonly associated with *Klippel-Feil syndrome.*

The Sprengel deformity will not improve with physical therapy. When the deformity and dysfunction are unacceptable, surgical intervention is necessary. However, because of the association with Klippel-Feil syndrome, the cervical spine should be assessed before any scapular surgery is undertaken. Congenital cervical fusions have been associated with hypermobility at adjacent unfused segments with resultant radiculopathy, myopathy, and quadriplegia.

Note: The presence of an osseous connection between the scapula and the cervical (or upper thoracic) vertebrae is referred to as an *omovertebral bone.*

References

Hall JE, et al.: Instability of the Spine and Neurologic Involvement in Klippel-Feil Syndrome. J Bone Joint Surg Am, 72:460–462, 1990.
Leibovic SJ, Ehrlich MG, Zaleske DJ: Sprengel Deformity. J Bone Joint Surg Am, 72:192–197, 1990.

47. **d** Progressive adduction. Surgical arthrodesis of the glenohumeral joint can yield significant functional improvement in children with brachial plexus palsies. A tendency for progressive radiographic loss of abduction after fusion has been noted by several authors. This loss of abduction has been attributed to asymmetric growth at the proximal humeral physis with resultant downward bending of the arm. Loss of abduction has not been a universal finding among children who have undergone glenohumeral arthrodesis for shoulder paralysis.

Reference

White JI, Hoffer MM, Lehman M: Arthrodesis of the Paralytic Shoulder. J Pediatr Orthop, 9:684–686, 1989.

48. **d** Zone of proliferation. Achondroplasia is a defect of endochondral ossification. The disease has its predominant effect at the *zone of proliferation,* where it causes a relative lack of cartilage production. The term *achondroplasia* is actually a misnomer because there is not a complete absence of cartilage production.

Intramembranous bone production, conversely, proceeds normally. Thus, the diaphyses of long bones have relatively normal width despite their altered length. The proximal segments of the limbs are most severely affected *(rhizomelic micromelia).*

49. **a** Figure-of-eight strap until the patient's discomfort resolves. The medial clavicular epiphysis does not appear until the age of approximately 18 to 20 years, and it does not fuse with the shaft until approximately 23 to 25 years of age. Because of the strong capsular attachments onto the medial clavicular epiphysis, most apparent "posterior sternoclavicular dislocations" in skeletally immature patients are, in fact, medial clavicular physeal injuries rather than dislocations.

Closed reduction should be attempted in all patients with acute (less than 10 days old) posteriorly displaced physeal injuries. However, if closed reduction is unsuccessful, these injuries may be treated conservatively, provided the patient has no symptoms suggesting mediastinal compromise. Most of the deformity associated with the injury will generally be eliminated as the clavicle grows and remodels.

Note: The medial clavicular epiphysis is the last epiphysis to ossify, and the medial clavicular physis is the last physis to close.

Reference

Wirth MA, Rockwood CA: Acute and Chronic Traumatic Injuries of the Sternoclavicular Joint. J Am Acad Orthop Surg, 4(5):268–278, 1996.

50. **a** It is the angle subtended by the physeal line of the lateral condyle and the long axis of the humerus. Refer to Fig. 9.18. The *Baumann angle* is a useful landmark for evaluating the adequacy of reduction of pediatric elbow fractures. In younger patients, the value of the Baumann angle approximates the carrying angle (the humeral-ulnar angle), but this similarity does not hold for older children.

Reference

Rockwood CA, Wilkins KE, Beaty JH, eds: Fractures in Children, 4th Ed. Philadelphia, Lippincott–Raven, 1996.

51. **e** 16 degrees. Based on the recommendations of Levine and Drennan, the cutoff value for diagnosing *Blount*

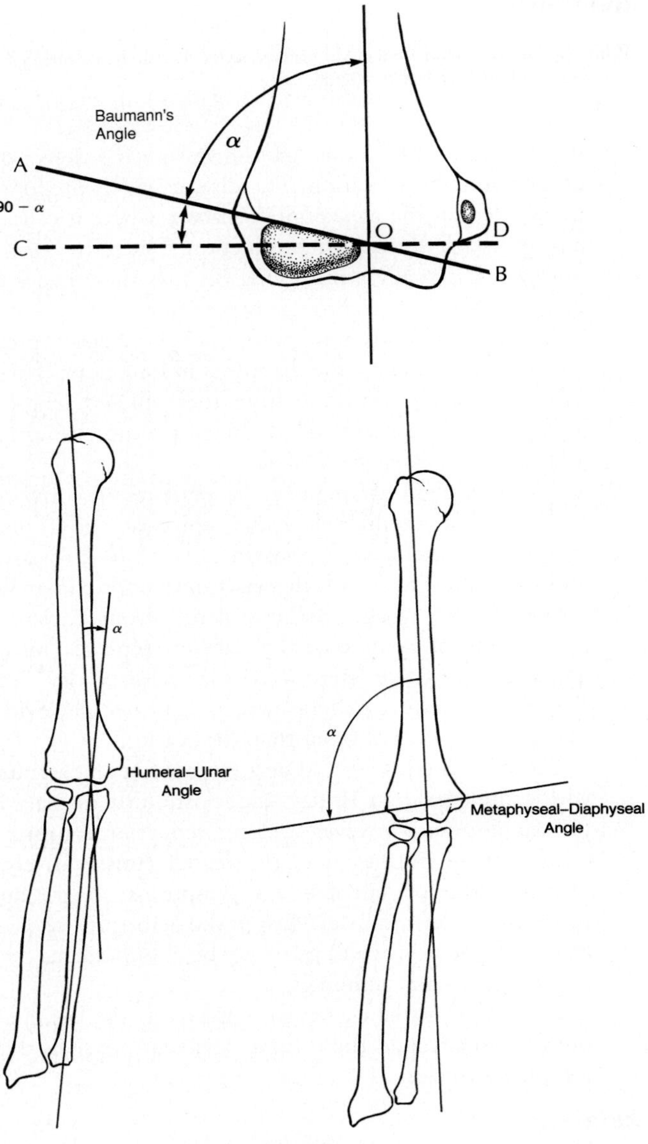

FIGURE 9.18

disease has traditionally been 11 degrees. However, a study by Feldman and Schoenecker demonstrated a 33% incidence of false-positive results and a 9% incidence of false-negative results when the threshold used was 11 degrees; 37% of the 179 extremities with physiologic bowing demonstrated a metaphyseal-diaphyseal angle of 11 degrees (or greater) at the time of presentation. A value of 16 degrees provided significantly improved accuracy (5% error). Using this value, only 5% of patients with physiologic bowing (as opposed to 33%) would receive bracing unnecessarily.

Note: According to the same investigation, a value of less than 9 degrees provided 95% accuracy in excluding the diagnosis of infantile Blount disease.

References

Feldman MD, Schoenecker PL: Use of the Metaphyseal-Diaphyseal Angle in the Evaluation of Bowed Legs. J Bone Joint Surg Am, 75:1602–1609, 1993.

Levine AM, Drennan JC: Physiological Bowing and Tibia Vara: The Metaphyseal-Diaphyseal Angle in the Measurement of Bowleg Deformities. J Bone Joint Surg Am, 64:1158–1163, 1982.

52. **a** Osteophyte formation at the margin of the pseudoacetabulum. Anatomic changes that may block reduction in this setting include the *hourglass deformity* in which the hip capsule becomes narrowed and forms an isthmus where the iliopsoas crosses. This was the most common intraoperative finding (52.4% of hips) in Scaglietti and Calandriello's classic article. The term *limbus* describes a coalescence of the inverted labrum and capsule. Other possible obstructions include hypertrophy of the pulvinar, ligamentum terres, and transverse acetabular ligament. Osteophyte formation is a late (degenerative) sequela that would be an uncommon finding in the dislocated hip of a 3-year-old child.

Reference

Scaglietti O, Calandriello B: Open Reduction of Congenital Reduction of the Hip. J Bone Joint Surg Br, 44(2):257–283, 1962.

53. **b** Hip spica cast for 4 to 6 weeks. Treatment of pediatric femur fractures is dictated by age. Between the ages of 0 and 2 years, treatment consists of a hip spica cast (preceded by 3 to 10 days of skin traction if the fracture is shortened more than 2 to 3 cm). Between the ages of 3 and 5 years, treatment is also a hip spica cast (preceded by skeletal traction if shortened more than 2 cm). Treatment of children between the ages of 6 and 11 years is controversial. Good results have been reported for spica casting, external fixation, flexible intramedullary nailing, and compression plating. Children 12 years old and older can be treated with femoral traction, a locked intramedullary nail, an external fixator, or a compression plate.

    Operative fixation is favored in instances when there is an associated closed-head injury or polytrauma. Treatment must be individualized, taking into account age, fracture type, social, and psychologic factors.

Reference

Beaty JH: Femoral-Shaft Fractures in Children and Adolescents. J Am Acad Orthop Surg, 3(4):207–217, 1995.

54. **c** Hindfoot valgus, abduction at the midtarsal joints, plantar flexion of the talus, and metatarsus adductus. *Scewfoot* is a variant of metatarsus adductus. This Z-shaped configuration is typically flexible. Operative correction is generally required.

Reference

Staheli LT: Rotational Problems in Children. J Bone Joint Surg Am, 75:939–949, 1993.

55. **b** Salter-Harris III on anteroposterior view; Salter-Harris II on lateral view. On the anteroposterior view, the epiphyseal fracture line is evident, but the metaphyseal fracture line is not typically visible because its plane is perpendicular to the direction of the beam. On the lateral view, the metaphyseal fracture line is evident, but the epiphyseal fracture line is not typically visible. Please refer to Fig. 9.19.

Reference

Rockwood CA, Wilkins KE, Beaty JH, eds: Fractures in Children, 4th Ed. Philadelphia, Lippincott–Raven, 1996.

Von Laer L: Classification, Diagnosis and Treatment of Transitional Fractures of the Distal Part of the Tibia. J Bone Joint Surg Am, 67:687–698, 1985.

56. **d** Foramen magnum stenosis. Achondroplasia is associated with decreased interpedicular distance and shortened pedicle length. These phenomena produce lumbar spinal stenosis. The defect in endochondral ossification may also produce stenosis of the foramen magnum. Resultant brainstem compression is a reported cause of paralysis, apnea, and potential death.

Note: Achondroplasia is not characteristically associated with atlantoaxial instability. This is an exception among the dwarfing conditions. C1-C2 instability is a common feature among most other forms of dwarfism (e.g., pseudoachondroplasia, metatrophic dysplasia, Kneist syndrome, Morquio-Brailsford syndrome, chondrodysplasia punctata, spondyloepiphyseal dysplasia, and metaphyseal chondrodysplasia).

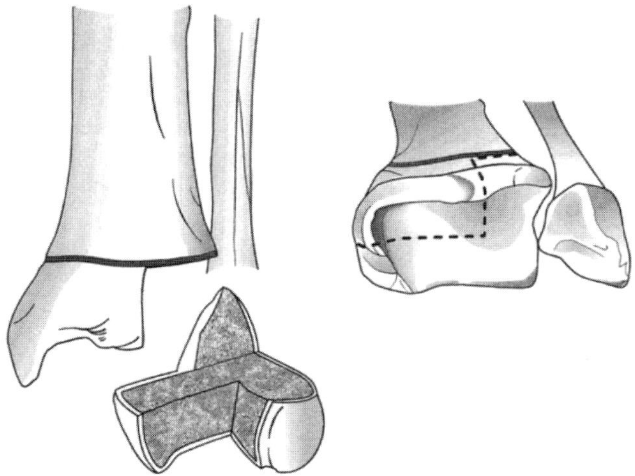

FIGURE 9.19

References

Pauli RM, et al.: Apnea and Sudden Unexpected Death in Infants With Achondroplasia. J Pediatr, 104:342, 1984.

Wynne-Davis R, et al.: Achondroplasia and Hypochondroplasia: Clinical Variation and Spinal Stenosis. J Bone Joint Surg Br, 63:508, 1981.

57. **b** Repetitive extension. The radiograph demonstrates *isthmic spondylolysis* with a grade I spondylolisthesis. Isthmic spondylolysis is produced by a stress fracture of the pars interarticularis. The putative mechanism of fatigue is repetitive hyperextension.

An increased incidence has been noted among female gymnasts, football linemen, and weightlifters. (These are the favorite activities of affected patients on standardized tests.)

Note: Chance fractures are produced by an acute combination of flexion and distraction. These are characteristically produced by rapid deceleration with seat-belt use.

Reference

Letts M, et al.: Fracture of the Pars Interarticularis in Adolescent Athletes: A Clinical-Biomechanical Analysis. J Pediatr Orthop, 6:40–46, 1986.

58. **a** Fusion *in situ*. Adolescents with symptomatic spondylolisthesis (pain or tight hamstrings) are at greater risk for experiencing progression than adolescents with asymptomatic spondylolisthesis. Other risk factors for progression include female gender, presentation at an early age, increased slip magnitude (higher than grade II), and dysplastic (as opposed to isthmic) spondylolisthesis. Affected patients require close radiographic and clinical follow-up until skeletal maturity.

Operative treatment is indicated when nonoperative measures (activity modification and bracing) fail. The preferred form of intervention for recalcitrant grade I slips consists of *in situ* arthrodesis. Fusion should consist of bilateral transverse process fusion from L5 to S1. Employing this technique, fusion rates exceed 90% without the assistance of instrumentation. Extension of the fusion to L4 is recommended for grade III or IV lesions that are associated with significant sagittal vertebral body rotation.

The *Gill procedure* consists of complete excision of the posterior spinal elements. This procedure should not be performed (in isolation) to treat adolescent spondylolisthesis because of its potential to increase instability.

Surgical reduction is associated with a significant risk of neurologic complications. Correction of the sagittal rotation and displacement may be considered for high-grade slips, but it is inappropriate for low-grade lesions.

Note: Wiltse et al. recommended that activities need not be restricted for asymptomatic grade I slips.

References

Hensinger RN: Spondylolysis and Spondylolisthesis in Children and Adolescents. J Bone Joint Surg Am, 71:1098–1106, 1989.
Wiltse LL, et al.: Fatigue Fracture: The Basic Lesion in Isthmic Spondylolisthesis. J Bone Joint Surg Am, 57:17–22, 1975.

59. **e** Congenital fusion of the odontoid to the atlas. *Morquio syndrome (mucopolysaccharidosis IV)* stems from a lysosomal hydrolase defect that causes an abnormal accumulation of glycosaminoglycans. The accumulation of glycosaminoglycans, in turn, alters normal cartilage and ligament formation. This causes ligamentous laxity and compromises growth. Faulty vertebral body growth produces platyspondyly and a characteristic anterior beaklike projection from involved vertebral bodies. Vertebral wedging, disc narrowing, and ligamentous laxity contribute to the propensity for thoracolumbar kyphosis.

    Congenital fusion of the odontoid to the atlas is not a described associated phenomenon. However, C1-C2 instability is common and potentially fatal. The atlantoaxial instability stems from odontoid dysplasia and laxity of the transverse ligament.

Reference

Milkes M, Stanton RP: A Review of Morquio Syndrome. Am J Orthop, 26(8):533–540, 1997.

60. **c** Osteogenesis imperfecta. Thin, gracile bones are characteristic of *osteogenesis imperfecta.* Pertinent characteristics of this disease include osseous fragility, growth retardation, blue sclerae, and ligamentous laxity. The osseous fragility leads to frequent fractures. The thin diaphyses are produced by "undertubulation" during remodeling. This defective periosteal appositional bone growth contrasts with the "overtubulation" seen in Gaucher disease, which produces abnormally wide (Erlenmeyer flask) metaphyses.

    Melorheostosis (Leri disease) is an uncommon, nonhereditary hyperostotic condition. Its radiographic hallmark is its flowing pattern of sclerotic cortical dysplasia that resembles melted wax dripping down the sides of a candle. Associated soft tissue abnormalities (including periarticular fibrosis or bone deposition) are common. It is typically unilateral and may either be monostotic or involve an entire limb, in which case it may produce a significant leg-length discrepancy.

    Osteopoikilosis (osteopathia condensans disseminata) typically manifests as multiple intraosseous, periarticular, sclerotic punctate foci. It is usually an incidental, asymptomatic finding. *Osteopathia striata (Voorhoeve disease)* is an asymptomatic condition marked by longitudinal dense osseous striations. Unlike melorheostosis, it is typically symmetric. Osteopathia striata can be seen in association with melorheostosis or osteopoikilosis, in which case the condition is termed *mixed sclerosing bone dystrophy.*

    Dysplasia epiphysealis hemimelica (Trevor disease) is an epiphyseal disorder that produces unilateral enlargement of a secondary ossification center. The *Sprengel deformity* is congenital anomaly of scapular elevation (see question 46).

References

Gertner JM, Root L: Osteogenesis Imperfecta. Orthop Clin North Am, 21:151, 1990.
Younge D, et al.: Melorheostosis in Children. J Bone Joint Surg Br, 61:415, 1979.

61. **d** Multiple epiphyseal dysplasia. Multiple epiphyseal dysplasia, achondroplasia, and Meyer dysplasia are all causes of waddling gait. *Multiple epiphyseal dysplasia* is a form of short-limbed disproportionate dwarfism characterized by bilateral delayed epiphyseal ossification of tubular bones. The ossific centers are often fragmented and flattened. This deformation leads to precocious osteoarthritis.

    Achondroplasia is also a form of short-limbed disproportionate dwarfism. However, it does not adversely affect the ossific nucleus of the femoral head. *Meyer dysplasia (dysplasia epiphysealis capitis femoris)* causes delayed appearance of the femoral head ossification centers, but his condition typically resolves in early childhood without adverse sequelae.

62. **d** Left subtrochanteric resection arthroplasty. Figure 9.11 demonstrates a left hip dislocation with an associated windswept deformity of the femurs.

    The left hip could conceivably be reduced by performing a femoral shortening with femoral derotational and pelvic osteotomies. However, this constellation of procedures would have a poor chance of providing long-term mobility, pain relief, and stability in this situation.

    Proximal femoral resection arthroplasty is an appropriate intervention for a nonambulatory spastic quadriplegic patient with a painful hip dislocation that poses a significant obstacle to nursing care. Hip arthrodesis would be less appropriate. If the left hip were fused in 90 degrees of flexion, the lower extremity would act as a lever arm when the patient was supine. Fusion of the nondislocated, nonadducted, painless right hip would be contraindicated. Fusion of either hip in full extension would preclude sitting. Analgesics would alleviate pain, but they would not rectify the nursing difficulties imparted by the stiff, windswept deformity.

63. **e** Fibrodysplasia ossificans progressiva. *Fibrodysplasia (myositis) ossificans progressiva* is a rare disorder of connective tissue characterized by congenital malformation

of the great toes and progressive soft tissue ossification. The frequently associated hallux valgus deformities stem from malformation of the great toe phalanges. Loss of spine motion occurs as a result of ossification of the paraspinal muscles. The intramuscular ossification consists of mature lamellar bone.

Sarcoidosis may also be associated with subcutaneous nodules. Associated radiographic abnormalities predominantly affect the phalanges. These include medullary widening, osseous sclerosis, tuft resorption, and "honeycomb" trabecular distortion. Sarcoidosis may also produce a granulomatous synovitis.

Behçet syndrome traditionally consists of the triad of ocular inflammation and recurrent oral and genital ulcerations. However, approximately 50% of affected patients also experience articular involvement (predominantly the knees).

References

Cohen RB, et al.: The Natural History of Heterotopic Ossification in Patients Who Have Fibrodysplasia Ossificans Progressiva. J Bone Joint Surg Am, 75:215–219, 1993.

Kaplan FS, et al.: The Histopathology of Fibrodysplasia Ossificans Progressiva: An Endochondral Process. J Bone Joint Surg Am, 75:220–230, 1993.

64. **a** Hemophilia. The radiograph (Fig. 9.12) demonstrates bilateral, symmetric joint space narrowing. This is a characteristic (albeit nonspecific) manifestation of inflammatory arthropathies. Recurrent hemarthroses in patient with *hemophilia* incite an inflammatory synovial response with resultant articular cartilage destruction. Additional radiographic features of hemophilia include widening of the intercondylar notch, squaring of the inferior pole of the patella, and overgrowth of the distal femoral and proximal tibial epiphyses. These features are nonspecific for hemophilic knee arthropathy. Juvenile rheumatoid arthritis may produce very similar findings.

Infantile cortical hyperostosis (Caffey disease) is typically a self-limited phenomenon. The underlying periostitis is idiopathic, and it is often associated with fever and soft tissue swelling. Caffey disease most commonly affects the mandible, clavicles, and ribs. Congenital syphilis is another source of extensive periostitis in childhood.

Radiographic hallmarks of fluorosis include ligamentous ossification and osteophyte formation, principally involving the axial skeleton. Another prominent feature of fluorosis is diffuse increased bone density. This feature assists in differentiating this condition from diffuse idiopathic skeletal hyperostosis. Childhood lead poisoning produces transverse sclerotic lines in the metaphyses of growing tubular bones.

Note: The joint which is most commonly affected by hemophilia is the knee.

Reference

Pettersson H, et al.: A Radiographic Classification of Hemophilic Arthropathy. Clin Orthop, 149:153, 1980.

65. **c** Scheuermann disease. *Scheuermann disease* is diagnosed by the following criteria: (1) structural kyphosis greater than 45 degrees; (2) 5 degrees or more of anterior wedging of at least three adjacent vertebrae; and (3) vertebral end-plate irregularities. The highest prevalence of Scheuermann disease is among adolescent males.

Acute leukemia is a potential source of back pain. Characteristic findings on plain radiographs include vertebral compression fractures from the associated osteopenia.

Intervertebral disc herniation occurs infrequently in adolescents. The lumbar spine is affected most frequently, and plain radiographs are typically normal. The signs and symptoms of acute disc herniation may be mimicked by a *slipped vertebral apophysis.* This condition also occurs most frequently in adolescent boys. Plain radiographs may demonstrate displacement of the ring apophysis into the vertebral canal. As with disc herniation, the lumbar spine is more commonly affected.

Discitis typically affects younger children. Plain radiographs are initially normal, but they subsequently reveal disc space narrowing and vertebral end-plate irregularities. (*Staphylococcus aureus* is the most commonly isolated source.)

Note: The thoracic hyperkyphosis of Scheuermann disease is associated with an increased incidence of L5 spondylolysis. This occurs because the compensatory lumbar lordosis subjects the L5 pars interarticularis to excessive shear force.

Reference

Thomson G: Back Pain in Children. J Bone Joint Surg Am, 75:928–938, 1993.

66. **a** Onset before 6 years of age. The earlier the onset of Legg-Calvé-Perthes disease, the better is the long-term prognosis. The less favorable prognosis associated with onset after 6 years of age has been attributed to decreasing remodeling potential.

An intact lateral column is a favorable prognostic sign. According to Herring et al., patients with collapse of the lateral epiphyseal pillar are at greater risk to suffer progressive flattening of the femoral head during reossification. Prolonged stiffness, lateral subluxation, hinged abduction, and a Gage sign (a radiolucent V on the lateral side of the epiphysis) have all been associated with a less favorable prognosis.

References

Skaggs DL, Tolo VT: Legg-Calvé-Perthes Disease. J Am Acad Orthop Surg, 4:9–16, 1996.

Wenger DR, et al.: Current Concept Review: Legg-Calve-Perthes Disease. J Bone Joint Surg Am, 73:778–788, 1991.

67. **c** Excision with extensor digitorum brevis interposition. The radiographs in Fig. 9.15 demonstrate a *calcaneonavicular coalition.* This finding is most evident on the oblique view. *Dorsal beaking* at the talonavicular joint (as seen on the lateral view) is a commonly associated finding. When conservative measures fail, recommended treatment consists of excision of the calcaneonavicular bar with interposition of the origin of the extensor digitorum brevis.

Triple arthrodesis has been recommended for talocalcaneal coalitions that involve more than 50% of the subtalar joint. Arthrodesis is also indicated as a salvage procedure for failed talocalcaneal bar excision.

Reference

Gonzalez P, Kumar SJ: Calcaneonavicular Coalition Treated by Resection and Interposition of the Extensor Digitorum Brevis Muscle. J Bone Joint Surg Am, 72:71–77, 1990.

68. **b** Decreased flexion and decreased internal rotation. In *slipped capital femoral epiphysis,* the femoral neck migrates anteriorly and superiorly relative to the femoral head. This produces a varus, retroverted deformity. Hence, physical examination of an affected hip classically demonstrates loss of internal rotation, flexion, and abduction.

Acute slips are associated with acute effusions. Thus, motion is restricted in all directions.

References

Aronsson DD, Karol LA: Stable Slipped Capital Femoral Epiphysis: Evaluation and Management. J Am Acad Orthop Surg, 4:173–181, 1996.

Crawford AH: Current Concepts Review: Slipped Capital Femoral Epiphysis. J Bone Joint Surg Am, 70:1422–1427, 1988.

69. **c** Spinal cord injury without radiographic abnormality is more common in skeletally immature persons than in adults. Most pediatric spine trauma occurs cephalad to C3. This is contrary to the distribution of damage to the adult spine. The reason is that the ratio of head size to neck length is greater in children. Thus, the fulcrum of head rotation is raised.

With congenital muscular torticollis, the head is tilted ipsilaterally and is rotated contralaterally to the side of sternocleidomastoid contraction. However, with atlantoaxial rotatory subluxation, the sternocleidomastoid contraction is not the source of the deformity. Rather, the contralateral sternocleidomastoid muscle contracts in an attempt to correct the deformity.

In general, the pediatric cervical spine is more mobile than the adult spine. This phenomenon is attributed to relative ligamentous laxity in children. This factor accounts for the higher incidence of spinal cord injury without radiographic abnormality among skeletally immature trauma victims. Immaturity of the spinal cord's vascular supply is believed to be another predisposing factor for spinal cord injury without radiographic abnormality.

Another manifestation of ligamentous laxity in the pediatric cervical spine is pseudosubluxation. Anterior subluxation of C2 on C3 of 4 mm is not necessarily a sign of posttraumatic ligamentous insufficiency. This amount of translation may be a normal finding in pediatric patients. In adults, the upper limit of normal ADI is 3.5 mm, whereas the maximum normal ADI value is 4.5 mm for children.

Reference

Jones ET, et al.: Injuries of the Cervical Spine. In Rockwood CA, Wilkins KE, Beaty JH, eds: Fractures in Children, 4th Ed. Philadelphia, Lippincott–Raven, 1996.

70. **e** Discoid meniscus. The images in Fig. 9.15 reveal that width and thickness of the lateral meniscus are markedly increased. This abnormal ("megahorn") shape is compatible with a diagnosis of discoid meniscus.

The patient's presenting symptoms suggest the possibility that this meniscus may be an unstable *(Wrisberg-type)* variant. The instability stems from deficient posterior attachment to the tibia. Under these circumstances, the only posterior attachment of the lateral meniscus is the ligament of Wrisberg.

Reference

Jordan M: Lateral Meniscal Variants: Evaluation and Treatment. J Am Acad Orthop Surg, 4:191–200, 1996.

FIGURE CREDITS

Figure 9.2. From Rockwood CA, Wilkins KE, Beaty JH, eds: Fractures in Children, 4th Ed. Philadelphia, Lippincott–Raven, p. 156, 1996, with permission.

Figure 9.4. From Craig EV: Clinical Orthopaedics. Philadelphia, Lippincott Williams & Wilkins, p. 591, 1999, with permission.

Figure 9.5. From Morrissy RT, Weinstein SL: Lovell and Winter's Pediatric Orthopaedics, vol 2, 4th Ed. Philadelphia, Lippincott–Raven, p. 652, 1996, with permission.

Figure 9.8. From Rockwood CA, Wilkins KE, Beaty JH, eds: Fractures in Children, vol 3, 4th Ed. Philadelphia, Lippincott–Raven, 1996, with permission.

Figure 9.10. From Morrissy RT, Weinstein SL: Lovell and Winter's Pediatric Orthopaedics, vol 2, 4th Ed. Philadelphia, Lippincott–Raven, p. 726, 1996, with permission.

Figure 9.11. From Morrissy RT, Weinstein SL: Lovell and Winter's Pediatric Orthopaedics, vol 2, 4th Ed. Philadelphia, Lippincott–Raven, p. 481, 1996, with permission.

Figure 9.13. From Morrissy RT, Weinstein SL: Lovell and Winter's Pediatric Orthopaedics, vol 2, 4th Ed. Philadelphia, Lippincott–Raven, p. 698, 1996, with permission.

Figure 9.17. From Rockwood CA, Wilkins KE, Beaty JH, eds: Fractures in Children, vol 3, 4th Ed. Philadelphia, Lippincott–Raven, p. 50, 1996, with permission.

Figure 9.18. From Rockwood CA, Wilkins KE, Beaty JH, eds: Fractures in Children, vol 3, 4th Ed. Philadelphia, Lippincott–Raven, p. 665, 1996, with permission.

Figure 9.19. From Rockwood CA, Wilkins KE, Beaty JH, eds: Fractures in Children, vol 3, 4th Ed. Philadelphia, Lippincott–Raven, p. 1411, 1996, with permission.

SUBJECT INDEX

Page numbers in bold refer to review questions; page numbers in italic refer to illustrations.

D

E

F

L

M

T